Orthodontics & Paediatric Dentistry

To my parents (Declan) and to Philly, Izzy, Ollie, Mum and Dad (Peter) for their enduring love and support.

For Elsevier
Content Strategist: *Alison Taylor*
Content Development Specialist: *Sally Davies*
Project Manager: *Louisa Talbott*
Designer/Design Direction: *Christian Bilbow*
Illustration Manager: *Lesley Frazier*

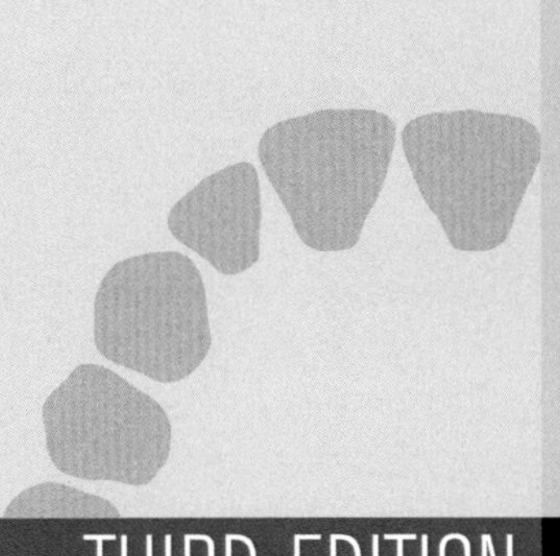

CLINICAL **PROBLEM SOLVING** IN DENTISTRY SERIES

THIRD EDITION

Orthodontics & Paediatric Dentistry

Declan Millett
BDSc DDS FDSRCPS(Glasg) FDSRCSEng DOrthRCSEng MOrthRCSEng FHEA
Professor of Orthodontics
Cork University Dental School and Hospital
University College Cork
Cork, Ireland

Peter Day
BDS PhD FDS(Paeds)RCSEng MPaedDent(RCSEng) MFDS(RCSEng) FRCD(Canada) FIADT PGCLTHE FHEA
Associate Professor and Consultant in Paediatric Dentistry
School of Dentistry at the University of Leeds and Bradford District Care NHS Foundation Trust Salaried Dental Service
Leeds, UK

With contributions from

Caroline Campbell
BDS MSc MPaedDent(Ed) MFDS RCPS(Glasg) FDSPaedDent(Glasg)
Consultant in Paediatric Dentistry, Honorary Senior Clinical Lecturer
Department of Paediatric Dentistry
Glasgow Dental Hospital and School
University of Glasgow
Glasgow, UK

Marie Therese Hosey
BDS MSc(MedSci) DDS FDS RCPS(Glas)
Professor of Paediatric Dentistry
Population and Patient Health Division
King's College London Dental Institute
London, UK

ELSEVIER

Edinburgh London New York Oxford Philadelphia St Louis Sydney Toronto 2017

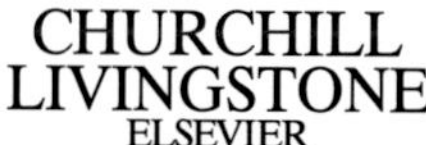

ISBN 978-0-7020-5836-3

Notices

Knowledge and best practice in this field are constantly changing. As new research and experience broaden our understanding, changes in research methods, professional practices, or medical treatment may become necessary.

Practitioners and researchers must always rely on their own experience and knowledge in evaluating and using any information, methods, compounds, or experiments described herein. In using such information or methods they should be mindful of their own safety and the safety of others, including parties for whom they have a professional responsibility.

With respect to any drug or pharmaceutical products identified, readers are advised to check the most current information provided (i) on procedures featured or (ii) by the manufacturer of each product to be administered, to verify the recommended dose or formula, the method and duration of administration, and contraindications. It is the responsibility of practitioners, relying on their own experience and knowledge of their patients, to make diagnoses, to determine dosages and the best treatment for each individual patient, and to take all appropriate safety precautions.

To the fullest extent of the law, neither the Publisher nor the authors, contributors, or editors, assume any liability for any injury and/or damage to persons or property as a matter of products liability, negligence or otherwise, or from any use or operation of any methods, products, instructions, or ideas contained in the material herein.

Printed in Great Britain

Last digit is the print number: 9 8 7 6 5

Contents

1 Median diastema and ectopic eruption of an upper first permanent molar 1

2 Unerupted upper central incisor 5

3 Absent upper lateral incisors 11

4 Crowding and buccal upper canines 16

5 Severe crowding 25

6 Palatal canines 36

7 More canine problems 46

8 Infraoccluded primary molars 51

9 Increased overjet 55

10 Incisor crossbite 62

11 Reverse overjet 66

12 Increased overbite 73

13 Anterior open bite 81

14 Posterior crossbite 87

15 Bilateral crossbite 91

16 Late lower incisor crowding 99

17 Prominent chin and TMJDS 102

18 Drifting incisors 109

19 Appliance-related problems 113

20 Tooth movement and related problems 118

21 Cleft lip and palate 125

22 Nursing and early childhood caries 130

23 High caries risk adolescents 135
by Caroline Campbell

24 Pain control and treatment planning for carious primary teeth 140

25 Facial swelling and dental abscess 146

26 The uncooperative child and adolescent 149
by Marie Therese Hosey

27 Children with disabilities and learning difficulties 157
by Marie Therese Hosey

28 Common medical problems in children 163

29 The displaced primary incisor 168

30 The fractured immature permanent incisor crown 171

31 The root fractured permanent incisor 175

32 The avulsed incisor 179

33 Disorders of eruption and exfoliation 184

34 Poor quality first permanent molars 187

35 Tooth discoloration, hypomineralization and hypoplasia 191

36 Mottled teeth 195

37 Multiple missing and abnormally shaped teeth 199

38 Amelogenesis imperfecta 203

39 Dentinogenesis imperfecta 206

40 Dental erosion 209

41 Gingival bleeding and enlargement 213

42 Oral ulceration 216

43 Mind Maps® 219

Appendices

A1 The index of orthodontic treatment need: dental health component 264

A2 Classification and definitions 265

A3 Orthodontic problems: referral guide 268

A4 Implications of some medical problems for orthodontics 269

A5 Lateral cephalometric analysis 271

A6 A structured dental trauma history form 273

Index 275

Preface to the third edition

The fondness of students for this problem-solving format and their encouraging feedback have led us to being asked by the publishers to do a third edition. The passage of time has brought a new co-author, Peter Day, to the Paediatric Dentistry section and a new contributing author, Marie-Therese Hosey. It is with great regret that Richard Welbury, who co-authored the first and second editions, was unable to continue in this role and we thank him most sincerely for his former involvement. We are indebted to our colleagues who have provided valuable suggestions regarding this revision.

The structure of the chapters remains unchanged, with the presentation of a clinical problem followed by a step-by-step lead-through assessment, diagnosis and treatment planning. All chapters and related Mind Maps®, where relevant, have been updated. Additional cases are included in several chapters to reflect the contemporary and changing face of orthodontic and paediatric dentistry clinical practice. Three new orthodontic appendices deal with classification and definitions, implications of common medical problems and referral guidelines. In addition, one new paediatric dentistry appendix provides a structured dental trauma history form. Two new chapters address management of the physically and medically compromised child. In promotion of evidence-based best practice and to direct further learning, reference lists have been updated throughout to include Cochrane reviews, where these have been developed.

It is our hope that this text will continue to be of use to undergraduates and to those in the early years of postgraduate training.

DTM
PFD
Cork and Leeds 2016

Preface to the first edition

Problem solving is a core skill which the dental undergraduate must develop and refine for examinations and everyday clinical practice. As orthodontics and paediatric dentistry interface broadly, combined clinical teaching and examinations in these disciplines are linked increasingly to encourage holistic problem solving of dental and occlusal problems in the child and adolescent patient.

This book aims, therefore, to address a range of common clinical problems encountered in orthodontic and paediatric dental practice. The format promotes a logical approach to problem solving through history taking, clinical examination and diagnosis, which underpin the principles of treatment planning for both disciplines. A short reference list is provided with each chapter to facilitate further directed learning.

Mind Maps® are also given for each topic to provide a focused framework for learning and revision. Each Mind Map® links key words, or key points, which are highlighted throughout the text, to create an overview of the subject and is designed to trigger information recall.

Intended primarily for the undergraduate, we hope this book will be of value also to the junior postgraduate and to those preparing for membership examinations.

DTM
RRW
Cork and Glasgow 2004

Acknowledgements

We are particularly grateful to Mrs K Shepherd and Mrs G Drake for their help and support in the preparation of photographic material. We would also like to thank especially Dr G McIntyre, Ms R Bryan, Mr J C Aird, Dr A Shaw, Miss D Fung, Dr T Ubaya, Dr C Campbell, Dr K O'Rourke, Dr P Murray, Dr T McSwiney, Dr P Murphy, Dr M Meade, Dr L Darby, Dr S McMorrow, Dr S Littlewood, Dr A Garry, Dr E Salloum, Dr D Morris, Dr S Fayle, Dr A Mighell and Cork University Dental School & Hospital for provision of some of the illustrations. Mr K Evans also kindly assisted with the production of the appliances shown in Figs 9.4 and 13.8. Ms N Kelly is thanked especially for the editing and compilation of photographic material. Thank you to students and staff who have undertaken some or all of the care on which the cases are based on. We are also grateful to Buzan Centres Ltd for the style for the Mind Maps®. Our gratitude is extended to the staff of Elsevier who have been very helpful throughout.

1

Median diastema and ectopic eruption of an upper first permanent molar

SUMMARY

Brian is almost 8 years of age. He presents with a gap between his upper front teeth and crooked lower front teeth (*Fig. 1.1*); an 'adult' upper back tooth also does not appear to be coming through properly. What are the causes of these problems and what treatment would you recommend?

History

Complaint

Brian's mother noticed the gap between his upper front teeth and the irregularity of his lower front teeth. She is anxious about his appearance and is keen for treatment to be provided. Recently she has also noticed that one of his new 'adult' upper back teeth is not coming through properly compared with his other upper back tooth on the opposite side.

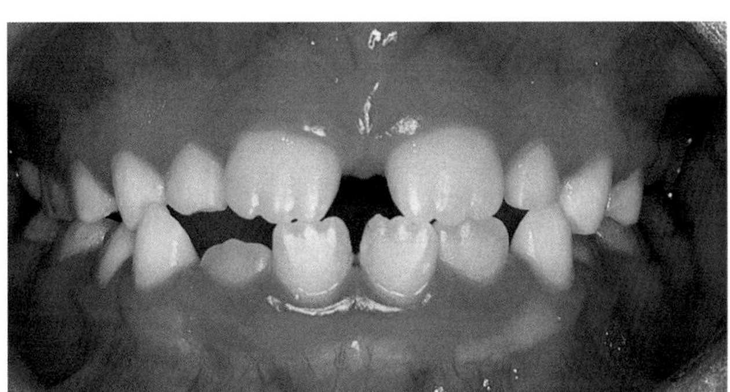

Fig. 1.1 Anterior occlusion at presentation.

History of complaint

Brian's primary front teeth had a pleasing appearance with a small midline space in the upper arch; the lower primary front teeth were not spaced. There is no history of trauma. The permanent incisors erupted in their present positions. Brian's permanent molars started to erupt over a year ago and there is no discomfort from any of them.

Medical history

Brian is fit and well.

Dental history

Brian attends his general dental practitioner every 6 months but has not required any treatment.

Family history

Brian's father had an upper midline space that was closed with a fixed appliance.

Examination

Extraoral examination

Brian has a Class I skeletal pattern with average FMPA and no facial asymmetry. Lips are competent with the lower lip resting at the incisal third of the upper central incisors. There are no temporomandibular joint signs or symptoms.

Intraoral examination

Soft tissues are healthy and the dentition is caries-free. The intraoral views are shown in **Figs 1.1** and **1.2**.

■ ***What do you observe?***

Low-lying maxillary labial frenum.

The following teeth are visible: $\dfrac{\text{6 E D C B 1} \mid \text{1 B C D}}{\text{6 E D C 2 1} \mid \text{1 2 C D E 6}}$

(note $\lfloor$E6 present, but $\lfloor$6 erupting into $\lfloor$E).

Mild lower labial segment crowding with distolabial rotations of $\overline{1|1}$; slight spacing distal of $\overline{2|2}$.

Upper median diastema with the crowns of $\underline{1|1}$ flared distally.

Class III incisor relationship.

Crossbites $\dfrac{\text{B} \mid \text{B}}{\text{C} \mid \text{C}}$.

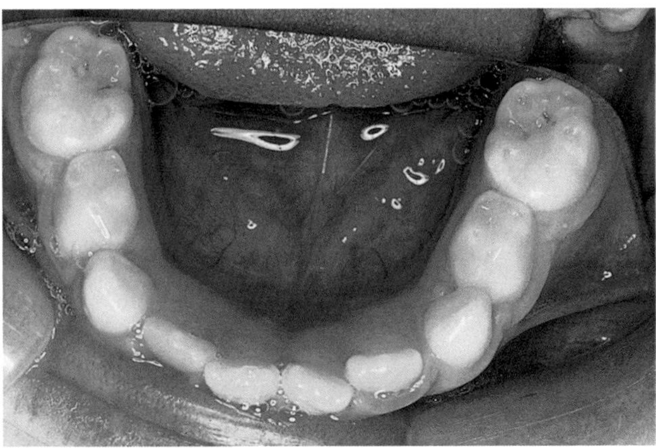

Fig. 1.2 Lower occlusal view (note $\overline{6|6}$ erupted but not shown).

■ ***What is the aetiology of the 1|1 rotations?***

Incisor rotations are usually a manifestation of inherent crowding in the arch, which is genetic in origin. The lack of primary lower incisor spacing reported by the child's mother is predictive of likely crowding of the permanent successors. Incisor rotations may also result from ectopic position of the tooth germs or from the presence of a supernumerary tooth.

■ ***What are the possible causes of the upper median diastema?***

These are listed in **Table 1.1**.

■ ***Is the dental and occlusal development normal?***

Dental development is normal. Eruption dates of the primary and permanent dentition are given in **Table 1.2**.

It is common for some crowding to be present as the lower incisors erupt, which usually manifests itself as slight lingual placement and/or rotation of the teeth, but the slight distal tilt and rotations of 1|1 may indicate inherent crowding. Also, there is no lower primate (anthropoid) space between the primary canines and first primary molars.

Spacing between the upper permanent central incisors (flared distally and formerly described as the 'ugly duckling' stage, terms best avoided with concerned parents) is also normal at this stage, but generalized spacing of the upper primary teeth including the upper primate spaces (located between the upper primary lateral incisors and the upper primary canines) should exist.

Although the primary incisor relationship is commonly edge-to-edge at 5–6 years with incisor attrition, it is not usual for the permanent incisor relationship to be similar. Rather a Class I incisor relationship should be present.

A crossbite should not exist on $\frac{B|B}{C|C}$.

The first permanent molars should normally be in a half-unit Class II relationship due to the 'flush terminal planes' relationship of the second primary molars.

Table 1.1 Causes of an upper median diastema

Causes	Comments
Developmental	Due to pressure of 2|2 on 1|1 roots (formerly referred to as 'ugly duckling' stage); tends to resolve by the time 3|3 erupt
Dentoalveolar disproportion	Small teeth in a large arch
Absent or peg-shaped 2's	
Supernumerary tooth/teeth in midline	
Proclination of 21|12	May be due to a digit sucking habit
Prominent labial frenum	Implicated where there is blanching of the incisive papilla on stretching the frenum and notching between 1|1 is seen on radiograph
Pathological	Cyst/tumour
	Juvenile periodontitis

Table 1.2 Eruption dates for primary and permanent teeth

Primary	Months	Permanent	Years
Upper		**Upper**	
Central incisor	6–7	Central incisor	7–8
Lateral incisor	7–8	Lateral incisor	8–9
Canine	18–20	Canine	11–12
First molar	12–15	First premolar	10–11
Second molar	24–36	Second premolar	10–12
		First molar	6–7
		Second molar	12–13
		Third molar	17–21
Lower		**Lower**	
Central incisor	6–7	Central incisor	6–7
Lateral incisor	7–8	Lateral incisor	7–8
Canine	18–20	Canine	9–10
First molar	12–15	First premolar	10–12
Second molar	24–36	Second premolar	11–12
		First molar	5–6
		Second molar	12–13
		Third molar	17–21

Key point

On eruption:

- Some crowding of 21|12 is usual.
- A median diastema between 1|1 is normal.

■ ***In the developing dentition, how is space created for the upper permanent incisor teeth?***

Space is obtained from three sources: the spacing which should exist between the primary incisors; an increase in intercanine width; and by the permanent upper incisors erupting more labially and proclined compared with their predecessors. On average, the upper and lower intercanine width increases by about 1–2 mm in the primary dentition; a further increase of around 3 mm occurs during the mixed dentition but is generally complete by about 9 years when the upper and lower permanent lateral incisors are fully erupted although some minor increase occurs until 13 years.

Key point

Intercanine width:

- Increases ~1–2 mm during primary dentition.
- Increases ~3 mm in mixed dentition.
- Is generally complete by ~9 years, with minor increase to ~13 years.

Investigations

■ ***What investigations would you undertake? Explain why.***

Clinical

- *Gently pull the upper lip upwards and observe if there is blanching of the incisive papilla from the frenal attachment.* This may implicate the frenum in the possible aetiology of the upper median diastema. In Brian's case, slight blanching of the incisive papilla was detected.

- *Check if there is a mandibular displacement associated with the crossbites on* $\frac{B|B}{C|C}$. If a displacement is detected, early crossbite correction is indicated. Brian, however, did not have a mandibular displacement, which was confirmed by the absence of a lower centreline shift.

Radiographic

A left bitewing radiograph could be taken to assess $\underline{|6}$ position/status of any root resorption of $\underline{|E}$ and an upper anterior occlusal radiograph to assess presence/absence of an upper midline supernumerary. Alternatively, a dental panoramic tomogram, which is easier for the child to cooperate with, could be taken initially, which will also allow you to ascertain the presence, position and form of all unerupted teeth.

If a supernumerary tooth/teeth or other pathology is observed or suspected on the dental panoramic tomogram in the anterior premaxilla, an upper anterior occlusal radiograph should be taken.

- ***The dental panoramic tomogram is shown in** Fig. 1.3**. What do you notice?***

Normal alveolar bone levels.

A normally developing dentition, which is consistent with the patient's chronological age.

Resorption of the distal root of $\underline{E|E}$.

Impaction of $\underline{|6}$.

Diagnosis

- ***What is the diagnosis?***

Mild Class III malocclusion in the early mixed dentition on a Class I skeletal base with average FMPA. Mild lower labial segment crowding; upper median diastema.

Crossbites $\frac{B|B}{C|C}$ with no mandibular displacement.

Impacted $\underline{|6}$.

- ***What is the IOTN DHC grade (see Appendix 1, p. 264)? Explain why.***

4t – due to a partially erupted and impacted $\underline{|6}$.

- ***What treatment would you advise for the labial segment problems? Explain why.***

No treatment is indicated at present. The mild lower labial segment crowding may reduce slightly by drift of $\overline{2|2}$ into the small existing spaces distal to them (**Fig. 1.4**). Further improvement in the lower incisor crowding is also likely until about 9 years of age as the intercanine width increases.

The upper median diastema is likely to reduce as the maxillary permanent lateral incisors and canines erupt. Brian's mother should be reassured about this. The attachment of the maxillary labial frenum, although initially to the incisive papilla during the primary dentition, moves to the labial attached mucosa as the permanent lateral incisors erupt and approximate the permanent central incisors (**Fig. 1.5**). In a spaced arch, this migration of the frenum is less likely. In contrast, where the upper arch is potentially crowded and the diastema is less than 4 mm, recession of the frenum and closure of the median diastema may be forthcoming eventually. However, in the present case, as Brian's father had an upper median diastema, there may be a tendency for the space to persist.

- ***How common is impaction of $\underline{6}$?***

This anomaly of eruption occurs in about 2–6% of children but has been reported in 20–25% of children with cleft lip and/or palate.

- ***What are the causes of impaction of $\underline{6}$?***

Impaction of $\underline{6}$ is indicative of crowding.

Both local and hereditary factors have been implicated (**Table 1.3**). A multifactorial mode of inheritance has been identified where both genetic and local factors act in combination.

- ***Describe the clinical features of ectopic eruption of $\underline{6}$ and classification of this anomaly.***

Ectopic eruption of $\underline{6}$ is manifested by eruption mesial of its normal path. Complete eruption of $\underline{6}$ is initially blocked by

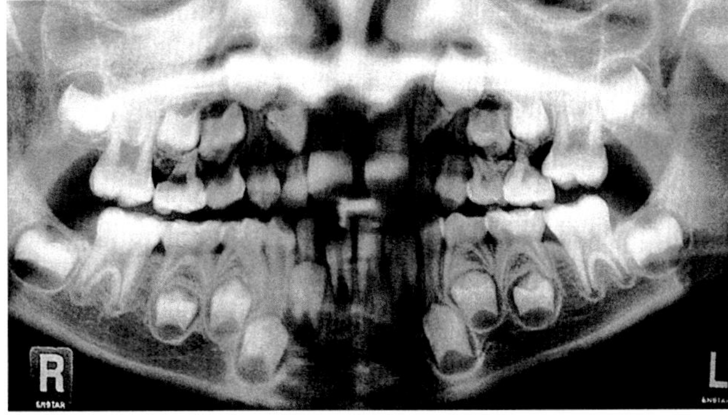

Fig. 1.3 Dental panoramic tomogram.

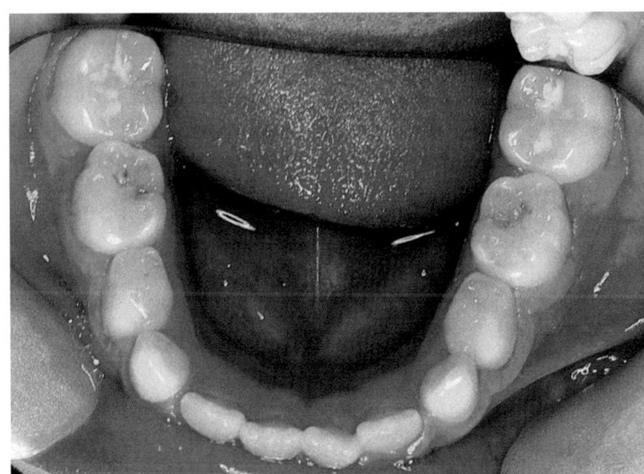

Fig. 1.4 Lower occlusal view 1 year after presentation.

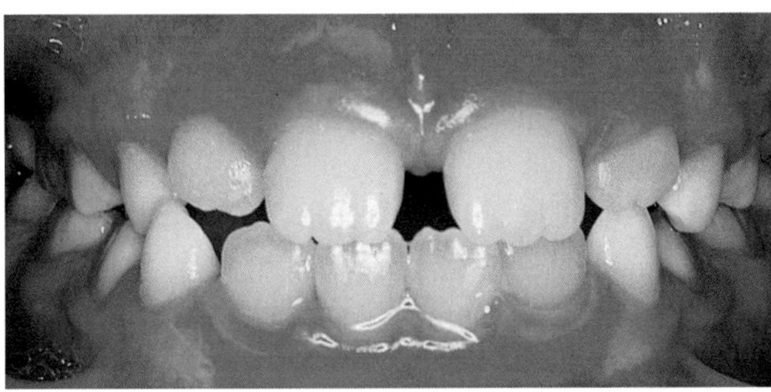

Fig. 1.5 Anterior occlusion following eruption of $\underline{2}$'s.

Table 1.3 Causes of impaction (ectopic eruption) of 6

Factor	Cause
Local	Significantly larger 6 and more pronounced mesial angle of eruption of 6
Hereditary	Familial tendency
	Small maxilla

the distal surface of E, which then, in response to tooth contact, undergoes resorption.

Ectopic eruption of 6 is described as 'reversible' if disimpaction and full eruption ensue spontaneously. After 8 years of age, this occurs rarely. If 6 remains impacted until treated or premature loss of E happens spontaneously, ectopic eruption of 6 is described as 'irreversible'.

Treatment

What treatment options are there for irreversible ectopic eruption of 6?

Without extraction of E Where impaction of 6 is mild, a brass wire separator may be tightened around the contact area of E and 6 over several visits; this will release 6 by displacing it distally. Discing the distal surface of E and the use of a separating spring have also been proposed.

If 6 exhibits marked mesial tipping, more active distal movement is required. This may be achieved by a spring soldered to a transpalatal bar uniting the D's. The spring acts against a composite stop bonded to the occlusal surface of 6.

With extraction of E If there is marked resorption or abscess formation of E, or if 6 cannot be disimpacted with a separating spring, or if 6 is carious and poor access impedes restoration, extraction of E is unavoidable. As 6 erupts with a mesial inclination, space loss occurs rapidly following loss of E. Consideration should be given to regaining space by distalizing 6 with a spring on an upper removable appliance in cases of unilateral loss of E. Where bilateral loss of E occurs, distal movement of 6's may be achieved by springs soldered to a transpalatal arch connecting both D's or by cervical traction to bands on 6's. Alternatively, management of the space loss resulting from extraction of E's can be deferred until the permanent dentition.

Key point

For impacted 6 consider:

- Brass wire separator.
- Discing distal surface of E.
- Move 6 distally.
- Extract E.

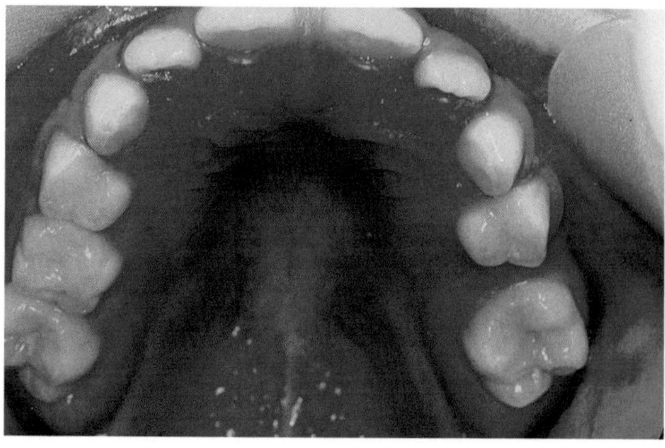

Fig. 1.6 Upper occlusal view following extraction of |E.

How will the orthodontist manage impaction of |6 in this case?

The various options regarding disimpaction of |6 should be discussed with Brian and his parents.

It should then be explained that if |E becomes abscessed, or attempts to disimpact |6 are unsuccessful, extraction of |E will be required. Treatment to deal with the resultant space loss will be required thereafter.

Brian was not keen for any orthodontic treatment and, therefore, it was decided to extract |E in view of the caries risk to |6. The consequent upper buccal segment crowding (**Fig. 1.6**) will be dealt with in the permanent dentition.

Impressions and a wax registration for study models should be recorded of the developing Class III malocclusion. This should then be monitored until the permanent dentition is fully established when treatment planning can be completed.

Primary resources and recommended reading

Bjerklin K, Kurol J, Valentin J 1992 Ectopic eruption of maxillary first permanent molars and association with other tooth and developmental disturbances. Eur J Orthod 14:369–375.

Foster TD, Grundy MC 1986 Occlusal changes from primary to permanent dentitions. Br J Orthod 13:187–193.

Huang WJ, Creath CJ 1995 The midline diastema: a review of its aetiology and treatment. Pediatr Dent 17:171–179.

Kurol J, Bjerklin K 1986 Ectopic eruption of maxillary first permanent molars: a review. ASDC J Dent Child 53:209–214.

For revision, see Mind Maps 1a and 1b, pages 220–221, and Appendices 2 and 3 pages 265–268.

2

Unerupted upper central incisor

SUMMARY

Neil, a 9-year-old boy, presents with 1| unerupted (Fig. 2.1). What are the possible causes and how would you manage the problem?

History

Complaint

Neil's mother is very concerned about the unerupted 1| as he is 9 years old and the tooth has not yet appeared; 2| is also erupting over B|, and she dislikes the appearance.

History of complaint

|A was lost at about 6 years of age, and |1 erupted normally at 6.5 years of age. Unfortunately, Neil fell over while playing soccer with his class team 4 months ago and fractured |1, exposing the pulp, which was treated by a coronal pulpotomy and placement of calcium hydroxide.

- ***Is there anything else you would wish to elicit from the history?***

Neil's mother should be asked about any history of trauma to the primary incisors, particularly intrusion of BA|.

There is no history of trauma to the primary dentition.

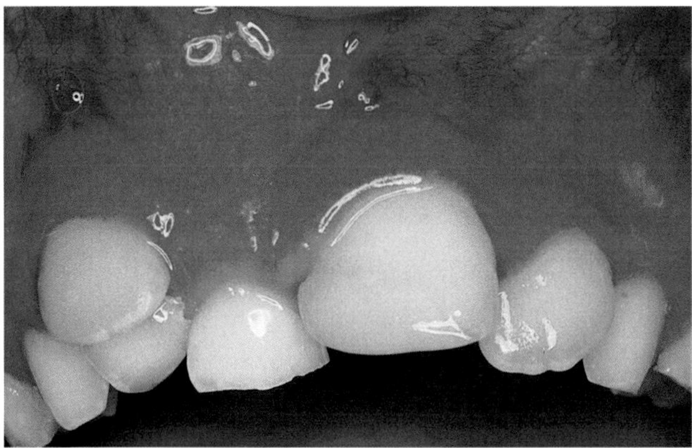

Fig. 2.1 Upper labial segment at presentation.

Medical history

Neil is fit and well.

Examination

Extraoral examination

Neil has a mild Class II skeletal pattern with slightly increased FMPA. His lips are competent. No facial asymmetry or abnormal temporomandibular joint signs or symptoms were detected.

Intraoral examination

- ***The appearance of the mouth is shown in*** *Figs 2.1* ***and*** *2.2*. ***What do you notice?***

Oral hygiene is fair – calculus is visible on the buccal aspect of 6|.

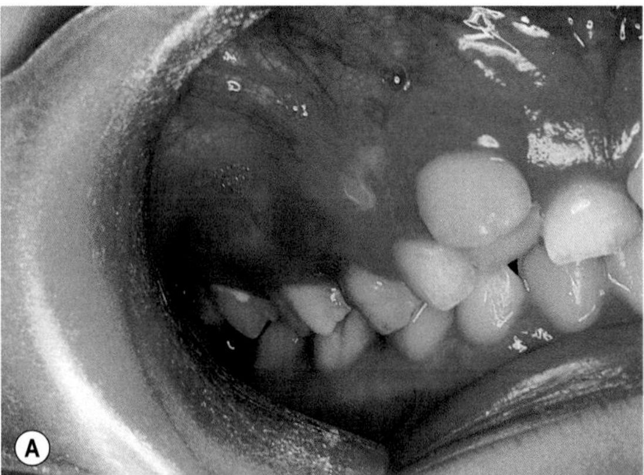

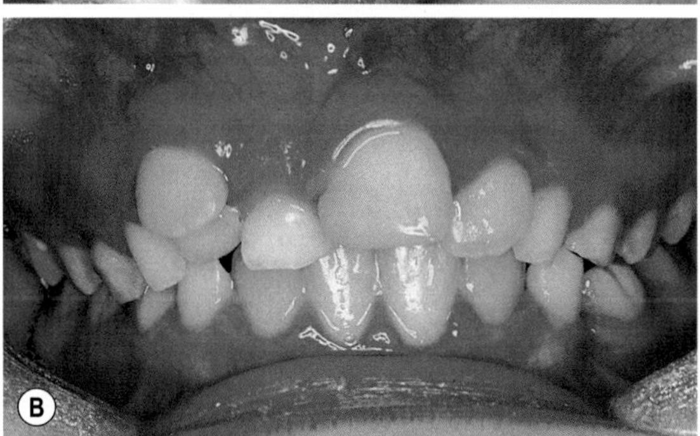

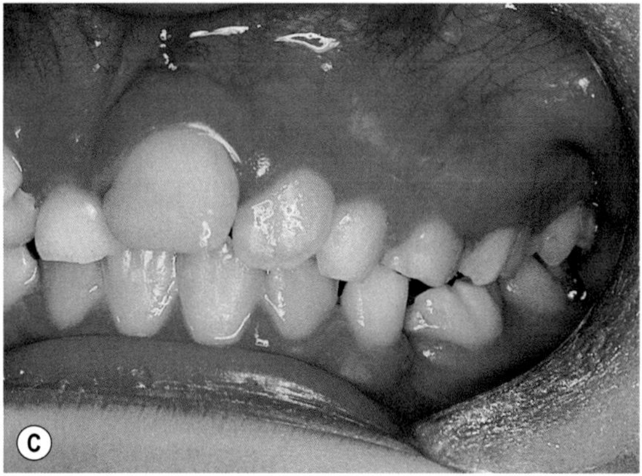

Fig. 2.2 **(A)** Right buccal occlusion. **(B)** Anterior occlusion. **(C)** Left buccal occlusion.

Mild plaque deposits on most teeth associated with marginal gingival erythema.

Early mixed dentition with $\begin{array}{c|c} 6EDC2BA & 12CDE6 \\ \hline 6EDC21 & 12CE6 \end{array}$ present.

Restored incisal edge of ⌊1, which also appears to be darker than the other incisors.

Class I malocclusion with mild lower and moderate upper labial segment crowding.

Upper centreline to the right; lower centreline to the left.

Potential crowding lower left quadrant.

Buccal segment relationship Class I bilaterally.

■ *Why are the centrelines displaced?*

An imbalance of upper anterior tooth size (the retained A⌋ is considerably smaller than an 1⌋) has promoted the upper centreline shift, but this has been aggravated by inherent upper arch crowding.

The lower centreline shift is due to early unbalanced loss of ⌈D in a potentially crowded arch.

■ *Could the lower centreline shift have been prevented?*

Following removal of ⌈D the lower centreline should have been monitored at review visits. D⌉ should have been extracted to balance for loss of ⌈D when the centreline appeared to be migrating.

■ *With unilateral loss of what other primary tooth, would you consider a balancing extraction to prevent a centerline shift?*

Where unilateral loss of a primary canine has occurred (or is planned as in the case of a palatally ectopic canine; see Chapter 6) and the contralateral tooth is not mobile, consideration should be given to its removal to prevent loss of the centreline. A balancing extraction of another second primary molar to prevent a potential centerline shift is unnecessary.

> **Key point**
>
> Always balance for unilateral loss/extraction of a primary canine.

■ *What are the possible causes of the unerupted 1⌋?*

These are listed in **Box 2.1**.

■ *How would you rate the likelihood in this case of each of the potential causes of unerupted 1⌋ listed in* Box 2.1*?*

Congenital absence of 1⌋ is highly unlikely. It would be very rare for 1⌋ to be absent without other congenitally missing teeth.

Avulsion of 1⌋ can be excluded as there is no history of 1⌋ having erupted or of incisor trauma.

Extraction of 1⌋ can be excluded also.

Ectopic position of the tooth germ is a possibility but is more likely to be secondary to some pathological cause or the presence of a supernumerary tooth.

Box 2.1 Causes of unerupted or missing upper permanent central incisor

Missing

- Congenitally absent.
- Avulsed.
- Extracted.

Present but unerupted

- Ectopic position of the tooth germ.
- Dilaceration and/or displacement due to trauma.
- Scar tissue.
- Supernumerary tooth.
- Crowding.
- Pathology, e.g. cyst, odontogenic tumour.

Box 2.2 Classification of supernumerary teeth (s/n) by morphology and effects on the dentition

- Conical or peg-shaped – most often lies between 1|1 and may produce no effect, a median diastema, incisor rotation or failure of 1 eruption (**Fig. 2.3A**); 75–78% of s/n.
- Tuberculate or barrel-shaped – most usually associated with unerupted 1; ~12% of s/n.
- Supplemental – resembles and lies adjacent to the last tooth of a series (2's, 5's, 8's); likely to produce crowding, centreline shift (**Fig. 2.3B**).
- Odontome – may be either compound or complex; compound is more common in the anterior maxilla; complex is more common in the premolar and molar areas; associated with unerupted/displaced teeth.

Dilaceration and/or displacement due to trauma can be excluded due to the absence of a relevant history.

Scar tissue can be excluded also as this would result from trauma.

A supernumerary tooth (**Box 2.2**) is the most likely cause of unerupted 1⌋. With an incidence of 1–3% in the premaxilla, supernumerary teeth (particularly the late-forming tuberculate type) are associated with delay or noneruption of an upper permanent central incisor.

Crowding is an unlikely cause. Although the upper labial segment is crowded, only very severe crowding would prevent 1⌋ erupting 2 years following its expected eruption time.

Pathology is also an unlikely cause. There is no evidence of alveolar expansion in the premaxilla, which would most likely be due to cyst formation possibly arising from 1⌋, a supernumerary or odontome. Other rarer lesions would need to be excluded.

> **Key point**
>
> A supernumerary tooth is the most common cause of failure of eruption of 1.

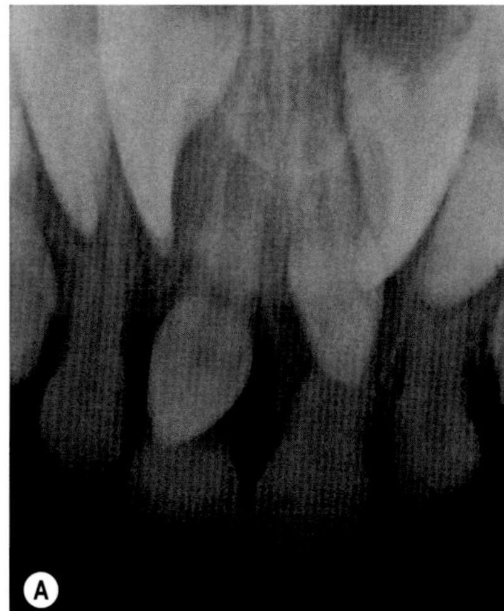

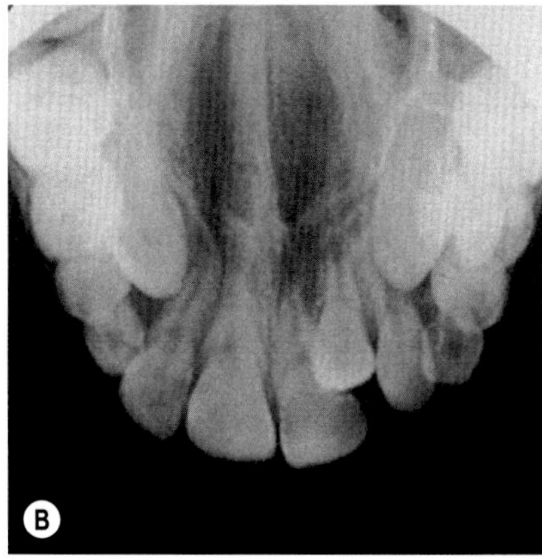

Fig. 2.3 (A) Two conical supernumerary teeth between 1⌋⌊1. **(B)** Supplemental ⌊2.

What is the aetiology of supernumerary teeth?

Although not entirely known, genetic factors seem to play a part with a male predilection. The cleft area is also frequently affected where the alveolus is involved. Dichotomy of the tooth bud and localized independent hyperactivity or fragmentation of the dental lamina have also been suggested; the latter is especially relevant to cleft lip and palate. Multiple supernumerary teeth rarely occur but are associated with cleidocranial dysplasia, Gardner syndrome and cleft lip and palate.

> **Key point**
>
> Supernumerary teeth are more common in males.

Investigation

What investigations are required? Explain why.

Clinical Palpation of the labial and palatal mucosae in the 1⌋ area to detect if the unerupted 1⌋ is present.

Sensibility testing of ⌊1 to assess pulpal status. ⌊1 was vital on sensibility testing to all stimuli, but as 1⌋ was unerupted, it was not possible to compare responses to that tooth. Comparison with the 2's indicated that ⌊1 had a diminished response to electric pulp testing.

Radiographic The following views are required to determine the presence/absence of 1⌋ and/or possible supernumerary teeth:

- *Dental panoramic tomogram* gives a general screen of the developing dentition allowing detection of the presence/absence of unerupted teeth.
- *Upper anterior occlusal or periapical views* provide greater detail of the anterior maxilla. In particular, the following can be assessed: the crown and root morphology of unerupted 1⌋, the presence of supernumerary teeth and/or other pathology and their relation to the incisor roots, the root and periapical status of traumatized ⌊1. On a panoramic radiograph these structures may be poorly defined due to superimposition of other anatomical features or by lying outside the focal trough of the tomogram. Periapical radiographs should include the roots of adjacent teeth to determine if they were damaged during previous trauma to ⌊1.

Used in combination and employing the principle of vertical parallax, the dental panoramic tomogram and the upper anterior occlusal or periapical views can be used to localize the position of any unerupted tooth and/or supernumerary relative to the dental arch.

> **Key point**
>
> - Two radiographic views are required to localize an unerupted tooth in the premaxilla using parallax.
> - *A lateral view* may be required to aid localization of a dilaceration, if visible on either the dental panoramic tomogram or on the upper anterior occlusal/periapical views.

How would you determine the position of an unerupted tooth in the anterior premaxilla using vertical parallax?

If the tooth moves in the same direction as the tube shift, it lies palatal to the arch; if it moves in the opposite direction to the tube shift, it lies buccal to the arch. Where there is no apparent shift in its position between the films, it lies in the line of the arch.

Neil's radiographs are shown in Fig. 2.4. What do these show?

The panoramic tomograph shows all permanent teeth to be present, including third molars. Dental development appears reasonably aligned with chronological age. There is a supernumerary tooth overlying 1⌋. Root resorption of the remaining first primary molars is advanced, and caries is evident in $\begin{array}{r|l} D & \\ \hline ED & E \end{array}$. Bitewing radiographs would be required for more accurate assessment of the extent of carious involvement of the primary molars.

The upper anterior occlusal view shows that root resorption of BA⌋ is advanced. 1⌋ has a normal crown and root form, and the root canal appears wide with an apical calcific bridge. A tuberculate supernumerary overlies the crown of 1⌋. The composite tip repair to ⌊1 is visible, and root formation is incomplete with apical narrowing.

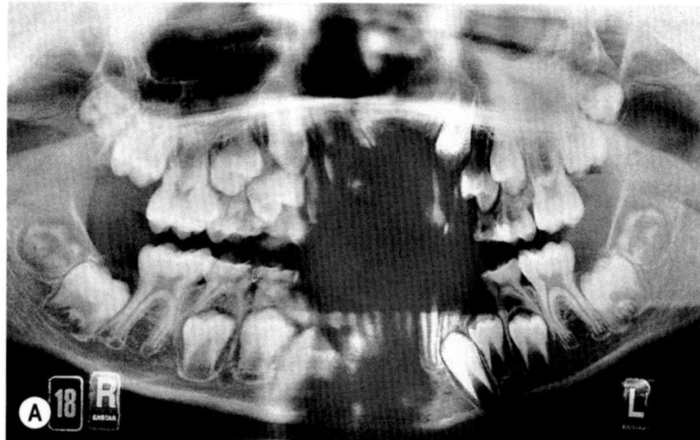

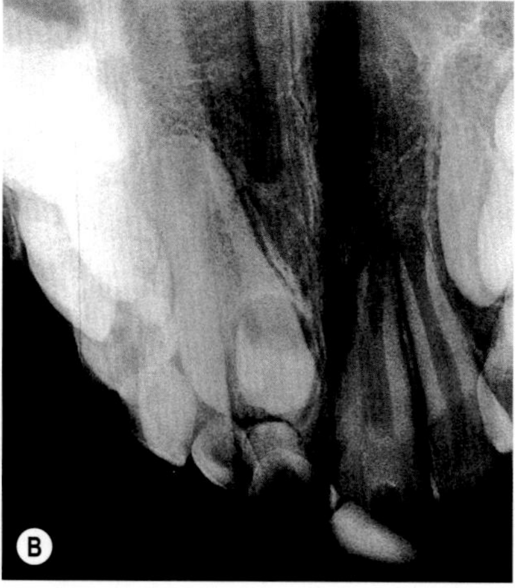

Fig. 2.4 **(A)** Dental panoramic tomogram. **(B)** Upper anterior occlusal radiograph.

Application of vertical parallax to these radiographs indicates that 1| and the supernumerary tooth are palatally positioned.

■ ***Is there any other alternative radiographic investigation you might consider? If so, why?***

Although a cone beam computed tomographic (CBCT) view may be considered in the assessment of unerupted tooth position, and if a supernumerary tooth, or teeth, is present, a risk/benefit analysis needs to be undertaken on a case-by-case basis. Only when conventional radiographic views fail to provide sufficient diagnostic information should CBCT be requested. In this case it was reckoned to be unnecessary based on the view shown in **Fig. 2.3**.

Diagnosis

■ ***What is your diagnosis?***

Class I malocclusion on a mild Class II skeletal base with slightly increased FMPA.

Generalized mild marginal gingivitis.

Caries in $\frac{D|}{ED|E}$; trauma to |1 involving the pulp.

Upper and lower arch crowding.

BA| retained; 2| erupting labially; 1| unerupted with associated tuberculate supernumerary.

Upper centreline shift to the right; lower centreline shift to the left.

Buccal segment relationship Class I bilaterally.

■ ***What is the IOTN DHC grade (see p. 264)? Explain why.***

5i – due to impeded eruption of 1| caused by the presence of a supernumerary tooth.

Treatment

■ ***What are your aims of treatment?***

- Restore gingival and dental health.
- Relief of crowding.
- Correction of centrelines.
- Alignment of 1|. Definitive restoration of |1.

■ ***What is your treatment plan?***

For treatment planning, you should make arrangements for Neil to be referred for joint consultation by an orthodontist, oral surgeon and paediatric dentistry colleague regarding management of unerupted 1|, associated supernumerary, the prognosis of |1 and the carious molars. The plan agreed was:

1. Oral hygiene instruction.
2. Dietary advice with the aid of a diet diary.
3. Provision of a custom-made mouthguard for soccer practice. The fit may need to be modified with regard to some aspects of the treatment given below.
4. Determine the prognosis of |1. The likelihood of apical closure was deemed to be good, and |1 was to be monitored radiographically at 3-month intervals.
5. Determine the prognosis of the second primary molars from bitewing radiographs. E's were deemed to be of reasonable prognosis, but Ē's require formocresol pulpotomy and stainless steel crowns or extraction in view of the pulpal carious involvement. More than half the root length of E|E remains, and in view of the space loss that already exists in the lower arch, it would be wise to minimize any further extractions except in an attempt to correct the centreline shift.
6. Open space for 1| and correct the upper centreline.
7. Taking the poor prognosis of $\frac{D|}{D|}$ into account, and to allow relief of upper arch crowding at this stage, to create space for centreline correction and for 1| to be accommodated, the following extractions are indicated $\frac{DCBA|CD}{D|}$.

   Removal of |D is required to balance the extraction of D|. Extraction of D| will balance the loss of |D and tend to encourage correction of the lower centreline shift.
8. The supernumerary tooth will also need to be surgically removed and an attachment with a length of gold chain should be bonded to 1|, followed by flap replacement (closed technique). 1| should not be surgically exposed with an open technique.
9. In this case it will be necessary to await further eruption of 2| following removal of BA| before moving 2| and |12 distally to create space for 1|.

■ ***How may space be created for 1|?***

Space may be created using an upper removable appliance or by a fixed appliance.

■ ***Are there any advantages to use of an upper removable appliance over a fixed appliance in this case and at this stage?***

A removable appliance has the following advantages in this case at this stage:

There are few permanent teeth erupted, and many of the primary teeth are to be extracted; this leaves very few teeth on which the appliance may be anchored. Although a fixed appliance could be bonded to the permanent incisors and bands placed on the first permanent molars, anchorage would need to be reinforced by means of linking the first molars on either side of the arch by means of a Nance transpalatal arch with an acrylic button which contacts the anterior vault of the palate. There will be long spans of the archwire unsupported and liable to distortion. As the baseplate covers the palate, anchorage is better with a removable appliance for the tooth movements required.

If desired, a prosthetic tooth could also be added when BA| have been removed and colour-matched to |1; this would enhance appliance aesthetics. It could be progressively trimmed as 1| is brought into alignment.

The appliance may also be removed for cleaning and for sports.

■ ***What design of upper removable appliance would you use to achieve the desired tooth movements?***

The appliance should be designed with the aid of the acronym ARAB (activation, retention, anchorage, baseplate) while the patient is still in the dental chair, so that nothing is overlooked.

- *Activation:* Palatal finger springs (0.5 mm stainless steel wire) to 2|12.
- *Retention:* Adams clasps (0.7 mm stainless steel wire) to 6|6. Recurved labial bow (0.7 mm stainless steel wire) from mesial of each E.
- *Anchorage:* From baseplate.
- *Baseplate:* Full palatal acrylic coverage (**Fig. 2.5**).

When space for 1| has been created, a hook may be soldered to the labial bow to allow attachment of the gold chain for 1| extrusion or the bow may be modified to create a buccal arm for this purpose.

Key point

Sequence in design of an upper removable appliance: ARAB acronym

- Activation.
- Retention.
- Anchorage.
- Baseplate.

■ ***Will an upper removable appliance achieve all the treatment objectives?***

An upper removable appliance will achieve the simple tooth movements (tipping and extrusion) required in this case at this stage. It is likely that further treatment, probably loss of a premolar unit from each quadrant and fixed appliance therapy, will be required at a later date, and then detailing of 1| position can be undertaken (**Fig. 2.6**).

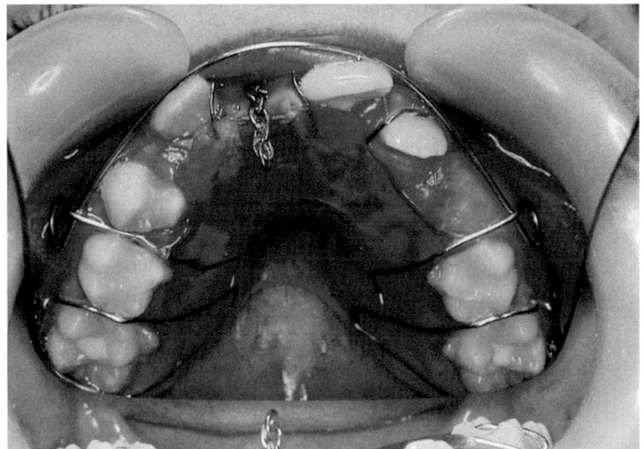

Fig. 2.5 Upper removable appliance to open space for 1|.

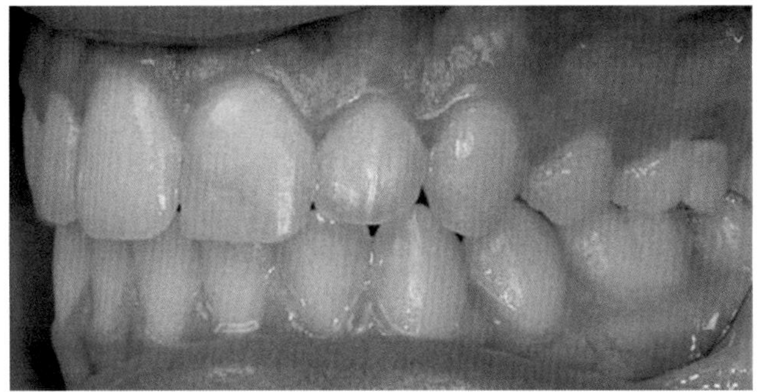

Fig. 2.6 Following extraction of four first premolars, fixed appliance therapy and further restorative treatment to |1.

■ ***What is the recommended root filling material for |1 during orthodontic tooth movement?***

When apical closure is evident on |*1*, no root canal treatment is required as the tooth has vital pulp tissue.

■ ***Does orthodontic tooth movement pose any risk to |1?***

There is an increased risk of root resorption. Neil and his mother should be warned about this during the informed consent process. |1 may also become non-vital and require endodontic treatment.

■ ***Are there any precautions you would take during orthodontic treatment to minimize this risk?***

As with all orthodontic tooth movement, excessive forces should be avoided. Sensibility testing and a periapical radiograph should be taken prior to starting treatment and subsequently, for monitoring, at 6 months into treatment. Neil and his mother should be informed of this also during the consent process. Neil should be advised to wear the mouthguard provided during contact sports to minimize the risk of repeat trauma.

|1 became non-vital nearing completion of 1| alignment and required endodontic treatment with gutta percha. This was completed uneventfully.

■ *How would you ensure long-term stability of 1| following alignment?*

Bonded palatal retention will be required to guarantee long-term alignment of 1|.

Labial gingivoplasty may be required at a later stage in relation to 1| to obtain coincidence of the gingival margins of 1|1.

Key point

Sequence in management of unerupted 1:

- Obtain oral surgical/orthodontic opinion (and possibly paediatric dental opinion); if prognosis for 1 alignment judged satisfactory then,
- Open space for unerupted 1 (may involve extractions of primary teeth).
- Remove supernumerary.
- Bond attachment to 1.
- Do not surgically expose 1.
- Align 1 with appropriate appliance.
- Maintain 1 correction with bonded retainer.
- Reassess malocclusion regarding further treatment needs.

Primary resources and recommended reading

Becker A, Brin I, Ben-Bassat Y et al 2002 Closed-eruption surgical technique for impacted maxillary incisors: a postorthodontic periodontal evaluation. Am J Orthod Dentofacial Orthop 122:9–14.

Fleming PS, Xavier GM, DiBiase AT et al 2010 Revisiting the supernumerary: the epidemiological and molecular basis of extra teeth. Br Dent J 208:25–30.

Kapila S, Conley RS, Harrell WE Jr 2011 The current status of cone beam computed tomography imaging in orthodontics. Dentomaxillofac Radiol 40:24–34.

Kindelan SA, Day PF, Kindelan JD et al 2008 Dental trauma: an overview of its influence on the management of orthodontic treatment. Part 1. J Orthod 35:68–78.

Mason C, Azam N, Holt RD et al 2000 A retrospective study of unerupted maxillary incisors associated with supernumerary teeth. Br J Oral Maxillofac Surg 38:62–65.

Yaqoob O, O'Neill J, Gregg T et al 2010 Management of Unerupted Maxillary Incisors. Faculty of Dental Surgery of the Royal College of Surgeons of England. Available at: http://www.rcseng.ac.uk/fds/publications-clinical-guidelines/clinical_guidelines/documents/ManMaxIncisors2010pdf.

For revision, see Mind Map 2, page 222.

3

Absent upper lateral incisors

SUMMARY

Sarah, aged 12 years, presents with spacing of her upper anterior teeth (*Fig. 3.1*). What are the possible causes, and how may it be treated?

History

Complaint

Sarah does not like the gaps between her upper front teeth. She has just moved to a new school and feels self-conscious about the appearance of her teeth.

History of complaint

All primary teeth were present and were lost normally. When her upper permanent front teeth erupted, there was considerable spacing between them, and this has not altered much since then. The permanent teeth erupted at a normal age, and none have been extracted or avulsed.

Medical history

Sarah is fit and well.

Dental history

Sarah attends her general dental practitioner regularly but has had no intervention other than placement of fissure sealants to her first permanent molars.

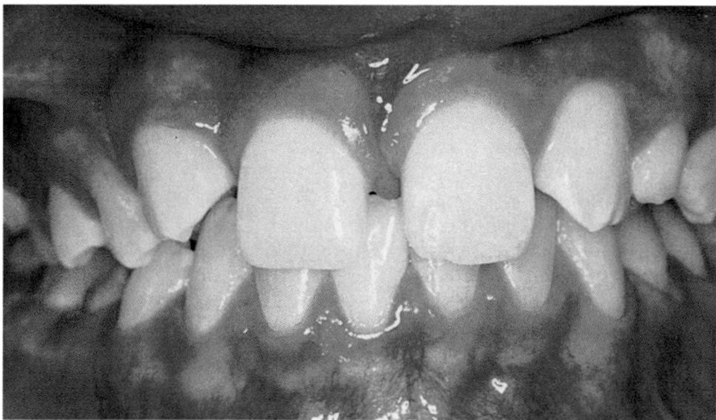

Fig. 3.1 Anterior occlusion at presentation.

Family history

Sarah's mother also has a small space between her upper front teeth due to one missing tooth (2┘).

Social history

Sarah is a keen clarinet player and is not motivated to wear a fixed appliance.

■ ***How will her instrument playing impact on orthodontic treatment?***

Wearing an orthodontic appliance will temporarily affect her musical performance, but with practice and motivation, most wind instrument players adjust. With a woodwind instrument such as a clarinet, it is likely that Sarah will adjust very quickly to wearing an orthodontic appliance and that playing will return to normal within a few weeks. It would, however, be advisable to avoid fitting an appliance close to dates of music exams, auditions or performances. Any orthodontic appliance, particularly fixed appliances, may rub the inside of the lips and cheeks when fitted, but wax may be applied to minimize this. As Sarah is not keen for a fixed appliance and provided treatment is possible with a removable appliance, this could be removed while playing. In advance of any orthodontic treatment, it would be useful for the orthodontist to ascertain how many hours Sarah practises per day, as leaving the appliance out for long periods is likely to impede treatment progress.

Examination

Extraoral

Sarah has a Class I skeletal pattern with average FMPA; there is no facial asymmetry. Her lips are competent with the lower lip covering the incisal third of the upper incisors. The temporomandibular joints are symptom-free.

Intraoral

■ ***The intraoral views are shown in* Figs 3.1 *and* 3.2*. What do these show?***

The soft tissues appear healthy and overall oral hygiene seems good, although there are small plaque deposits labially on the lower incisors. All teeth are of good quality, and no caries is evident.

The following teeth are present:

7 6 5 4 3 1	1 3 C 4 5 6 7
7 6 5 4 3 2 1	1 2 3 4 5 6 7

There is a retained fragment of E┐.

There is mild imbrication of the lower incisors; the upper arch is spaced.

The incisor relationship is Class I with a complete overbite.

The lower centreline is shifted slightly to the left.

The buccal segment relationship is half unit Class II bilaterally.

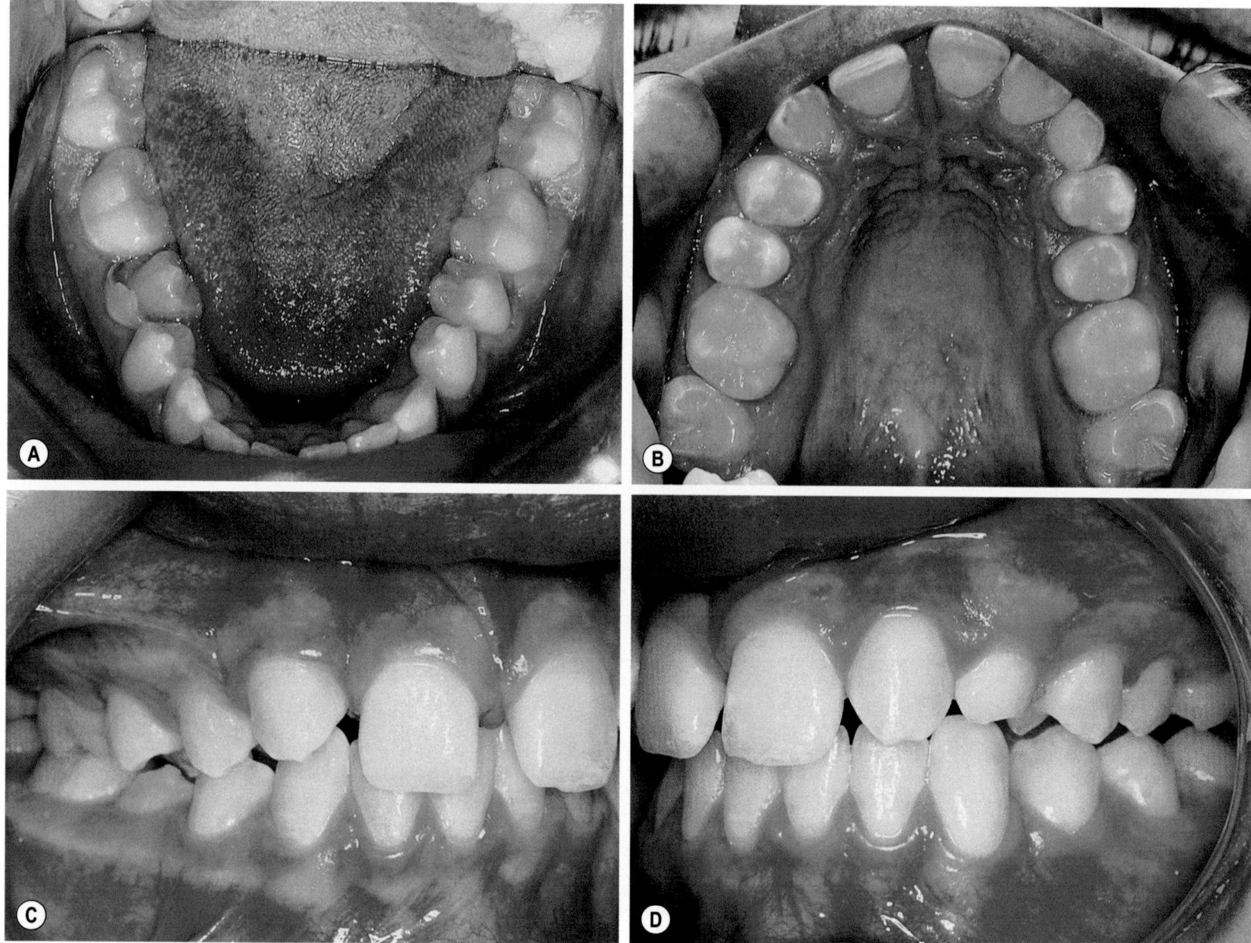

Fig. 3.2 (A) Lower occlusal view. **(B)** Upper occlusal view. **(C)** Right buccal occlusion. **(D)** Left buccal occlusion.

■ ***What other clinic assessment would you undertake?***

The labial and palatal mucosae in the $\underline{2}$ area should be palpated for the presence of an unerupted tooth or any pathology.

■ ***What are the possible causes of the upper labial segment spacing?***

These are listed in **Table 3.1**.

■ ***What is the most likely cause in this case?***

Congenital absence of $\underline{2|2}$ is most likely. This is more common in females than males. The genetic linkage is indicated by Sarah's mother, who has absence of $\underline{2|}$.

Table 3.1 Possible causes of the upper labial segment spacing

Cause	Aetiology
Absence of $\underline{2\|2}$	Hypodontia (affects ~2% of Caucasians) – also associated with cleft lip and palate, Down syndrome and ectodermal dysplasia Avulsion Extraction
Failure of/delayed eruption of $\underline{2}$'s	Crowding Ectopic position Supernumerary tooth Scar tissue Dilaceration Cyst/tumour

Key point

Congenital absence of $\underline{2}$'s is more common in females.

Investigations

■ ***What further investigations would you undertake?***

Clinical

- Mobility testing of the retained upper primary canine ($\underline{|C}$) is required. Grade 1 mobility was detected.

Radiographic

- A dental panoramic tomogram is required to determine the presence/absence of $\underline{2}$'s, 8's, supernumerary teeth or any pathology.

Sarah's dental panoramic tomogram showed:

- Normal alveolar bone height.
- Absence of $\underline{2|2}$ and third molars; short root on $\underline{|C}$.
- No pathology associated with any erupted or unerupted teeth.

Occlusal

- Impressions and a wax registration should be taken for study models to allow further assessment of the occlusion.

What genes have been linked to hypodontia?

MSX1 and PAX9 have been linked.

How would you rate the severity of the hypodontia?

Sarah has missing 2's and thus has mild hypodontia (one or two teeth missing). Moderate or severe hypodontia indicates three to five or more than six teeth missing, respectively.

Are there other facial/dental/occlusal features associated with hypodontia?

Reduced lower facial height, delayed dental development, retained primary teeth, small teeth and an increased overbite have been associated. Thinning of the hair and absence of palmar sweat glands are features of anhidrotic ectodermal dysplasia, which is associated with severe hypodontia (see Chapter 37).

Diagnosis

What is your diagnosis?

Class I malocclusion on a Class I skeletal base with average FMPA. Well cared for mouth. Mildly imbricated lower incisors but otherwise uncrowded lower arch; spaced upper arch with absent 2|2 and retained |C. Buccal segment relationship is half-unit Class II bilaterally.

What is the IOTN DHC grade (see p. 264)? Explain why.

4h – due to absence of 2|2.

Treatment

What are the treatment options?

These are:

1. Accept the spacing – not a realistic option as Sarah is concerned by it.
2. Build up the mesiodistal width of 1's and 3's with composite or by veneering to reduce the spacing, but not to close it completely. The median diastema is too large for restorative build up of 1|1 to look aesthetic. Some recontouring of the cusp tips of 3's would also be required to improve the final appearance.
3. Orthodontic space closure. This would require a considerable amount of tooth movement along with |C extraction, the wearing of a fixed appliance and reverse headgear or the placement of TADs may be considered to assist space closure.
4. Orthodontic space opening (this would require extraction of |C) for replacement of 2's on resin-retained bridges, by fixed bridgework or by implants in late teenage years. Replacement of 2's by autotransplantation of lower premolars (see Chapter 2) is not a viable consideration as (i) the lower arch does not warrant premolar extractions and (ii) root formation on lower premolars is in advance of the ideal stage (two-thirds to three-quarters complete).

As option 2 will only partly address Sarah's concerns it has to be ruled out. The choice then is between the two orthodontic options.

> **Key point**
>
> Management options with absent 2's are to
>
> - Maintain or close 2 space.
> - Open space for 2 replacement.

What factors would you consider in deciding between space closure or space opening?

Sarah should be seen with a restorative colleague who will provide input regarding the restorative implications of each treatment option. Then, it is often wise to undertake a trial set-up of the optimal treatment option using duplicate study models and to show this to the patient, to allow a fuller appreciation of the likely treatment outcome.

The following factors should be considered:

The patient's attitude to orthodontic treatment. If the patient is not keen to wear fixed appliances, it may necessitate a change in treatment plan.

The anteroposterior and vertical skeletal relationships. In Class II cases with an increased overjet, space closure is desirable as it will eliminate the overjet, whereas in Class III cases this would tend to worsen the incisor relationship. Space opening is optimal in Class III cases where proclination of the incisors is likely to correct an anterior crossbite. Where the FMPA is reduced, space opening is preferable to space closure, and the converse is true where an increased FMPA exists.

The colour, size, shape and angulation of the canine and incisor teeth. Where the maxillary canine is considerably darker than the incisors and/or it has a marked canine form, space closure is not advisable as considerable recontouring of 3's will be required to enable them to resemble 2's. Where the canine and incisor teeth are so angulated that it is possible to reposition them into their desired locations by tipping movements, a removable rather than a fixed appliance may be used.

Whether the arches are spaced or crowded, and the buccal segment occlusion. In uncrowded or mildly crowded arches, where the buccal segment occlusion is Class I or at most half-unit Class II, space opening is best. Space closure is preferable where more crowding exists and the buccal segment relationship is a full-unit Class II.

In this case it was decided to proceed with space opening for replacement of 2|2, ultimately on resin-retained bridges. This required an initial phase of distal movement of the upper buccal segments to achieve a Class I molar relationship, extraction of |C, followed by retraction of 3's to a Class I relationship with 3's and space opening for 2's replacement. Importantly, overbite reduction was also undertaken in conjunction with these tooth movements to provide space for the metal framework of the resin-retained bridges.

Ideally, a fixed appliance would be indicated to achieve these objectives, but as Sarah was not keen for this form of treatment, an acceptable though not optimal outcome was deemed achievable by upper removable appliance therapy.

Could treatment time have been shortened by an earlier interceptive measure?

Removal of C's is a useful interceptive measure in the early mixed dentition when space closure is planned as it encourages 3's to erupt more mesially. In this case, however, space opening for 2's replacement was planned. Hence removal of |C at age 10 is likely to have allowed |3 to erupt in a more distal position than it is now but would also have encouraged mesial drift of the upper left buccal segment. So on balance, this extraction at an earlier stage is unlikely to have shortened treatment time.

> **Key point**
>
> With absent 2's consider:
>
> - Patient's attitude to orthodontic treatment.
> - Skeletal relationships.
> - Colour, size, shape and angulation of 3 and 1.
> - Crowding/spacing.
> - Buccal segment occlusion.

■ *How could the upper buccal segments be moved distally using a removable appliance to achieve a Class I molar relationship?*

An upper removable appliance with bilateral screws to move 6 5 4| and |4 5 6 distally is an option. Anchorage needs to be reinforced by allowing provision for headgear to be attached to the appliance. The appliance should also incorporate:

- Adams clasps (0.7 mm stainless steel wire) with headgear tubes soldered to 6's clasp bridges; Adams clasps (0.7 mm stainless steel wire) to 4's also.
- Short labial bow 3| to |3 (0.7 mm stainless steel wire).
- Flat anterior biteplane to half the crown height of 1|1 and extended 3 mm further palatally than the maximum overjet measurement.

When there is evidence of full-time appliance wear, headgear should be fitted for anchorage with an upward direction of pull to prevent the appliance becoming dislodged when the headgear is being worn.

■ *What force and duration of headgear wear is required for anchorage?*

A force of 250–350g per side for 8–10 hours per day is required.

■ *What precautions must be adhered to when prescribing headgear?*

Two safety mechanisms must be fitted to the headgear assembly, preferably a safety release spring mechanism attached to the headcap and a facebow with a locking device. Verbal and written safety instructions must be issued to both patient and parent(s)/guardian. The headgear should be checked at each visit.

When compliance with headgear wear is evident, then Sarah should be instructed to turn each screw once per week. |C should be extracted and acrylic relieved to allow for potential distal drift of |3 as the buccal segments are retracted to Class I. Some over-retraction is advisable to allow for any slight anchorage slip during the next phase of treatment when 3's will be retracted to a Class I relationship with 3's; 1's will be approximated and overbite reduction will be maintained.

■ *What design of upper removable appliance would you consider for these tooth movements?*

Palatal finger springs to 31|13 (0.5 mm stainless steel wire).

Adams clasps 6|6 (0.7 mm stainless steel wire) with headgear tubes soldered to the clasp bridges.

Long labial bow with 'U' loops (0.7 mm stainless steel wire) from 4| to |4.

Flat anterior biteplane to half the crown height of 1|1 and extended 3 mm further palatally than the maximum overjet measurement. This is an important component of the appliance to ensure that overbite reduction is maintained, creating sufficient interocclusal clearance for placement of the metal framework on the resin-bonded bridges.

■ *When space has been created for 2|2, what should be done?*

The patient should be seen again with a restorative colleague to ensure that the tooth movements achieved will allow restorative treatment to proceed as planned. Then a removable retainer should be fitted for 6 months carrying replacement 2|2 and ensuring that space for them is maintained by placing wire spurs in contact with the adjoining teeth (**Fig. 3.3**).

> **Key point**
>
> - Always place wire spurs on the removable retainer, to the teeth adjoining the 2 space after space opening.
> - Retain for 6 months before replacing 2 on resin-retained bridge (underline 2).

■ *What design of resin-retained bridge is required?*

Maintenance of closure of the median diastema requires permanent retention. A bonded palatal retainer framework linking 1|1 together is indicated along with resin-retained bridges with single wing, off 3|3. It is better that 1|1 are retained as a separate unit rather than risk the retention integrity and success of the bridges by incorporating 1|1 retention in the bridge design.

Implant replacement of 2|2 later is unlikely as the roots of 31|13 are tipped toward the 2|2 space, compromising access for implant positioning. The final result with 2|2 replaced on adhesive bridgework is shown in **Fig. 3.4**.

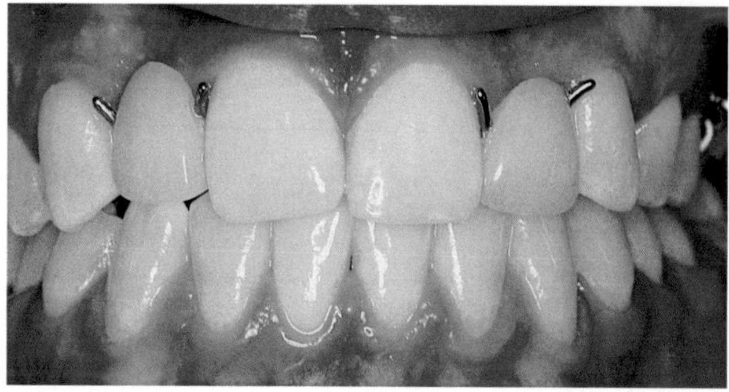

Fig. 3.3 Upper removable appliance retainer with replacement 2's.

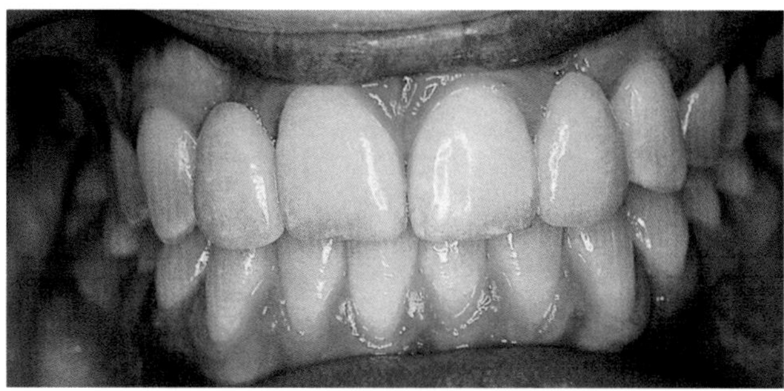

Fig. 3.4 Final restorations.

What additional factors would need to have been considered if replacement of 2's by implants was the preferred plan?

It would be necessary to wait until facial growth has reduced to adult levels. In a girl, growth of the maxilla is complete by about 15 years of age and mandibular growth usually 2 years later, whereas in boys maxillary growth usually continues to about 17 years of age and mandibular growth until 19 years or later. This is especially important as an implant has no eruptive potential and will be left behind if eruption of adjacent teeth is still continuing, compromising aesthetics.

Aside from sufficient distance between the roots of the adjacent teeth, space must also exist between the tooth crowns with sufficient interocclusal clearance. Additionally, ample buccopalatal width and height of the alveolar bone is required in the 2 area.

Primary resources and recommended reading

British Orthodontic Society 2007 Advice for musicians. Available at: www.bos.org.uk/orthodonticsandyou/orthodonticsforschools/adviceformusicians.htm.

Carter NE, Gillgrass TJ, Hobson RS et al 2003 The interdisciplinary management of hypodontia: orthodontics. Br Dent J 194:361–366.

Harrison JE, Bowden DE 1992 The orthodontic/restorative interface. Restorative procedures to aid orthodontic treatment. Br J Orthod 19:143–152.

Khalaf K, Miskelly J, Voge E, et al 2014 Prevalence of hypodontia and associated factors: a systematic review and meta-analysis. J Orthod 41:299–316.

Kohich KO Jr, Kinzer GA, Janakievski J, 2011 Congenitally missing maxillary lateral incisors: restorative replacement. Am J Orthod Dentofac Orthop 139:435–445.

Mossey PA 1999 The heritability of malocclusion: part 2. The influence of genetics in malocclusion. Br J Orthod 26:195–203.

Qadri S, Parkin NA, Benson PE 2016 Space closing versus space opening for bilateral missing upper laterals - aesthetic judgments of laypeople: a web-based survey. J Orthod 43 (2):137–146.

Robertsson S, Mohlin B 2000 The congenitally missing upper lateral incisor. A retrospective study of orthodontic space closure versus restorative treatment. Eur J Orthod 22:697–710.

Silveira GS, De Almeida NV, Pereira DMT et al 2016 Prosthetic replacement vs space closure for maxillary lateral incisor agenesis: A systematic review. Am J Orthod 150, 228–237.

Zachrisson BU, Rosa M, Toreskog S 2011 Congenitally missing maxillary lateral incisors: canine substitution. Am J Orthod Dentofac Orthop 139:434–444.

For revision, see Mind Map 3, page 223.

4

Crowding and buccal upper canines

CASE 1

SUMMARY

Gemma, an 11-year-old girl, attends for a 6-month dental assessment at your practice with both upper permanent canines erupting buccally** (Fig. 4.1)**. What is the cause, and how may it be treated?

History

Complaint

Gemma does not like the 'squint' appearance of her top and bottom teeth, in particular the position of the upper eye teeth, which she says 'look like fangs'.

History of complaint

The crookedness of Gemma's teeth has been getting worse for the past year. The appearance of her upper teeth has become of more concern to her in recent months when both upper eye teeth started to erupt. She is now teased at school and called 'Fangs', which annoys her.

Gemma's mother reports that her daughter's baby teeth were also slightly crooked. Both she and Gemma are very keen for treatment.

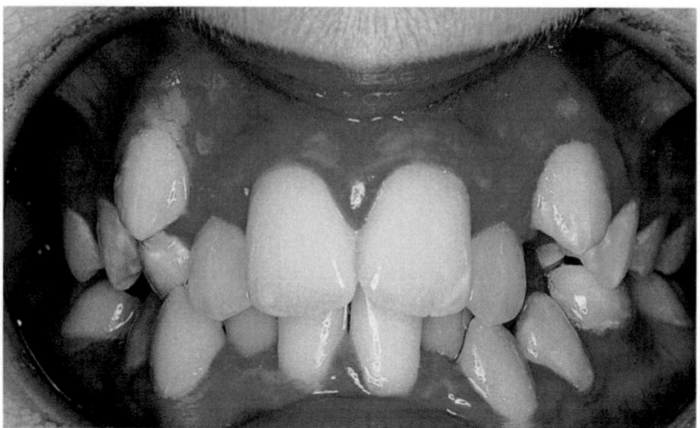

Fig. 4.1 Anterior occlusion at presentation.

Medical history

Gemma has had asthma since she was 5 years of age and uses a salbutamol (Ventolin) inhaler; otherwise she is fit and well.

■ ***What are the implications for orthodontic treatment with asthma?***

These are summarized in Appendix 4.

Dental history

Gemma has attended for routine dental examinations since she was 3 years old but has not undergone any active dental treatment.

Examination

Extraoral

Gemma has a Class I skeletal pattern with average FMPA. There appears to be slight facial asymmetry with the chin point deviated mildly to the right. The lips are competent.

No temporomandibular signs or symptoms were detected or reported.

Gemma and her mother were unaware of Gemma's slight facial asymmetry and have noticed no change in her facial appearance over recent years.

■ ***Would you be concerned by the mild facial asymmetry?***

A mild degree of facial asymmetry is normal, and as facial appearance is reportedly unaltered for several years, there is no cause for concern.

Intraoral

■ ***Gemma's intraoral views are shown in** Figs 4.1 **and** 4.2**. What do you notice?***

Generalized marginal gingival erythema.

Plaque deposits visible on several teeth, notably both 3's.

There are no restorations, and there is no obvious caries.

Gemma is in the late mixed dentition stage with the following teeth present: $\frac{6\,5\,4\,C\,3\,2\,1 | 1\,2\,3\,4\,5\,6}{7\,6\,5\,4\,3\,2\,1 | 1\,2\,3\,4\,E\,6\,7}$ (note 5⌉ and 7⌋⌊7 are partially erupted).

The lower labial segment is moderately crowded with 2⌉⌈2 bodily displaced lingually and 1⌉⌈1 slightly mesiolabially rotated.

3⌉ is distally angulated; ⌈3 is mesially angulated.

The lower right buccal segment is also crowded with insufficient space for 5⌉; the lower left buccal segment is uncrowded with ⌈E present.

The upper labial segment is moderately crowded with 1⌋⌊1 slightly mesiolabially rotated and 3⌋⌊3 erupting buccally; C⌋ is present.

3⌋ is upright and ⌊3 is slightly distally angulated.

The upper buccal segments are aligned.

In occlusion, there is a Class I incisor relationship.

The overbite is average and complete.

The lower centreline is slightly to the right.

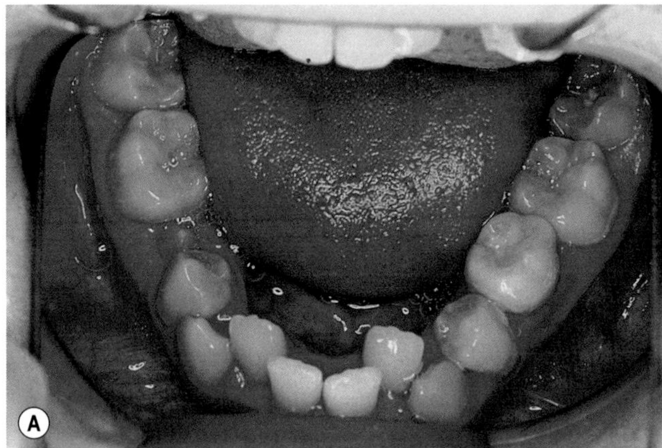

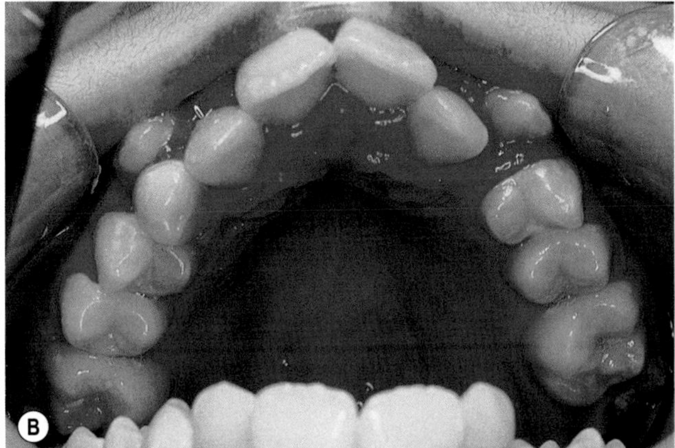

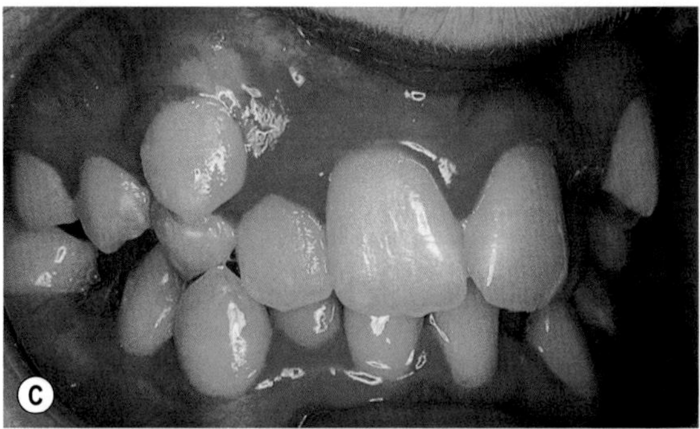

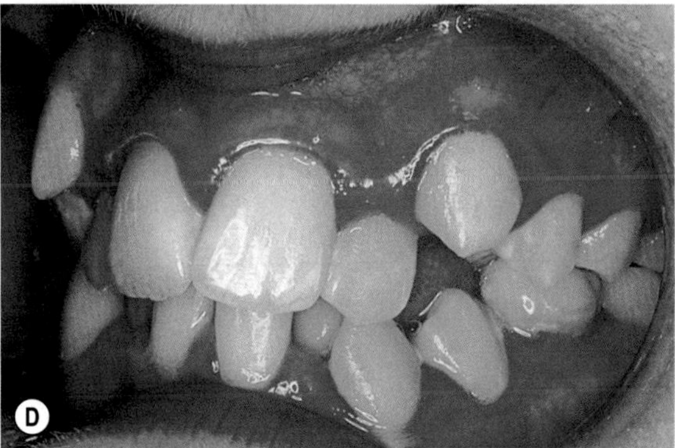

Fig. 4.2 **(A)** Lower occlusal view. **(B)** Upper occlusal view. **(C)** Right buccal occlusion. **(D)** Left buccal occlusion.

The right molar relationship is Class III, and the left molar relationship is Class I.

- ***What are the possible reasons for 3's erupting buccally?***

  - *Crowding* – buccal displacement of 3's is often a manifestation of inherent crowding in the upper arch. A contributory factor is 3 being the last tooth to erupt anterior to the first permanent molars.

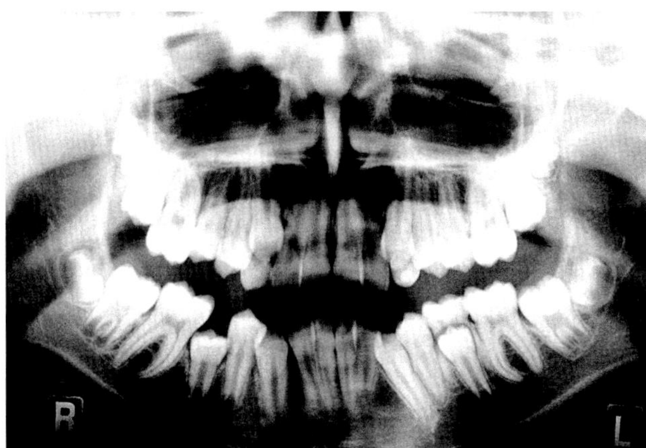

Fig. 4.3 Dental panoramic tomogram.

  - *Retention of the primary canine* – this usually leads to slight buccal displacement of 3.

Key point

Buccal displacement of 3 is more usual in a crowded arch.

Investigations

- ***What investigations would you request and why?***

A dental panoramic tomogram is required to provide a general view of the developing dentition and to confirm the presence and position of all unerupted permanent teeth.

- ***Gemma's dental panoramic tomogram is shown in*** *Fig. 4.3*. ***What do you notice?***

  Alveolar bone level is normal.

  Presence of a full complement of developing permanent teeth, including third molars.

  All teeth appear caries-free.

Diagnosis

- ***What is your diagnosis?***

  Class I malocclusion on a Class I skeletal base with average FMPA, with the chin point displaced slightly to the right.

  Generalized marginal gingivitis.

  Moderate upper and lower arch crowding with the lower centreline shifted slightly to the right.

  Right molar relationship is Class III; left molar relationship is Class I.

- ***What is the IOTN DHC grade and why (see p. 264)? Explain why.***

4d – due to severe displacements of teeth, greater than 4 mm.

Treatment

- ***What treatment is likely to be required in this case? Explain why.***

Extractions are required to relieve the moderate crowding. Fixed appliance therapy is indicated in view of the distal angulation of most canines, the rotations of the central incisors, the bodily lingual displacement of $\overline{2}$'s and the centreline shift.

What would you do now?

Explain to the patient the likely plan for correction of her malocclusion.

Arrange for several visits of oral hygiene instruction by the practice hygienist, and assuming that oral hygiene improves satisfactorily, take upper and lower impressions and a wax registration for study models.

Arrange referral to an orthodontist and enclose the study models and dental panoramic tomogram.

Write a referral letter to the orthodontist (**Fig. 4.4**).

What aims of treatment do you think will be proposed by the orthodontist?

Relief of crowding.

Upper and lower arch alignment.

Correction of lower centreline.

Correction of right molar relationship.

Closure of any residual spacing.

Describe how you would approach treatment planning.

1. *Consider the lower arch first and plan the lower labial segment.* As the latter is in a narrow zone of soft tissue balance between the lips and the tongue, it is best to consider this sacrosanct. First the alignment of the labial segment must be assessed, and if it is crowded, as in Gemma's case, the degree of crowding must be assessed to ascertain if this is sufficient to warrant extractions.

Practice address

Date

Dear

Re [patient's name, address, date of birth]

I would be grateful if you could see Gemma for orthodontic assessment and treatment.

Gemma is very concerned about the crowding of her teeth. Apart from using a salbutamol (Ventolin) inhaler for asthma, she is in good health.

Gemma's oral hygiene is improving following several visits to our hygenist. She has a caries-free dentition. She is very keen for treatment and is prepared to wear fixed appliances.

She has a Class I malocclusion on a Class I skeletal base with average FMPA and the chin point slightly to the right. The upper and lower arches are moderately crowded and the lower centreline is slightly to the right. The right molar relationship is Class III; the left molar relationship is Class I.

I enclose current study models and a recent dental panoramic tomogram.

Yours sincerely

Fig. 4.4 Example of a referral letter.

As Gemma has moderate lower labial segment crowding, space will be required to achieve alignment.

What possible means are there of creating space?

Extractions.

Arch expansion (laterally and/or anteroposteriorly).

Distal movement of the molars.

Enamel stripping.

Any combination of the above.

Expansion of the lower intercanine width is unstable as is forward movement of the lower labial segment (with a few exceptions which will be dealt with elsewhere); distal movement of the lower first permanent molars is difficult without extraction of lower second permanent molars and is undertaken rarely. Enamel stripping is usually only considered in adults to gain 1–2 mm of space in total. In view of these considerations, extractions are the only realistic option of gaining space in Gemma's case.

Key point

Always consider the lower arch first in treatment planning.

What factors govern the choice of extraction?

Prognosis of teeth.

Site of crowding.

Degree of crowding.

Individual tooth position, e.g. grossly displaced or ectopic teeth.

In this case there are no lower teeth of poor prognosis, and in view of the site and degree of crowding, the lower first premolars would be the teeth of choice for extraction.

Why are first premolars commonly chosen for extraction?

They are in the middle of the arch and, therefore, provide space for relief of moderate labial and buccal segment crowding.

The contact point between the canine and second premolar is as good as between the canine and the first premolar.

If a canine is mesially angulated, considerable scope exists for spontaneous alignment of the labial segment as the canine uprights into the extraction space. For maximum spontaneous improvement, it is best to extract the first premolars as the permanent canines are erupting.

Any residual space is not at the front of the mouth and is likely to close further with mesial drift of the buccal segments.

2. *Imagine the corrected position of $\overline{3}$.* $\overline{|3}$ is mesially angulated and will upright spontaneously following removal of $\overline{|4}$, thereby providing space for labial segment alignment; $\overline{3|}$, however, is distally angulated and will require bodily retraction with a fixed appliance.
3. *Mentally reposition $\underline{3}$ to be in a Class I relationship with the corrected position of $\overline{3}$.* Space is required in Gemma's case for this. Extraction of both upper first premolars should provide adequate space for retraction of $\underline{3}$'s. As

3⌋ is upright and ⌊3 is distally angulated, fixed appliance therapy is indicated to effect this movement.

4. *Plan the upper labial segment.* The incisors are mildly crowded and slightly rotated, so fixed appliance therapy is required to produce ideal alignment.
5. *Decide on the final molar relationship.* As upper and lower first premolar extractions are planned, the final molar relationship should be Class I. Closure of residual buccal segment spacing following the extractions will require fixed appliance therapy.
6. *Assess the anchorage needs.* As almost all of the upper first premolar extraction spaces will be required for relief of upper arch crowding, and retraction of the upright/distally angulated $\underline{3}$'s is needed, anchorage would be best reinforced with a palatal arch attached to bands on $\underline{6}$'s or temporary anchorage devices (TADs).
7. *Plan retention.* The prognosis is favourable, but bonded retention to the lower labial segment would be wise in view of the bodily lingual displacement of $\overline{2|2}$. Upper and lower vacuum-formed retainers should also be provided to be worn at night for the first 12 months following debond; the lower is designed to fit over the bonded retainer. Thereafter, retention should continue on a night-only basis, reducing to alternate nights for another year and then to twice weekly. Gemma's responsibility with regard to retention should be explained before treatment starts.

Key point

- Always plan anchorage at the treatment planning stage.
- The amount of space and type of intended tooth movement influence anchorage demands.
- Always consider retention in the treatment plan.

■ *What is the final orthodontic treatment plan likely to be?*

No appliance therapy would be considered until Gemma has demonstrated that she is capable of maintaining a high standard of oral hygiene. Then the orthodontic plan would be:

8. Fit palatal arch for anchorage or place TADs (see Chapter 5).
9. Extraction of four first premolars (provided there is satisfactory cooperation with wear of the palatal arch). TADs could be placed, instead of the palatal arch, at the time of the upper arch extractions.
10. Upper and lower fixed appliance therapy.
11. Lower canine to canine bonded retainer with upper and lower vacuum-formed retainers.

■ *What risks should the patient be warned of regarding fixed appliance orthodontic treatment?*

The patient should be warned of the risk of:

Enamel demineralization.

Root resorption.

Loss of tooth vitality.

Relapse.

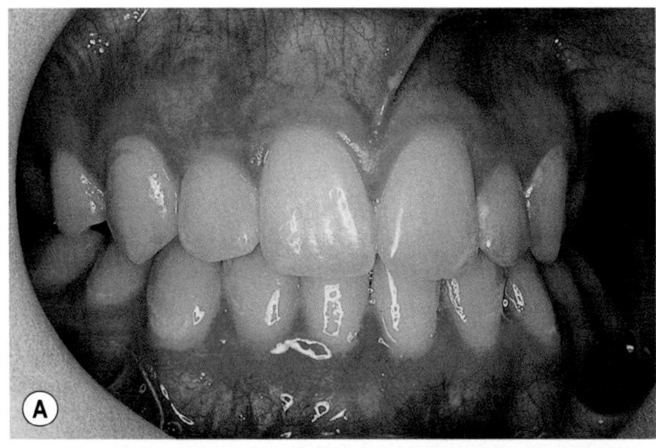

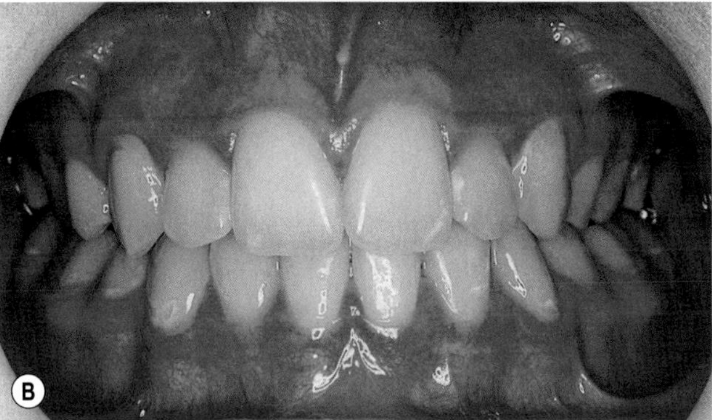

Fig. 4.5 (A) Post-treatment: right buccal occlusion. **(B)** Post-treatment: anterior occlusion.

■ *Gemma's final occlusion is shown in* Fig. 4.5. *What undesirable sequelae of treatment are visible?*

Several teeth are affected by white spot lesions or demineralization, indicating early carious involvement.

■ *How common is this with fixed appliance therapy and which teeth are affected mostly?*

The reported prevalence is between 2% and 96%. Upper lateral incisors and lower canines are affected most commonly.

■ *How may the problem be prevented or minimized?*

Careful patient selection; ensure a high standard of oral hygiene pre-treatment.

Advise the patient that fizzy drinks and sugary foods should not be consumed between meals.

The teeth should be brushed with a fluoridated dentifrice after each meal.

Regular surveillance of oral hygiene and oral hygiene instruction should be undertaken by a hygienist throughout treatment.

Daily use of a fluoride mouthrinse (0.05% sodium fluoride) is recommended during treatment.

Moderate quality evidence exists that application of a fluoride (0.1% fluoride) varnish around the brackets on a 6-weekly basis is effective.

■ *How may these 'white spots' be managed?*

Usually, following removal of the appliances, the white spots regress slightly as maintenance of an improved standard of oral hygiene is facilitated. Application of high-concentration fluoride varnish is inadvisable at this stage as it leads to hypermineralization of the lesions, which makes them more obvious.

Where the white spot lesions are extensive and pose an obvious aesthetic insult, acid-pumice abrasion with 0.2% hydrofluoric acid may be carried out. In rare severe cases, veneers or composite restorations are likely to be required.

> **Key point**
>
> Demineralization with fixed appliances:
> - Is common (2–96% prevalence).
> - Mostly affects $\underline{2}$'s and $\overline{3}$'s.
> - Is best prevented by careful patient selection and dietary advice.

CASE 2

SUMMARY

Aoife, a 12-year-old girl, presented with crowded upper teeth. Her mother reported a possible nickel allergy.

■ ***How would you deal with the history of a possible nickel allergy?***

Aoife should be referred to a dermatologist for assessment and patch testing.

Fortunately, no allergy to nickel was reported.

■ ***How common is nickel allergy?***

Nickel allergy is more common in females (10–30%) than males (~2%), possibly due to increased contact from nickel-containing jewellery.

■ ***What implications does a nickel allergy have for orthodontic management?***

These are summarized in Appendix 4.

> **Key point**
>
> A suspected nickel allergy:
> - Should be assessed by a dermatologist.
> - Is more common in females.
> - May require use of nickel-free appliance components.

■ ***What do you notice on the radiographs shown in** Fig. 4.6**?***

The dental panoramic tomogram shows:

Normal alveolar bone height.

7 6 5 4 C 2 1 | 1 2 3 4 5 6 7
7 6 5 4 3 2 1 | 1 2 3 4 5 6 7 erupted.

Four third molars developing.

All permanent teeth of good quality; some root shortening of C| but of reasonable length.

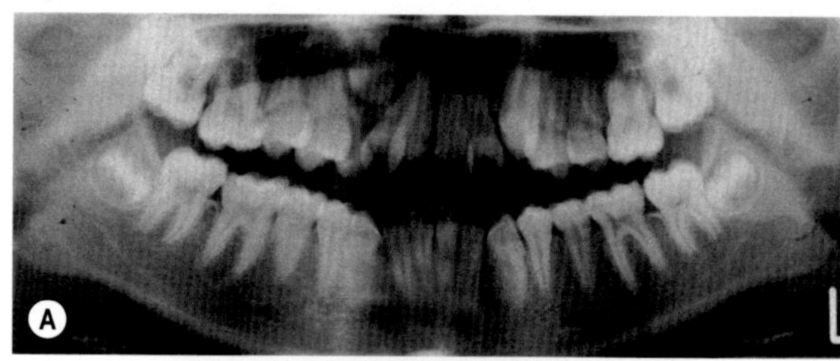

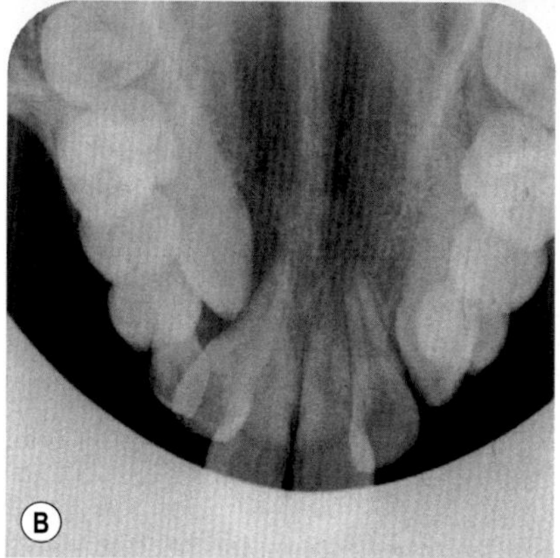

Fig. 4.6 (A) Dental panoramic tomogram. **(B)** Upper anterior occlusal radiograph.

The upper anterior occlusal radiograph reveals:

Tapered roots of the upper incisors.

3| to be in contact with 2| root which is distally angulated.

■ ***Where is 3| located? Explain how this assessment is made and your reasoning.***

3| is buccally placed. This assessment is made by comparing the position of 3| on the panoramic film and the occlusal film using vertical parallax. The x-ray tube has moved up between the panoramic (taken at −10° to the occlusal plane) and the occlusal (taken at 65–70° to the occlusal plane). This would be a 75–80° tube shift. The position of 3| relative to the adjacent 2| is then assessed. An object closer to the x-ray beam (buccally placed) will seem to move in the opposite direction as the tube shift. This is evident for 3|.

■ ***What do you notice in** Fig. 4.7**?***

Right buccal occlusion showing:

Mild marginal gingival erythema with apparent bulge over 2|.

No caries.

Crowded lower arch with mesially angulated $\overline{3}$| (lower arch was overall moderately crowded).

Spacing between 4| and 2| but insufficient for 3|; 2| distally angulated and mesiopalatally rotated.

Class 1 incisor and molar relationship; average overjet; overbite average (1| covers half lower incisor crown) and complete.

■ ***What are the aims of treatment?***

The aims of treatment are to:

Improve oral hygiene.

Relieve upper and lower arch crowding with alignment of 3|.

Closure of residual spaces.

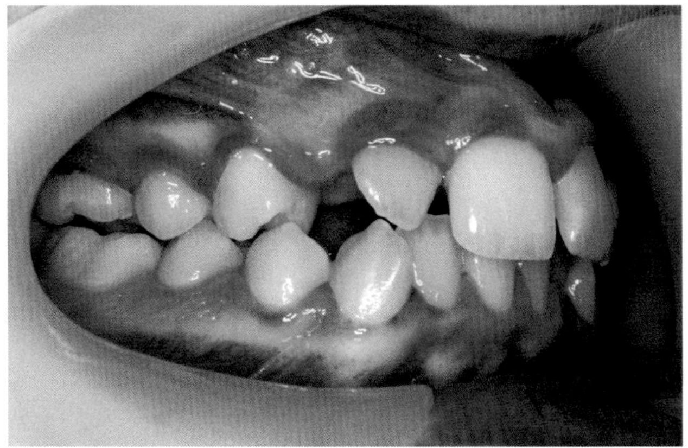

Fig. 4.7 Right buccal occlusion at presentation.

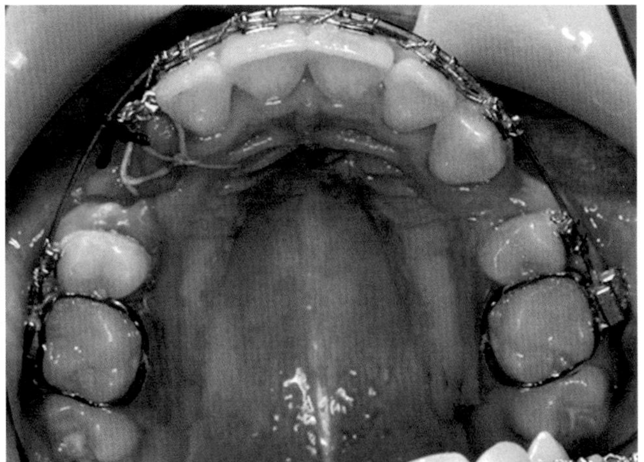

Fig. 4.8 Upper occlusal view following extraction 4|4 and closed surgical exposure of 3|.

Four first premolars were extracted followed by fixed appliance mechanics.

3| remained unerupted 9 months after extraction of 4|. How would you manage 3|?

It would be advisable to assess 3| with an oral surgeon and discuss surgical exposure.

■ ***What types of surgical exposure are there for a buccally positioned canine?***

Open or closed exposure are the possible surgical options. With open exposure, an apically repositioned flap would be required. With closed exposure, a buccal flap is raised and an attachment with gold chain bonded to 3| to facilitate traction, followed by replacement of the flap. Due to operator preference, a closed exposure was agreed upon (**Fig. 4.8**).

■ ***How may 3| be aligned?***

Initially, 3| may be aligned partially by attaching the gold chain to the base archwire; a bracket will then need to be bonded to 3| and a light (typically 0.012-in or 0.014-in nickel titanium) archwire 'piggy-backed' to the base archwire to improve alignment until 3| can be fully engaged in a 0.019 × 0.025-in stainless steel wire (assuming an 0.022 × 0.028-in slot).

The final occlusion is shown in **Fig. 4.9**.

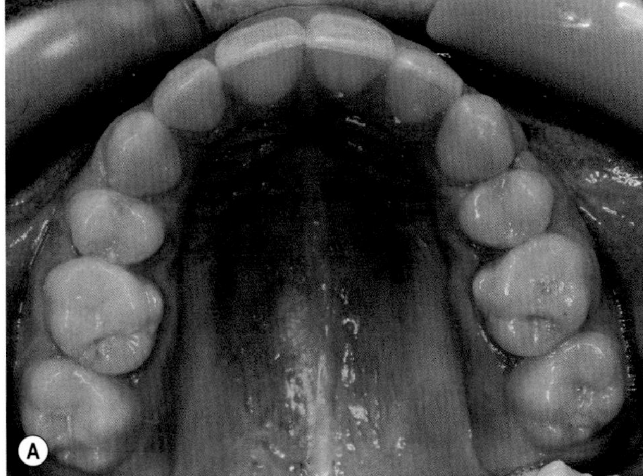

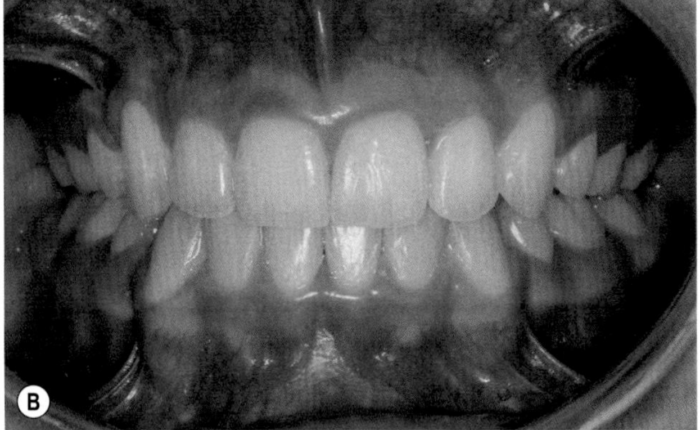

Fig. 4.9 **(A)** Post-treatment: upper occlusal view. **(B)** Post-treatment: anterior occlusion.

CASE 3

SUMMARY

Triona, a 13-year-old girl, presents with 3| and |3 erupting buccally. How will you manage the problem?

■ ***What do you notice in** Fig. 4.10**?***

Mild generalized marginal gingiva erythema; caries-free dentition with fissure sealants in all first permanent molars.

Mild lower arch crowding; severe upper arch crowding with 3| and |3 erupting buccally. (Cusp tip of |3 just visible.)

Lower incisors appear slightly retroclined and upper incisors appear upright to retroclined.

Class III incisor relationship; with 21|1 in crossbite (reverse overjet was 1 mm on 1|); minimal overbite (~1 mm measured clinically on 1|).

Centreline shift (upper was 3 mm to the left clinically).

Right molar relationship slightly Class II; left molar relationship slightly Class III with |5 erupting potentially in crossbite.

■ ***Is it possible to make a reliable assessment of the incisor inclination to the underlying dental bases from intraoral images of the dentition in occlusion?***

It is not possible to tell the upper and lower incisor inclination reliably from intraoral clinical images as there are no reference planes visible (Frankfort or maxillary and

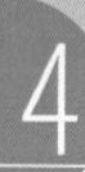

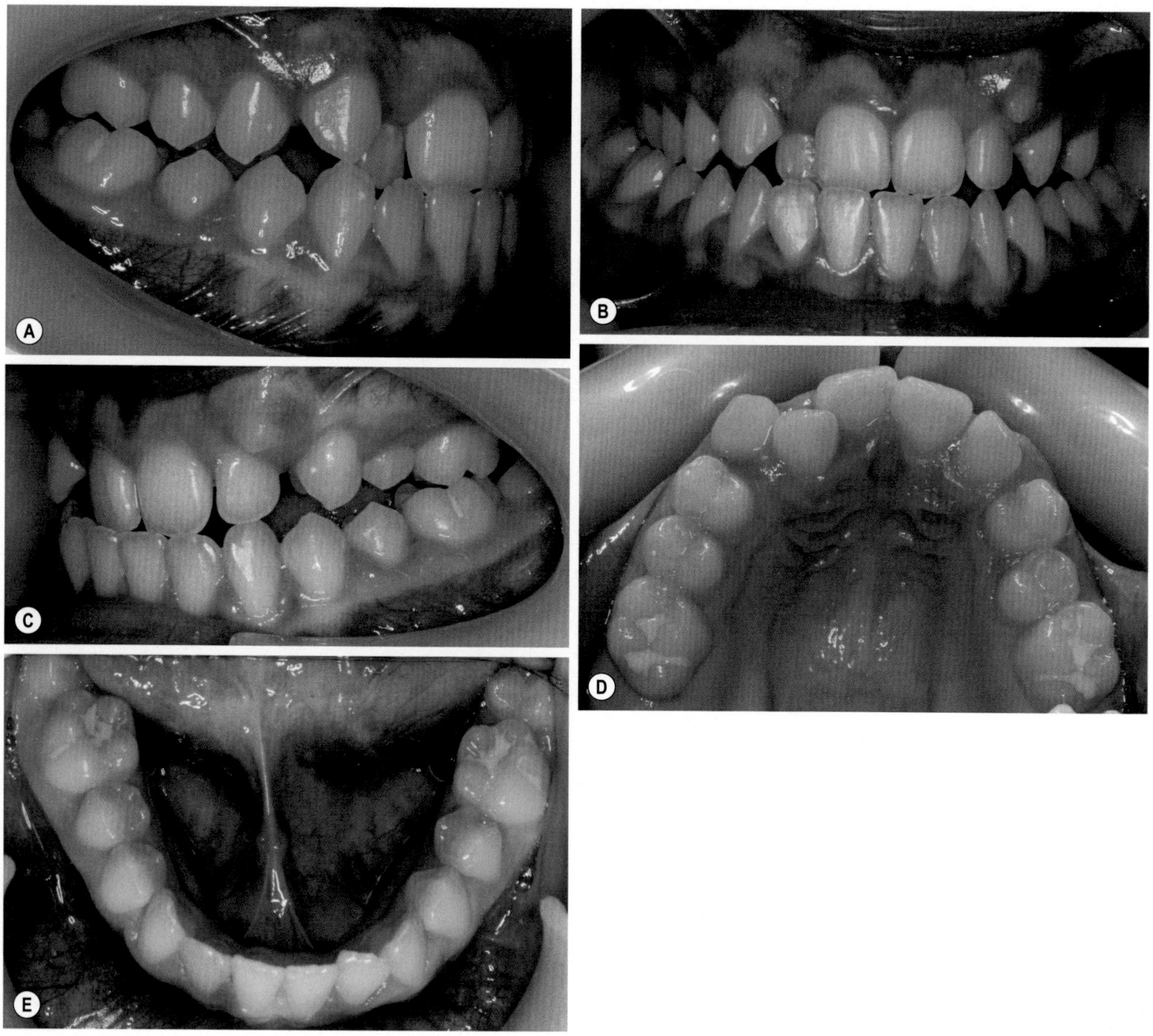

Fig. 4.10 **(A)** Right buccal occlusion. **(B)** Anterior occlusion. **(C)** Left buccal occlusion. **(D)** Upper occlusal. **(E)** Lower occlusal.

mandibular planes respectively). Only in the broadest sense may comment be made regarding how the inclination of the incisors 'appears'.

■ ***What clinical assessment should you undertake of* $\lfloor\underline{2}$*?***

$\lfloor\underline{2}$ should be checked for mobility in case it is being resorbed by $\lfloor\underline{3}$. If this is suspected, sensibility tests should also be undertaken.

Investigations

■ ***The patient presented with a dental panoramic radiograph taken 6 months previously by her general dental practitioner. What radiographic investigations would you request and why?***

It is not necessary to repeat the panoramic film. This revealed all permanent teeth to be developing normally and to be of good quality. The root status of $\lfloor\underline{2}$ also appeared to be sound with no evidence of root resorption from $\lfloor\underline{3}$.

As 6 months has elapsed since the last radiograph was taken of $\lfloor\underline{2}$, it would be sensible to take two periapical radiographs of $\lfloor\underline{2}$ to ensure that the root status remains unchanged.

This was found to be the case.

A lateral cephalometric radiograph is required to provide more information about the severity of the Class III malocclusion and the extent of any dentoalveolar compensation.

■ ***What is your interpretation of the following cephalometric findings?***

SNA = 81°; SNB = 79.5°; SN-maxillary plane = 8°; $\underline{1}$ to maxillary plane = 105°; $\overline{1}$ to mandibular plane = 90°; maxillary mandibular planes angle (MMPA) = 28°; facial proportion = 57%.

The skeletal pattern is mildly Class III (ANB = 1.5°; SNA-SNB) due to very slight mandibular prognathism. Compared with mean values, the upper and lower incisors are somewhat retroclined, but within the normal range, and the $\overline{1}$ angle is not compensating for the MMPA (should be 120–28° = 92°). Both the MMPA and facial proportion are slightly increased from normal values, but both are within the normal range.

Diagnosis

■ *What is your orthodontic diagnosis?*

Class III malocclusion on a mild Class III dental base with slightly increased facial proportions.

Mild marginal gingivitis. Mild lower arch and severe upper arch crowding with |3 excluded buccally.

Upper centreline shift of 2 mm to the left.

Right molar relationship is slightly Class II, and left molar relationship is slightly Class III.

■ *What is the IOTN DHC grade? Explain your reasoning.*

4d – due to severe displacement of teeth greater than 4 mm (between 2's and 3's bilaterally).

Treatment

■ *What are your aims of treatment?*

Improve oral hygiene.

Relief of upper and lower arch crowding.

Establish a positive overjet and overbite.

Correction of the upper centreline.

Correction of the molar relationships to Class I.

Retain the correction.

Monitor third molars.

■ *What possible options are there to relieve the upper arch crowding and correct the upper centreline?*

Space is required in order to address these treatment aims. Possible means to provide this are:

- *Extractions* – removal of a premolar on either side of the upper arch. Removal of 5|5 is usually considered in Class III camouflage, but anchorage would need to be reinforced (with either a palatal arch or TADs) if their removal was considered. Removal of 4|4, situated right beside where space is needed, would facilitate alignment of 3|3, and although not all the 4| space is required for relief of crowding in the upper right quadrant, the residual space will be utilized for upper centreline correction. With both extraction options, the upper arch would be aligned inside the lower.
- *Arch expansion* – both anteroposterior and lateral expansion of the upper arch would correct the anterior crossbites as well as the tendency to buccal crossbite. It will also provide further space for |3, which may erupt. Care is required as arch expansion may cause the palatal cusps of the maxillary molars to tip buccally, which will compromise the already tenuous overbite. A potential advantage of this approach is that extractions are delayed while further mandibular growth is observed when it will become more apparent whether orthodontic correction is possible or not. Such a 'therapeutic diagnosis' approach to treatment is often advisable in a Class III malocclusion where the extent of further mandibular growth is unknown.
- *Arch expansion and extractions* – expansion will reduce the need to extract 4|4, so 5|5 may be considered.
- *Arch expansion and distal movement of the left buccal segment* – the former is as previously outlined; the latter may be achieved by placing a TAD between and pushing against it with coil spring on a fixed appliance to move |4 5 6 distally.

Triona's mother was keen to avoid extractions, if possible. Following consideration of all options, it was agreed to proceed with an initial non-extraction 'therapeutic diagnosis' approach (**Fig. 4.11**).

■ *What appliance is shown in* Fig. 4.11A*? How is it constructed and how is it activated?*

This is a quadhelix appliance and has been custom-made in the laboratory; preformed types, however, also exist. The quadhelix is attached to bands cemented to a molar on each side of the arch. For a custom-made appliance, an impression must be taken with the bands in place, then the bands are removed and located carefully in the impression before being disinfected and sent to the laboratory. For the preformed types, attachments are welded to the palatal surfaces of the bands into which slot the arms of the quadhelix; this facilitates removal for adjustments. Both appliance types are made of 1 mm stainless steel wire. Typically, activation is achieved by 'expanding' the appliance around half a tooth width on each side. Although activation may be achieved intraorally with triple-beak pliers, it is difficult to gauge the amount of activation by that mean; it is usually preferable to remove the appliance every second visit and activate it extraorally.

■ *What is the most likely initial aligning archwire shown in* Fig. 4.11C*? What favourable properties has it got for alignment?*

This is most likely a nickle–titanium archwire of small diameter, probably 0.012-in. Its properties include flexibility without undergoing deformation, and it exerts a light force when tied into displaced teeth.

■ *How would you re-evaluate treatment progress following upper arch expansion and alignment?*

Interim records should be taken for further treatment planning. These are clinical photographs (extraoral and intraoral views), study models, and a lateral cephalometric radiograph.

The lateral cephalometric measurements should be compared with those taken at the start of treatment. Any change in SNB, ANB and MMPA should be noted. The incisor inclinations should also be assessed relative to the maxillary and mandibular planes respectively. 1 inclination will indicate how much their inclination has changed during upper arch alignment, and 1 inclination when considered with the ANB and MMPA angles will indicate if any dentoalveolar compensation has occurred since treatment started and whether further orthodontic compensation is feasible or desirable. If there has been minimal/no change in SNB, ANB and MMPA then the prospect of orthodontic correction is good. Otherwise any attempt at orthodontic camouflage should be considered with caution due to the likely guarded prognosis;

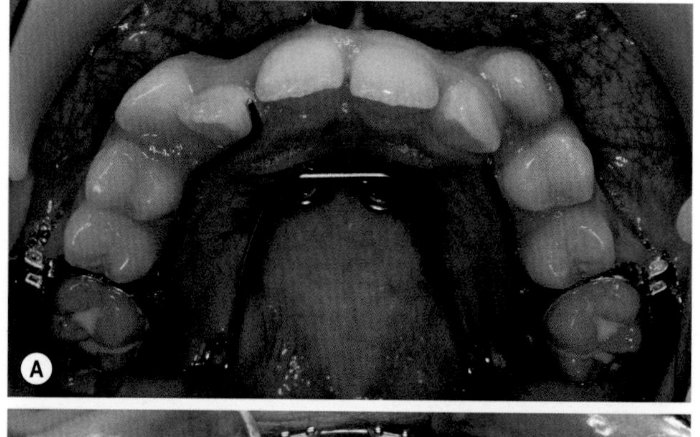

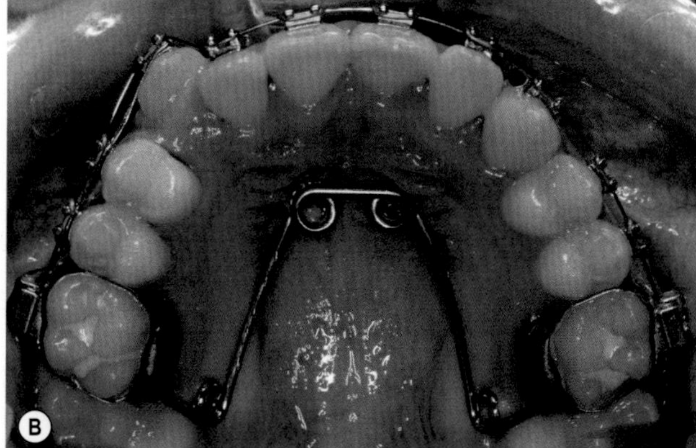

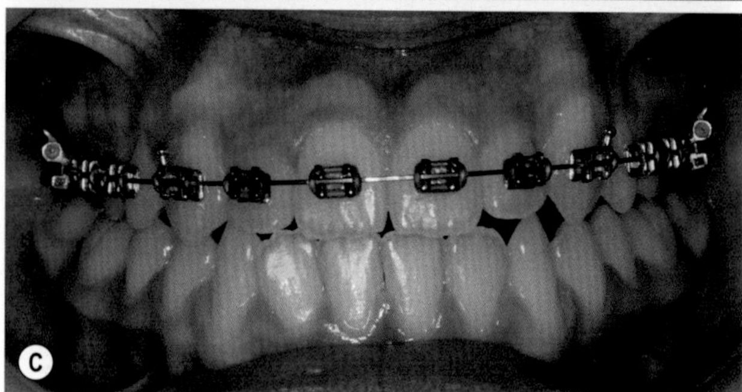

Fig. 4.11 (A) Mid-treatment: upper occlusal view; note eruption of 3|. **(B)** Mid-treatment: initial aligning archwire. **(C)** Mid-treatment: upper arch alignment.

in such circumstances, it would be wise to delay any further intervention and review at a later stage when growth is complete.

When is mandibular growth completed?

Mandibular growth is usually complete by about 17 years of age in girls and about 2 years later in boys.

As reassessment revealed that growth had not been adverse, it was decided to proceed with lower fixed appliance therapy and orthodontic camouflage on a non-extraction basis. The final occlusion is shown in **Fig. 4.12**.

What will determine whether the correction remains stable?

The amount of overbite and the buccal segment interdigitation will determine the stability of the anterior and posterior crossbites respectively, but both will also be greatly influenced by the extent and direction of further mandibular growth. The latter will have the final say with regard to long-term stability.

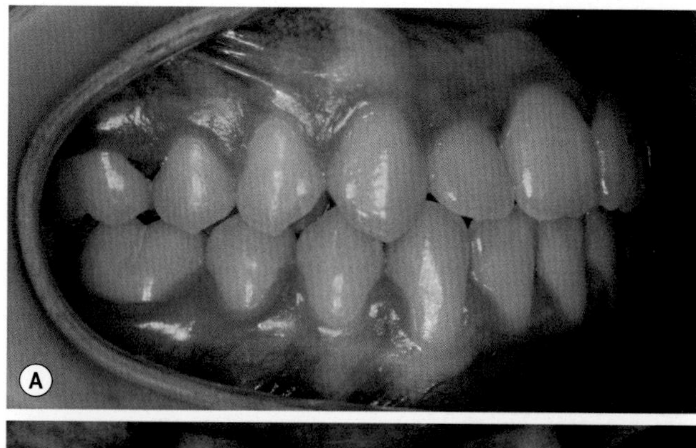

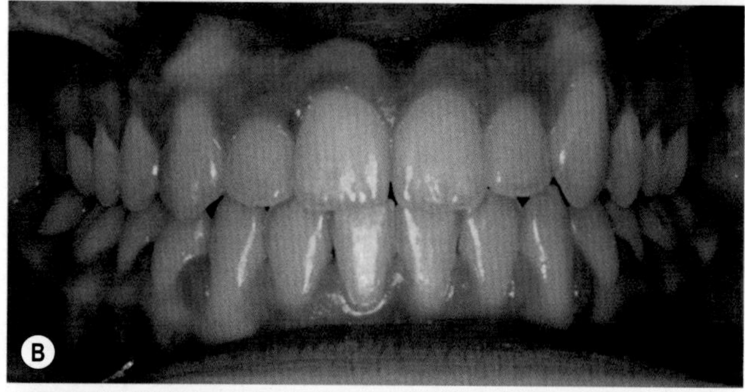

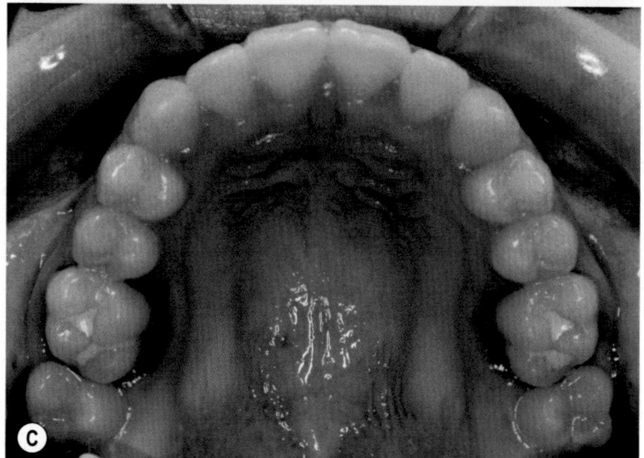

Fig. 4.12 (A) Post-treatment: right buccal occlusion. **(B)** Post-treatment: anterior occlusion. **(C)** Post-treatment: upper occlusal view.

Primary resources and recommended reading

Benson PE, Parkin N, Dyer F et al 2013 Fluorides for the prevention of early tooth decay (demineralised white lesions) during fixed brace treatment. Cochrane Database of Syst Rev Issue 12. Art No: CD003809. DOI: 10.1002/14651858.CD003809.pub3.

Hafez HS, Shaarawy SM, Al-Sakiti AA et al 2012 Dental crowding as a caries risk factor: a systematic review. Am J Orthod. Dentofacial Orthop 142:443–450.

Little RM, Wallen TR, Reidel RA 1981 Stability and relapse of mandibular anterior alignment-first premolar extraction cases treated by traditional edgewise orthodontics. Am J Orthod 80:349–365.

Mitchell L 1992 Decalcification during orthodontic treatment with fixed appliances – an overview. Br J Orthod 19:199–205.

Rahilly G, Price N 2003 Nickel allergy and orthodontics. J Orthod 30:171–174.

Stephens CD 1989 The use of natural spontaneous tooth movement in the treatment of malocclusion. Dent Update 16:337–338, 340–342.

For revision, see Mind Map 4, page 224.

5

Severe crowding

CASE 1

SUMMARY

Amy, an almost 11-year-old girl, presents with marked space shortage for both unerupted 3's (Fig. 5.1). What has caused this problem and how may it be treated?

History

Complaint

Amy does not like the appearance of the upper 'side teeth' being beside her upper front teeth; the 'side teeth' she thinks 'look like two rows of teeth'. She also does not like the crookedness of her lower front teeth.

History of complaint

Amy has become aware of the worsening appearance of her teeth over the past year. In that time, she has lost some baby teeth and the new teeth have come through crooked.

Amy's mother reports that her daughter's baby teeth looked good with only mild irregularity of the lower front teeth. Both she and Amy are keen for treatment.

Medical history

Amy's mother reports that her daughter had a heart murmur as a baby and attended a cardiologist at the local hospital.

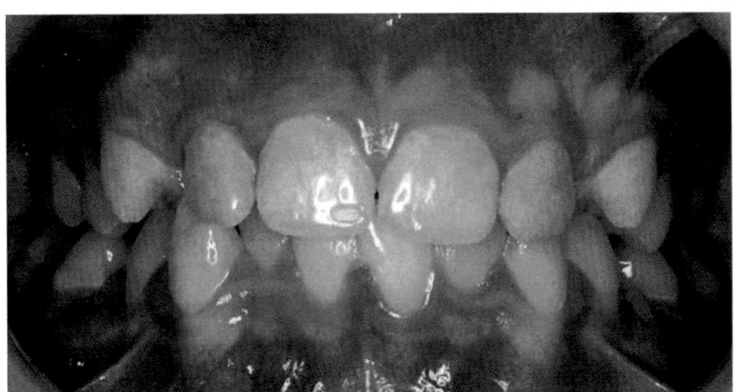

Fig. 5.1 Anterior occlusion at presentation.

She fractured her right wrist in a fall from her mountain bike 4 months ago and has been attending for physiotherapy at the local hospital since the cast was removed. Mobility is almost back to normal now, but she has difficulty with some procedures, such as toothbrushing. Otherwise she is fit and well.

■ ***What implications does the medical history have for any proposed orthodontic treatment?***

Amy's cardiologist should be consulted regarding the cardiac status and the possible need for antibiotic prophylaxis for procedures likely to produce bacteraemia because of the potential risk of infective endocarditis. The National Institute for Health and Clinical Excellence (NICE, which governs clinical practice in England and Wales) guidelines (2016) do not recommend routine antibiotic prophylaxis for those undergoing dental procedures; the American Heart Association (AHA) recommends antibiotic cover only for those at high risk.

Amy's cardiologist confirmed that her cardiac murmur had fully resolved and that antibiotic prophylaxis was not required prior to any dental or orthodontic (separator placement, fitting/removal of bands) procedures.

As excellent oral hygiene is essential with any orthodontic treatment, the impact of lack of optimal wrist mobility on oral hygiene should be assessed. Assistance with toothbrushing by a parent may be required until wrist mobility is fully restored; compared with manual brushes, powered brushes with a rotation oscillation action provide better plaque removal in the short term and better protection against gingivitis in the short and long term.

Amy's mother is already assisting with her daughter's toothbrushing using a powered toothbrush.

Dental history

Amy is a regular attender at her general dental practitioner. She had several of the baby back teeth extracted a few years ago and has some fissure sealants placed in the first permanent molars. She brushes her teeth twice per day, but her mother says that she needs reminding about toothbrushing, with which her mother currently assists her.

Examination

Extraoral

Amy has a Class I skeletal pattern with average FMPA, average lower facial height and no facial asymmetry. Her lips are competent with the lower lip resting in the midlabial third of the upper central incisors.

No abnormal temporomandibular joint signs or symptoms were detected.

Intraoral

■ ***The intraoral views are shown in** Figs 5.1 **and** 5.2**. Describe what you see.***

Poor oral hygiene with plaque deposits visible on several teeth and associated generalized marginal gingival erythema.

Stained occlusal fissures in 6|, brown staining on the mesial of |6 and decalcification at the gingival margin level on the

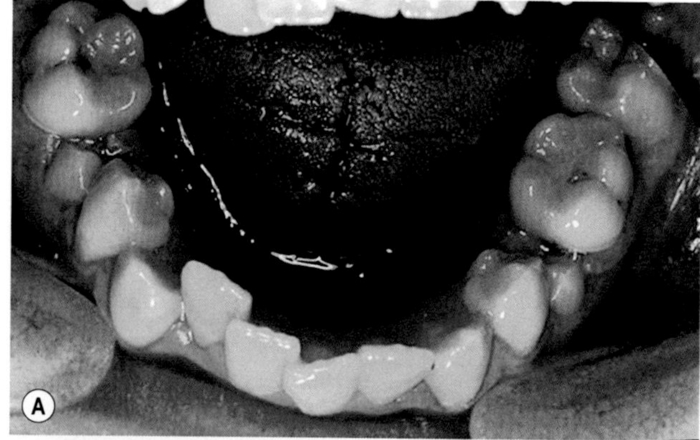

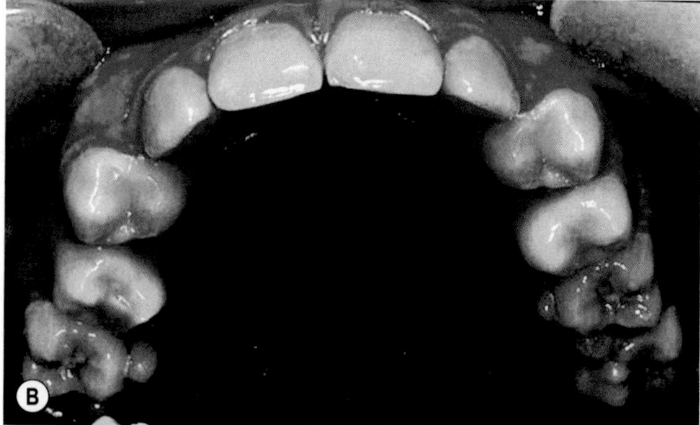

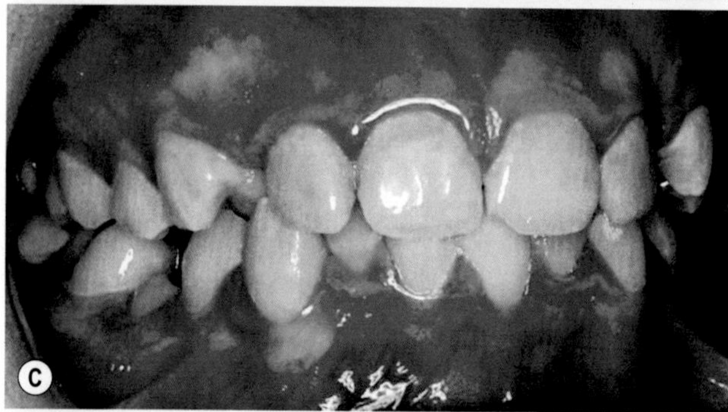

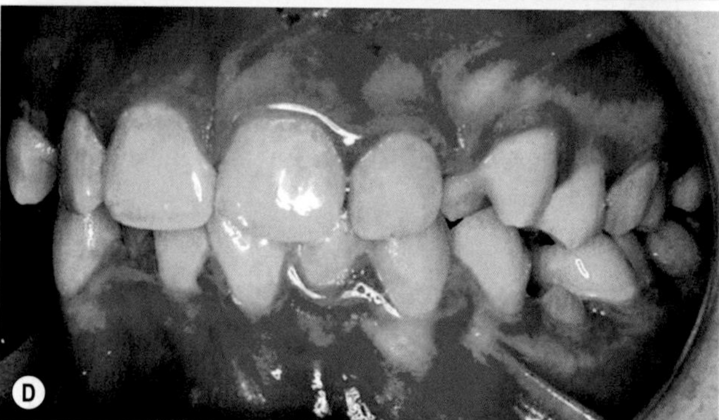

Fig. 5.2 **(A)** Lower occlusal view. **(B)** Upper occlusal view. **(C)** Right buccal occlusion. **(D)** Left buccal occlusion.

buccal aspects of 6⌉⌈6; fissure sealants are visible in the occlusal surface of the first permanent molars. 5⌋ has a mildly hypoplastic palatal cusp (this was non-carious).

All permanent teeth present from the second permanent molar to the second permanent molar in the lower arch (5̄'s are partially erupted); in the upper arch, all permanent teeth (except 3's) erupted from second permanent molar to second permanent molar.

Table 5.1 Factors affecting the rate of space loss following early loss of a primary molar

Factor	Effect*
Age at loss	The younger the age at loss, the greater the potential for space loss
Degree of crowding	The more crowded the arch, the more space that will be lost
Tooth extracted	Early loss of an E, rather than of a D, is likely to lead to more space loss (see below regarding arch). 5's may erupt and be excluded palatally/lingually or be impacted; 5 may be in crossbite; centreline shift if asymmetrical extraction and in case of E, if early loss before age 7
Arch from which tooth is lost	Greater loss is likely in the upper, rather than in the lower arch, as mesial drift tendency is greater in the former
Type of occlusion	Less space loss will occur where good buccal interdigitation exists

*The effects listed above are those that are, in general, likely to result from each of the factors given. Individual variation with regard to outcome is, however, possible.

Mild lower labial segment crowding with 1⌉ distolabially rotated; 3⌉ slightly mesially inclined and ⌈3 upright.

Lower right and left buccal segments exhibit mild crowding.

Overall, summing the labial and buccal segments, the lower arch has moderate to severe crowding.

Severe upper labial segment crowding; 2's very slightly mesiolabially rotated; both 3's are about to erupt buccal to the line of the arch.

Upper buccal segments are not crowded; there is mesiopalatal rotation of 5⌋ and distopalatal rotation of 4⌋; small amount of space on either side between the premolar teeth and between the first premolars and lateral incisors.

Class I incisor relationship; overbite is average and complete; lower centreline shifted slightly to the right.

Class I molar relationship on right and left.

What is the likely cause of the enamel hypoplasia on 5⌋?

This is most likely due to pulpal pathology in the overlying E⌋, affecting amelogenesis, often referred to as a Turner's tooth or Turner's hypoplasia.

What are the likely causes of the severe upper arch crowding?

- Inherent dentoalveolar disproportion – this is genetically determined and represents a mismatch in tooth size and the size of the alveolus. Added to this, the maxillary canines are the last permanent teeth to erupt anterior to the first permanent molars and are often squeezed buccally in a crowded arch.
- Early loss of primary teeth – this leads to mesial drift of the buccal segments and aggravates crowding.
- Supernumerary teeth and megadont teeth are other causes of crowding but are not relevant in this case.
- Any combination of the previously mentioned causes.

What factors influence the rate of space loss following early loss of a primary molar? What are the effects of early loss of a primary molar?

These are given in **Table 5.1**.

> **Key point**
>
> On average, space loss is greater following extraction of a primary molar:
> - The younger the age at extraction.
> - In the upper rather than the lower arch.
> - In a crowded arch.
> - Where the second rather than the first primary molar is extracted.
> - Where there is poor occlusal interdigitation.

What are the likely causes of the upper premolar rotations?

Developmental – where the tooth germ is rotated in its crypt, which could be a manifestation of inherent crowding.

Acquired – due to early loss of the primary predecessor, most likely due to caries, which removes its main guidance into occlusion and allows the premolar to initially rotate in the tooth crypt, and become characteristically mesiopalatally rotated later due to mesial drift pressure of the first permanent molars.

A retained primary molar or its root fragment may also induce rotation of the successor if it fails to erupt in the correct position.

Investigations

What investigations would you request and why?

A dental panoramic tomogram is required to determine the presence and position of all unerupted teeth. Bitewing radiographs would be advisable in view of the fissure and mesial surface staining observed related to 6⌉ and ⌈6, respectively. These will also allow the status of 5⌉ to be assessed.

The presence of all permanent teeth including third molars was confirmed; enamel caries was detected in 6⌉ and ⌈6 (this had not progressed through to dentin).

Diagnosis

What is your diagnosis?

Class I malocclusion on a Class I skeletal base with average FMPA.

Generalized marginal gingivitis; enamel caries in $\overline{6|6}$.

Moderate to severe lower arch crowding; severe upper arch crowding with $\underline{3}$'s unerupted but positioned buccally; lower centreline displaced slightly to the right.

Class I molar relationship on right and left.

What is the IOTN DHC grade (see p. 264)? Explain why.

5i – due to the impacted maxillary canines.

Treatment

What are the aims of treatment?

To improve oral hygiene and restore dental health.

To relieve crowding.

To align upper and lower arches.

To correct the lower centreline.

To close residual buccal segment spacing, maintaining Class I incisor and molar relationships.

What is your treatment plan?

1. Provide oral hygiene instruction and dietary advice.
2. Topical fluoride (Duraphat) application to early enamel lesions on lower first permanent molars.
3. Composite restoration of the palatal aspect of 5⌋.
4. Referral, with the recently taken radiographs, to an orthodontist for further assessment and management of the severe crowding.

Explain the treatment options for Amy's severe upper arch crowding and moderate to severe lower arch crowding. What are the implications of each option?

Although Amy's principal concern relates to her upper arch crowding, it is essential that treatment planning begins in the lower arch. (See p. 18 for an explanation of this and options for relief of crowding.) Based on the assessment of the overall severity of the lower arch crowding, extraction of first premolars will be required. This will relieve impaction of the second premolars and provide space for the canines to move distally to facilitate labial segment alignment. The latter is more likely to occur spontaneously on the right side due to the uprighting of the slightly mesially angulated 3⌉. Provided oral hygiene has improved sufficiently, fixed appliances will then be required because of the angulation of ⌈3, rotation of ⌈1, the need for centreline correction and space closure.

Following on the same scheme given on pages 18–19 for treatment planning, after you:

Imagine the corrected position of $\overline{3}$ (in this case taking the need to move the lower centreline to the left), the next step is to

Mentally reposition $\underline{3}$ *to be in a Class I relationship with the corrected position of* $\overline{3}$. For Amy, space is required to achieve this.

How would you assess the space required in the upper arch?

As space is at a premium, the distance from the distal of the lateral incisor to the mesial of the first permanent molar should be measured with fine pointed stainless steel dividers.

This measured 16 mm on the right and left sides.

Is this sufficient to achieve the treatment objectives?

Removal of both upper first premolars will provide space for alignment of $\underline{3}$'s, but it will be insufficient to achieve this completely and obtain a Class I canine relationship with the $\overline{3|3}$ positions corrected unless *all* the space from the upper arch extractions is maintained. No space loss is permissible. Anchorage reinforcement is required. It is important to realize that removal of an upper first premolar creates usually 7 mm of space, but the average mesiodistal width of the permanent maxillary canine is 8 mm – so generally, on average, 15 mm of space is required to accommodate $\underline{3}$ and $\underline{5}$. Fortunately, in Amy's case, there is a small amount of space present in the upper premolar areas which will assist correct positioning of $\underline{3}$'s with the aligned $\overline{3}$'s.

Removal of both upper canines is another possibility; if they erupt buccal to the line of the arch in a few months' time, they could be extracted, or if not, surgical removal could be undertaken. Upper fixed appliance therapy would then be required to rotate the first premolars slightly mesiopalatally to hide the palatal cusp and occupy a greater mesiodistal width akin to that of the extracted canine; the palatal cusp of 4's should also be ground to avoid interferences in lateral excursions. Bonded retention would also be needed to maintain the final position of 4's.

Removal of upper 4's addresses Amy's concern and is likely to give the better final appearance.

> **Key point**
>
> An upper first premolar extraction space will not accommodate an upper permanent canine.

Finalize your treatment planning.

The next steps are:

Plan the upper labial segment. The mild rotation of 2's is best dealt with by fixed appliance therapy.

Decide on the final molar relationship. With four first premolar extractions, this should be Class I; residual space closure in the lower arch will necessitate fixed appliance therapy.

Assess the anchorage needs. The high anchorage demands in the upper arch have already been identified. Options are a space maintainer with anchorage support (headgear), headgear alone, Nance palatal arch with/without transpalatal arch or temporary anchorage devices (TADs). Anchorage demands in the lower arch are modest; there is no need for anchorage reinforcement.

Plan retention. Upper and lower vacuum-formed retainers (Essix retainers) should be adequate to be worn night-time only for 1 year followed by a second year of every second night wear.

What is the final orthodontic treatment plan?

Assuming that Amy's oral hygiene improves and is maintained at a high standard following instruction, then the plan would be as follows:

1. Anchorage reinforcement in the upper arch by one of several means (see above).
2. Extraction of four first premolars.
3. Upper and lower fixed appliances.
4. Upper and lower Essix retainers.

> **Key point**
>
> Where anchorage is at a premium, always reinforce anchorage before any extractions for relief of crowding.

If an upper removable appliance space maintainer were to be considered, what would be your design? What instructions would you issue regarding appliance wear?

Activation: there are no active components.

Retention: Adams clasps 6|6 (0.7 mm stainless steel wire) with headgear tubes soldered to the 6's clasp bridges; flat stops distal of 2|2.

Anchorage: full palatal acrylic coverage; also headgear to be added to fit into the molar clasp tubes.

Baseplate: full palatal acrylic coverage.

The upper removable appliance should be worn full-time except for contact sports and after meals when it should be removed for cleaning. Sticky and hard foods as well as fizzy drinks should be avoided when the appliance is worn. Details regarding headgear force and wear for anchorage reinforcement as well as safety precautions necessary are given on page 14.

Describe the alternatives to this appliance.

Space could be maintained with headgear alone fitted to bands on the upper first permanent molars, with a force of 200–250 g per side, worn 10–12 hours per day. Should the headgear not be worn as required in this case, then mesial drift of the second premolar and first permanent molar will compromise space required for 3's.

A Nance button palatal arch soldered to bands on the upper first permanent molars is an alternative (**Fig. 5.3**), but as space is critical in this case, soldering a transpalatal arch also to the molar bands may support anchorage further (**Fig. 5.11**). The Nance button palatal arch provides anchorage through mucosal contact of the acrylic button with the anterior vault of the palate while the palatal arch maintains the intermolar distance, preventing mesial drift and molar tipping. This is assisted further by the addition of a transpalatal arch, straight across the palate, linking 6| to |6. Another option is to place a TAD distal to the 6's on either

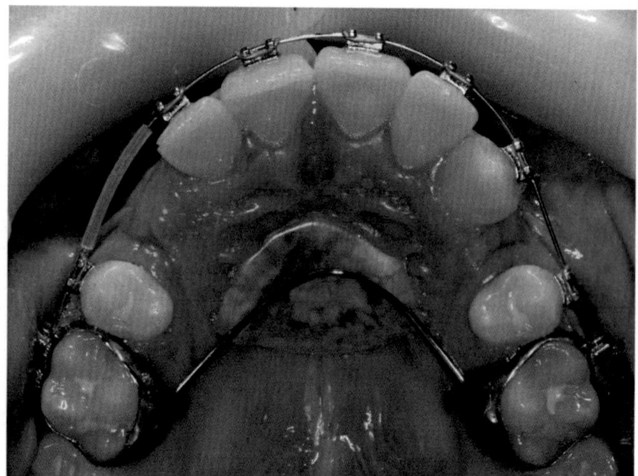

Fig. 5.3 Nance button palatal arch.

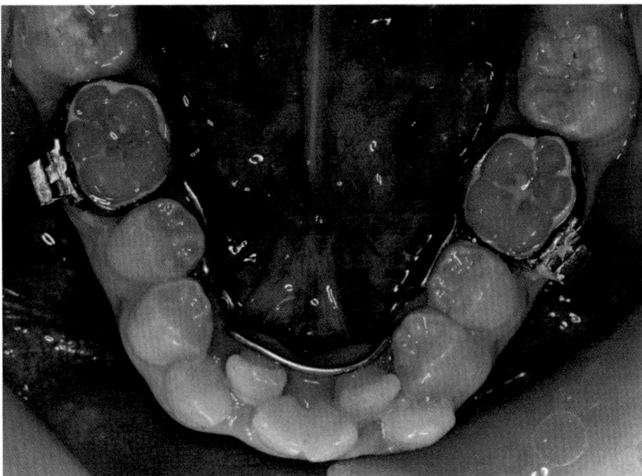

Fig. 5.4 Lingual arch.

side and use it to keep the $\underline{6}$'s and second premolars from moving mesially.

If all the space from lower premolar extractions had been required for lower labial segment alignment, how could anchorage have been reinforced there?

A lower removable appliance is not well tolerated due to encroachment on tongue space, interference with speech and difficulty with achieving good appliance retention due to the lingual inclination of the molars. A lower lingual arch soldered to bands on the first permanent molars is a better option (**Fig. 5.4**). Alternatively, the second permanent molars could be bonded or banded and ligated to the first permanent molars. Another option is to place a TAD into the retromolar area on each side and use it to keep the first permanent molars and second premolars from moving mesially while providing anchorage for canine retraction.

> **Key point**
>
> Options for reinforcing anchorage in upper arch:
> - Upper removable appliance space maintainer with headgear support.
> - Headgear to molar bands.
> - Nance button palatal arch (with/without transpalatal arch).
> - TAD.
>
> Options for reinforcing anchorage in lower arch:
> - Lingual arch.
> - Bond/band $\overline{7}$'s and ligate to $\overline{6}$'s.
> - TAD.

How effective are TADs at reinforcing anchorage? How do they compare to other methods of anchorage reinforcement?

Evidence indicates that TADs are an effective, non-compliant means of reinforcing anchorage or of moving upper first permanent molars distally. A recent randomized clinical trial compared anchorage supplementation with headgear or Nance button palatal arch or TADs, in cases that required maximum anchorage support; there was no difference in effectiveness between the appliances in terms of anchorage support, but there were more problems reported with headgear and Nance buttons than with TADs.

Are there any risks with TADs?

Risks include:

- Screw breakage during insertion (5%).
- Root contact during placement (should heal uneventfully).
- Failure necessitating TAD replacement/removal (~14%).
- Infection (unlikely if the area around the screw is brushed gently with a small headed toothbrush and fluoride toothpaste and chlorhexidine mouthrinse (0.2%) is used for first 5 days after insertion).
- Screw loosening (may be replaced in original or different position).

If Amy were issued an upper removable space maintainer with headgear support, how would you know at her 2-week review whether the appliances were being worn as instructed?

Amy should be speaking normally with the upper removable appliance in place; she should also be able to remove and insert the appliance unaided by a mirror. The baseplate should have lost its shine; there should be evidence of mild gingival erythema along the palatal margins of the appliance and at the posterior extension of the baseplate (if the appliance had a bite platform, there would be marks from the occlusion also). She should also be able to insert, assemble and remove the headgear easily. If it is being worn as instructed, the headcap will have signs of wear and the headgear tubes in the removable appliance should be free of any food debris from insertion of the facebow.

The occlusion following appliance wear with headgear support and extraction of four first premolars is shown in **Fig. 5.5**. The lower centreline shift corrected without appliance treatment. At this stage, Amy indicated that she was sufficiently pleased with the improvement in her dental appearance that she did not wish to proceed to further fixed appliance therapy. This was fortunate as she was not keen on assisted tooth brushing by her mother and had struggled, due to continuing problems with right wrist mobility, to maintain a high standard of oral hygiene during removable appliance treatment, despite the use of a powered toothbrush.

An Essix retainer was fitted in the upper arch only; Amy was instructed to wear this at night-time only for 12 months initially. Arrangements were made to review her occlusion at that stage.

What is an Essix retainer, and what are its potential advantages over a Hawley retainer in the upper arch? Aside from the usual advice regarding retainers, what specific advice should the patient be given regarding this retainer?

An Essix retainer is a clear vacuum-formed thermoplastic retainer. Some of its potential advantages over a Hawley retainer are:

- Better aesthetics.
- Less difficulty with speaking.
- Cheaper.
- Easier to make.

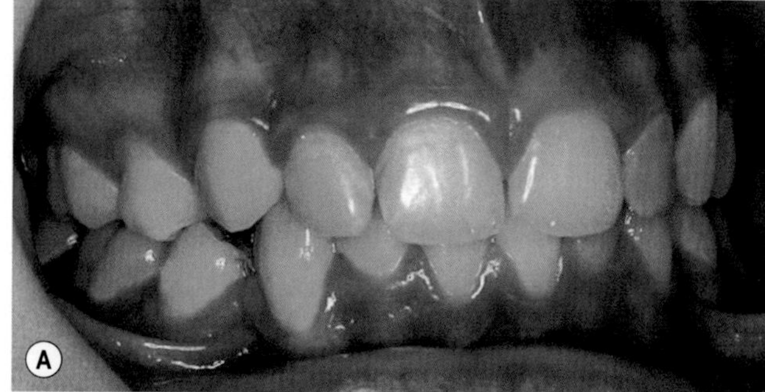
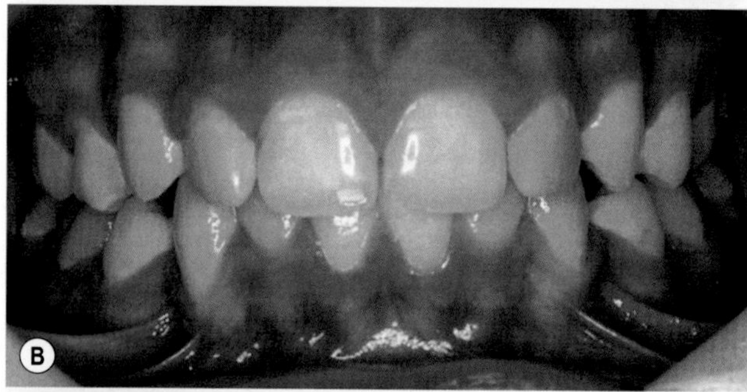
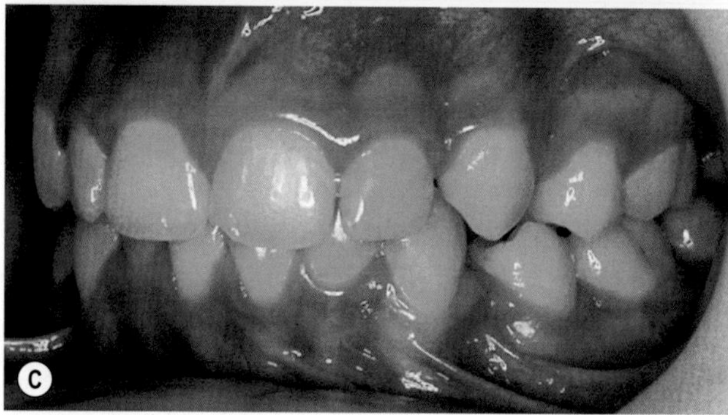

Fig. 5.5 (A) Post-treatment: right buccal occlusion. **(B)** Post-treatment: anterior occlusion. **(C)** Post-treatment: left buccal occlusion.

Vacuum-formed retainers appear more effective than Hawley retainers at maintaining correction of the upper and lower labial segments, with greater effectiveness in the upper than the lower arch.

The retainer must not be worn while eating and must never be worn while consuming beverages, especially carbonated drinks, as with these there is a high risk of enamel demineralization.

CASE 2

SUMMARY

Roger has recently relocated to your area from another country. He presents with a tooth erupting in his palate and an impacted 3⌉. What are the causes of these problems, and how may they be managed?

Roger has a Class I skeletal pattern with average FMPA and lower facial height; there is no facial asymmetry.

■ *What do you notice in* Fig. 5.6*?*

Poor oral hygiene with plaque deposits on most teeth.

Generalized marginal gingival erythema.

7654321|1234567
7654321|1234567 visible (note 3⌉ cusp tip).

Caries-free dentition.

Moderate lower arch crowding with 3⌉ impacted but erupting.

Severe upper arch crowding; 5⌋ excluded palatally with 6⌋ and 4⌋ in contact; 6⌋ rotated mesiopalatally; median diastema ~2 mm; ⌊3 buccal and mesially inclined.

Class I incisor relationship; overjet 2 mm (measured clinically); overbite average and complete; centreline shift (lower was ~4 mm to the right).

Right molar relationship is Class II; left molar relationship is Class I.

Crossbite 6⌋ (5⌋ also in crossbite).

■ *What is the IOTN (DHC) grade (see p. 264)? Explain why.*

4d – due to contact point displacement between 5⌋ and 4⌋, or between ⌊3 and ⌊4. Although 3⌉ is impacted, it is partially erupted and so would score 4t and not 5i (if 4 mm or less between 4 and 2.5i).

■ *What are the possible causes of the crowding and tooth displacements in the upper and lower arches?*

The palatal exclusion of 5⌋ is most likely due to early loss of E⌋ in an inherently crowded arch. Space closure has been complete with 6⌋ and 4⌋ in contact. Factors influencing the rate of space closure have been given in **Table 5.1**. Note the characteristic mesiopalatal rotation of 6⌋ following early loss of E⌋.

Roger's mother confirmed that E⌋ had been extracted at age 5 due to caries.

⌊3 is the last tooth to erupt in the upper left quadrant and is buccally displaced due to the inherent crowding.

The lack of space for 3⌉ may be linked to the lower centreline shift (see possible causes below). Note the distal tilt of 2⌉. Early loss of lower primary molars appears unlikely due to the reasonably aligned buccal segments.

■ *Why has 6⌋ rotated mesiopalatally?*

As the palatal root is the largest, the tooth rotates around this rather than around either of the buccal roots.

■ *What is unusual about the eruption pattern in the lower arch?*

Usually the canines erupt before the premolars (the opposite is true in the upper arch) so it is unusual that 3⌉ is impacted. See Chapter 1 for the average eruption dates of teeth.

■ *What is the likely cause of the lower centreline shift?*

Premature loss of C⌉ due to inherent crowding is a likely cause. Early unbalanced loss of C⌉ or D⌉ due to caries is another possibility as E⌋ was lost early due to caries. No lower primary teeth had been extracted.

Other causes of a centreline shift are given in Chapter 14, Box 14.1, page 88.

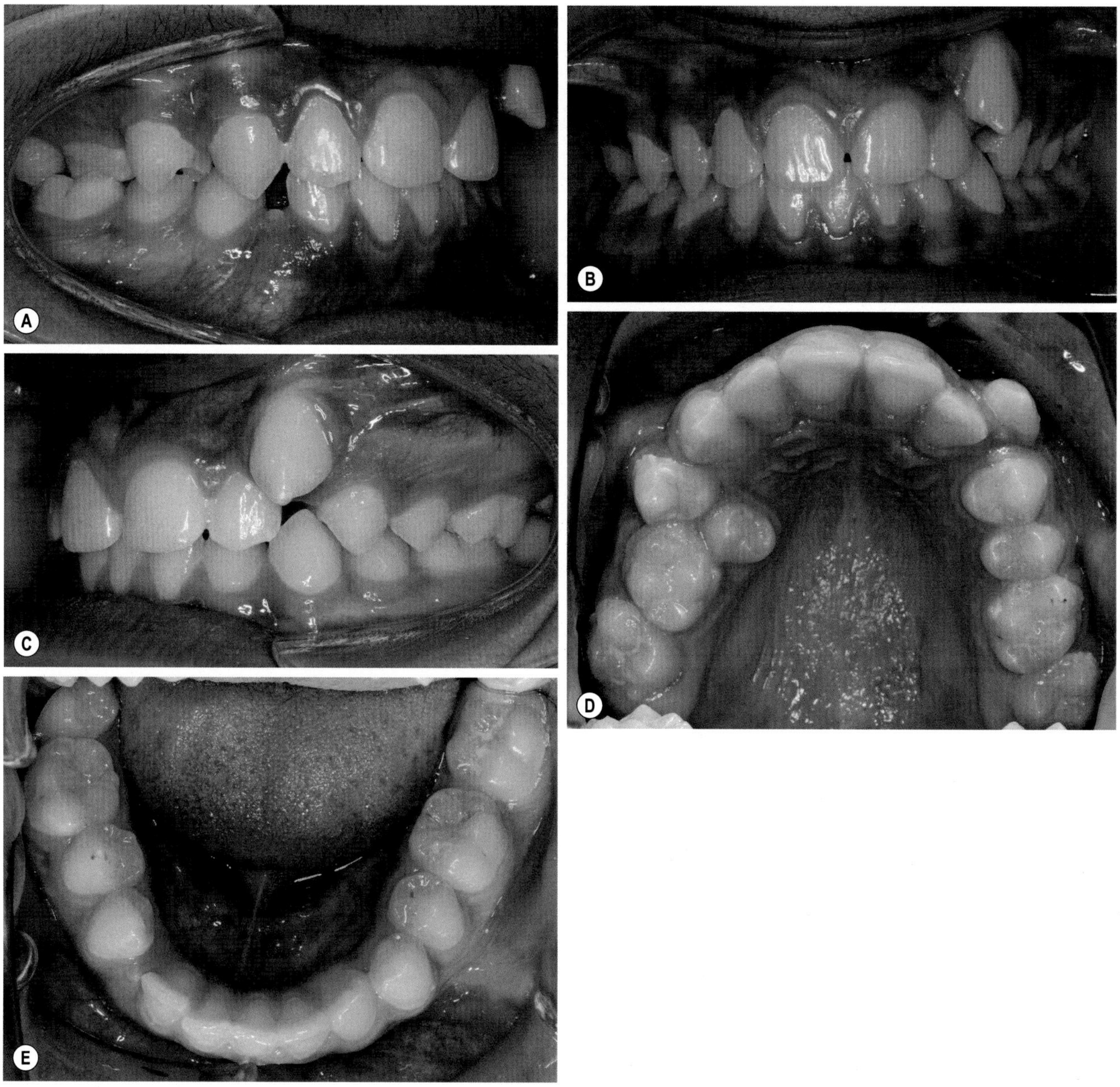

Fig. 5.6 **(A)** Right buccal occlusion. **(B)** Anterior occlusion. **(C)** Left buccal occlusion. **(D)** Upper occlusal view. **(E)** Lower occlusal view.

> **Key point**
>
> 6̲ rotates mesiopalatally with mesial drift following early loss of E̲.

Investigations

■ ***A dental panoramic tomogram (DPT) was taken by Roger's previous dental practitioner a few months ago. You request this by email. What do you notice in** Fig. 5.7**?***

The DPT shows:

Normal alveolar bone height.

All erupted permanent teeth sound.

5⌋ overlapping 4⌋; impacted 3⌉.

Four third molars developing.

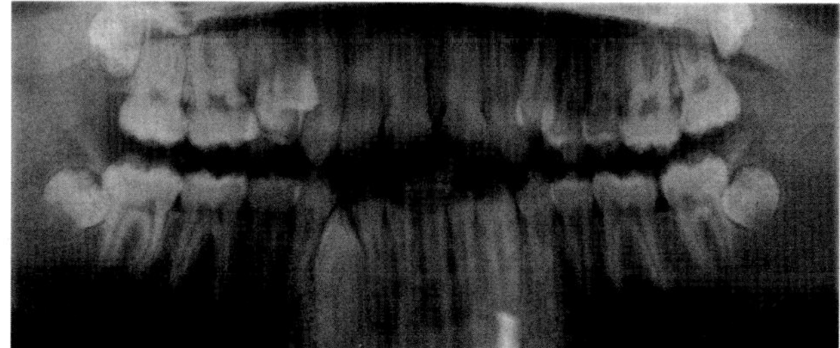

Fig. 5.7 Dental panoramic tomogram.

■ ***Do you require any further radiographs?***

It is not possible to see the roots of 5⌋ and 4⌋ clearly; two periapical radiographs with a tube shift could be taken to assess this more completely and to exclude any resorption. Should the intraoral views not provide sufficient information, a CBCT could be taken.

Periapical views indicated no root resorption of either premolar.

Diagnosis

■ ***What is your diagnosis?***

Class I malocclusion on a Class I skeletal base with average FMPA.

Generalized mild marginal gingivitis.

Moderate lower and severe upper arch crowding with the lower centreline shifted to the left.

Right buccal segment relationship is Class II; left buccal segment relationship is Class I.

Buccal crossbite 6⌋ and 5⌋.

Treatment

■ ***What are your aims of treatment?***

Establish good oral hygiene.

Relief of crowding.

De-rotation and crossbite correction of 6⌋.

Correction of lower centreline.

Establish Class I right and left molar relationships.

Retain.

■ ***What is your treatment plan?***

1. Oral hygiene instruction.
2. Correct the crossbite on 6⌋ and derotate 6⌋.
3. Extract $\frac{5|4}{4|4}$.
4. Upper and lower fixed appliances.
5. Upper and lower vacuum-formed retainers.

■ ***How could the crossbite be corrected on 6⌋ and 6⌋ be derotated?***

The crossbite may be corrected by cementing bands to 6⌋ and 6⌉ and running cross-elastics from an attachment on the palatal of 6⌋ band to the hook on the buccal of 6⌉ band. In order to facilitate band placement and to ensure that movement of 6⌋ is not obstructed by 5⌋, it would be sensible to have 5⌋ extracted prior to band placement. The cross-elastics should be worn full-time, including at meals. Crossbite correction is likely to take a short time, following which the elastics should be discontinued for a month to assess stability. Derotation of 6⌋ will likely occur with increasing diameter of the archwires when the remainder of the fixed appliances has been placed.

An alternative is to use a quadhelix appliance and adjust it to both derotate 6⌋ and to move it buccally. There is, however, likely to be some reciprocal unwanted buccal movement of ⌊6 by this means.

Roger was a keen rugby player, and although he wanted to improve the appearance of his teeth, he was not prepared to wear fixed appliances.

■ ***Is there another option you could consider to address his wishes?***

An extraction-only plan could address several issues. Removal of 5⌋⌊4 and 4⌉ will relieve crowding and allow ⌊3 to align and 3⌉ to erupt. The mesial angulation of ⌊3 is favourable to allow it to move distally following ⌊4 extraction, and it should align considerably under cheek pressure. Although this may be incomplete, it will improve ⌊3 position greatly. This plan accepts the lower centreline shift and the very mild crowding of the lower left buccal segment. These shortcomings must be explained to Roger and his parents should he wish to proceed. A digitally simulated image of the potential outcome of this plan is shown in **Fig. 5.8**.

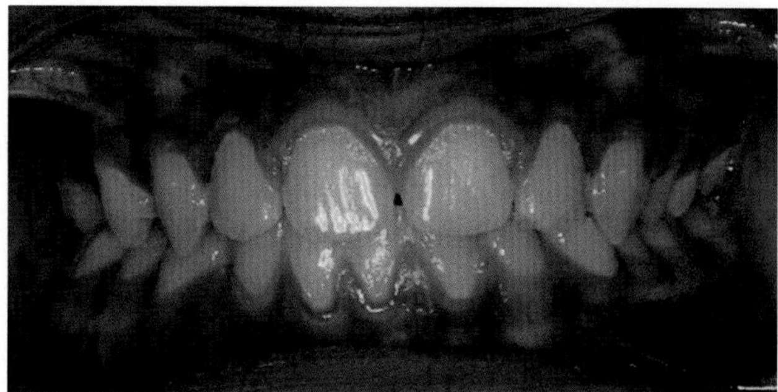

Fig. 5.8 Digital simulation of potential outcome following extractions and ⌊3 alignment.

CASE 3

SUMMARY

Conal, a 12-year-old boy, presents complaining about the crowding of his upper and lower front teeth. He is keen for treatment. What has caused this problem and how may it be treated?

Conal has a mild Class III skeletal pattern with slightly increased FMPA and lower facial height; there is no facial asymmetry. His lips are competent and no temporomandibular joint signs or symptoms were recorded.

■ ***What do you notice in*** *Fig. 5.9****?***

Mild marginal gingival erythema.

6⌋ has an amalgam restoration. 6⌉⌈6 are fissure sealed.

Severe lower and upper arch crowding with all canines erupting buccally.

Class III incisor relationship; reduced and complete overbite; centreline shift (lower was 3 mm to the left and upper was 1 mm to the right).

6⌋ and ⌊2 in crossbite.

Buccal segment relationship is Class I bilaterally.

■ ***What should you check for with the crossbite on the 2's?***

You should check if there is a mandibular displacement present on closing.

No mandibular displacement was detected.

■ ***What is the likely cause of the upper and lower arch crowding?***

Inherent dentoalveolar disproportion is the most likely cause.

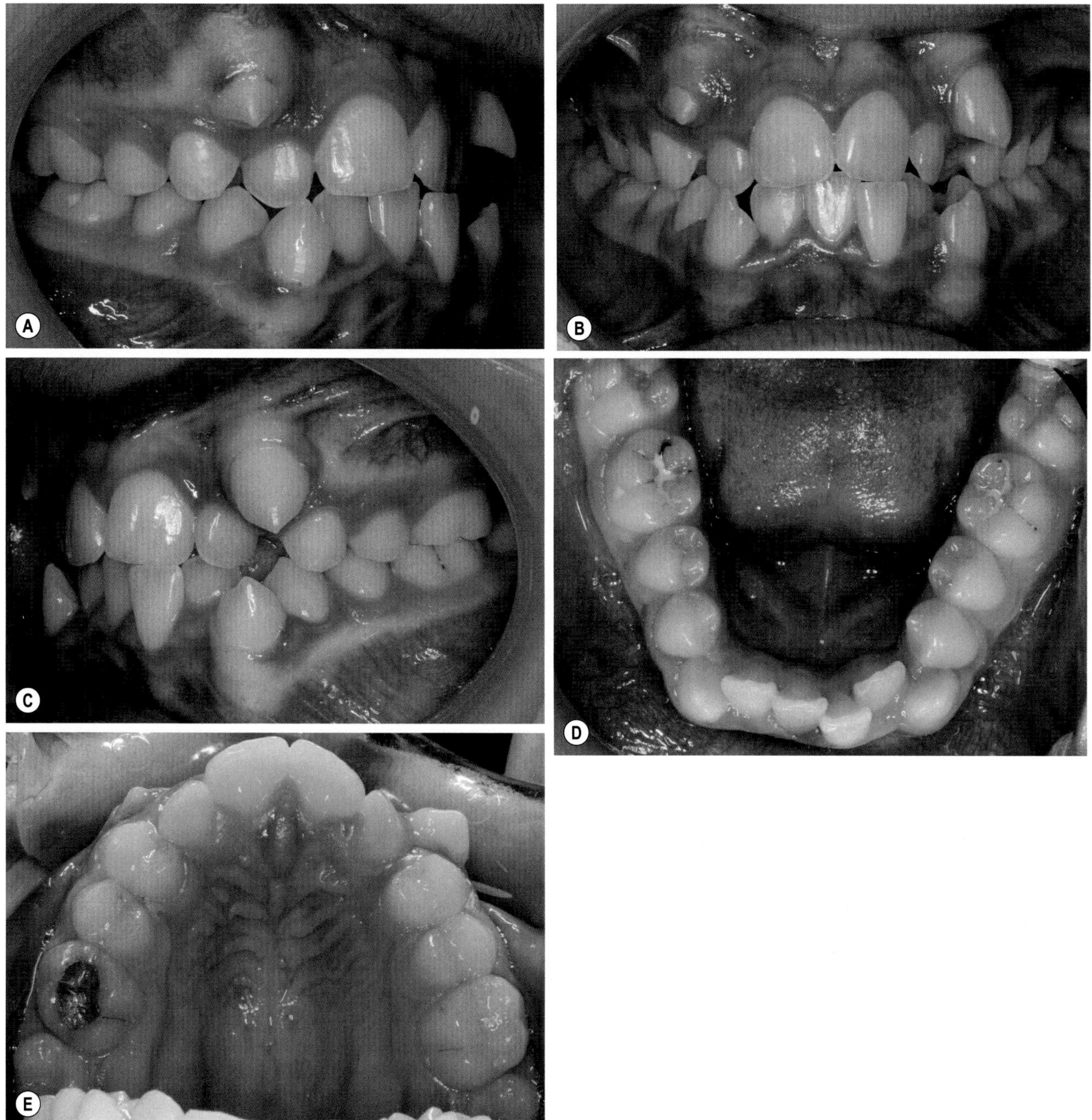

Fig. 5.9 **(A)** At presentation: right buccal occlusion. **(B)** Anterior occlusion. **(C)** Left buccal occlusion. **(D)** Lower occlusal view. **(E)** Upper occlusal view.

■ ***What is the IOTN (DHC) grade (see p. 264)? Explain why.***

4d – due to contact point displacement >4 mm (present on several teeth, but greatest with $\underline{|3}$ and adjacent teeth).

Investigations

■ ***What investigations would you request and why?***

A dental panoramic view would be advisable to check the condition of all erupted teeth and to ascertain if third molars are developing.

This revealed all teeth including third molars to be developing normally and in the correct positions with no apparent resorption of the $\underline{2}$'s by $\underline{3}$'s. The restoration in $\underline{6|}$ was deep. A subsequent periapical radiograph of $\underline{6|}$ indicated secondary caries.

A lateral cephalometric film is also required to assess more fully the Class III skeletal pattern and the angulations of the upper and lower incisors to their respective dental bases. This revealed the following: SNA = 81°; SNB = 81°; SN-maxillary plane = 5°; MMPA = 29°; $\underline{1}$ to maxillary plane = 112°; $\overline{1}$ to mandibular plane = 91°; interincisal angle = 130°; facial proportion = 58%.

■ ***How would you assess the long term prognosis of $\underline{6|}$?***

As the patient's general dental practitioner, you should check the clinical notes regarding the last time $\underline{6|}$ was restored. This should have recorded whether an indirect pulp cap was undertaken or whether the pulp was exposed during the restorative procedure. You should also ask Conal if he is having any symptoms associated with $\underline{6|}$, then check the buccal sulcus for any swelling or sinus related to $\underline{6|}$, as well as the restoration for integrity of the margins, and assess whether 6| is tender to percussion.

The clinical notes recorded a pulp exposure and a direct pulp cap, so although the tooth has been symptom-free, the prognosis would be somewhat guarded.

■ *What is your interpretation of the cephalometric findings?*

Relative to Caucasian norms, SNA is average and SNB is slightly increased, indicating mild mandibular prognathism. The skeletal pattern is mildly Class III (SNA – SNB = ANB = 0°). SN to maxillary plane is slightly less than average; MMPA is slightly increased; $\underline{1}$ to maxillary plane is slightly increased, and $\overline{1}$ to mandibular plane is slightly reduced. The interincisal angle is reduced and facial proportion is increased. The $\overline{1}$ angulation is compensating for the mildly increased MMPA (120° – 91° = 29°).

Diagnosis

■ *What is your diagnosis?*

Class III malocclusion on a mild Class III skeletal base with slightly increased FMPA.

Generalized mild marginal gingivitis.

Restored 6| with guarded long-term prognosis.

Severe upper and lower arch crowding with upper and lower centreline shifts (lower 3 mm to the left, upper 1 mm to the right).

Crossbite of 2| and |2 with no associated mandibular displacement.

Molar relationship is Class I bilaterally.

Treatment

■ *What are the aims of treatment?*

Improve oral hygiene.

Relieve crowding.

Align upper and lower arches.

Correct centrelines.

Maintain Class I buccal segment relationship.

■ *If 6| is removed in view of its guarded prognosis, what implications will that have for treatment and the final outcome?*

Anchorage demands are already high in the upper arch and extraction of 6| rather than 4| will increase that further on the upper right side as both premolars will require retraction before 3| can be aligned. So although 6| is a larger tooth mesiodistally than 4|, the space created is further from the site where space is required and its removal will make treatment more complex. If 6| is extracted, the cusp tip of 5| should occlude with the buccal groove of $\overline{6}$ at the end of treatment.

■ *What is your treatment plan?*

1. Reinforce upper and lower arch anchorage.
2. Extract $\frac{6|4}{4|4}$.
3. Upper and lower fixed appliances.
4. Upper and lower vacuum-formed retainers.
5. Monitor third molars.

■ *How may anchorage be reinforced in the upper and lower arches?*

Means to reinforce anchorage in the upper and lower arches have been outlined on page 29.

A lingual arch and a Nance palatal arch with transpalatal bar from 7| to |6 were placed (**Figs 5.10** and **5.11**).

■ *Are there any means by which anchorage demands may be reduced in the upper arch?*

Extraction of 4| in addition to 6| would reduce anchorage demands in the upper right buccal segment.

■ *Does this option have any other potential benefits? Are there any risks?*

It would make alignment of 3| much easier, as the 4| extraction space is adjacent. 7| should also end up in a Class I relationship with $\overline{6}$|.

As the incisor relationship is mildly Class III, closure of three extraction spaces (64|4) in the upper arch may run the risk of bringing the incisors to an edge-to-edge relationship or even into a slight reverse overjet.

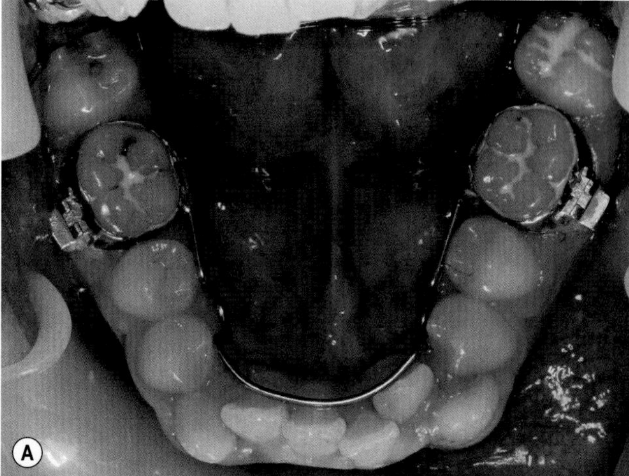

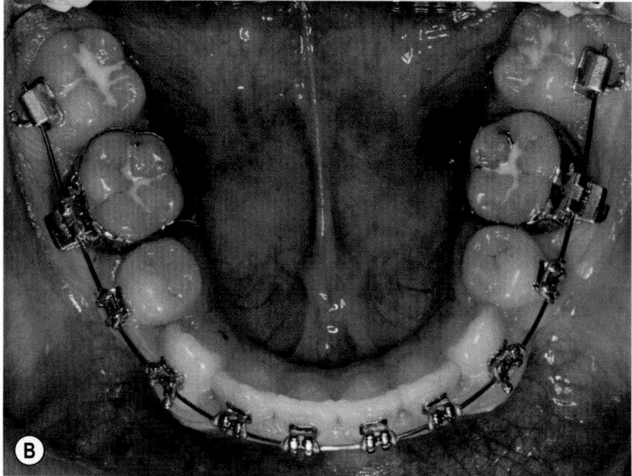

Fig. 5.10 **(A)** Lingual arch. **(B)** After the removal of 4|4 (note small amount of space remaining).

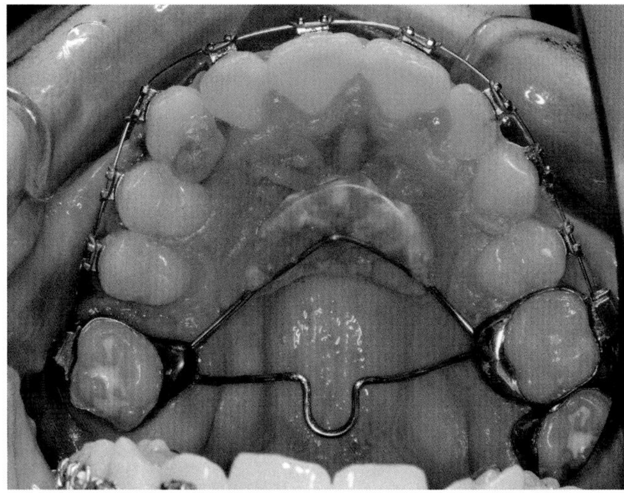

Fig. 5.11 Nance palatal arch with transpalatal arch (following removal of 6|4 and retraction of 5 4 3|3; note minimal residual space).

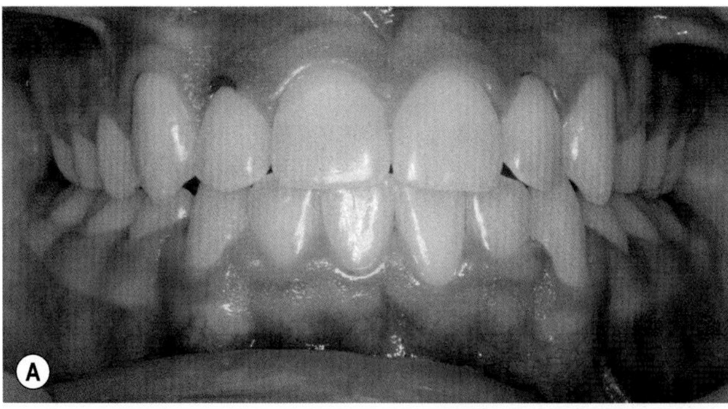

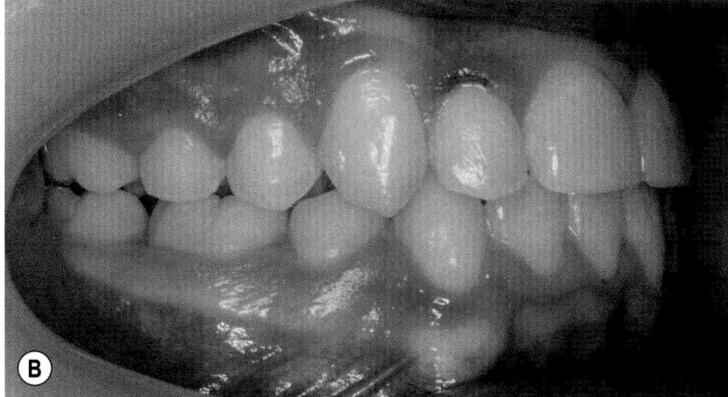

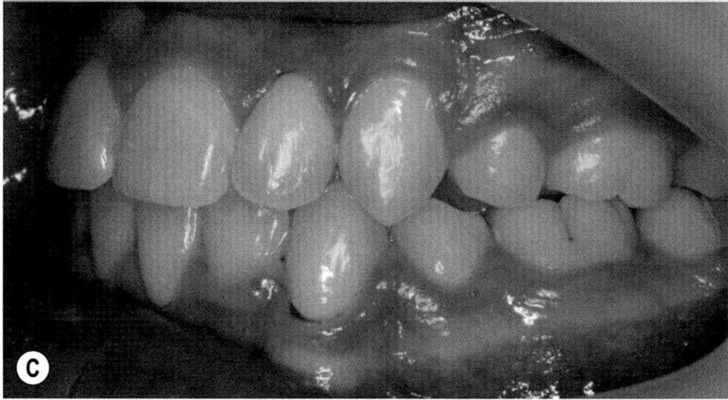

Fig. 5.12 (A) Post-treatment: anterior occlusion. **(B)** Right buccal occlusion (note position of 5|). **(C)** Left buccal occlusion.

Key point

Extraction of a first permanent molar in an upper arch with severe labial segment crowding will complicate anchorage requirements.

The occlusion following canine retraction and alignment is shown in **Fig. 5.11**. The final occlusion is shown in **Fig. 5.12**.

Primary resources and recommended reading

British Orthodontic Society 2009 Patient Information Leaflet: Orthodontic Mini-Screws. London: British Orthodontic Society.

Jambi S, Walsh T, Sandler J et al 2014 Reinforcement of anchorage during fixed brace treatment with implants or other surgical methods. Cochrane Database of Syst Rev Issue 8. Art No: CD005098. DOI: 10.1002/14651858.CD005098.pub3.

Rowland H, Hitchens L, Williams A et al 2007 The effectiveness of Hawley and vacuum-formed retainers: a single-center randomized controlled trial. Am J Orthod Dentofacial Orthop 132:730–737.

Sandler J, Murray A, Thiruvenkatachari B et al 2014 Effectiveness of 3 methods of anchorage reinforcement for maximum anchorage in adolescents: a 3-arm multicenter randomized clinical trial. Am J Orthod Dentofacial Orthop 146:10–20.

Thornhill MH, Dayer M, Lockhart PB et al 2016 A change in the NICE guidelines on antibiotic prophylaxis. Br Dent J 221:112–114.

Yaacob M, Worthington HV, Deacon SA et al 2014 Powered versus manual toothbrushing for oral health. Cochrane Database of Syst Rev Issue 6. Art No: CD002281. DOI:10.1002/14651858.CD002281.pub3.

For revision, see Mind Map 5, page 225.

6

Palatal canines

CASE 1

SUMMARY

Diane, a 15-year-old girl, presents with both upper primary canines retained (*Fig. 6.1*). What is the cause and what treatment possibilities are there?

History

Diane is concerned about the size of the baby upper 'eye' teeth that are present and by the spaces on either side of her upper two front teeth. She is not bothered by the small space between the upper front teeth. C| is also slightly loose, and she is worried in case it is lost, producing a big space.

History of complaint

Diane has been aware that the baby 'eye' teeth should have been lost a few years ago. Her previous general dental practitioner, who retired last year, advised her that these teeth would eventually fall out by themselves and that when the new 'eye' teeth came through, she would then need a brace to close the spaces between her top teeth. There is no history of trauma to C|C areas, and all other primary teeth were lost naturally. All permanent teeth have erupted on schedule.

She has noticed that C| has been loose intermittently for the past 18 months. It does not appear to have got looser in recent months. Diane is very keen to improve the appearance of her upper teeth.

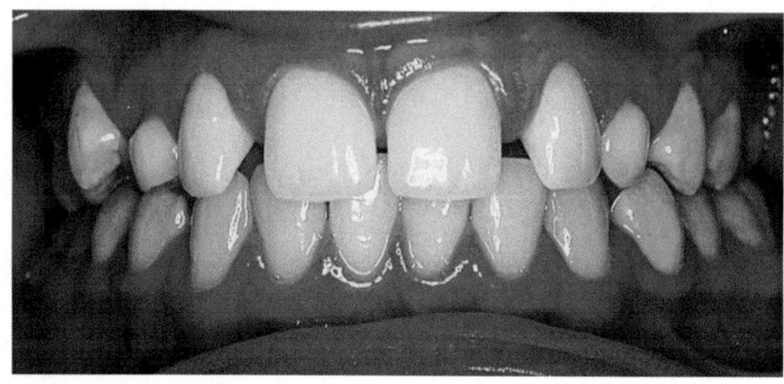

Fig. 6.1 Anterior occlusion at presentation.

Medical history

Diane is fit and well.

Dental history

Diane is a regular attender at her general dental practitioner but has never had any dental treatment.

Examination

Extraoral

Diane has a Class I skeletal pattern with average FMPA and lower facial height and no facial asymmetry. Her lips are competent with the lower lip at the level of the incisal third of the upper incisors.

There is a slight lateral mandibular displacement to the left on closure on $\frac{4|}{4|}$.

Intraoral

■ ***The intraoral views are shown in** Figs 6.1 **and** 6.2**. Describe what you see.***

Oral hygiene is fair with mild marginal gingival erythema related to 2|2 and the upper left buccal segment teeth.

No obvious buccal swellings in the C areas, but there seem to be mucosal swellings palatal to C2|2C, perhaps indicating the position of unerupted 3's.

Slight enamel demineralization buccally on 6|6.

$\frac{7654C21|12C4567}{7654321|1234567}$ erupted.

Mild lower labial segment crowding; 1|1 very slightly mesiolingually rotated; lower buccal segments spaced.

Upper arch uncrowded; spacing in the upper labial segment.

Class I incisor relationship with a centreline shift (clinically the lower centreline was 1.5 mm to the left).

Buccal segment relationship is Class I bilaterally; lingual crossbite of 4| with 4|; buccal crossbite of |6 with |6.

■ ***What are the potential causes of C's being retained?***

Absence of 3's – this is highly unlikely (0.3% of Caucasians).

Ectopic position of 3's – this is the most likely cause (1–2% in Caucasians with 8% of these being bilateral).

■ ***What factors are implicated in palatal canine ectopia?***

The aetiology of palatal canine ectopia is obscure but most probably multifactorial. Possible causative factors are:

1. Genetic – palatally displaced 3 appears to result from a polygenic mode of inheritance, with associated anomalies including incisor-premolar hypodontia, peg-shaped 2 (see below), infraoccluded primary molars, impacted 6, other ectopic teeth and transposition (see Chapters 1, 7 and 8). Class II division 2 malocclusion is also associated with an increased incidence of palatal 3. Lending further support to a genetic aetiology is that palatal 3 has a predilection for those of European origin as well as those with a familial tendency, with females

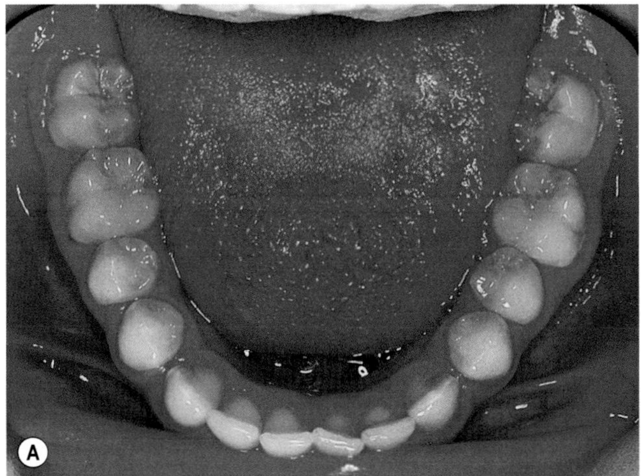

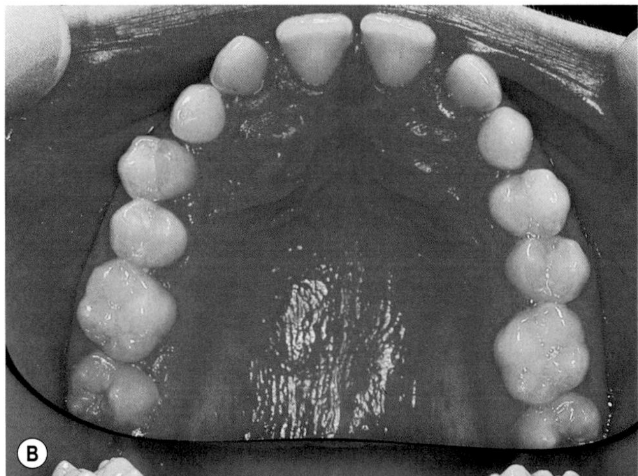

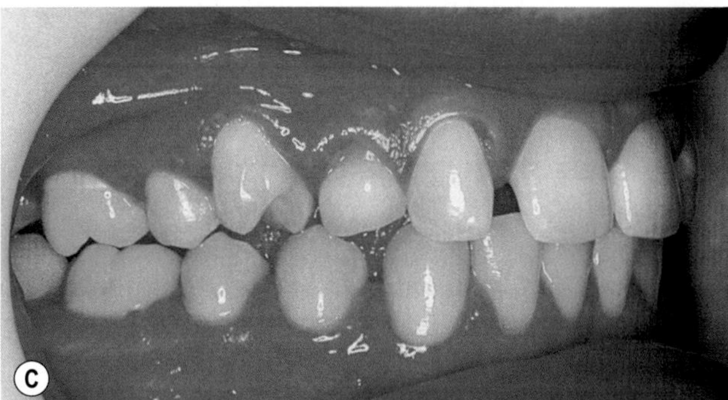

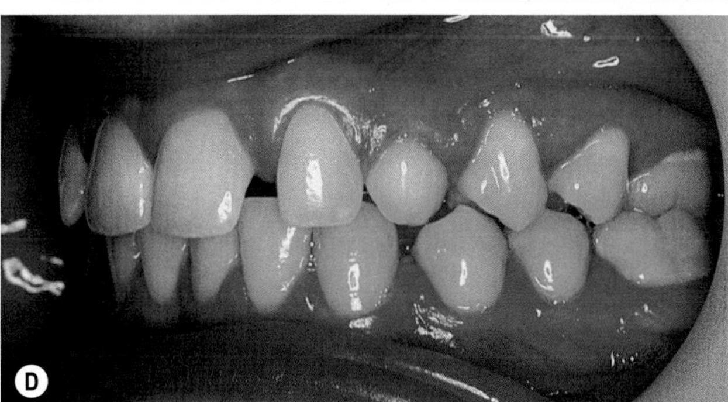

Fig. 6.2 **(A)** Lower occlusal view. **(B)** Upper occlusal view. **(C)** Right buccal occlusion. **(D)** Left buccal occlusion.

affected more than males and occurrence being more common on both sides of the maxillary arch than one would envisage.

2. Crypt displacement – where the position of 3 is grossly displaced, this may be an aetiological factor.
3. 3 has the longest path of eruption of any permanent tooth.
4. Arch length discrepancy – palatal displacement of 3's has been mostly associated with an uncrowded or spaced arch. Note the spacing present in Diane's upper arch.
5. Trauma to the maxillary anterior area at an early stage of development – this has been suggested, but there is no history of trauma in this case.
6. Peg-shaped, short-rooted 2's or absent 2's – guidance for 3 is reduced where these features are evident, doubling the incidence of palatal impaction of 3.

Key point

Palatal displacement of 3:

- Affects Europeans, females and both sides of the arch more commonly.
- Is more common in an uncrowded arch.
- Is associated with small, absent or abnormal formation of 2's, hypodontia, impacted 6 infraoccluded primary molars, other ectopic teeth and Class II division 2 malocclusion.

Note in Diane's case, the mesiodistal width of 2's were the same as those of 2's, indicating that 2's are smaller than average and that a tooth-size discrepancy (TSD) or Bolton discrepancy exists between the upper and lower labial segment teeth.

■ ***What is the prevalence of TSD, and which teeth are most commonly affected?***

Between 5% and 14% of the population have a significant overall TSD, whereas 20–30% have a significant anterior TSD (see below). Although a TSD is most commonly due to a size anomaly of the upper lateral incisor, premolars or other teeth may also be responsible.

■ ***How would you assess for a TSD?***

Quick-check method

- For anterior TSD: compare the width of the upper and lower lateral incisors; if the upper lateral incisor is not wider than the lower, a TSD exists.
- For posterior TSD: compare the width of the upper and lower second premolars; these should be about equal size.

Computational method A tooth-size analysis, often referred to as a Bolton analysis after its developer, may also be performed. The mesiodistal width of each permanent tooth, excluding second and third molars, is measured and then the summed widths of the maxillary to mandibular teeth are compared with a standard table. This allows calculation of Bolton anterior (canine to canine) and overall (first molar to first molar) ratios as follows:

(Sum mandibular anteriors)/(sum maxillary anteriors) × 100 = anterior ratio (%)

(Sum mandibular 6–6)/(sum maxillary 6–6) × 100 = overall ratio (%)

Bolton obtained an anterior ratio of 77.2 ± 1.65% and an overall ratio of 91.3 ± 1.91%.

Discrepancies greater than 2SDs (2 standard deviations) beyond these mean values have been regarded as clinically relevant to treatment planning. Tooth-size analysis may also be undertaken using digital models; the measurements are as accurate and reliable as those obtained from plaster models.

■ ***What are the implications of a TSD?***

The teeth must be proportional in size to ensure good occlusion. Rarely is a TSD of less than 1.5 mm of significance with regard to treatment planning, but where larger discrepancies exist, adjustment of the mesiodistal tooth width through either addition to the enamel (e.g. composite build-ups or porcelain veneers) or enamel removal (e.g. interdental enamel stripping/reproximation) may be required to close or open spaces in the opposing arch.

Key point

TSD:

- May be assessed comprehensively by a Bolton analysis: mean anterior ratio is 77.2 ± 1.65%; mean overall ratio is 91.3 ± 1.91%.
- Is rarely significant if <1.5 mm.
- Clinically significant for treatment planning if >2SDs beyond Bolton mean values.

Investigations

■ ***What investigations would you undertake regarding the retained C's? Explain why.***

It would be essential to determine if 3's are present and to localize their position. Initial assessment should be clinical, and where suspicion of 3 displacement exists, radiographic examination should follow.

Clinical

Palpation of the buccal sulci and palatal mucosae in the upper canine regions, as well as observation of the 2 inclination, usually provides a reasonable guide to the probable position of an unerupted 3. Labial displacement of 2 crown indicates 3 to be lying high and buccal over 2 root, or low and palatal.

Radiographic

Two films taken with either a vertical or a horizontal tube shift are required to assess accurately the location of unerupted 3's. Alternatively, cone beam computed tomography (CBCT) may be used, but its use is generally confined to cases where there is speculation of root resorption of adjacent teeth or where uncertainty remains regarding 3 position, having screened initial conventional radiographs. A dental panoramic tomogram (DPT) gives a general good assessment of 3 position, although its potential for alignment is presented more favourably as 3 appears at a more obtuse angle to the occlusal plane and less close to the midline. The root length of C, the vertical and mesiodistal position of 3 relative to the incisor roots and the axial angulation and apex location should be assessed. An upper anterior occlusal radiograph or a periapical film of each 3 is useful for detecting incisor resorption and determining the prognosis of the C's. Either of these views, used in combination with the panoramic view and application of parallax (a palatal 3 moves with the tube shift), can be used to locate the 3's. Localization of a palatally impacted canine, however, has been shown to be best undertaken using the combination of an occlusal and a periapical radiograph allowing horizontal parallax. A lateral cephalometric radiograph is not indicated in Diane's case, but where it is justified on clinical grounds, it provides valuable information about the position of 3's, when used in combination with the panoramic view.

Three-dimensional evaluation of the canine position and any suspected resorption to the roots of other teeth is provided by CBCT, which could in time, replace the radiographic views given above for canine localization (**Fig. 6.3**). The recent development of a low dose protocol (~50% less) for CBCT of the anterior maxilla with an impacted canine in paediatric dentistry may facilitate this. Using CBCT, the incidence of incisor root resorption from an impacted maxillary canine has been estimated to be as high as 68%, more than five times higher than that reported from conventional radiographs. A more robust research base for orthodontic application of this technique, however, is required before it can be advocated more widely.

Key point

Using CBCT:

- Incidence of incisor root resorption associated with an ectopic maxillary canine may be five times higher than with conventional radiographs.

■ ***Does CBCT have any other uses in orthodontics aside from assisting with the localization of unerupted teeth and any associated pathology?***

CBCT also assists appraisal of alveolar bone height, width and volume, which may be beneficial for cases requiring combined surgical–orthodontic management, cleft lip and palate for alveolar bone grafting, and orthodontic–restorative care for implant planning. In certain other cases, it may also be useful for assessment of the airway or the temporomandibular joint.

■ ***How does the radiation dose from CBCT compare with that of a DPT?***

Although the effective radiation dose is less (generally 50–500 µSv) than that of a conventional CT, one exposure equates to about 2–8 conventional panoramic radiographs (3–24 µSv).

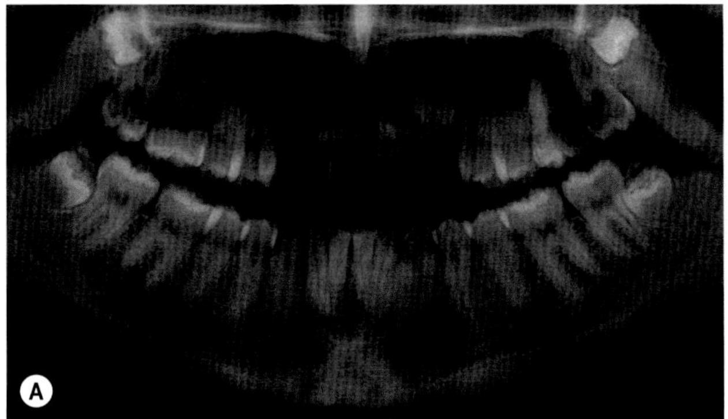

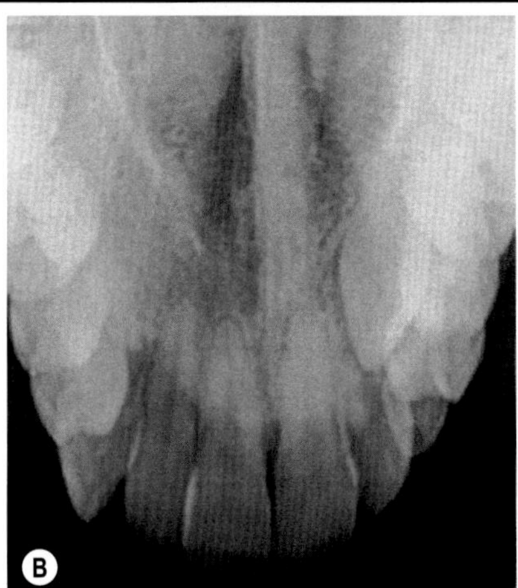

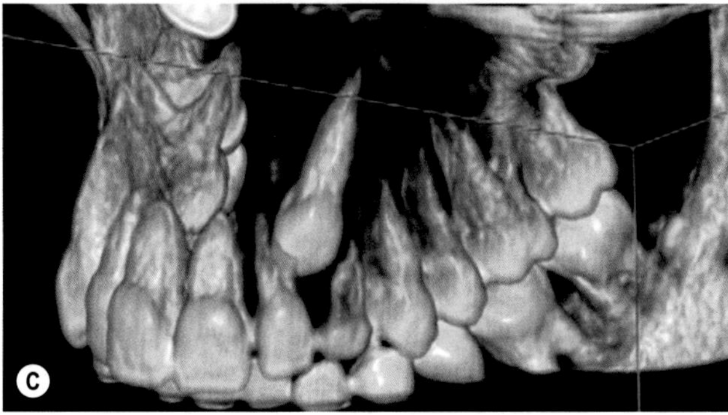

Fig. 6.3 (A) Another case: dental panoramic tomogram showing ⌊3 overlying ⌊2. **(B)** Upper anterior occlusal radiograph indicating ⌊3 to be slightly palatal with possible resorption of ⌊2. **(C)** CBCT image showing ⌊3 to be palatal to ⌊2 and indicating the site and extent of resorption of ⌊2.

Are there any other disadvantages to CBCT in orthodontics?

Currently, CBCT units are costly and considerable time must be allocated to view, and report on, all the data obtained, in line with medicolegal requirements.

Diane's DPT and upper anterior occlusal radiograph are shown in *Fig. 6.4*. ***What are the features of note?***

- Four developing third molars.
- Presence of 3|3, which are palatal.
- Resorption of the roots of C|C.

How may palatal ectopia of 3 be intercepted?

Early detection of an abnormal eruption path of 3 is essential in order to provide, if appropriate, an opportunity for interceptive measures to be undertaken. If 2 is peg-shaped, small or absent, then extra vigilance is required from age 8 in view of the association of palatal 3's with these anomalies. From 9 years of age, palpation for unerupted 3's should be carried out routinely. Importantly, the position of 3 must be localized before considering any interceptive extractions. Radiographic investigation is required when a difference is detected on clinical palpation of the upper buccal sulcus between opposite sides of the arch.

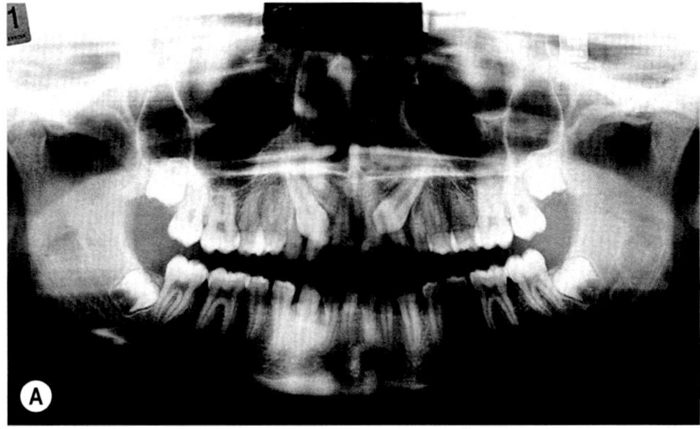

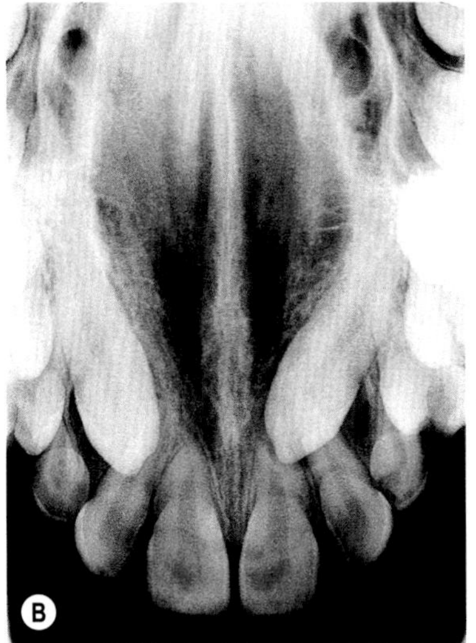

Fig. 6.4 (A) Dental panoramic tomogram. **(B)** Upper anterior occlusal radiograph.

Where 3 is displaced palatally in an uncrowded arch, in a child aged 10–13 years old, removal of C may lead to 3 reverting to a normal path of eruption. The amount of improvement depends on the degree of overlap of 3 over 2 root, with a better prognosis when 3 overlies the distal rather than the mesial half of 2 root. Although improvement in 3 position may occur even where 3 is markedly displaced, specialist advice must be obtained before removal of C. Consideration must be given to balancing the extraction of C with removal of the opposite C to prevent a centreline shift. Normally, following extraction of C, clinical and radiographic re-evaluation should be undertaken at 6-monthly intervals. If no improvement in 3 position is observed on a DPT within 12 months, alternative treatment is required.

How strong is the evidence to support extraction of C's as an interceptive measure for palatally displaced canines?

Clinical experience indicates that there is evidence to support this intervention. However, a Cochrane review concluded that currently there is no firm research base from controlled clinical trials on which to base this practice.

Key point

Removal of C's between 10 and 13 years of age may encourage improvement in the position of a palatally ectopic canine, although there is no firm research base for this.

When 3 displacement is associated with crowding, elimination of crowding and space maintenance, if required, may stimulate 3 position to improve.

Key point

In planning treatment for a palatally ectopic canine, assess the following on radiograph:

- The root length of C and root status of incisors.
- The vertical and mesiodistal position relative to the incisor roots.
- The axial angulation.
- The apex location.

Diagnosis

■ ***What is your diagnosis?***

Class I malocclusion on a Class I skeletal base with average FMPA.

Lateral mandibular displacement on closure on $\frac{4|}{4|}$.

Marginal gingivitis related to 2's and upper left buccal segment teeth; enamel demineralisation buccally on 6's.

Mild lower labial segment crowding but spaced buccal segments; uncrowded upper arch with C's retained (3's unerupted and displaced palatally); lower centreline shift to the left.

Class I molar relationship bilaterally; lingual crossbite of 4| with |4; buccal crossbite of 6| with |6.

■ ***What is the IOTN DHC grade (see p. 264)? Explain why.***

5i – due to impeded eruption (owing to palatal ectopia) of 3's.

Treatment

■ ***What management options are there for Diane's unerupted 3's? What are the indications for each option?***

These are summarized in **Table 6.1**.

Key point

Surgical exposure and orthodontic alignment of a palatal 3 requires a well-disposed patient with good oral hygiene and dentition.

■ ***Which option would you favour?***

As Diane is a highly motivated patient with a high standard of general dental care and the roots of C's are resorbing, with the 3's in reasonably favourable positions for orthodontic alignment, surgical exposure of 3's and orthodontic alignment would be optimal.

■ ***What are the ideal aims of treatment?***

Alignment of 3's.

Build up 2's to increase mesiodistal width.

Correction of crossbites on 4|6.

Correction of lower centreline shift.

Table 6.1 Management options, with indications, for palatally displaced unerupted 3's*

Option	Indications	Comments
Early removal of C's	See comments in the text in relation to interceptive treatment	Not a viable option in this case as Diane is 15 years old
Retain 3 and observe	Patient not keen for treatment	Need to monitor radiographically the unerupted 3 for cystic degeneration and/or root resorption of incisors
	Pathology or resorption of adjacent teeth not evident	
	Good aesthetics/prognosis of C's or 2 and 4 in good contact	
	3 severely displaced with no associated pathology evident	
Surgical exposure of 3's and orthodontic alignment	Highly motivated patient with excellent general dental health	Prognosis is good: the nearer 3 is to the occlusal plane, 3 overlaps at most the distal half of 1 root, when 3 long axis is ≥30° to the midsagittal plane, when root of 3 is not dilacerated or ankylosed or 3 apex is not more distal than 5. Bond gold chain, bracket or magnet to 3 at surgery; alignment of 3 may commence with removable appliance but fixed appliance required to align 3 apex
	Spaced arch or possible to create space; vertical, anteroposterior and transverse position of 3 crown and root favourable	
Remove 3	Patient not keen for alignment of 3 and radiographic evidence of associated cystic degeneration	Prosthetic replacement of C required when lost
	Hopeless prognosis for alignment of 3, 2 and 4 in good contact, or good root length on C with good aesthetics, or patient willing to undergo fixed appliance therapy to substitute 4 for 3. Early resorption of adjacent teeth	
Transplant 3	Adequate space in arch for 3	Prognosis best if root of 3 is 50–75% formed, minimal handling of 3 root at surgery, and rigid splinting is avoided
	Intact removal of 3 possible	
	Adequate buccal/palatal bone	

*May need to address any associated TSD.

For treatment planning, Diane should be seen by an orthodontist, oral surgeon and restorative colleague to discuss management of 3's and 2's. Orthodontic alignment of 3's, following their surgical exposure, was agreed. Build-up of 2's mesially was to precede this. Mid-treatment, after 3's were across the occlusion, build-up of 2's distally was planned. Diane, however, decided not to have 2 mesial build-ups, and the likely effect of this on the final result was explained to her.

The need for lower centreline correction should be reassessed following crossbite correction on $\frac{4|}{4|}$.

■ ***How would you proceed with treatment?***

Create space for 3's alignment. This will be obtained by moving 2|2 slightly mesially. As they are distally angulated, mesial tipping only is required. These movements, as well as palatal movement of 4| and buccal movement of |6, could be accomplished easily by upper removable appliance therapy. Alternatively, a fixed appliance may be used for these movements.

■ ***Detail the design of a suitable removable appliance.***

Activation

Palatal finger springs (0.5 mm stainless steel wire to move 2's mesially).

Buccally approaching spring (0.7 mm stainless steel wire) with 'u' loop to 4|.

Screw section to move |6 buccally.

Retention

Adams clasps 6|6 (0.7 mm stainless steel wire).

Southend clasp 1|1 (0.7 mm stainless steel wire).

Anchorage

From baseplate.

Baseplate

Full palatal acrylic coverage.

Posterior bite platforms ~2 mm in thickness to facilitate crossbite correction on 4|6. The acrylic needs to be relieved palatal and occlusal to 4|.

■ ***What instructions would you give the patient regarding turning of the screw?***

It should be turned one quarter turn once per week (this is ~0.25 mm).

■ ***When the crossbites on 4|6 have been corrected, what would you do?***

Reduce the posterior capping to half its height at one visit and then remove it completely at the following visit to allow the posterior occlusion to settle. It would then be advisable to place an upper fixed appliance unless this was placed at the outset for the initial movements outlined above. A transpalatal arch, attached to bands on 6's, should be cemented for anchorage. Brackets should be bonded to all other upper teeth except 7C|C7 and alignment continued until a rectangular stainless steel stabilizing archwire (0.019 × 0.025-in stainless steel in an 0.022 × 0.028-in slot) can be placed.

Then arrange for surgical exposure of 3's. If temporary anchorage devices (TADs), rather than a palatal arch, are used for anchorage, these could be placed at the same time as surgical exposure of 3's.

■ ***What methods of surgical exposure are there?***

Three methods exist:

1. Open surgical exposure followed by spontaneous eruption. 3 needs to be of correct angulation for this to succeed.
2. Open surgical exposure of 3 with packing.
3. Closed surgical exposure of 3 with attachment bonded during surgery.

With open exposure, the palatal mucosa overlying 3 is excised and a surgical pack is sutured in place for 7–10 days. Following removal of the pack, 3 can be allowed to erupt for usually up to 3 months before bonding an attachment to commence traction. 3 is then aligned orthodontically above the mucosa.

With closed exposure, after uncovering 3, an eyelet attachment with a gold chain is bonded to either the buccal or palatal aspect of 3, depending on ease of access. 3 is then moved orthodontically beneath the mucosa into alignment.

■ ***What is the evidence regarding open versus closed exposure of palatally displaced 3's?***

A recent multicentre randomized clinical trial found no difference in periodontal health of palatally displaced canines treated with an open or closed surgical technique. Surgical exposure produced a small aesthetic impact, but this did not differ between open or closed techniques.

Key point

Surgical exposure of 3, whether by open or closed technique, has no significant effect on:

- Periodontal health.
- Dental aesthetics.

■ ***How may the 3's be aligned?***

Elastic traction may be applied from the attachment bonded to 3's to the archwire (**Fig. 6.5**) or to a TAD. Light forces (20–60 g) should be used. When movement of 3's is evident, C's should be extracted. Once 3's are close to the line of the arch, a bracket should be bonded to the mid-buccal aspect of each tooth. It is essential that the roots of 3's are adequately torqued to finalize their positioning.

■ ***What factors may you consider for retaining 3's in their corrected positions?***

Aside from full correction of torque, early correction of rotations should be undertaken, followed by circumferential fibreotomy to 3's and then the provision of a bonded retainer.

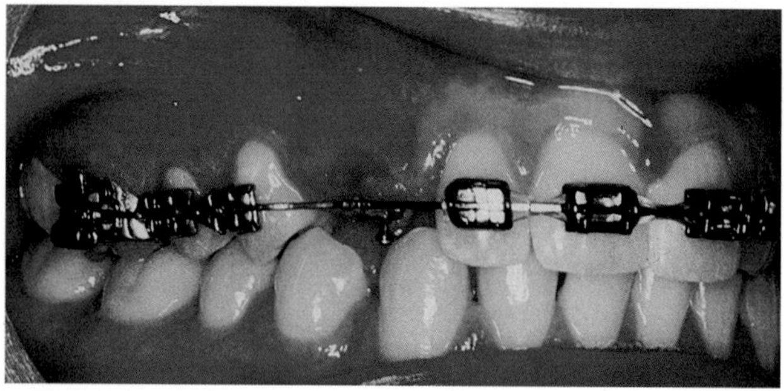

Fig. 6.5 Mid-treatment view.

CASE 2

SUMMARY

Paula, an 11-year-old girl, presented with |3 unerupted. How will you manage the problem?

■ ***The intraoral views at presentation are shown in*** *Fig. 6.6* ***and the radiographs in*** *Fig. 6.7*. ***Describe what you see.***

Generalized slight gingival erythema.

Caries-free dentition.

654321	12456	visible.
654321	123456	

Moderate lower arch crowding/moderate upper arch crowding with 3| erupting buccally; 2|2 mesiolabially rotated.

Class II division 2 malocclusion; deep and compete overbite; upper centreline shift slightly to the left.

Buccal segment relationship appears to be almost Class I bilaterally; (both, however, were half Class II clinically).

The dental panoramic tomogram and maxillary anterior occlusal radiograph show:

- Normal alveolar bone height.
- All teeth including third molars to be present.
- Caries-free dentition.

|3 palatal; roots of 1|1 appear narrow.

■ ***What risk factor is evident for 3 being palatal?***

Paula has a Class II division 2 malocclusion.

■ ***What aspects of Class II division 2 malocclusion have been proposed as predisposing to this risk?***

Class II division 2 malocclusion has a strong genetic linkage and is associated with multiple dental anomalies including palatal 3. The anterior transverse width of the upper arch, especially in the canine/first premolar area, is wider in Class II division 2 malocclusion than in other malocclusions and affords 3 greater scope to wander in the anterior maxilla. In addition, due to their retroclination, the guidance to 3 provided by the root of 2 is lacking.

■ ***Is the position of |3 favourable for orthodontic alignment?***

The position of |3 is reasonably favourable for alignment (see **Table 6.1**). The crown of |3 only extends marginally beyond the mesial aspect of |2 root, and the root apex does not go beyond |5 root. |3 crown lies in the mid to apical third of |2, and the angulation of |3 to the midsagittal plane is >30°.

■ ***What other investigations would you require for treatment planning?***

A lateral cephalogram is required to provide further information on the skeletal pattern and to assess more fully the incisor angulations.

■ ***What is your interpretation of the following cephalometric findings?***

SNA = 78°; SNB = 75°; ANB = 3°; SN-Max plane = 7°; MMPA = 22°; $\underline{1}$ to maxillary plane = 99°; $\overline{1}$ to mandibular plane = 88°; interincisal angle = 151°.

Relative to Caucasian mean values, SNA and SNB are reduced but within the normal range. ANB indicates a Class 1 skeletal pattern, but application of the Eastman correction, as the SN to Maxillary plane angle, is within the range of 8° ± 3°, indicating a mild Class II skeletal pattern (3° + 1.5° = 4.5°; 1.5° arises from half the difference of SNA from the average SNA value of 81°). Compared with Caucasian norms, the MMPA angle is reduced; upper and lower incisor inclinations are decreased indicating retroclination. The $\overline{1}$ incisor angle is more retroclined than it should be for the MMPA; the $\overline{1}$ incisor angle should be 98° (120° – 22°). The interincisal angle is increased indicating a deep overbite.

■ ***What is your diagnosis?***

An 11-year-old girl with a Class II division 2 malocclusion on a mild Class II skeletal base with decreased MMPA. Generalized mild marginal gingivitis. Moderate upper and lower arch crowding with |3 unerupted and palatally displaced. The upper centreline is slightly to the left. Buccal segment relationship is mildly Class II bilaterally.

■ ***What is the IOTN (DHC) grade (see p. 264)? Explain why.***

5i – due to the impacted |3.

Treatment

■ ***What are your aims of treatment?***

- Improve oral hygiene.
- Relieve upper and lower arch crowding.
- Reduce the overbite.
- Align the arches, including |3.
- Correct the upper centreline.
- Correct the molar and incisor relationships to Class I.
- Retain and monitor third molars.

Paula and her mother were keen on avoiding extraction of any permanent teeth, if possible.

■ ***How would you relieve lower and upper arch crowding?***

In Class II division 2 malocclusion, a non-extraction approach is favoured (see Chapter 12). Fitting an upper removable appliance with a flat anterior bite plane would free the anterior occlusion and allow the lower incisors to

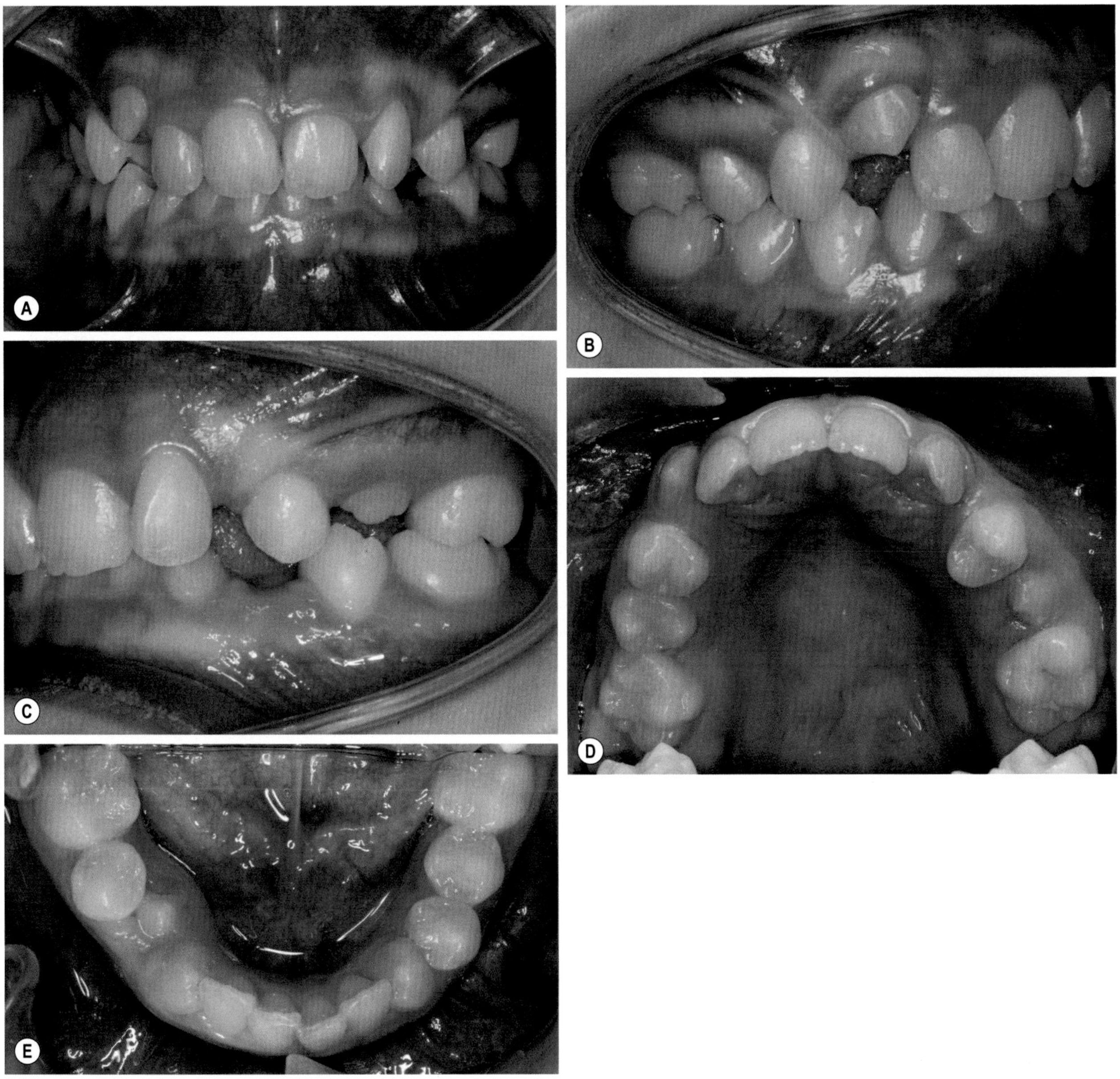

Fig. 6.6 (A) Anterior occlusion at presentation. **(B)** Right buccal occlusion. **(C)** Left buccal occlusion. **(D)** Upper occlusal view. **(E)** Lower occlusal view.

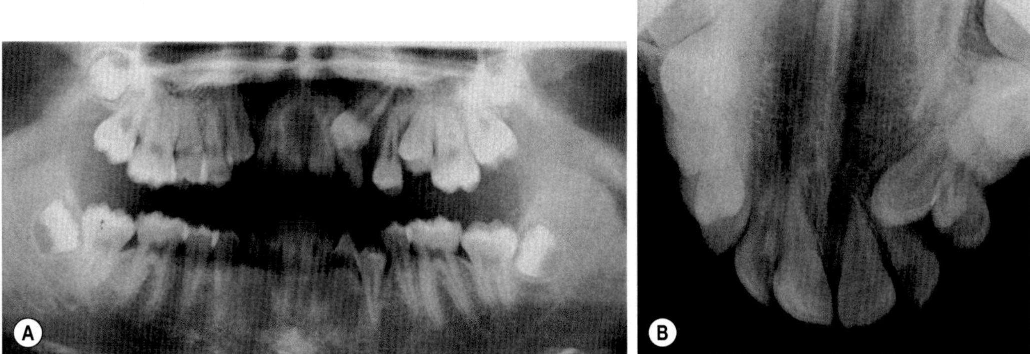

Fig. 6.7 (A) Dental panoramic tomogram at presentation. **(B)** Upper anterior occlusal radiograph.

procline unrestrained by the upper incisors. This will provide some space for relief of lower arch crowding, but the alignment of the teeth will require a fixed appliance.

As a non-extraction approach is being adopted in the lower arch, a similar strategy should be considered for the upper arch.

■ *How could you create space for ⌊3 alignment?*

This would involve distalizing the upper first permanent molars initially followed by retraction of the premolars to open space for ⌊3. This could be accomplished by headgear, TADs or headgear in combination with a removable (Ten Hove appliance; **Fig. 6.8A**) or fixed appliance (**Fig. 6.8B**).

■ *When should ⌊3 be surgically exposed?*

The typical treatment sequence would be to firstly create space for ⌊3 and then to organize for surgical exposure of ⌊3, followed by a 2–3-month period to allow ⌊3 eruption prior to the application of traction to align ⌊3. However, in this case, as no extractions are planned for the upper arch, it would be beneficial to have ⌊3 surgically exposed at the start of treatment so ⌊3 can then erupt while other aspects of the treatment are progressing. Open or closed exposure should be discussed with the surgeon.

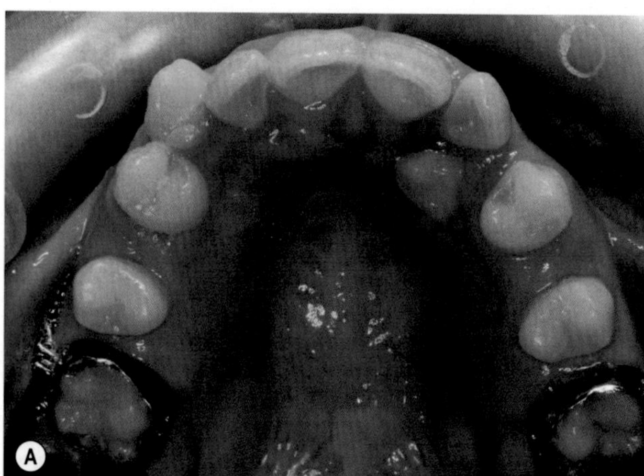

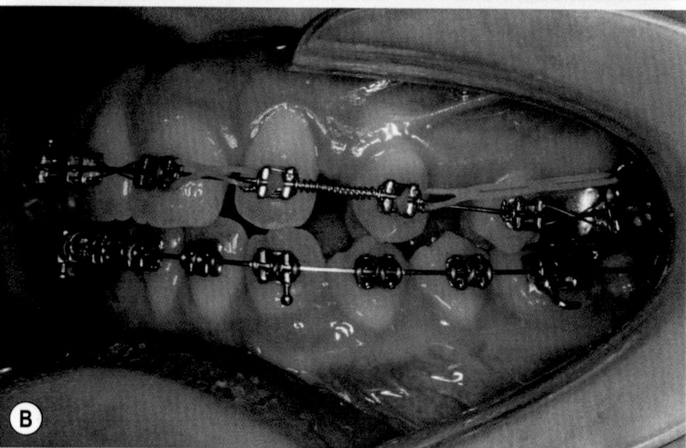

Fig. 6.8 (A) Upper occlusal view showing space created by distalization of 6's by Ten Hove appliance and headgear. (Note: ⌊3 erupting following open surgical exposure). **(B)** Left buccal view showing space for ⌊3 then being created by retraction of ⌊4 with elastomeric chain as further space is opened with nickel–titanium coil spring. (Note anchorage was supported by maintenance of headgear wear at night-time).

■ *What procedure would you prefer?*

Current evidence indicates that it is a matter of personal preference whether to use an open or closed surgical technique. In this case, after discussion between the orthodontist and oral surgeon, open exposure was favoured.

■ *How may ⌊3 be brought across the occlusion?*

When sufficient space has been created for ⌊3 and a minimum of an 0.018-in stainless steel archwire has been in place (assuming an 0.022 × 0.028-in slot), orthodontic traction may be applied to ⌊3 either by an auxillary wire attached over the base archwire or by elastic chain (**Fig. 6.9A**). The former involves 'piggy-backing' an 0.012-in or 0.014-in nickel–titanium archwire on an 0.018-in stainless steel wire, or one of greater dimensions.

It will also be necessary to disengage the occlusion to allow ⌊3 to be free of occlusal interference during movement across the lower arch. This can be achieved by one of the following *short-term* measures: provision of a lower removable appliance with buccal capping of 2–3 mm to 'clip over' the lower fixed appliance; bonding of glass ionomer cement to the occlusal surfaces of the first permanent molars or bonding of stainless steel 'bite turbos' to the palatal aspect of the upper central incisors (**Fig. 6.9B**). The last option given is the most favourable in this case as it does not compromise overbite reduction.

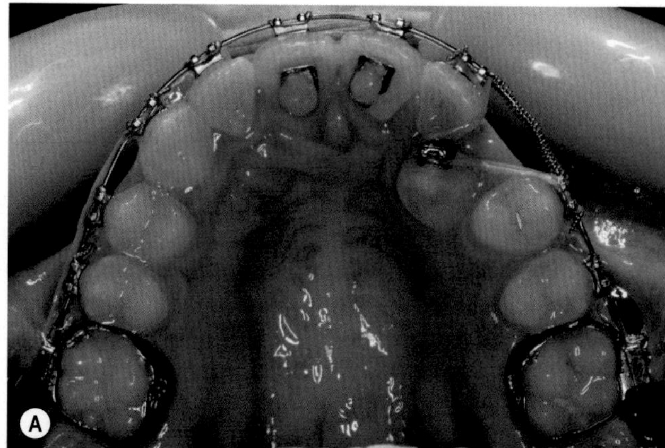

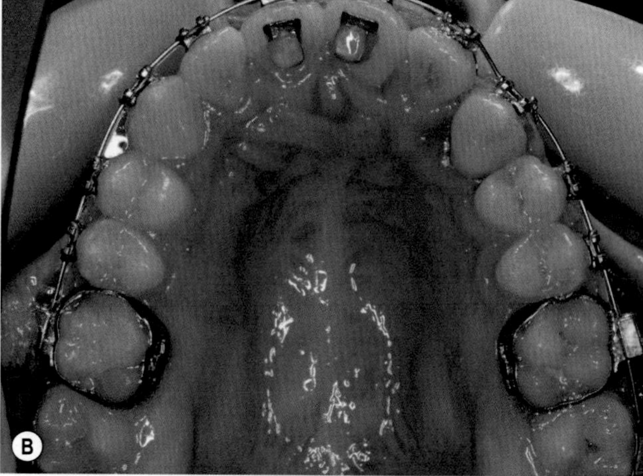

Fig. 6.9 Upper occlusal views: **(A)** showing elastomeric traction to ⌊3 with bite turbos bonded palatal to 1|1; **(B)** with ⌊3 moved across the occlusion.

What are the advantages of nickel–titanium archwires in ⌊3 alignment?

Nickel–titanium archwires offer greater flexibility and greater resistance to deformation than stainless steel archwires. Furthermore, even if the archwire is deflected several millimetres, as in this case to engage the attachment on ⌊3, a light force is applied without deforming the wire.

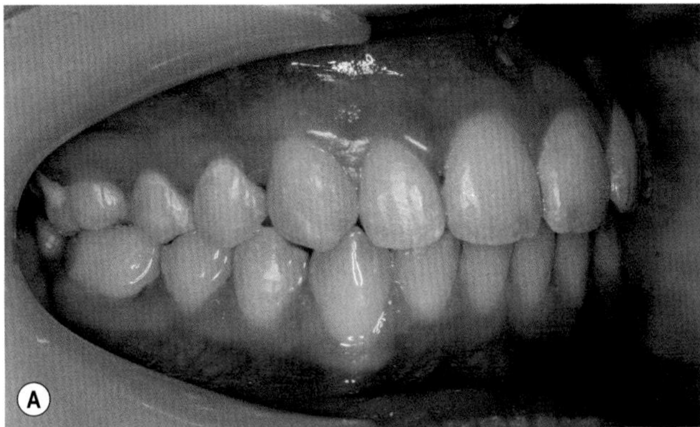

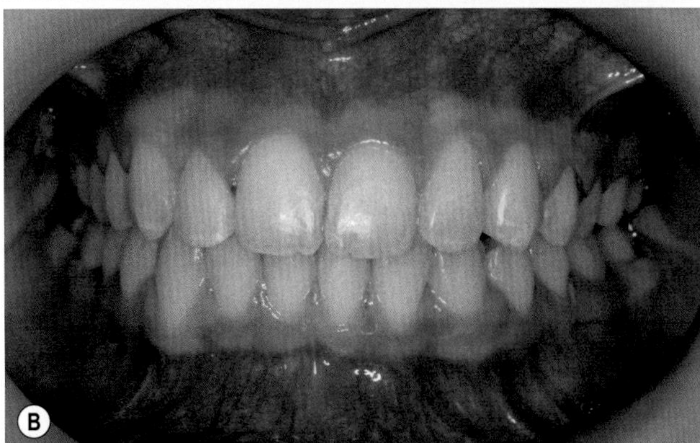

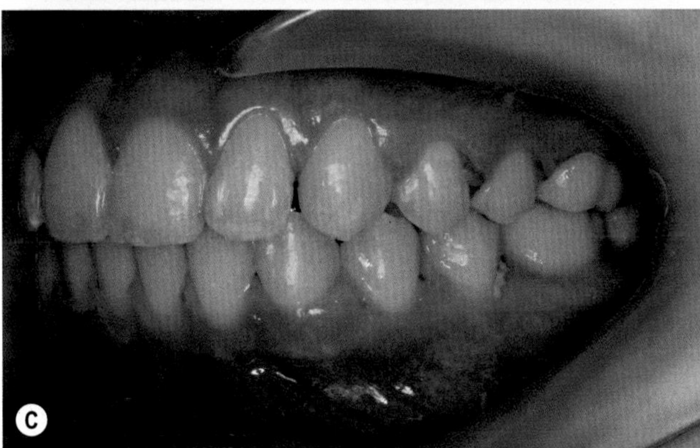

Fig. 6.10 Post treatment. **(A)** Right buccal occlusion. **(B)** Anterior occlusion. **(C)** Left buccal occlusion.

What type of retainer would you consider?

A lower bonded retainer from 3⌉ to ⌈3 and an upper bonded retainer from 2⌋ to ⌊2 should be placed in view of the planned proclination of the lower labial segment and the initial rotations on 2⌋ and ⌊2. This should be supported by provision of an upper Hawley retainer with a flat anterior bite plane to be worn at night only and a lower vacuum formed retainer also to be worn at night only; both of these retainers should fit over the fixed retainers.

The occlusion following alignment of ⌊3 is shown in **Fig. 6.10**.

Primary resources and recommended reading

Fleming PS, Sharma PK, DiBiase AT 2010 How to … mechanically erupt a palatal canine. J Orthod 37:262–271.

Hidalgo Rivas JA, Horner K, Thiruvenkatachari B et al 2015 Development of a low-dose protocol for cone beam CT examinations of the anterior maxilla in children. Br J Radiol 1054:20150559.

Husain J, Burden D, McSherry P 2010 Management of the palatally ectopic maxillary canine. Faculty of Dental Surgery of the Royal College of Surgeons of England. Available at: http://www.rcseng.ac.uk/fds/publications-clinicalguidelines/clinical_guidelines/index.html.

Isaacson KG, Thom AR, Atack NE et al 2015 Orthodontic Radiographs: Guidelines, 4th ed. British Orthodontic Society, London.

Kokich VG, Spear FM 1997 Guidelines for managing the orthodontic-restorative patient. Semin Orthod 3:3–20.

Noar J, Pabari S 2013 Cone beam computer tomography – current understanding and evidence for its orthodontic applications? J Orthod 40:5–13.

Othman SA, Harradine NW 2006 Tooth-size discrepancy and Bolton's ratios: a literature review. J Orthod 33:45–51.

Parkin N, Benson P 2011 Current ideas on the management of palatally displaced canines. Fac Dent J 2:24–29.

Parkin N, Furness S, Shah A et al 2012 Extraction of primary (baby) teeth for unerupted palatally displaced permanent canine teeth in children. Cochrane Database Syst Rev Issue 12. Art. No.: CD004621, DOI:10.1002/14651858.CD004621.pub3.

Parkin NA, Milner RS, Deery C et al 2013 Periodontal health of palatally displaced canines treated by open or closed surgical technique: a multicenter, randomized controlled trial. Am J Orthod Dentofacial Orthop 144:175–184.

Parkin NA, Freeman JV, Deery C et al 2015 Esthetic judgements of palatally displaced canines 3 months postdebond after surgical exposure with either a closed or an open technique. Am J Orthod Dentofacial Orthop 147:173–181.

For revision, see Mind Map 6, page 226.

7

More canine problems

CASES 1 AND 2

SUMMARY

Two similar canine-related problems are shown. What is the cause of each, and how may they be managed?

■ ***What do you notice in** Fig. 7.1**?***

Fair oral hygiene with marginal gingival erythema related to several teeth.

654321⌋⌊1

7654321⌉⌈12 visible with 3⌉ erupting mesial of 2⌉.

Uncrowded upper and lower arches: space mesial to 3⌉; 2⌉ bodily displaced lingually and tilted distally; 3⌉ rotated distobuccally; space between 1⌋⌊1; Class I incisor relationship.

Molar relationship is slightly Class III; 3⌉ in crossbite with 2⌋.

■ ***What do you notice in** Fig. 7.2**?***

Mild marginal gingival erythema related to most teeth, more marked interproximally.

654C21 | 12

654321 | 123 visible with 4⌋ erupted forward of 3⌋ and displaced palatally.

Moderate lower and upper arch crowding; mesiopalatal rotation of 3⌋; distopalatal rotation of 2⌋; mesiolabial rotation of 1⌋. Class I incisor relationship.

Molar relationship is Class I (4⌋ was in buccal crossbite with 4⌉).

■ ***What is the term used to describe the anomaly in position of the canine teeth? How common is this?***

The term used is transposition (positional interchange of two adjacent teeth or tooth development/eruption in a position normally occupied by a non-adjacent tooth). In the general population, prevalence remains under 1% but varies according to the sample investigated.

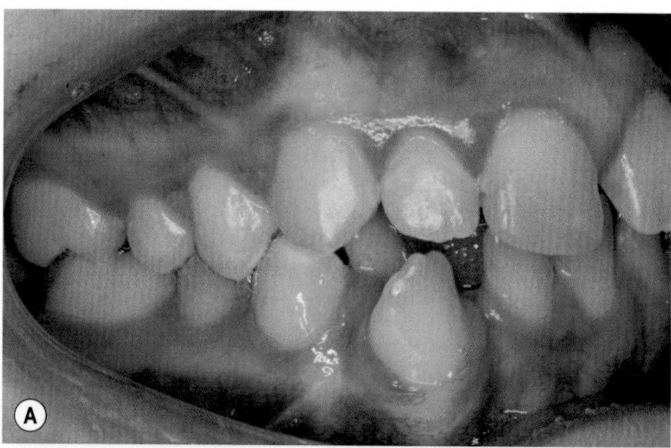

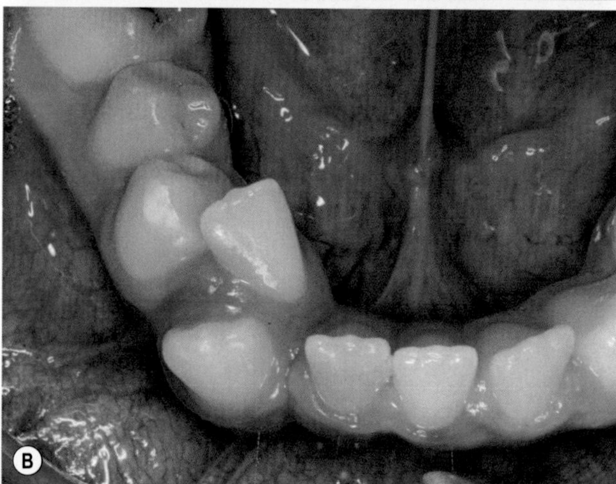

Fig. 7.1 (A) Case 1 at presentation: right buccal occlusion. **(B)** Case 1 at presentation: lower sectional occlusal view.

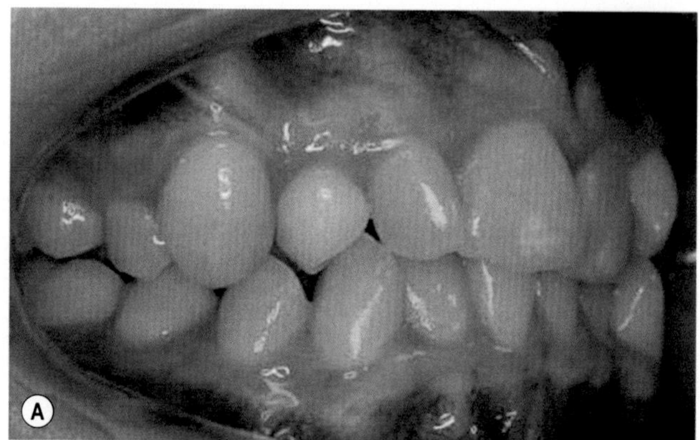

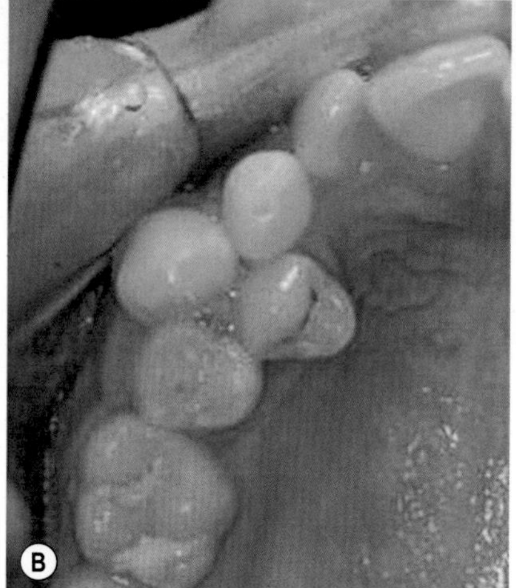

Fig. 7.2 (A) Case 2 at presentation: right buccal occlusion. **(B)** Case 2 at presentation: upper sectional occlusal view.

■ ***Which arch and which teeth are affected mostly? Is there a gender difference in incidence?***

Transposition is more common in the upper arch, where it most commonly affects the canine and first premolar, followed by the canine and lateral incisor. In the lower arch, it seems to affect exclusively the canine and lateral incisor. The left side seems to be favoured in the upper arch and the right side in the lower arch.

A female predilection has been highlighted in some studies, whereas others have indicated either no difference in gender prevalence or a male predilection.

■ ***What is the aetiology of this anomaly?***

Although several theories have been proposed – interchange of developing tooth buds, altered eruption paths, presence of retained primary teeth, trauma – the aetiology is now suggested to be multifactorial with involvement of complex relationships between genetic and environmental factors. There is evidence of associated gender predilection, hypodontia, peg-shaped maxillary lateral incisors and retained primary teeth.

Key point

Transposition:

- In maxilla: more commonly affects $\underline{3}$ and $\underline{4}$ than $\underline{3}$ and $\underline{2}$.
- In mandible: affects $\overline{3}$ and $\overline{2}$ almost exclusively.
- Prevalence: less than 1%.
- Aetiology: genetic and environmental.

■ ***Could you classify this anomaly?***

The transposition may be partial or complete, the apices of the affected teeth being transposed in the latter.

■ ***What factors would you consider in treatment?***

These are given in **Table 7.1**.

■ ***What are the treatment options?***

These are as follows:

Interceptive treatment: if detected early (on average, between 6 and 8 years of age), extraction of primary teeth may be undertaken in an attempt to guide the transposed teeth to their normal positions while ensuring that space is maintained by either an upper removable appliance/palatal bar or lingual arch. This approach is only possible where the teeth affected are tilted so their roots are near the desired positions (sometimes called pseudotransposition).

Acceptance: especially if transposition and root formation are complete, followed by reshaping of incisal/occlusal surfaces and/or composite additions to camouflage for tooth position.

Extraction of the most displaced tooth: this strategy has been recommended where the arch is crowded or for caries; appliance therapy may be required thereafter.

Orthodontic alignment: whether the affected teeth are aligned in their transposed positions or whether these are corrected, depends on the relative position of the root apices.

Table 7.1 Factors to consider in treatment planning for transposition

Factor(s)	Reason(s)
Underlying malocclusion, facial aesthetics, degree of crowding	These will influence need for extraction(s)
Stage of dental development and position of root apices	When root development is complete, interception (by extraction of primary teeth) is unlikely to lead to spontaneous improvement in tooth position
	With complete transposition and root apices closed, acceptance of transposition may be best due to the root resorption and periodontal risks (e.g. gingival recession, alveolar dehiscence) involved in correction
Dental morphology	If transposition is to be maintained, reshaping is necessary to disguise for incorrect tooth position
Occlusal considerations	Judicious grinding of the palatal cusp of a maxillary first premolar will be required where it is aligned in the canine position

Key point

Management options for transposition:

- Intercept.
- Accept/tooth reshaping.
- Extract most displaced tooth.
- Align orthodontically: consider relative position of root apices.

■ ***How would you manage Case 1 and Case 2?***

Request a periapical radiograph of the transposed teeth to determine position of the root apices.

- Case 1: this indicated that the apex of 2⌉ was slightly ahead of the long axis of 3⌉; root formation was nearing completion. No root resorption was observed.
- Case 2: this indicated that half the root length of C⌋ was remaining; root apices of 4⌋ were marginally ahead of 3⌋ root; no root resorption was visible.

Treatment options are to align the transposed teeth in their transposed position or to correct the transpositions.

- Case 1: in view of the relation of the 2⌉ apex to the 3⌉ root, it was decided to proceed with orthodontic alignment, correcting the transposition.
- Case 2: a periodontal specialist's opinion deemed that as 4⌋ was quite markedly palatal (almost in line with the palatal cusp of 5⌋), there was adequate alveolar bone to align 3⌋ in its correct position without risk of gingival recession/alveolar dehiscence. To encourage 3⌋ to move mesially, C⌋ was removed initially and an upper removable space maintainer was fitted. It was decided to commence treatment on a non-extraction basis and to review need for extractions based on further cephalometric evaluation of profile and incisor inclinations when the arches were aligned.

■ ***What appliance type will be required? Explain why.***

Fixed appliance therapy is indicated in both cases in view of the need for bodily movement. These are: Case 1: the

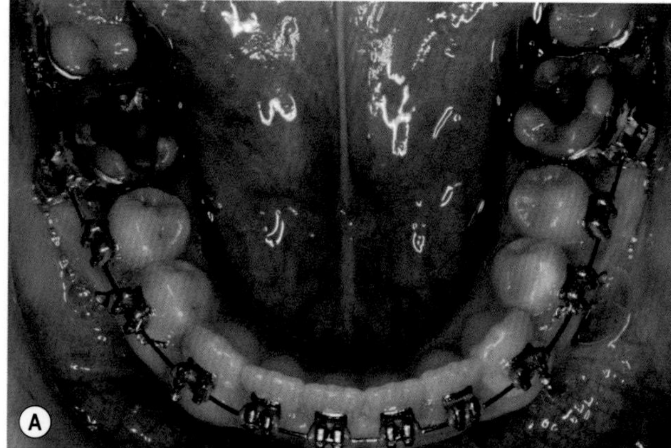

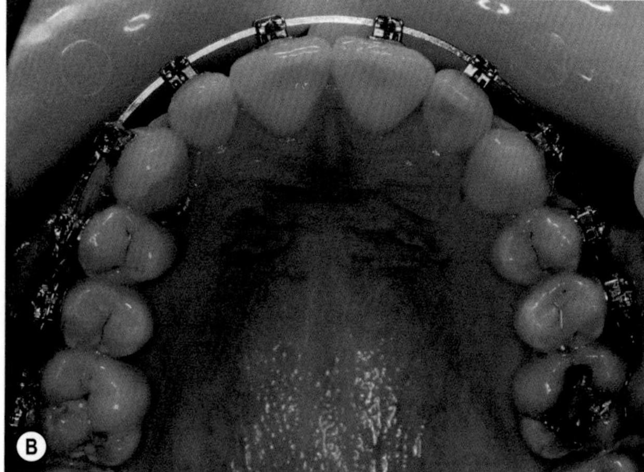

Fig. 7.3 (A) Case 1 following fixed appliance alignment. **(B)** Case 2 following fixed appliance alignment.

positions of 3| and 2| to be corrected; rotational correction of 3|; space closure. Case 2: positions of 43| to be corrected; rotational correction of 321|; correction of incisor relationship; space closure.

In Case 1, the upper arch also required fixed appliance therapy to close the median diastema. In Case 2, the lower arch required fixed appliance alignment.

■ ***How would you check that the positions of the corrected transposed teeth are optimal?***

Palpate the labial/buccal sulci for root position of the corrected teeth (Case 1: 3| and 2|; additional labial crown torque may be required in a rectangular steel or TMA archwire to maximize root positions; Case 2: 4| and 3|; additional buccal root torque may be required to 4| and palatal root torque to 3| in rectangular steel or TMA wires for maximum correction).

Take a *periapical radiograph* to check root alignment and any root resorption of the corrected teeth.

Check *functional occlusion*, lateral and protrusive movements, to ensure no occlusal interferences.

The occlusion following fixed appliance alignment for Case 1 and Case 2 is shown in **Fig. 7.3A** and **B**, respectively.

An example of a case where the transposition of |3 and |2 was accepted is shown in **Fig. 7.4**.

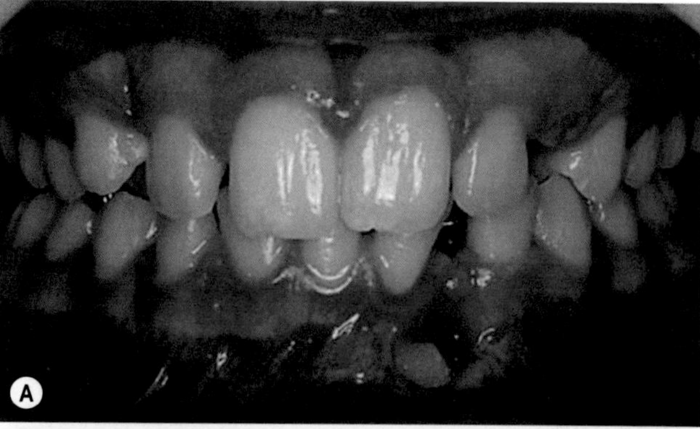

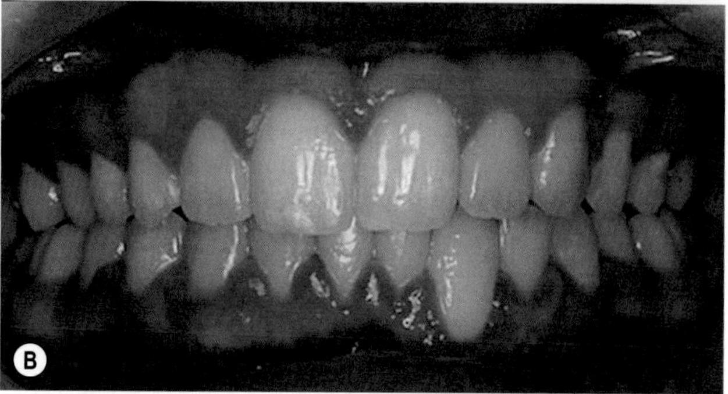

Fig. 7.4 (A) Pre-treatment following surgical exposure of |3. **(B)** Following fixed appliance alignment accepting the transposed positions of |3 and |2.

CASE 3

SUMMARY

Adrienne, an 11.5-year-old girl, presents with mobile 2's and C's with 3's unerupted and not palpable buccally** (Fig. 7.5)**. You order a dental panoramic tomogram and upper anterior occlusal radiograph.

■ ***What do you notice in** Fig. 7.5**?***

Mild marginal gingival erythema.

654C21|12C456
654321|123456.

Attrition of C's.

Uncrowded upper and lower arches.

Class I (tending toward Class III) incisor relationship.

Molar relationship Class I bilaterally.

■ ***Why are radiographs requested?***

To localize the position of the unerupted 3's and to determine the cause of mobility of 2's.

■ ***What do you notice on the radiographs** (Fig. 7.6)**?***

Normal alveolar bone height.

All permanent teeth present except for third molars; all erupted permanent teeth appear to be caries-free with possible exception of |6.

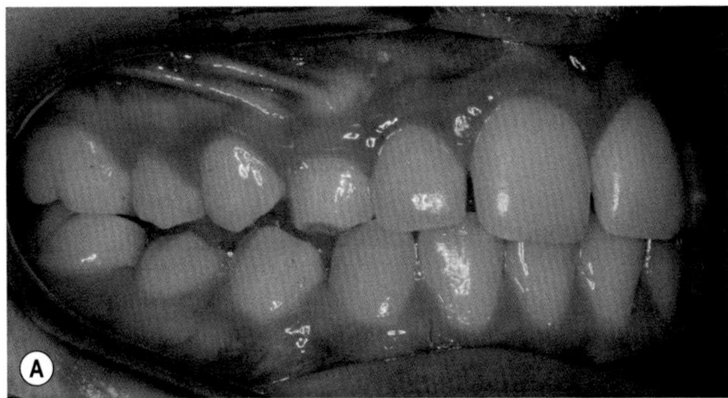
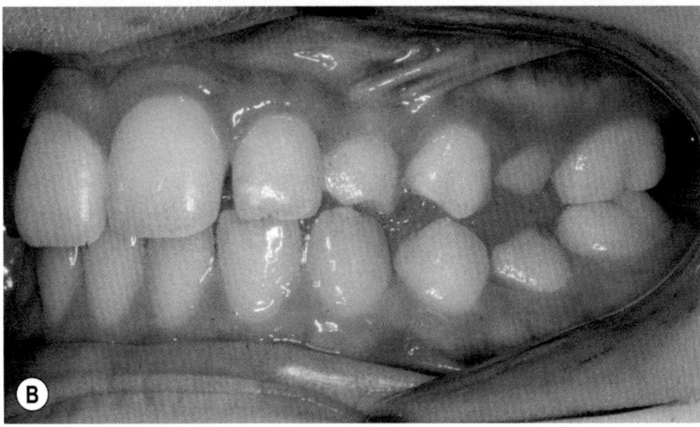

Fig. 7.5 **(A)** Case 3 at presentation: right buccal occlusion. **(B)** Case 3 at presentation: left buccal occlusion.

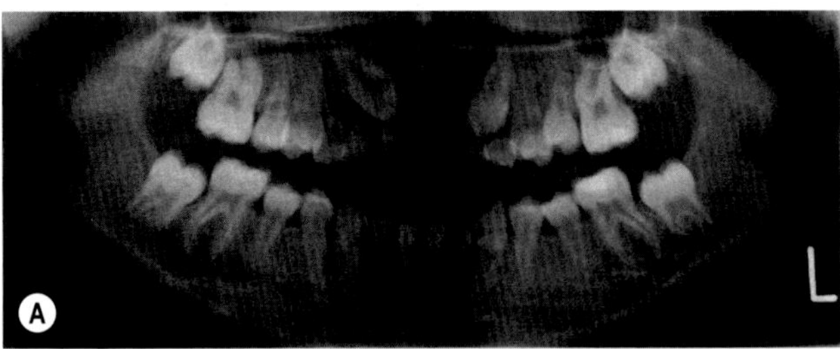

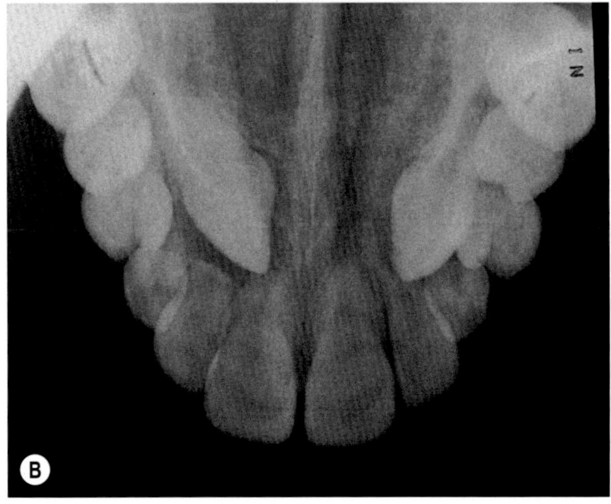

Fig. 7.6 **(A)** Case 3 at presentation: dental panoramic tomogram. **(B)** Case 3 at presentation: upper anterior occlusal radiograph.

Root resorption of C21|2C with less than half the root length of 2| remaining; slight pipette root morphology of 1| and apical curvatures developing on 5|45.

3's palatally positioned (3| much more so than |3 by parallax; see p. 7 and p. 38).

What is the most likely cause of root resorption of the incisors?

It is probably caused by a combination of inherent pressure due to migration of the displaced, erupting canines and their physical contact with the incisor roots.

What is the incidence of root resorption of 2's by ectopic 3's? What sites are most commonly affected? Is there a gender predilection?

Depending on the modality of diagnosis and population sampled, an incidence of between 12% and 68% has been reported, with the apical and middle thirds of the incisor roots most commonly affected. It is more common in females.

How accurate is the information regarding resorption of 2's from the radiographs?

Due to superimposition of the malpositioned canine, especially when it is buccal or palatal to the incisor root, the true extent of the injury may be obscured. If, however, the angulation of 3 to the midline is greater than 25°, the risk of incisor resorption increases by 50%.

Even without overlapping teeth, intraoral radiographs make it difficult to detect resorption on the palatal side.

Key point

Incisor resorption by an ectopic maxillary canine:

- Has an incidence of 12–68%.
- Is more common in females.
- Risk increases by 50%, if angulation of 3 to the midline is greater than 25°.

How may more detailed information regarding 2's resorption be obtained?

Cone beam computed tomography (CBCT; see p. 38) has proved useful.

Key point

Detection of incisor root resorption may be:

- Difficult on conventional radiographs.
- Facilitated by CBCT.

What other investigations would you do in relation to 2's?

Sensibility tests and periodontal assessment (pocket depths/bleeding on probing/attachment loss) should be undertaken. It would also be wise to enquire regarding bruxing habits.

Both 2's were vital on electric pulp testing; aside from mild bleeding on probing consistent with slight marginal gingivitis, no periodontal pocketing of >2 mm or loss of attachment was noted; no bruxing habits were reported.

What are the treatment options in relation to 2's?

Accept and monitor: this is not advisable as the resorption of 2's is likely to worsen due to presence of 3's impinging on their roots. Swift intervention is required as the progression of incisor resorption can be rapid.

Extraction of C2|2C: both 3's may erupt spontaneously, or |3 may erupt and 3| may require surgical exposure. In view of the lack of upper arch crowding, it would be difficult to then close the upper labial segment spacing by fixed appliance therapy without creating a reverse overjet; opening space for the lateral incisors, to be replaced with resin-retained bridges or by implants at a later stage, would likely be a better option.

Extraction of C's and surgical exposure of 3's: orthodontic alignment by fixed appliance therapy would then be required; lower arch fixed appliance therapy may also be required to detail the occlusion.

There is a risk of further root resorption to 2's by aligning 3's; however, if this occurs and prognosis of 2's is deemed hopeless, retaining 2's for as long as possible will preserve alveolar bone for possible implant placement later. Otherwise 2's may be replaced on resin-retained bridges.

After discussion with Adrienne and her mother, they decided to proceed with the last option. They were both warned in relation to the possible resorption risk to several other teeth due to their root morphology.

Key point

Swift intervention is required for incisor resorption by an ectopic 3.

How would you minimize and monitor resorption of the upper incisors during orthodontic treatment?

This is dealt with on page 120.

What is the short- to medium-term prognosis of 2| with the markedly resorbed root?

From the limited evidence available in the literature, this should be reasonable. In a Swedish study, even in cases of severe resorption, the incisor roots showed good healing when assessed at a mean time of 3.5 years (range 2–10 years) after treatment with fixed appliances. Such healing was observed in most cases after management of the ectopic canine, either by surgical exposure and orthodontic alignment or by surgical removal. The resorbed incisors were incorporated in the orthodontic appliance system, and endodontic treatment was not indicated to arrest further root resorption.

Key point

Severely resorbed maxillary incisors:

- May heal after management of the associated ectopic canine.
- May be incorporated in an orthodontic appliance.
- Do not require endodontic treatment to arrest further root resorption.

Radiographic follow-up during treatment (**Fig. 7.7**) showed minimal change in 2| root resorption after surgical

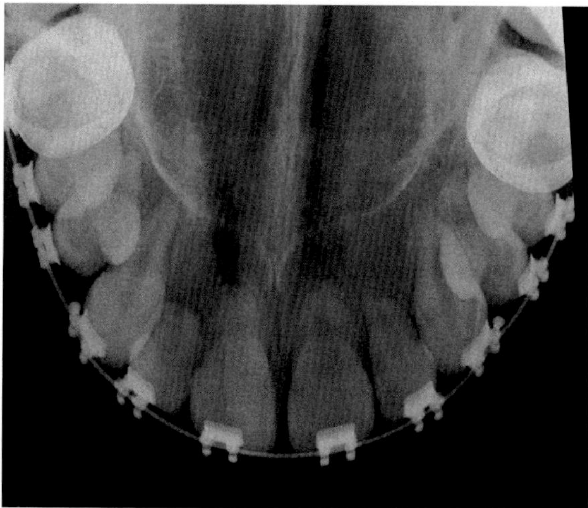

Fig. 7.7 Case 3: upper anterior occlusal radiograph mid-treatment.

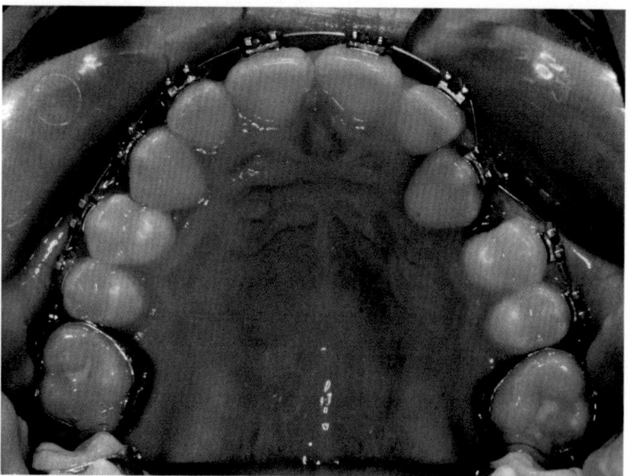

Fig. 7.8 Case 3: occlusal view following surgical exposure of 3's and during fixed appliance alignment.

exposure and fixed appliance alignment of 3's (**Fig. 7.8**). There was minor further resorption of the other upper incisors.

Primary resources and recommended reading

Alqerban A, Jacobs R, Lambrechts P et al 2009 Root resorption of the maxillary lateral incisor caused by impacted canine: a literature review. Clin Oral Investig 13:247–255.

Bjerklin J, Bondemark L 2008 Ectopic maxillary canines and root resorption of adjacent incisors. Does computed tomography (CT) influence decision-making by orthodontists? Swed Dent J 32:179–185.

Ciarlantini R, Melsen B 2007 Maxillary tooth transposition: correct or accept? Am J Orthod Dentofacial Orthop 132:385–394.

Ely NJ, Sherriff M, Cobourne MT 2006 Dental transposition as a disorder of genetic origin. Eur J Orthod 28:145–151.

Falahat B, Ericson S, Mak D'Amico R et al 2008 Incisor root resorption due to ectopic maxillary canines: a long-term radiographic follow-up. Angle Orthod 78:778–785.

Peck S, Peck L 1995 Classification of maxillary tooth transpositions. Am J Orthod Dentofacial Orthop 107:505–517.

For revision, see Mind Map 7, page 227.

8

Infraoccluded primary molars

SUMMARY

Aileen is 11 years old. She is referred by her general dental practitioner for infraoccluded lower primary molars (*Fig. 8.1*). What is the cause, and how would you treat it?

History

Complaint

Aileen is unconcerned by the position of her back teeth.

History of complaint

Aileen and her mother were unaware of any problem with her molars until this was brought to their attention recently by their general dental practitioner. There is no discomfort associated with these teeth and they are not loose.

Medical history

Apart from a possible latex allergy, Aileen is fit and well.

■ ***What implications does this have for her management?***

Aileen should be referred to a clinical immunologist, allergist or dermatologist for testing. If a latex allergy is confirmed, the clinical team and radiographers should be informed. To reduce exposure, more frequent cleaning of the surgery with a protein wash and changing of the air filters is recommended. Latex-free products should be kept separately in a screened area away from latex products. Emergency drugs and resuscitation equipment should also be latex-free. Specifics regarding orthodontic management are summarized in Appendix 4.

Fortunately, Aileen was deemed not to require any specific precautions.

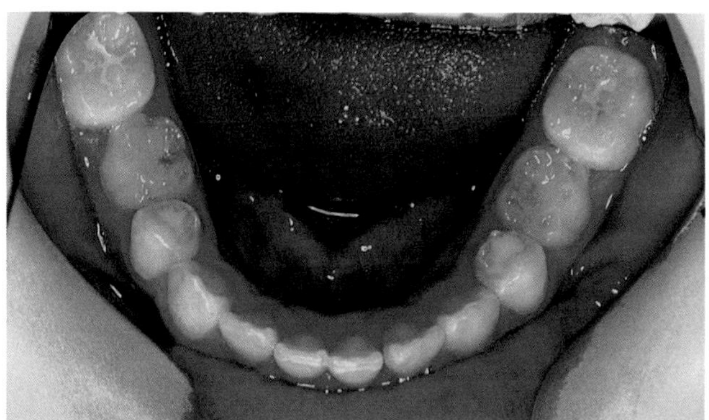

Fig. 8.1 Lower occlusal view at presentation.

Dental history

She is a regular attender at the family's general dental practitioner. No dental treatment has been required to date.

Family history

Aileen's mother has several permanent teeth missing, and these have been replaced by bridgework.

Examination

Extraoral examination

Aileen has a mild Class II skeletal pattern with average FMPA and no facial asymmetry. The lips are incompetent with the lower lip lying at the incisal edges of the upper incisors. There are no temporomandibular joint signs or symptoms.

Intraoral examination

Soft tissues of the tongue, floor of mouth, palate/oropharynx and the oral mucosa are healthy. The intraoral views are shown in **Figs 8.1** and **8.2**.

■ ***What do you see?***

Plaque deposits on many teeth with associated marginal gingival erythema.

Dentition appears caries-free; fissure sealants are present occlusally in the first permanent molars.

6E4321|1234E6
6E4321|1234E6 erupted.

Uncrowded lower labial segment; E|E infraoccluded; uncrowded upper arch.

Mild Class II division 1 incisor relationship (overjet is 4.5 mm measured clinically); overbite slightly increased and complete.

Lower centreline to the right.

First molar relationship: right half unit Class II with 6E| in crossbite; left Class I.

■ ***What is the prevalence of infraocclusion of primary molars?***

Between 1% and 9% of children seem to be affected, but prevalence estimates vary.

■ ***What is the aetiology of infraocclusion of primary molars? Is it linked to any other anomalies?***

Current epidemiological evidence suggests a genetic link and an association with palatally displaced canines (see Chapter 6), ectopic eruption of first permanent molars (see Chapter 1) and absent premolars.

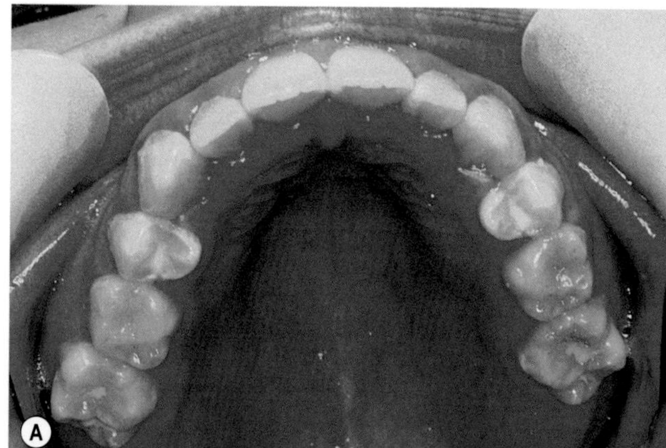

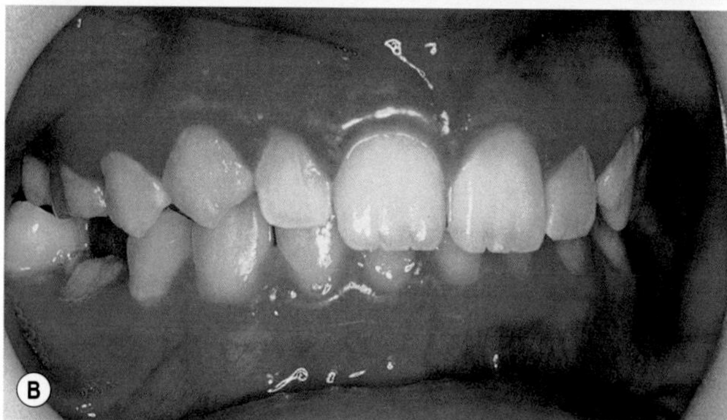

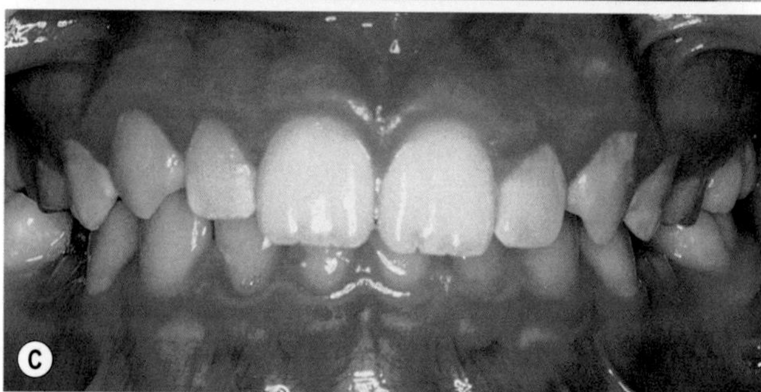

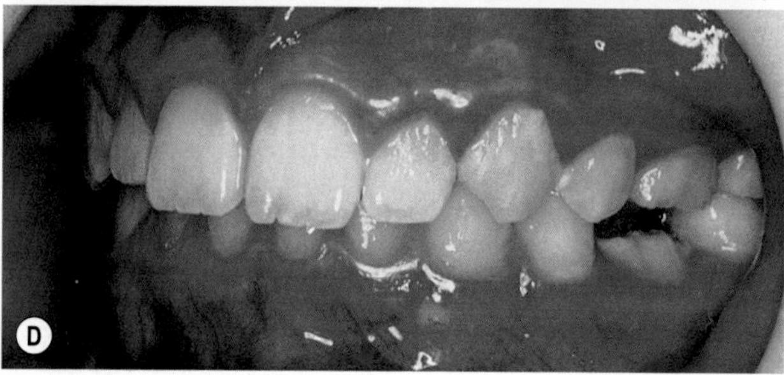

Fig. 8.2 **(A)** Upper occlusal view. **(B)** Right buccal occlusion. **(C)** Anterior occlusion. **(D)** Left buccal occlusion.

■ ***Why does infraocclusion of primary molars occur?***

Separate phases of resorption and repair occur in the exfoliation of primary teeth. Although resorption predominates in most cases, sometimes repair prevails temporarily leading to ankylosis of a primary molar. As alveolar growth and eruption of the adjacent teeth continue, the tooth infraoccludes.

> **Key point**
>
> Infraocclusion of a primary molar is due to ankylosis of the tooth while alveolar growth and eruption of the adjacent teeth continues.

Investigations

■ ***What investigations would you undertake? Explain why.***

Clinical

Assess:

1. Mobility of $\overline{E}$'s – if these are mobile, this tends to indicate that they are close to exfoliation and that the permanent successors are present.
2. Extent of infraocclusion of $\overline{E}$'s – if these teeth are in danger of submerging below gingival level, their removal is indicated.
3. If $\overline{E}$'s are ankylosed – typically a 'tin-can' sound is audible when the occlusal surface is percussed with the stainless steel handle end of a dental mirror and the sound compared with that obtained from percussion of adjacent fully erupted teeth.
4. Overeruption of opposing teeth – this could lead to interferences in functional occlusion and present difficulties if prosthetic replacement of $\overline{E}$'s spaces is required in the absence of $\overline{5}$'s.

> **Key point**
>
> With infraoccluded $\overline{E}$'s, assess:
>
> - Mobility of $\overline{E}$'s.
> - Extent of infraocclusion.
> - If $\overline{E}$'s are ankylosed.
> - Overeruption of opposing teeth.
> - If $\overline{5}$'s are present.

Radiographic

1. A dental panoramic tomogram – to determine if unerupted teeth are present, in normal developmental position and of normal form and size.
2. A lateral cephalometric radiograph may be required later if fixed appliance therapy is planned and the patient is keen to proceed. It would allow more accurate determination of the skeletal pattern in the anteroposterior and vertical dimensions and for the incisor inclinations to be assessed.

Both $\overline{E}$'s were found to be non-mobile and were not infraoccluded below gingival level, but clinically both were ankylosed.

■ ***The dental panoramic tomogram is shown in** Fig. 8.3**. What are the findings of note?***

- Dental development corresponds with chronological age.
- Extensive resorption of the roots of $\underline{E}$'s; short roots on $\overline{E}$'s.
- Absent $\overline{5}$'s and all third molars.
- Absence of periodontal ligament space related to $\overline{E|E}$.

■ ***What is the prevalence of hypodontia in the permanent dentition? Which teeth and gender does hypodontia affect most commonly?***

A recent systematic review found the prevalence of hypodontia in the permanent dentition to be around 6% with a

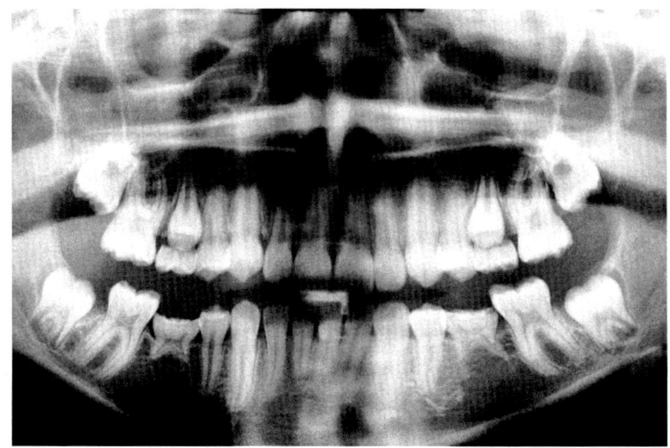

Fig. 8.3 Dental panoramic tomogram.

significant difference between continents; it is highest in Africa (~13%) and lowest in Latin America (~4%), with a prevalence in Europe of 7%. In Caucasians, third molars are most commonly affected (20–30%) followed by $\overline{5}$ (3%), then $\underline{2}$ (2%) and $\underline{5}$ (less than 2%). Females are affected more than males, and tooth size in the remainder of the dentition tends to be reduced.

> **Key point**
>
> Hypodontia:
>
> - Prevalence: ~6% in permanent dentition and differs significantly by continent.
> - Frequency: 8's, then $\overline{5}$, $\underline{2}$, $\underline{5}$.
> - Females more than males.

Following perusal of the panoramic tomogram and preliminary discussion of treatment options with Aileen and her mother, a lateral cephalometric radiograph was taken. Analysis revealed the following:

SNA = 82°; SNB = 76.5°; ANB = 5.5°; $\underline{1}$ to maxillary plane = 112°; $\overline{1}$ to mandibular plane = 92°; MMPA = 26°; facial proportion = 55%.

■ ***What do these values tell you (see p. 270)?***

They confirm the clinical impression of a mild Class II skeletal pattern with average FMPA. Incisor inclinations to their underlying dental bases are also within the normal range.

Diagnosis

■ ***What is your diagnosis?***

Mild Class II division 1 malocclusion on a mild Class II skeletal base with average FMPA.

Generalized marginal gingivitis, uncrowded lower arch with infraoccluded $\overline{E}$'s.

Uncrowded upper arch. First molar relationship right half unit Class II with $\underline{6E|}$ in crossbite; left Class I.

Hypodontia of $\overline{5}$'s and third molars.

■ ***What is the IOTN (DHC) grade (see p. 264)? Explain why.***

4h – due to absent $\overline{5}$'s.

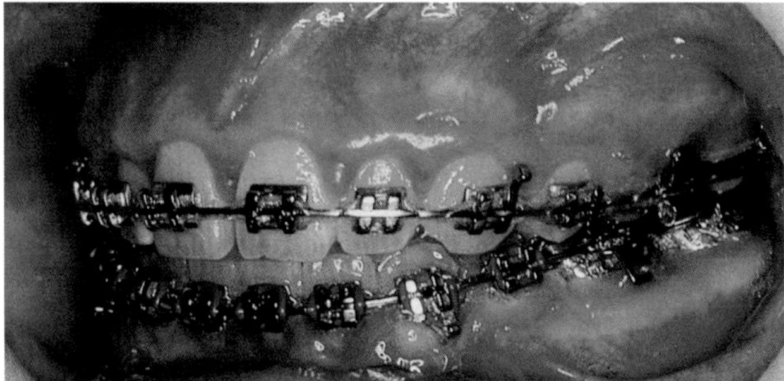

Fig. 8.4 Fixed appliances.

Treatment

■ ***What treatment options are there for the lower arch? Explain why.***

In view of the lack of crowding:

1. Accept the position and status of $\overline{E|E}$, realizing their poor long-term prognosis due to the short root length, but build up $\overline{E|E}$ with occlusal onlays in composite to bring them into occlusion. This procedure has been shown to improve longevity of infraoccluded molars. Maintaining $\overline{E|E}$ rather than extracting them also preserves alveolar bone. When eventually they are lost, resin-bonded or conventional bridgework or implants may be used to replace the missing units. Aileen and her mother would need to be aware of the implications of this treatment proposal over the lifetime of the dentition, including the need for replacement of any prosthesis as required.
2. Extract $\overline{E|E}$ in view of their poor long-term prognosis and as infraocclusion is likely to progress with the absence of $\overline{5}$'s. Then, close the extraction spaces with a lower fixed appliance. This has the advantage of removing the need for a prosthesis, but a retainer would need to be worn post-treatment for several years at night to minimize the likelihood of space opening. Alternatively bonded retainers could be placed on the buccal aspects of $\overline{64|46}$ to maintain space closure.

■ ***What implications do these options have for the upper arch?***

If $\overline{E}$'s are retained, the slight overjet increase could be accepted as the teeth are aligned, provided the patient is in agreement.

If $\overline{E}$'s are to be extracted and a lower fixed appliance planned, it would be sensible to resort to an upper premolar extraction on either side in the upper arch (probably $\underline{5}$'s in view of the small overjet and absence of crowding, although it will be necessary to await their eruption) and proceed to fixed, appliance therapy to achieve Class I molar and incisor relationships.

Following several visits to the hygienist, Aileen's oral hygiene improved, and having considered all options, she decided to proceed with fixed appliance therapy (**Fig. 8.4**).

■ ***What type of fixed appliance is shown in** Fig. 8.4**? What means are there to close premolar extraction spaces with this appliance type? What method is most effective?***

This is a pre-adjusted edgewise appliance. Space closing sliding mechanics with this appliance may be undertaken

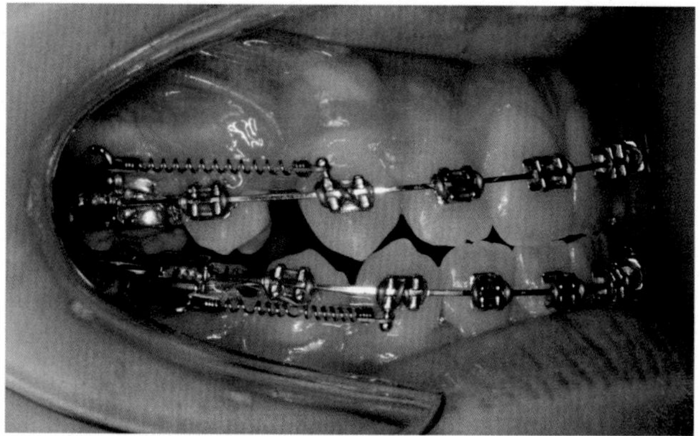

Fig. 8.5 Another case with Ni-Ti coils used for the closure of premolar extraction spaces.

in each quadrant by one of the following methods, each of which is attached from the first molar band hook to the hook on the canine bracket or to a soldered hook on the archwire (so-called posted archwire):

- Polyurethane powerchain – narrow spaced polyurethane powerchain is stretched to about double its resting length.
- Active ligatures – a grey elastic module is stretched by a ligature to double its resting length (otherwise known as a Berman ligature).
- Nickel-titanium (NiTi) springs attached as for the active ligatures (**Fig. 8.5**).

A force of 100–200 g has been recommended. Class II elastics may also be used to assist with closure of upper and lower premolar extraction spaces.

A randomized clinical trial compared the three options listed above. The most rapid rate of space closure was achieved with NiTi springs and was considered the treatment of choice. Elastic chain, however, was as effective and is cheaper. The addition of Class II elastics did not seem to affect the rate of space closure.

The occlusion following removal of $\underline{E|E}$, then $\underline{5|5}$ and $\overline{E}$'s and fixed appliance therapy is shown in **Fig. 8.6**.

■ ***If $\overline{5}$'s had been present radiographically, what would have been your treatment plan?***

Ankylosis of $\overline{E}$'s is likely to be temporary when permanent successors exist, and $\overline{E}$'s should exfoliate within a normal time frame. The position of $\overline{E}$'s should be monitored until then, and if the infraocclusion progresses, extraction is recommended, particularly if the crown of $\overline{E}$ moves to lie below gingival level (reinclusion) and/or apical closure is almost complete on $\overline{5}$.

Key point

Management options for infraoccluded $\overline{E}$:

- $\overline{5}$ present, no reinclusion: allow $\overline{E}$ to exfoliate.
- $\overline{5}$ present, and reinclusion: extract or surgically remove $\overline{E}$.
- $\overline{5}$ absent: retain and place onlay:
  - extract and space close.
  - extract and prosthetic replacement.

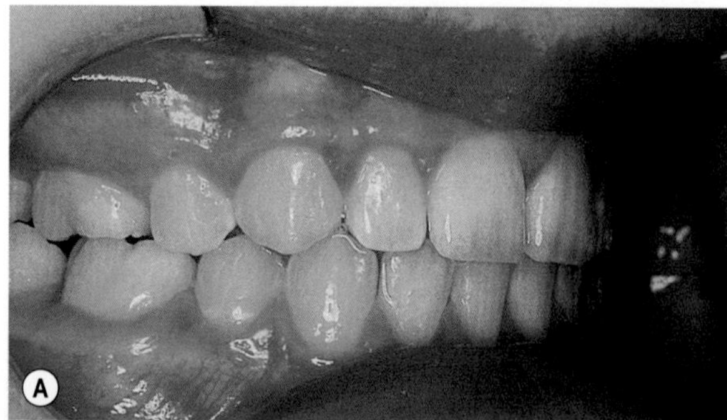

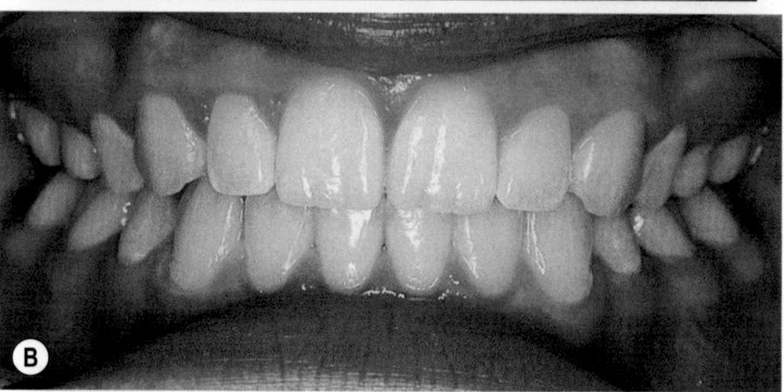

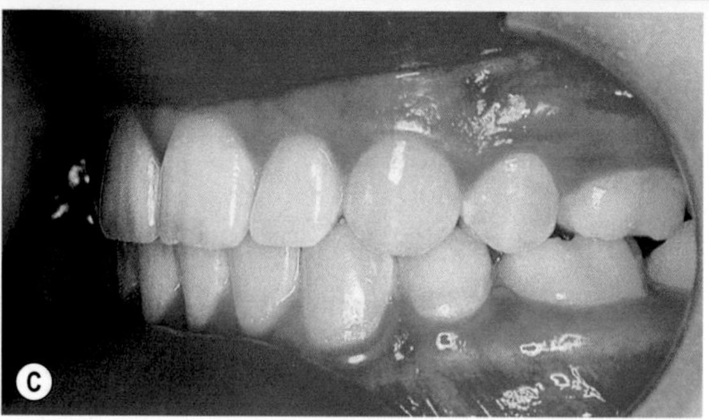

Fig. 8.6 **(A)** Post-treatment: right buccal occlusion. **(B)** Post-treatment: anterior occlusion. **(C)** Post-treatment: left buccal occlusion.

Primary resources and recommended reading

Bjerklin K, Al-Najjar M, Karestedt H et al 2008 Agenesis of mandibular second premolars with retained primary molars: a longitudinal radiographic study of 99 subjects from 12 years of age to adulthood. Eur J Orthod 30:254–261.

Dixon V, Read MJF, O'Brien KD et al 2002 A randomized clinical trial to compare three methods of orthodontic space closure. J Orthod 29:31–36.

Hudson AP, Harris AM, Morkel JA et al 2007 Infraocclusion of primary molars: a review of the literature. SADJ 62:114, 116,118–122.

Khalaf K, Miskelly J, Voge E et al 2014 Prevalence of hypodontia and associated factors: a systematic review and meta-analysis. J Orthod 41:299–316.

Kurol J, Koch G 1985 The effect of extraction of infraoccluded deciduous molars: a longitudinal study. Am J Orthod 87:46–55.

Patel A, Burden DJ, Sandler J 2009 Medical disorders and orthodontics. J Orthod 36:1–21.

For revision, see Mind Map 8, page 228.

9

Increased overjet

SUMMARY

Emma, aged 11, is teased at school about her prominent upper front teeth (Fig. 9.1). What are the possible causes, and how may it be treated?

History

Complaint

Emma's upper front teeth stick out. Her mother is very concerned about her daughter's appearance and is anxious for her to be treated.

History of complaint

The upper front teeth have always been prominent, even when the primary incisors were present. Emma is teased about her teeth at school, and the teasing is upsetting her. She recently fell in the school yard and hit her two upper front teeth on the ground. Fortunately there was only minimal incisal enamel damage to $\underline{1|1}$.

■ ***Is teasing the same as bullying?***

Teasing is sometimes confused with bullying, but they are not the same. Teasing has been described as ambiguous social exchange that may be friendly, neutral or negative, whereas bullying is demarcated by repeated aggressive behaviour or intentional harm over time and is characterized by an imbalance of power.

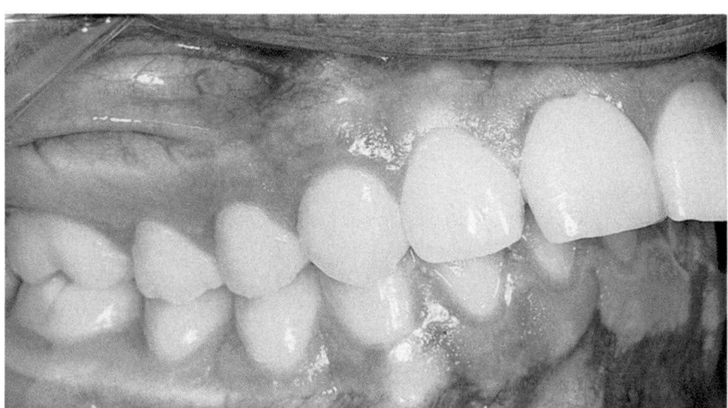

Fig. 9.1 Right buccal occlusion at presentation.

■ ***How common is bullying among school children? What influence do prominent teeth have, and does bullying have any long-term consequences?***

Using a validated measure, the prevalence of bullying among 8–18-year-olds in 11 European countries was found to be 20.6%. In a recent UK study, nearly 13% of children aged 10–14 who were assessed for orthodontic treatment had been bullied due to their malocclusion, and bullying was significantly associated with an increased overjet. The negative impact on self-esteem and oral health–related quality of life was also reported by those who had been bullied. Long-term effects of bullying into adulthood have also been reviewed and have indicated impacts on physical and mental well-being.

■ ***What is the risk of trauma with an increased overjet?***

For an overjet of 3–4 mm, the risk is doubled and increases for an overjet of 5–7 mm.

■ ***What is the significance of the history of teasing and incisor trauma?***

It would be important to ascertain the intensity of the teasing and whether Emma is bullied at school about her teeth. If so, it would be prudent not to delay treatment especially as $\underline{1|1}$ have also suffered trauma. There is a risk of teeth with a history of trauma becoming non-vital in the future. This should be assessed before, and monitored during, any orthodontic treatment. Traumatized teeth also have a greater risk of root resorption during orthodontic treatment. Although suggested as a risk factor for orthodontically-induced tooth reabsorption, previous trauma seems an unlikely cause (see p. 120). Emma and her mother should be advised accordingly as part of informed consent prior to treatment.

Medical history

Emma has had asthma since she was 4 years old. This is managed with a salbutamol inhaler (Ventolin).

> **Key point**
>
> An increased overjet increases the risk of incisor trauma and may predispose a child to teasing.

Examination

Extraoral

Emma's full facial and profile views are shown in **Fig. 9.2**.

■ ***How would you assess Emma's skeletal pattern?***

The skeletal pattern is the relationship of the mandibular to the maxillary dental base in all three planes of space – anteroposterior, vertical and lateral. Assessment should be made with Emma seated upright in the natural head position (the position in which the head is supported naturally when looking straight ahead at a distant object); the lips should

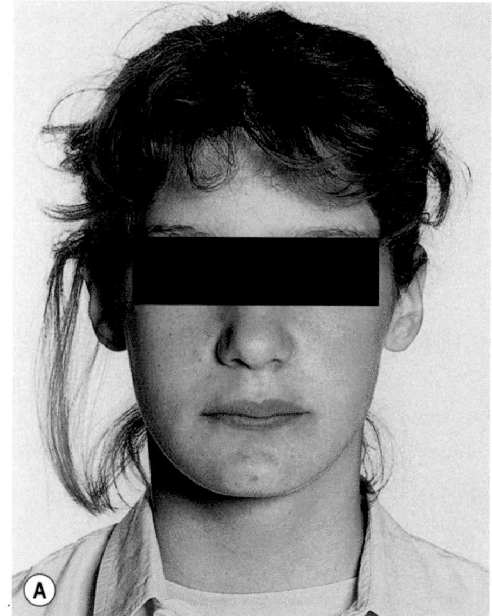

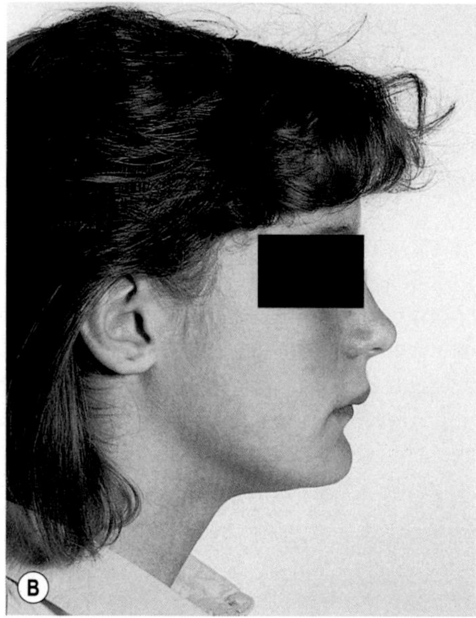

Fig. 9.2 **(A)** Full face view. (B) Profile.

be at rest and the teeth in maximum interdigitation. Assessment should be as follows:

1. *Anteroposterior.* Viewing the soft tissue facial profile in most cases allows the following classification to be made:

   Class I: the mandible lies 2–3 mm behind the maxilla.

   Class II: the mandible lies more than 2–3 mm behind the maxilla.

   Class III: the mandible lies less than 2–3 mm behind the maxilla.

   Due to variation in lip thickness, this method is not always reliable and palpation of the alveolar bases over the apices of the upper and lower incisors in the midline has been claimed to give a better estimate of skeletal pattern.

   Two other assessments may also be made:

   1. The relationship of the lips to zero meridian (a true vertical from soft tissue nasion): the upper lip should be on, or slightly ahead, and the chin just behind.
   2. The angle of facial convexity of the middle (mid-eyebrow to base of nose) to lower (base of nose to front of chin) facial thirds; this may be increased (Class II; convex profile), average (12° $\pm$ 4°; Class I) or reduced (Class III; concave).

   Emma has a Class II skeletal pattern.

2. *Vertical.*

   Lower facial height. The distance from the mid-eyebrow level to the base of the nose (upper facial height) should equal that from the base of the nose to the inferior aspect of the chin (lower facial height). The lower facial height is reduced when the latter measurement is reduced, and the converse is true when this distance is increased.

   Frankfort-mandibular planes angle (FMPA). With a finger along the lower border of the mandible and a ruler placed along the Frankfort plane (lower border of the orbit to the superior aspect of the external auditory meatus), project both of these lines backwards in the imagination to estimate the FMPA. The FMPA is then classified as average (both lines intersect at the back of the skull, occiput), reduced (both lines meet beyond occiput) or increased (both lines meet anterior to occiput).

   Emma has a slightly reduced lower facial height and FMPA.

3. *Transverse.* Stand directly behind the patient and look down across the face, checking the coincidence of the midlines of the nose, upper and lower lips and midpoint of the chin. Alternatively assess the face from the front. It is important to note that slight facial asymmetry is common. The location (upper, middle or lower facial third) and extent of any asymmetry should be recorded. Emma's chin point is marginally to the right. As this is very mild and has not been noticed by her or her mother before now, and as a slight degree of facial asymmetry is regarded as normal, there is no cause for concern.

   No mandibular deviation on closure or temporomandibular signs/symptoms were detected.

   The lips are habitually competent with the lower lip tending to lie under the upper incisors at rest (**Fig. 9.2B**).

Intraoral

■ ***The intraoral views are shown in** Figs 9.1 **and** 9.3**. What do these show?***

There are plaque deposits on several teeth and overall mild marginal gingival erythema.

All teeth appear to be of good quality.

Emma is in the permanent dentition with

6 5 4 3 2 1 | 1 2 3 4 5 6
6 5 4 3 2 1 | 1 2 3 4 5 6 present. (Note 7|7 are erupting.)

The upper and lower arches are uncrowded.

There is a Class II division 1 incisor relationship with increased overjet (measured 7 mm clinically); the overbite is increased and complete. The buccal segment relationship is a half-unit Class II bilaterally. There is a lingual crossbite (scissors bite) affecting |4.

■ ***What are the causes of an increased overjet?***

These are given in **Table 9.1**.

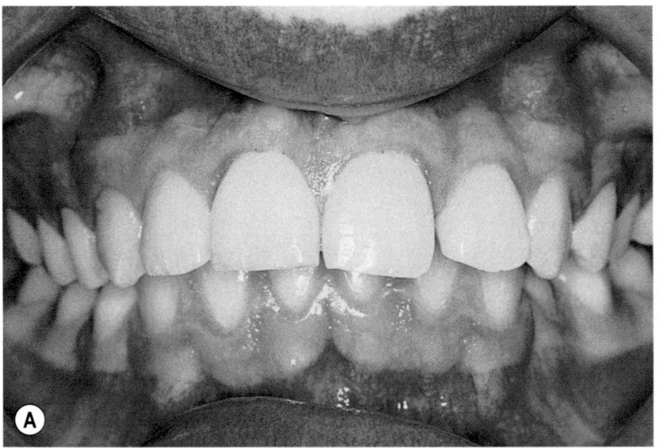

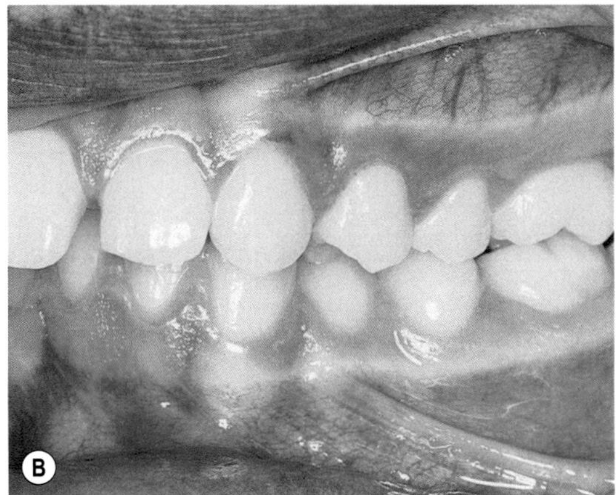

Fig. 9.3 **(A)** Anterior occlusion. **(B)** Left buccal occlusion.

Table 9.1 Causes of an increased overjet

Cause	Aetiology
Skeletal pattern	May be Class I, II or III
	If Class II, mandibular deficiency is almost entirely the primary cause but may be excessive horizontal maxillary growth or a combination of the two factors
Soft tissues*	Lower lip lying under the upper incisors to create an anterior oral seal will procline the upper incisors and retrocline the lower incisors (likely if there is a Class II skeletal pattern, reduced lower facial height and lip incompetence)
	Hyperactive lower lip will retrocline the lower incisors
	Primary atypical swallowing pattern (endogenous tongue thrust) will tend to procline upper (but also lower) incisors
Digit sucking habit	If present for more than 6 hours out of 24, it will procline upper incisors, retrocline lower incisors, create an anterior open bite and a tendency to buccal segment crossbite
	Overjet increase is often asymmetrical due to digit positioning
Crowding	Labial displacement of upper incisors and/or lingual displacement of lower incisors
Any combination of the above	

*Effects determined principally by the skeletal pattern, and thereafter by the manner in which an anterior oral seal is produced.

Investigations

What radiographs are indicated?

A dental panoramic tomogram is required to check the presence, position, developmental stage and any abnormalities of crown and root of unerupted teeth. Untreated caries should also be noted and bitewing radiographs requested, if necessary. In view of the history of trauma to the upper incisor area, a periapical view or an upper anterior occlusal radiograph should be taken and examined for possible apical pathology.

A lateral cephalometric radiograph is indicated as there is an anteroposterior and a vertical skeletal discrepancy. In addition, anteroposterior movement of the incisors is planned.

The findings of the cephalometric analysis are:

SNA = 82°; SNB = 76°; SN to maxillary plane = 9°; MMPA = 22°; $\underline{1}$ nomenclature to maxillary plane = 114°; $\overline{1}$ to mandibular plane = 92°; facial proportion = 52%.

What do these indicate (see p. 270)?

ANB value of 6° (SNA minus SNB) indicates a Class II skeletal pattern.

Reduced MMPA and facial proportion.

Relative to mean Caucasian values, the upper incisors are proclined (but within the normal range) and the lower incisors are slightly retroclined. Although within the normal range the $\overline{1}$ to mandibular plane must be considered with the MMPA as there is an inverse relationship between the two values. $\overline{1}$ to mandibular plane (93°) and MMPA (27°) should total 120° or, alternatively, $\overline{1}$ to mandibular plane angle should be 120° – MMPA. Hence in this case, the $\overline{1}$ to mandibular plane angle should be 120° – 22° = 98°. At 92°, it is retroclined.

What other important information regarding growth potential may be obtained from the lateral cephalometric film? How is this assessed?

It may also be used to determine skeletal maturity. This is assessed by the cervical vertebral maturation (CVM) index which has five stages, each with morphological changes in the second, third and fourth cervical vertebrae. The peak in mandibular growth occurs between CVM stage II and CVM stage III; CVM stage V occurs 2 years after the peak.

How valid and reliable is the CVM index?

CVM has been shown to have high validity and reproducibility.

Would you consider any other investigations?

It would be wise to do sensibility tests of $\underline{1|1}$. These proved positive for all tests, with no marked difference in recordings between teeth.

Diagnosis

What is the diagnosis?

Emma has a Class II division 1 malocclusion on a mild Class II skeletal base with reduced FMPA.

There is generalized marginal gingivitis.

$\underline{1|1}$ have suffered recent trauma.

There is no crowding of the upper and lower arches.

The buccal segment relationship is a half-unit Class II bilaterally with a lingual crossbite of $\overline{|4}$.

■ ***What is the IOTN (DHC) grade (see p. 264)? Explain why.***

4a – due to overjet >6 mm but ≤9 mm.

Treatment

■ ***What factors other than increased overjet predispose to upper incisor trauma?***

The risk is doubled where the overjet exceeds 9 mm.

Lip incompetence – due to the absence of lip protection.

Gender of the patient – boys experience more upper incisor trauma than girls.

■ ***What are the aims of treatment?***

To reduce the overbite and overjet to establish a Class I incisor relationship.

To correct the buccal segment relationship to Class I.

To correct the crossbite on $\left|\frac{4}{4}\right.$.

■ ***What treatment would you advise? Explain why.***

Emma's malocclusion should be amenable to correction by growth modification with functional appliance therapy. Favourable features are that Emma is likely to be growing and is approaching the pubertal growth spurt. The skeletal pattern is mildly Class II due to mandibular retrusion rather than maxillary protrusion. The arches are uncrowded and aligned; the lower incisors are slightly retroclined; the buccal segment relationship is a half-unit Class II, so a modest shift of the arch relationship is required for it to be corrected to Class I.

Functional appliances are usually contraindicated where the lower incisors are proclined, as they induce further proclination through generation of Class II intermaxillary traction. Following functional appliance therapy, fixed appliances may be required to detail the occlusion. It would be advisable then to retain the result by night-only wear of a functional appliance until growth is complete.

Key point

A functional appliance:

- Aims to 'modify' growth.
- Is only effective in growing children, preferably just prepubertal.

■ ***Should Emma have been treated earlier? What evidence is available regarding this?***

A recent Cochrane review compared the effects of orthodontic treatment for children with prominent upper front teeth when treatment is started between 7 and 11 years compared with treatment started in early adolescence. Evidence suggests that earlier treatment reduces the incidence of incisor trauma but *does not offer* any other advantages compared with treatment in early adolescence. Emma has recently suffered upper incisor trauma, and starting treatment earlier may have averted this; however, she is still within the scope of the ages deemed 'early treatment'. Although this review reported no psychosocial benefits of early or later treatment, recent longitudinal data from a UK study on bullied children found that interceptive treatment for an increased overjet reduced the prevalence of bullying and improved oral health–related quality of life.

■ ***What types of functional appliances are there? Which is the most popular?***

Functional appliances may be classified as tooth-borne (e.g. Twin-Block appliance, medium opening activator, Herbst) or soft tissue borne (e.g. Frankel). The Herbst is a fixed functional appliance; all others are removable, although the Twin-Block appliance may also be cemented in place. In the UK, the Twin-Block appliance is most popular, but the Herbst appliance is favoured in North America.

■ ***Describe the records you would take to allow fabrication of a Twin-Block appliance?***

The records required are well-extended upper and lower alginate impressions as well as a wax registration taken with the mandible postured forward, usually to an edge-to-edge incisor relationship, the bite open about 8 mm in the premolar areas with no appreciable shift in the upper and lower dental midlines. This 'working bite' may be recorded by softening several layers of wax in warm water, forming this to a horseshoe shape indexed firmly over the upper teeth and finally guiding the mandible to the correct antero-posterior, vertical and lateral position by checking the relationship of the centrelines and the incisal opening. Alternatively, layers of wax may be adapted to a proprietary bite registration fork, which has graduated markings to facilitate assessment of the postured mandibular position. The wax registration should then be chilled, examined for adequate dental registration and re-checked for accuracy in the mouth before forwarding with the impressions to the laboratory. Where the overjet is large, the mandible may be advanced to 70–80% of maximum protrusion to facilitate patient comfort.

■ ***On issuing the Twin-Block appliance, what instructions would you give Emma?***

The instructions would be as follows:

- The appliance should be worn full-time, including at mealtimes, from insertion. The only times it is removed are after meals for cleaning and for contact sports, during which times it should be stored in the hard plastic tub provided.
- Speaking and eating will be difficult for the first few days but will improve if you persevere.
- Avoid eating hard or sticky foods or consuming fizzy drinks while wearing the appliance as these are likely to damage the appliance and/or your teeth. The appliance and the teeth should be cleaned thoroughly after every meal.
- Mild jaw discomfort and muscle tenderness are common for the first few days but reduce after that. It may be

necessary to take a mild analgesic, as required, during this 'settling-in' period.

- Should a sore spot develop or there be any breakage of the appliance, you should contact us immediately by telephone to arrange an appointment to have any adjustments carried out.

How does a Twin-Block work and what effects does it produce?

The Twin-Block appliance consists of upper and lower appliances incorporating buccal blocks with interfacing inclined planes (at about 70°), which posture the mandible forward on closure (**Fig. 9.4**). This appliance works by using the forces generated by the orofacial musculature, tooth eruption and dentofacial growth. The upper midline expansion screw is usually adjusted once per week by the patient until the arch widths are coordinated with the mandible postured forward in a Class I incisor relationship. In this case, no expansion was required in view of the scissors bite on $\frac{|4}{|4}$. The effects are usually as follows:

Skeletal (~20–30%)

Forward growth of the mandible.

Increase in lower anterior facial height.

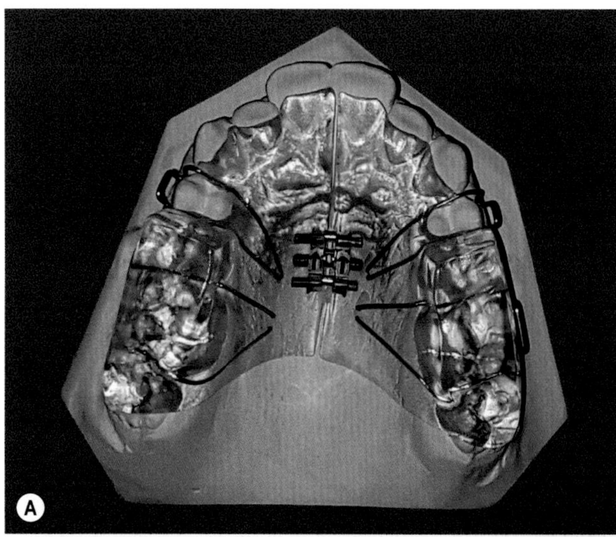

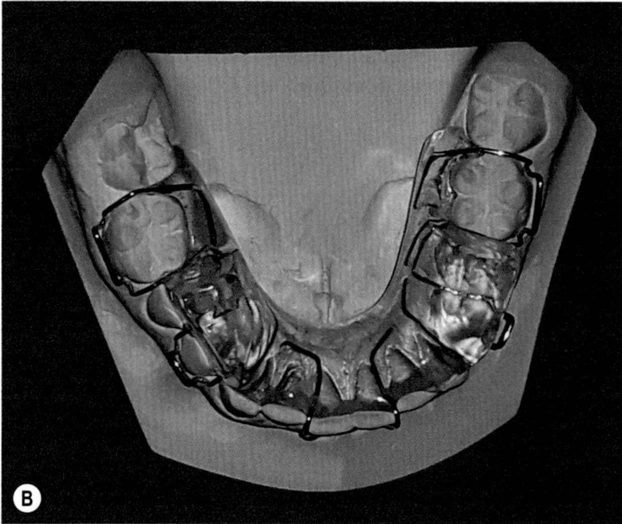

Fig. 9.4 Twin-block appliance. **(A)** Upper occlusal view. **(B)** Lower occlusal view. The design is modified from the original developed by Clark.

Dentoalveolar (~70–80%)

Retroclination of upper incisors/proclination of lower incisors.

Promotion of mesial and upward eruption of lower posterior teeth (see below).

Distal movement of the upper molars.

Upper arch expansion.

> **Key point**
>
> A functional appliance for Class II correction:
>
> - Postures the mandible downward and forward.
> - Generates intermaxillary traction.
> - Uses, removes or modifies forces of the orofacial musculature, tooth eruption and dentofacial growth.

How do the effects produced by a Twin-Block appliance differ from those of other functional appliances?

The recent Cochrane review also assessed the effect of orthodontic treatment for prominent upper front teeth when undertaken by different orthodontic appliances. Functional appliance treatment, irrespective of type, in early adolescence appears to produce some minor beneficial skeletal changes. When the Twin-Block was compared with other appliances, there was no difference in overjet, but the Twin-Block produced a statistically significant greater reduction in ANB, although this was small. There were no advantageous effects of other functional appliances compared with the Twin-Block.

Following overjet correction by Twin-Block therapy, what occlusal anomaly is usually manifest posteriorly in the dental arches?

A posterior open bite is usually present bilaterally due to the buccal blocks.

How may this be corrected?

There are three possible means available to allow for correction of the posterior open bite by eruption of the buccal segment teeth:

- The patient may be instructed to proceed to part-time wear of the appliance.
- The Adams' clasps on the lower molars may be removed initially and then acrylic trimmed progressively over a period of a few months, from the undersurface of the lower block and the lower surface of the upper block, until a posterior occlusion is established.
- Wear of the Twin-Block appliance may be ceased and the patient fitted with an upper Hawley retainer (Adams clasps 0.7 mm on $\underline{6|6}$, labial bow 0.7 mm $\underline{3|}$ to $\underline{|3}$) with a 'steep and deep' anterior inclined biteplane, which aims to maintain overjet correction by posturing the mandible forward while encouraging eruption of the lower buccal segment teeth. Full-time wear of the appliance is required, except for contact sports and teeth cleaning, until a well-interdigitating posterior occlusion is established. Then night-only wear of the appliance, until growth has ceased or until a second phase of treatment commences, is permissible.

■ ***If there is no progress at 6 months, what action would you take?***

Lack of overjet correction could be due to poor patient response to the appliance, improper design or poor compliance. Treatment should be discontinued and a re-evaluation made. The patient's standing height should be recorded and compared with the pre-treatment measurement. This will give an indication of growth over the intervening period. Provided Emma remains keen for orthodontic treatment, new records, including a progress cephalometric radiograph, should be taken and analysed to allow for a new treatment plan to be devised.

■ ***What other treatment options are there?***

If a *design problem* with the appliance is identified as the cause of lack of treatment progress, then remaking the appliance to incorporate appropriate design modifications could be undertaken and treatment recommenced.

If *poor compliance* is to blame for no progress, then the reason(s) should be ascertained from discussion with the child. If lack of motivation or interest in treatment is the cause, it would be prudent to avoid any further appliance therapy until such time as the child has a change of heart regarding orthodontic treatment.

Orthodontic camouflage – by retraction of the upper incisors into first premolar extraction spaces, accepting the Class II skeletal pattern. Importantly, this treatment should not be detrimental to facial aesthetics. Although some amount of tipping movement of the upper incisors is permissible, fixed appliances would be required to ensure an optimal interincisal angle is created. A useful rule of thumb with tipping movement is that each millimetre of upper incisor retraction approximates to a 2.5° change in angulation. With an original overjet of 7 mm and a target overjet of 3 mm (representing a 4 mm reduction), this would equate to a 10° change producing a final incisor angulation of 104°. This value is just within the normal range (109° ± 6°), and the incisors would be quite upright. An upper incisor angulation of 95° to the maxillary plane is regarded as the limit for acceptable retraction by tipping movements.

■ ***What factors govern stability of the corrected overjet?***

For the best prospects of stability the interincisal angle should be within normal limits (135° ± 10°) and the overjet completely reduced with the incisors in soft tissue balance, i.e. no tongue thrust and the lower lip covering at least one-third of the labial surface of the upper incisors. A period of retention will nonetheless be required, and this should extend until growth is complete following functional appliance therapy. Most patients, however, usually proceed directly to a second phase of fixed appliance therapy to detail the occlusion followed by retention.

Key point

After functional appliance therapy with or without subsequent fixed appliance therapy:

- Ensure the upper incisors are in soft tissue balance and controlled by the lower lip.
- Retain until growth is complete.

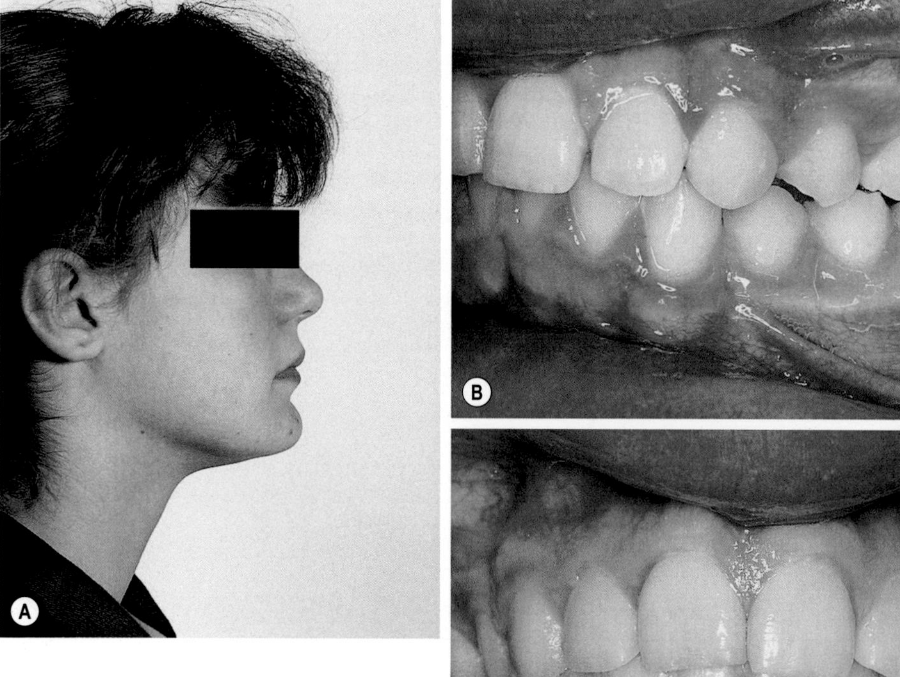

Fig. 9.5 **(A)** After functional appliance therapy: profile. **(B)** After functional appliance therapy: left buccal occlusion. **(C)** After functional appliance therapy: anterior occlusion.

The profile and occlusion following functional appliance therapy are shown in **Fig. 9.5**.

Primary resources and recommended reading

Baccetti T, Franchi L, McNamara JA Jr 2005 The cervical vertebral maturation (CVM) method for the assessment of optimal treatment timing in dentofacial orthopaedics. Semin Orthod 11:119–129.

Clark W 2010 Design and management of Twin Blocks: reflections after 30 years of clinical use. J Orthod 37:209–216.

DiBiase AT, Sandler PJ 2001 Malocclusion, orthodontics and bullying. Dent Update 28:464–466.

Fleming PS, Scott P, DiBiase AT 2007 How to … manage the transition from functional to fixed appliances. J Orthod 34:252–259.

Petti S 2015 Over two hundred million injuries to anterior teeth attributable to large overjet: a meta-analysis. Dent Traumatol 31:1–8.

Seehra J, Fleming PS, Newton T et al 2011 Bullying in orthodontic patients and its relationship to malocclusion, self-esteem and oral health-related quality of life. J Orthod 38:247–256.

Shah AA, Sandler J 2009 How to … take a wax bite for a Twin Block appliance. J Orthod 36:10–12.

Thiruvenkatachari B, Harrison JE, Worthington HV et al 2013 Orthodontic treatment for prominent upper front teeth (Class II malocclusion) in children. Cochrane Database of Syst Rev Issue 11. Art No: CD003452. DOI: 10.1002/14651858.CD003452.pub3.

Wolke D, Lereya ST 2015 Long-term effects of bullying. Arch Dis Child 100:879–885.

For revision, see Mind Map 9, page 229.

10

Incisor crossbite

SUMMARY

Matthew is 8 years old. He presents with an upper incisor in crossbite (*Fig. 10.1*). What is the cause, and how would you manage it?

History

Complaint

Matthew's mother is concerned that her son's upper front teeth are not straight and is anxious for treatment to be undertaken soon.

History of complaint

1⌋ erupted inside the lower teeth. There is no history of a fall or other trauma to the primary predecessor or to 1⌋. A⌋ was lost over a year ago, a little later than ⌊A.

Medical history

Matthew is in good health.

Dental history

D⌉ was extracted uneventfully under local anaesthesia 8 months ago.

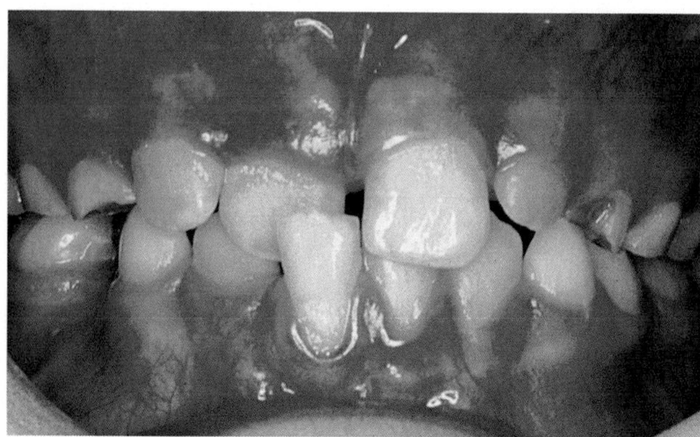

Fig. 10.1 Anterior occlusion at presentation.

Examination

Extraoral

The skeletal pattern is Class I with an average FMPA. There is no facial asymmetry. The lips are competent.

There are no abnormal temporomandibular joint signs or symptoms.

Intraoral

■ ***What features are visible on the intraoral views (*Figs. 10.1* and *10.2*)?***

Oral hygiene is fair. Marginal gingival erythema is evident related to the incisor teeth. There is marked attrition of C⌋⌊C, with carious involvement of ⌊C mesially and D⌋⌊D distally. With the exception of the lower right quadrant where D⌉ has been lost, 6EDC21 are present in each quadrant.

Gingival recession appears to be evident on the labial aspect of 1⌉. 1⌉ is displaced labially; the lower arch appears uncrowded. 2⌋⌊2 are rotated mesiolabially; 1⌋ is displaced

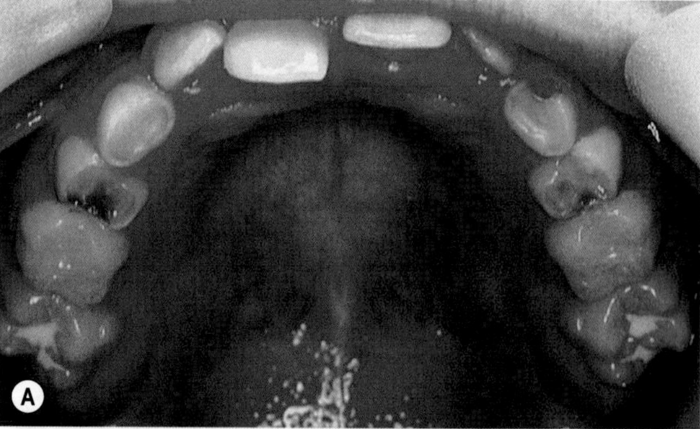

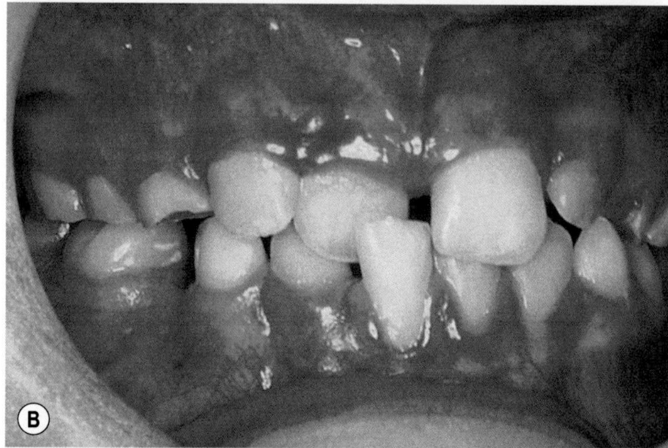

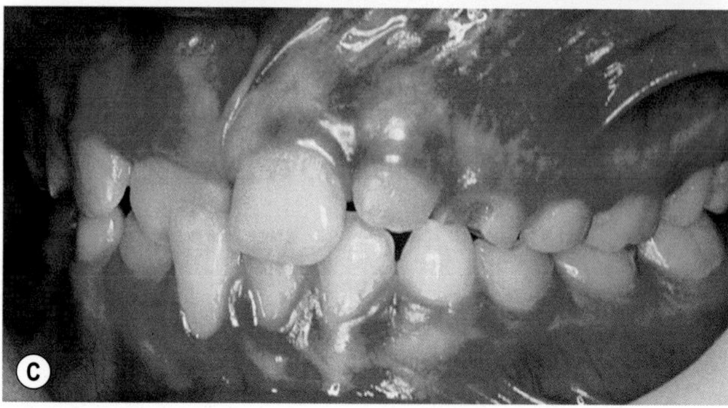

Fig. 10.2 **(A)** Upper occlusal view. **(B)** Right buccal occlusion. **(C)** Left buccal occlusion.

slightly palatally, and there is a small median diastema. Otherwise the upper arch appears uncrowded. The incisor relationship is Class I and 1⌋ is in crossbite; ⌊2 is partially erupted with the distoincisal aspect in crossbite with ⌈C.

What is the prevalence of anterior crossbite reported in the literature?

Depending on the racial group, age at assessment and if an edge-to-edge incisor relationship was included or not, the reported prevalence varies from 2.2–11.9%.

What specific features would you check? Explain why.

1. *The periodontal status of* 1⌉ – degree of mobility and pocket probing depth associated with 1⌉ should be assessed to determine its prognosis as it is being displaced labially by deflecting occlusal contact (see below) and gingival recession is present. 1⌉ exhibited grade 2 mobility, but probing pocket depth was less than 2 mm, indicating good periodontal prognosis in the event the crossbite relationship is corrected.
2. *Is it possible to achieve an edge-to-edge relationship on* 1|/1|? If so, this indicates that only a small amount of labial movement of 1⌋ is required to correct the crossbite relationship. An edge-to-edge relationship of 1|/1| was easily achievable.
3. *Is there a mandibular displacement on closure?* If the mandible is shifted anteriorly or laterally on closure from initial tooth contact, on 1|/1| or |2/|C into maximum interdigitation, early treatment to eliminate the displacement is indicated on dental health grounds. The rationale for this approach is that in susceptible individuals, mandibular displacement on closure due to premature tooth contact(s) may lead eventually to temporomandibular joint dysfunction syndrome. A 3 mm anterior mandibular displacement on closure was detected from initial contact on 1|/1|; there was no lateral mandibular displacement associated with the crossbite affecting |2/|C.
4. *The amount of overbite on 1⌋* – as the amount of overbite post-treatment is a major factor governing stability of incisor crossbite correction and as overbite reduces when the incisor edge is moved upwards and forward during incisor proclination, a deep overbite pre-treatment is a favourable feature. In this case, the overbite was 3.5 mm on 1⌋ and there is a good prospect of adequate overbite following crossbite correction.
5. *The inclination of 1⌋* – an upper incisor that is upright or retroclined (1⌋) is better for proclination than an incisor that is already labially inclined. Further proclination of the latter may not be possible or could result in unfavourable occlusal loading.
6. *The amount of space required to procline 1⌋* – space already exists in the upper incisor area, and there is no need for any extractions.

Key point

Where an incisor crossbite is present, check:

- Periodontal status of lower incisors.
- If an edge-to-edge incisor occlusion is achievable.
- If mandibular displacement is present.
- Amount of overbite.
- Incisor inclination.
- Amount of space required for correction.

Investigations

What special investigations would you request? Why?

As a dental panoramic tomogram taken 6 months prior to this visit by a previous general dental practitioner (see below) was available for inspection, a repeat film of this nature was not indicated on clinical grounds. From this radiograph it was possible to check the presence/absence of permanent teeth and whether there was a supernumerary tooth present in the upper midline. Should there have been any suspicion of the latter, a maxillary anterior occlusal view would be indicated to note the relation of the supernumerary tooth to the roots of the upper incisors. No supernumerary tooth was evident in the upper midline. A periapical radiograph of the lower central incisors is not required as the clinical examination does not lend significant cause for concern to the prognosis of these teeth.

Bitewing radiographs should be taken to diagnose accurately the extent of carious involvement of the primary molars.

The dental panoramic tomogram taken 6 months prior to this visit is shown in *Fig. 10.3*. **What does it show?**

Normal alveolar bone height, except for apparent angular bone defects related to the mesial aspects of 6⌉6. (Both teeth, however, were not mobile, and pocket depths were <2 mm on the mesial and distal aspects of 6⌉6.)

D⌉ absent; caries in D|CD / E|DE.

All permanent teeth (except 8's) present, of normal size and in normal developmental positions.

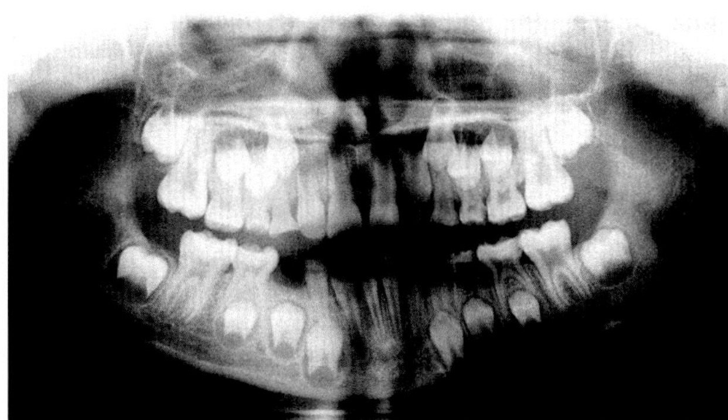

Fig. 10.3 Dental panoramic tomogram.

Diagnosis

■ ***What is your diagnosis?***

Matthew has a Class I malocclusion on a Class I skeletal base with average FMPA.

Mild marginal gingivitis related to the incisor teeth.

Gingival recession related to 1⌉ labially.

Caries in D|CD / E|DE.

Crossbite on 1⌋ with associated mandibular displacement.

Misalignment of upper and lower labial segments.

■ ***What is the IOTN DHC grade (see p. 264)? Explain why.***

4c – due to mandibular displacement >2 mm between the retruded contact position (RCP) and the intercuspal position (ICP).

■ ***What would you deem to be the prognosis for the labial recession related to 1⌉?***

For accurate assessment of the extent of the labial recession, the soft tissues should be healthy, and at present gingival inflammation is evident. There appears, however, to be some attached gingiva labially, and the recession does not extend to the sulcus reflection. It is also not associated with a frenal pull. At this stage, provided oral hygiene improves and the crossbite is corrected, the gingival recession should not worsen, although the width of attached gingiva will not increase.

■ ***Why is 1⌋ in crossbite?***

This is most likely due to a slightly palatal ectopic position of 1⌋ tooth bud.

Treatment

■ ***What treatment would you provide and why?***

1. *Oral hygiene instruction* – this is required to improve gingival health and to remove the plaque insult to the gingival recession related to 1⌉.
2. *Caries management* – a diet diary should be completed over 3 consecutive days (one of which should be a weekend day) and then appropriate dietary advice should be given based on the findings (see Chapter 22). Although several primary molars are carious, none have associated symptoms. Restorative management of carious primary teeth is dealt with in Chapters 22 and 24.
3. *Upper removable appliance therapy to procline 1⌋* – due to the mandibular displacement that is producing periodontal trauma to 1⌉, correction of the crossbite on 1⌋ is required urgently.
4. *Monitor the lower centerline* – consider removal of ⌈D if a centreline shift develops.

■ ***Describe the appliance design you would use to align 1⌋.***

The appliance would have the following design:

Activation: Z spring (0.5 mm stainless steel wire) to procline 1⌋.

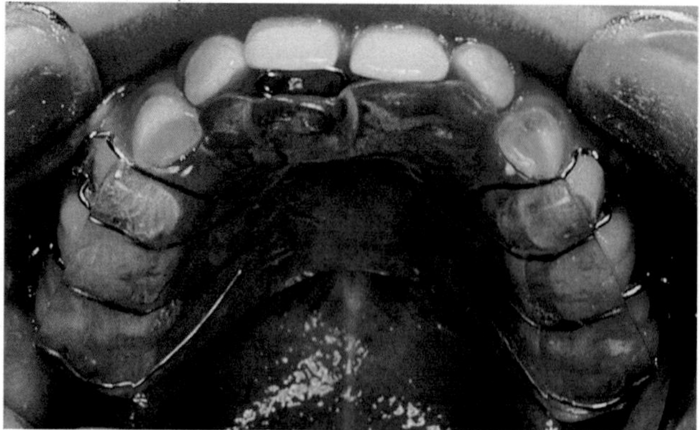

Fig. 10.4 Upper removable appliance to procline 1⌋.

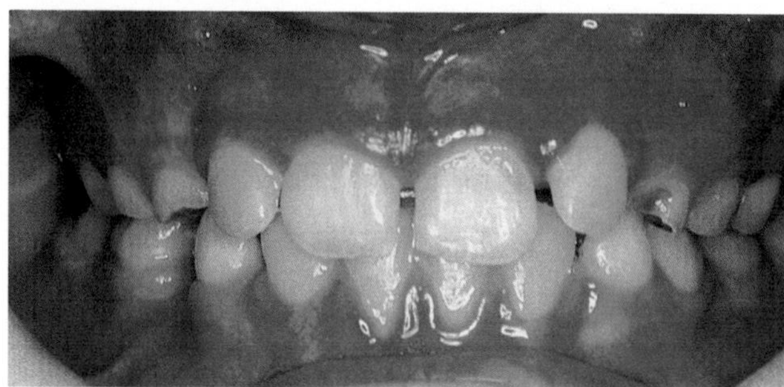

Fig. 10.5 Post-treatment.

Retention: Adams clasps 6D|D6 (clasps on 6|6 in 0.7 mm stainless steel wire; clasps on D|D in 0.6 mm wire).

Anchorage: from baseplate.

Baseplate: acrylic baseplate with full palatal coverage incorporating posterior capping (~2 mm in height).

The appliance is shown in **Fig. 10.4**.

■ ***What will determine stability of crossbite correction on 1⌋?***

Provided there is 2–3 mm of overbite on 1⌋ following proclination, the prospect of stability is good. Subsequent mandibular growth must also be favourable.

The occlusion following crossbite correction on 1⌋ is shown in **Fig. 10.5**.

> **Key point**
>
> Early treatment of an incisor crossbite is advisable if there is associated mandibular displacement and/or periodontal trauma.

■ ***What other treatment possibilities are there? What evidence is there in relation to their effectiveness?***

Other treatment options include fixed appliances incorporating the incisors and first permanent molars ('2 × 4'; although ⌊2 is only partly erupted presently and will need to have the bonded attachment repositioned as treatment progresses), use of an inclined composite slope bonded to the opposing lower incisor (at about a 45° incline and 3–4 mm in height), a combination of these techniques, elastics attached to bonded brackets/buttons or modified functional appliances. A systematic review published in 2011 indicated that the evidence level was low with regard to anterior crossbite correction, but evidence favoured the use of fixed appliances. A recent randomized controlled trial conducted in Sweden found minimal differences between fixed and removable appliances for anterior crossbite correction; treatment duration was slightly shorter (1.4 months) with a fixed appliance (brackets bonded to the maxillary incisors, primary canines, primary first molar or first premolar, if erupted) than with a removable appliance, but the latter treatment cost more. At 2-year follow-up, stability was similar in both groups.

Primary resources and recommended reading

Borrie F, Bearn D 2011 Early correction of anterior crossbites: a systematic review. J Orthod 38:175–184.

Gravely JF 1984 A study of the mandibular closure path in Angle Class III relationship. Br J Orthod 11:85–91.

Joss-Vassalli I, Grebenstein C, Topouzelis N et al 2010 Orthodontic therapy and gingival recession: a systematic review. Orthod Craniofac Res 13:127–141.

McComb JL 1994 Orthodontic treatment and isolated gingival recession: a review. Br J Orthod 21:151–159.

Wiedel A, Bondemark L 2014 Fixed versus removable orthodontic appliances to correct anterior crossbite in the mixed dentition – a randomized controlled trial. Eur J Orthod 37:123–127.

For revision, see Mind Map 10, page 230.

11

Reverse overjet

CASE 1

SUMMARY

Alistair, 8.5 years old, presents with a reverse overjet on all of the upper incisors (Fig. 11.1). What is the cause, and how may it be treated?

History

Complaint

Alistair is not bothered about the way his teeth bite together and is not concerned about any aspect of his facial appearance. His father, however, feels that Alistair's chin is somewhat prominent and gives the boy an aggressive-looking appearance. Sometimes Alistair is teased about his chin at school.

History of complaint

Alistair's permanent upper front teeth erupted behind his lower teeth. His mother's recollection is that the bite of his 'milk' teeth was similar. Alistair is not bothered by the occasional teasing he gets about his chin.

Alistair's parents are keen for treatment, if possible, at this stage to correct his bite and reduce the prominence of his chin, which would remove the source of teasing at school.

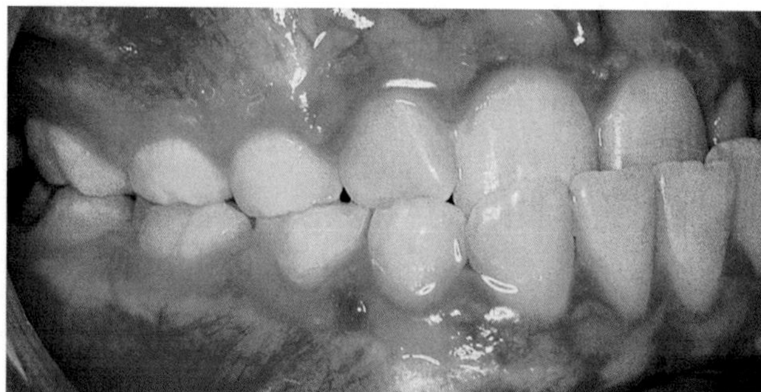

Fig. 11.1 Right buccal occlusion at presentation.

Medical history

Alistair is fit and well.

Family history

Alistair's father reports that his own teeth meet in a manner similar to his son's, and he also has a slightly prominent chin but is unconcerned by it. He had orthodontic treatment with extraction of two lower teeth and fixed appliances when he was a teenager to correct the bite of his front teeth. His bite changed a lot after he stopped wearing the retainers.

Examination

Extraoral

Alistair has a mild Class III skeletal pattern with average FMPA (**Fig. 11.2**) and no facial asymmetry.

■ ***What other features would you check for?***

- Presence/absence of a mandibular displacement on closure.
- Temporomandibular joint signs/symptoms.

Alistair could just achieve an edge-to-edge incisor relationship.

A 3 mm anterior mandibular displacement on 1|1 was detected from RCP to ICP. No temporomandibular joint signs were noted, and Alistair reported no temporomandibular joint symptoms. There was no masticatory muscle tenderness.

Intraoral

■ ***What are your observations from the intraoral views (Figs 11.1 and 11.3)?***

The soft tissues appear healthy with the exception of mild marginal gingival erythema related to the incisor teeth. Oral hygiene is fair. The dentition appears caries free. 6EDC21 are present in each quadrant.

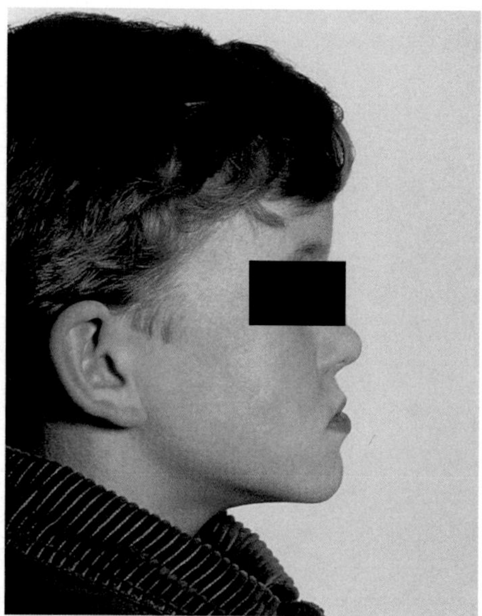

Fig. 11.2 Profile.

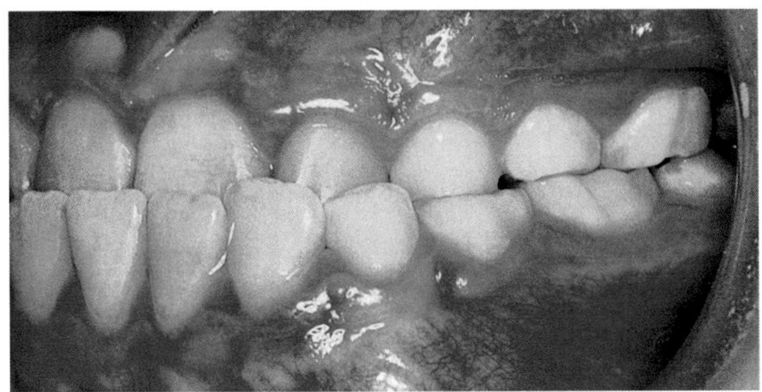

Fig. 11.3 Left buccal occlusion.

Table 11.1 Causes of reverse overjet

Cause	Aetiology
Skeletal	Usually Class III due to any of the following: long mandible; forward placement of glenoid fossa positioning the mandible more anteriorly; short and/or retrognathic maxilla; short anterior cranial base
Anterior mandibular displacement on closure	A premature contact may displace the mandible forward on closure into maximum interdigitation
Retained primary upper incisors	These may deflect the eruption path of their successors palatally into crossbite
Pattern/excessive mandibular growth	Forward pattern of mandibular growth will exacerbate a Class III skeletal pattern
	Excessive mandibular growth may be due to excess growth hormone resulting from a pituitary adenoma
Restraint of maxillary growth	Found in repaired cleft lip and palate and attributed to the effect of post-surgical scar tissue

Upper and lower incisors are very mildly crowded and in crossbite. The overbite is average to slightly increased and complete. Upper and lower centrelines are displaced. The buccal segment relationship is Class III bilaterally.

■ ***What are the possible causes of the reverse overjet?***

These are listed in **Table 11.1**.

■ ***What radiographic investigations would you request and why?***

A dental panoramic tomogram would be required to account for the presence and position of all the remaining permanent teeth.

A lateral cephalometric radiograph is indicated to assess more accurately the magnitude of the Class III skeletal pattern and the incisor inclinations, which will facilitate treatment planning. It will also form a baseline from which treatment progress/growth changes can be evaluated by comparison with future cephalometric films.

The panoramic radiograph showed all permanent teeth to be developing.

■ ***What is your interpretation of the following cephalometric findings?***

SNA = 80°; SNB = 82°; $\underline{1}$ to maxillary plane = 106°; $\overline{1}$ to mandibular plane = 97°; maxillary mandibular planes angle = 25°; facial proportion = 53%.

The skeletal pattern is Class III (SNA – SNB = ANB = –2°) due to mild maxillary retrognathism and mandibular prognathism. The upper incisors are slightly retroclined relative to the mean (109°) but are within the normal range. Taking account of the MMPA, the $\overline{1}$ angle should be 120° – 25° = 95° but is 2° proclined at 97°. The MMPA and facial proportions are slightly reduced from average values but are within the normal range.

Diagnosis

■ ***What is your orthodontic diagnosis?***

Alistair has a Class III malocclusion on a Class III skeletal pattern with slightly reduced facial proportions. There is an anterior mandibular displacement on closure on $\underline{1|1}$. Marginal gingivitis related to the upper and lower incisors. Upper and lower arches exhibit mild incisor crowding; the upper incisors are in crossbite. Upper and lower centrelines are slightly displaced. The buccal segment relationship is Class III bilaterally.

■ ***What is the IOTN (DHC) grade (see p. 264)? Explain why.***

4c – due to >2 mm mandibular displacement between the RCP and ICP.

■ ***What dental health reasons are there for orthodontic treatment?***

Mandibular displacement on closure may increase the likelihood of temporomandibular joint dysfunction in susceptible individuals. In addition, displacing occlusal contacts may lead to lower incisor mobility and contribute to gingival recession.

■ ***What factors would you assess in orthodontic treatment planning?***

These are given in **Table 11.2**.

Treatment

■ ***What orthodontic treatment would you undertake and why?***

In view of the already apparent Class III skeletal pattern, the ability of the patient to just achieve an edge-to-edge incisor relationship, the inherent tendency for downward and forward mandibular growth and the family history, a sensible option would be to accept the malocclusion for the present and reassess in the light of further mandibular growth. Alistair has not yet entered the pubertal growth spurt, which is likely to exacerbate the Class III malocclusion and chin prominence as mandibular growth proceeds. On average, mandibular growth continues until 19 years of age in boys, but it may progress for longer.

Key point

Class III malocclusion in the mixed dentition is likely to worsen with mandibular growth, especially in boys.

As the parents are keen for treatment if possible, to try to reduce any further teasing at school, another option to consider would be growth modification by functional appliance therapy (Fränkel III or FR III, where FR stands for

Table 11.2 Factors to assess in treatment planning

Factor	
Degree of anteroposterior and vertical skeletal discrepancy	Most important factor
	Reflected directly in facial and dental appearance; patient's perception of these will influence complexity of treatment undertaken
Potential direction and extent of future facial growth	Assess relevant family history, age and gender of the patient and vertical facial proportions
	Reverse overjet is likely to worsen with a forward growth rotation and horizontal pattern of mandibular growth, usually observed when the anterior facial height is reduced or average
	The converse is likely where there is an increased vertical facial height
Incisor inclinations	If dentoalveolar compensation is already marked, further orthodontic compensation is unlikely to be stable or to produce an aesthetic result
Amount of overbite	The deeper the overbite, the better the likelihood of stable correction of the reverse overjet
Ability to achieve edge-to-edge incisor contact	If this is not possible, correction of the incisor relationship by simple means is unlikely
Degree of upper and lower arch crowding	Delay upper arch extractions until the reverse overjet is corrected, as this may provide space for relief of mild/moderate crowding
	If extractions are undertaken in the upper arch only, the reverse overjet may worsen by the upper labial segment moving palatally
	If mid upper arch extractions are necessary, extraction of 4|4 is usually advisable to allow for correction of the incisor relationship

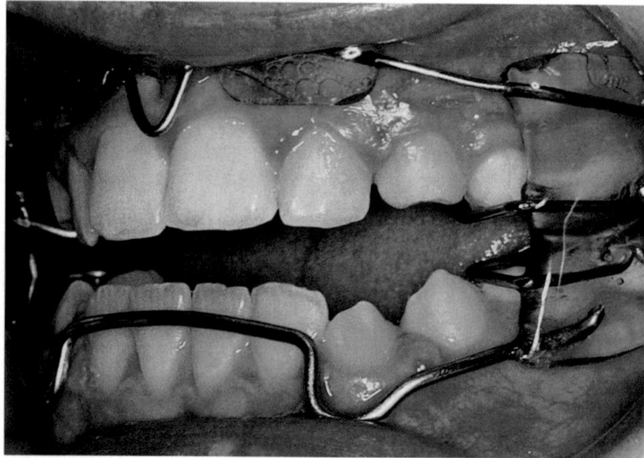

Fig. 11.4 Fränkel III appliance.

Function Regulator; **Fig. 11.4**) to correct the incisor relationship because:

- Skeletal pattern is mildly Class III.
- An anterior mandibular displacement exists on closure, i.e. Alistair can achieve edge-to-edge incisor contact.
- MMPA is slightly reduced.
- Upper incisors are not proclined.
- Lower incisors are very mildly proclined.
- Overbite is average to slightly increased.

It is essential, however, that Alistair and his parents are aware of the need for prolonged retention during continuing growth and of the need for reassessment in the light of ensuing growth. This form of treatment should only be undertaken by a specialist and only when Alistair's oral hygiene has improved.

■ *How would you take a wax registration for this appliance?*

The mandible is rotated downward and backward until the incisors are brought to an end-to-end relationship or better, with the bite open about 2 mm. Alistair may be instructed to place the tip of his tongue at the back of the hard palate and to maintain it there while closing slowly into a horseshoe of softened wax placed over the upper teeth until the desired position is reached. This wax registration should then be chilled in cold water and its accuracy re-checked in the mouth before forwarding to the laboratory with impressions of the dental arches to allow for appliance construction.

■ *How much should Alistair wear this appliance?*

He should build up wear over the first week so that it is worn for at least 14 hours out of 24. Encouragement should be given to increase wear to full-time with the exception of mealtimes and during sports, although this may prove difficult for some children. As its name implies, the Function Regulator was designed with the intention of altering function of the circumoral and masticatory musculature. For this reason, the patient should be instructed to 'exercise' these muscles by gently opening and closing into the appliance. Alistair should be given a time sheet to allow him to record the number of hours of wear per day. This should be inspected at each visit and used to encourage progress.

■ *What effects will this appliance have?*

The response is a downward and backward rotation of the mandible accompanied by an increase in facial height. Evidence suggests that mandibular growth may be constrained by the FR3 but it does not promote forward maxillary growth. The lower incisors are uprighted, and the upper incisors may be proclined slightly. The upper molars should erupt more than the lower ones.

> **Key point**
>
> The FR3 appliance for correction of Class III malocclusion:
>
> - May constrain mandibular growth.
> - Does not promote forward maxillary growth.
> - Produces mostly dentoalveolar changes.

■ *What other treatment options are there?*

An alternative approach to try to modify growth where mandibular excess exists is by chincup therapy. This requires specialist management. The line of force application should be oriented below the condyle to produce downward and backward rotation of the chin. As a result, lower anterior facial height is increased but chin prominence is reduced simultaneously. In essence, the appliance works in exactly the same way as functional appliances for mandibular prognathism. As a significant amount of force from the chincup is transferred to the base of the lower alveolar process, the lower incisors are also uprighted.

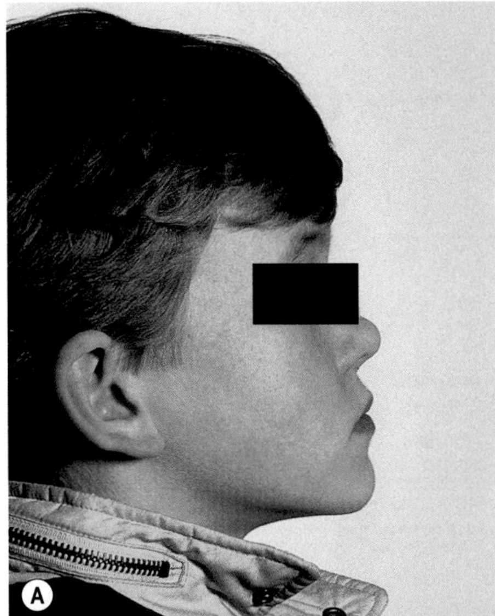

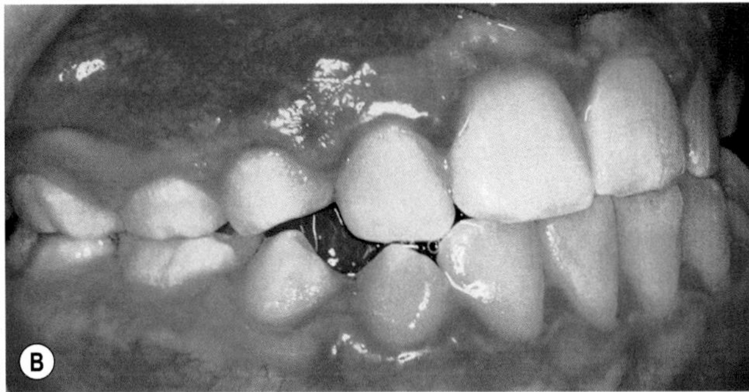

Fig. 11.5 **(A)** Post-treatment: profile view. **(B)** Post-treatment: occlusion.

If the patient is not keen to try growth modification or the parents express concern about the need for prolonged retention of the corrected incisor relationship, the malocclusion should be accepted for the present. Arrangements should be made to review occlusal development and to monitor facial growth. In Alistair's case it would be wise to review his occlusion in 18 months (at age 10) to check particularly on the position of the unerupted permanent maxillary canines and to measure the reverse overjet.

Once the permanent dentition is established, provided the reverse overjet has not worsened markedly and the chin prominence has not increased greatly, consideration could be given to removal of 4|4 only, in conjunction with upper and lower fixed appliance therapy to correct the incisor relationship. If the upper arch is crowded, 5|5 may be removed also, but it is wise to delay the decision regarding the need for any upper arch extractions until the reverse overjet has been corrected. It is important to assess the pattern of mandibular growth from an updated cephalometric radiograph prior to this treatment approach, and if there is any concern about it, treatment should be delayed until growth is almost complete.

If the reverse overjet increases considerably with further growth, a combined orthodontic and surgical approach may be required for correction, depending on the patient's concerns. This treatment would not be undertaken until mandibular growth is complete in the late teens.

Prognosis

■ ***What factors will influence stability of the corrected incisor relationship?***

The amount of overbite is important in the short term, but the pattern of facial growth, in particular the magnitude and direction of mandibular growth, will influence longer-term stability.

The profile and occlusion following crossbite correction are shown in **Fig. 11.5**.

CASE 2

SUMMARY

Daniel, a 9.1-year-old boy, presents with all of the upper incisors in crossbite. Daniel is unconcerned by this. He is in good health. His mother is keen for treatment to correct Daniel's bite.

History

History of complaint

All of the permanent upper front teeth erupted inside the lower teeth; the 'baby' teeth had the same bite.

Medical history

Daniel is in good health.

Dental history

He has not had any previous dental treatment.

Examination

Extraoral

Daniel has a Class III skeletal pattern with average FMPA and no facial asymmetry. The Class III pattern appears to be mostly maxillary rather than mandibular in origin, with midface flattening rather than a prominent chin. Lips are competent. There is no mandibular displacement on closure and no abnormal temporomandibular joint signs or symptoms.

■ ***What do you notice in** Fig. 11.6?*

Oral hygiene is poor with plaque deposits on most teeth and associated generalized mild marginal gingival erythema. The dentition appears caries-free. EDC21 are visible in each quadrant. (6's were erupted but not shown).

Upper and lower incisors are very mildly crowded and in crossbite as is the mesial aspect of C|. The overjet is reversed (measured 2 mm); the overbite is average to slightly reduced and appears complete on 2|. The buccal segment relationship is slightly Class III.

■ ***What radiographic investigations would you request and why?***

A dental panoramic tomogram should be requested to ascertain the presence and position of all the unerupted permanent teeth.

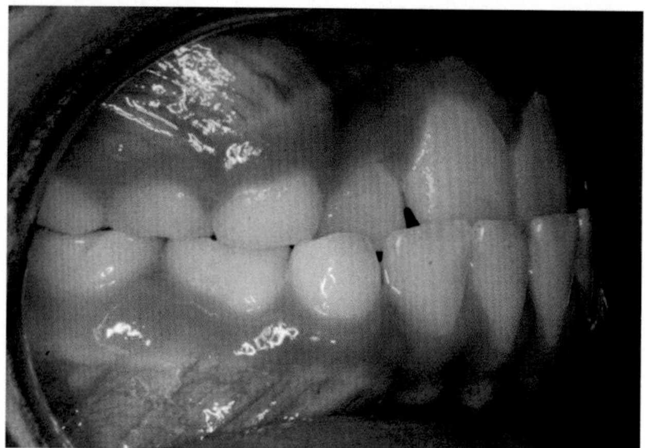

Fig. 11.6 Pre-treatment: right buccal occlusion.

This showed all permanent teeth to be present.

A lateral cephalometric film would also be required to inform the diagnosis more fully with regard to the skeletal components of the Class III skeletal pattern and the extent of any compensation exhibited by the incisor inclinations; both these factors will help treatment planning.

- ***As Daniel is of mixed-race origin, how valuable would cephalometric data be?***

The cephalometric findings should only be compared with appropriate racial norms. Daniel's mother was Caucasian, but his father was African. As there are no norms available for this racial mix to which comparison can be made, comparison to Caucasian norms is not appropriate. As clinical assessment takes precedence and is more valuable than any cephalometric analysis, treatment planning should be based on the clinical findings.

A cephalometric radiograph was taken to act as baseline from which to monitor mandibular growth.

- ***What is your interpretation of the following cephalometric findings?***

SNA = 78°; SNB = 79°; $\underline{1}$ to maxillary plane = 105°; $\overline{1}$ to mandibular plane = 89°; maxillary mandibular planes angle = 26°; facial proportion = 54%.

Interpretation can only be in the broadest sense due to Daniel's mixed racial background. With that in mind, the following should be interpreted with great caution. Based on the values given and considering Caucasian norms, the skeletal pattern is Class III (SNA – SNB = ANB = –1°) due to the slightly more maxillary retrognathism than mandibular prognathism. Relative to the mean value (109°), the upper incisors are slightly retroclined but are within the normal range. Taking into account the MMPA, the $\overline{1}$ angle should be 120° – 26° = 94° but is 5° retroclined at 89°. The MMPA and facial proportions are only slightly reduced from average values but are within the normal range.

Diagnosis

- ***What is your diagnosis?***

Daniel has a Class III malocclusion on a Class III skeletal base with average FMPA and no mandibular displacement.

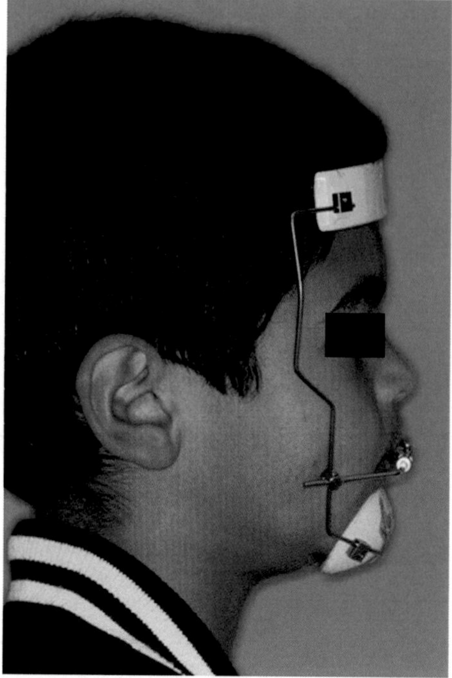

Fig. 11.7 Delaire-type facemask.

Mild marginal gingivitis. Upper and lower arches are mildly crowded, and the buccal segment relationship is slightly Class III.

Treatment

- ***What treatment would you consider? Explain why?***

Protraction (reverse-pull) headgear, otherwise known as facemask, treatment would be suitable. This treatment is most appropriate with mild to moderate Class III skeletal problems due to maxillary retrusion, in the early mixed dentition (and preferably no later than 10 years) as it attempts to stimulate growth at the maxillary sutures to bring the maxilla forward. Daniel satisfies all these criteria.

- ***What is the design of the protraction headgear appliance?***

Several designs are commercially available and are adjustable at the chair-side. All incorporate forehead and chin pads. The Delaire-type has two vertical rods located to the lateral aspects of the head which connect to the pads and allows adjustment vertically for optimal fit. **(Fig. 11.7)** If the plastic pads produce skin irritation, padding may need to be added or ventilation holes drilled in the chin pad.

The adjustable midline crossbow is connected via elastics to vestibular hooks (located in the region of $\underline{D|D}$) on a maxillary splint which is either cemented or bonded, usually to $\underline{6ED|DE6}$; the appliance may or may not incorporate an expansion screw (**Fig. 11.8**). Although it was formerly advised that rapid maxillary expansion be carried out simultaneously with facemask treatment, this has now been shown not to be necessary.

An alternative, rail-style design of facemask is more streamlined, easier to adjust and appears to be more comfortable for sleeping **(Fig. 11.9)**.

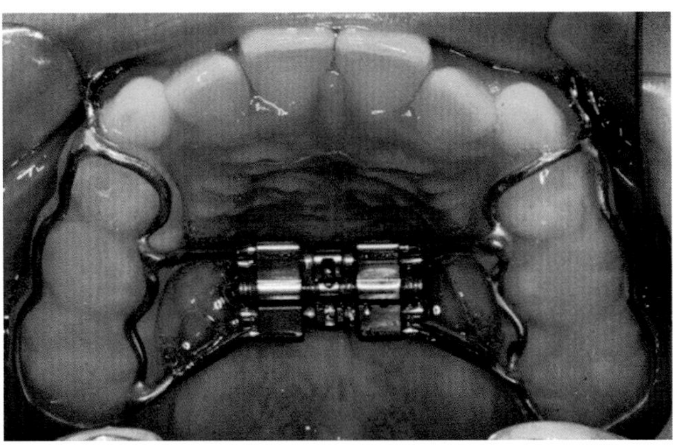

Fig. 11.8 RME appliance.

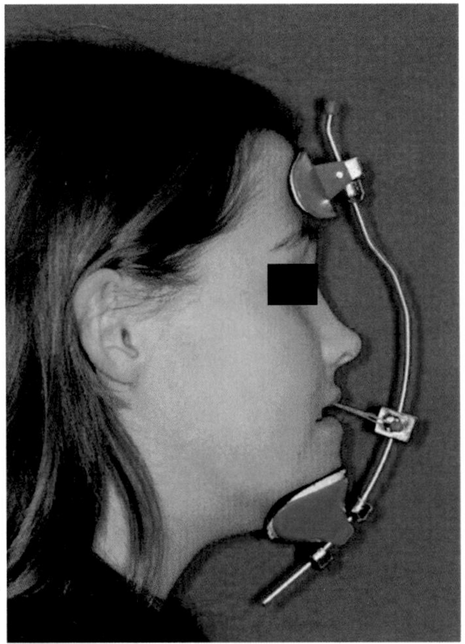

Fig. 11.9 Rail-style facemask.

Key point

Facemask (reverse pull headgear) treatment may be considered for:

- Mild to moderate Class III malocclusion due to maxillary retrusion.
- ≤10 years.

How does this work?

Forces of about 400 g per side are applied by elastics for 14 hours per day from the vestibular hooks on the bonded maxillary splint/expander to the crossbow of the facemask. These pull at 30° in a downward and forward direction to advance the maxilla.

What effects does it have?

Cephalometric findings indicate that, compared with an untreated control group, facemask treatment produces a small amount of maxillary protraction (mean SNA change 1.4°), slight backward movement of the mandible (mean SNB change 0.7°) with an overall mean skeletal change (ANB) of about 2°. The occlusal plane rotates upward and forward with a downward and backward rotation of the maxilla. Dentally, the overjet is increased and the lower incisors are retroclined by about 5°.

The facial and occlusal outcomes shown 7 months later and at 1-year follow-up are shown in **Figs 11.10** and **11.11**, respectively.

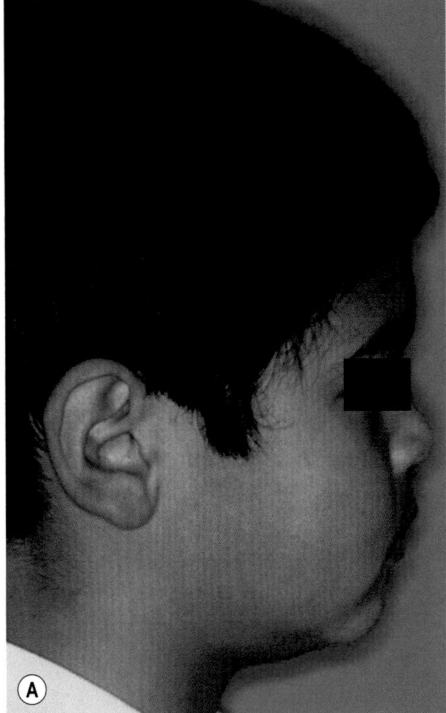

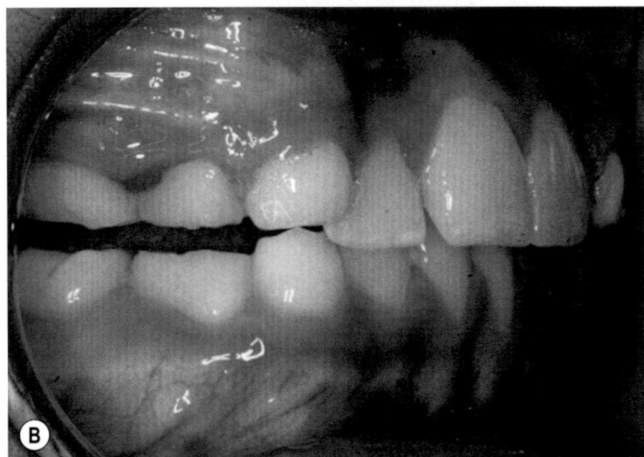

Fig. 11.10 Seven months later on removal of RME **(A)** profile and **(B)** right buccal occlusion.

Does treatment pose any risk to the jaw joints? Are there any psychological benefits?

In the one randomized controlled trial that recorded temporomandibular joint signs and symptoms with facemask treatment compared with an untreated control group, no adverse effects were reported at 15-month and 3-year follow-up. The same trial found no improvement in the child's self-esteem at either point in time. At 15-month review, a significant reduction was recorded in the impact of malocclusion scores relative to controls, which alludes to less unease about dental appearance, but this effect was not present at 3-year review.

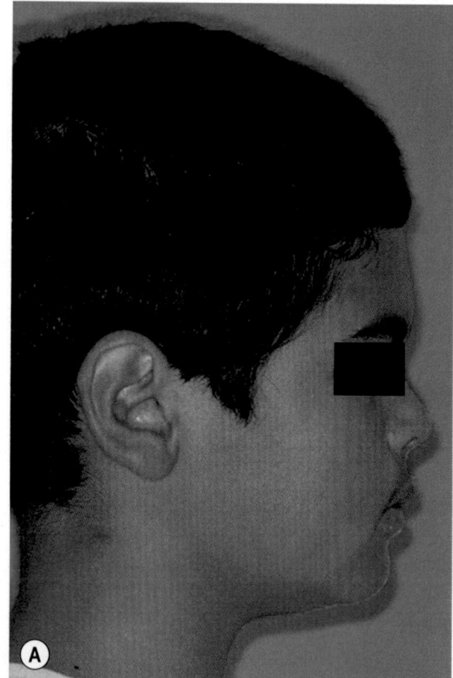

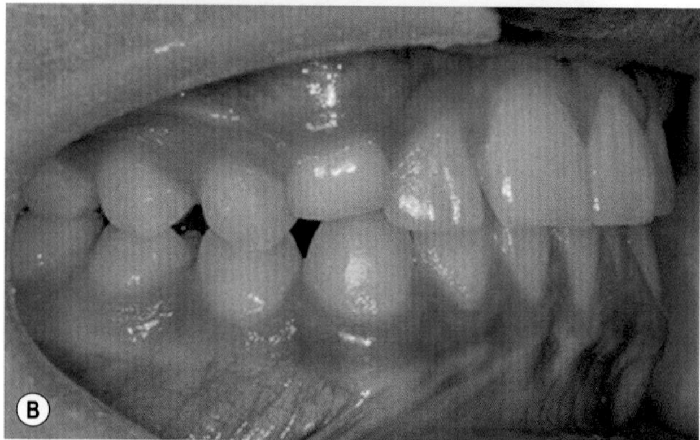

Fig. 11.11 At 1-year review: **(A)** profile and **(B)** right buccal occlusion.

How successful is facemask treatment for Class III malocclusion in the short term?

Facemask treatment appears to be 70% successful at 15-month and 3-year follow-up.

What is the long-term success rate of this treatment?

The longest follow-up to date has been for 6 years for patients treated in the trial mentioned above. Almost 70% of those treated by protraction facemask maintained a positive overjet. Panel consensus indicated that 36% of those treated by protraction facemask needed orthognathic surgery versus 66% of the control group. Patients in the control group were 3.5 times more likely to need surgery. Self-esteem, however, did not differ significantly between the groups.

> **Key point**
>
> Facemask treatment for Class III malocclusion in the early mixed dentition:
>
> - Is 70% successful at 3 year follow-up.
> - Has no adverse effect on the TMJs.
> - Reduces the need for orthognathic surgery.

Are there any alternatives to facemask treatment that may produce the same, or greater, outcome?

Greater maxillary protraction has been reported by the following means:

Application of the facemask to miniplates placed either posteriorly in the maxilla at the base of the zygomatic arch or anteriorly in the maxilla above the incisors.

Application of Class III intermaxillary elastic traction from miniplates located at the base of the zygomatic arch to screws positioned in the anterior mandible, usually mesial to the canines. This is known as bone anchored maxillary protraction (BAMP).

What are the advantages and disadvantages of BAMP?

The major advantages are that full-time elastic traction is possible with no need for an extraoral appliance. In addition, although more effective than treatment by conventional facemask therapy with more skeletal movement than from a facemask attached to miniplates in the anterior maxilla, both placement and removal of the miniplates requires a surgical procedure.

Primary resources and recommended reading

Battagel JM 1993 The aetiological factors in Class III malocclusion. Eur J Orthod 15:347–370.

Cevidanes L, Baccetti T, Franchi L et al 2010 Comparison of two protocols for rapid maxillary protraction: bone anchors versus face mask with rapid maxillary expansion. Angle Orthod 80:799–806.

Jamilian A, Cannavale R, Piancino MG et al 2016 Methodological quality and outcome of systematic reviews reporting on orthopaedic treatment for Class III malocclusion: Overview of systematic reviews. J Orthod 43:102–120.

Levin AS, McNamara JA Jr, Franchi L et al 2008 Short-term and long-term treatment outcomes with the FR-3 appliance of Frankel. Am J Orthod Dentofacial Orthop 134:513–524.

Mandall N, Cousley R, DiBiase A et al 2016 Early class III protraction facemask treatment reduces the need for orthognathic surgery: A multi-centre, two-arm parallel randomised, controlled trial. J Orthod 43:164–175.

Mandall NA, Cousley R, DiBiase A, et al 2012 Is early class III protraction facemask treatment effective? A multicentre, randomised, controlled trial: 3-year follow-up. J Orthod 39:176–185.

Watkinson S, Harrison JE, Furness S et al 2013 Orthodontic treatment for prominent lower front teeth (Class III malocclusion) in children. Cochrane Database of Syst Rev Issue 9. Art No: CD003451. DOI: 10.1002/14651858.CD003451.pub2.

Yang X, Li C, Bai D et al 2014 Treatment effectiveness of Fränkel function regulator on the Class III malocclusion: a systematic review and meta-analysis. Am J Orthod Dentofacial Orthop 146:143–154.

For Revision See Mind Map 11, page 231.

12

Increased overbite

CASE 1

SUMMARY

Harry, aged 10 years and 6 months, presents with crowded upper teeth and a deep traumatic overbite (*Fig. 12.1*). What has caused these problems, and how may they be treated?

History

Complaint

Harry does not like the appearance of his upper teeth and has recently complained about the gum behind his upper front teeth being sore. His mother is keen for treatment.

History of complaint

His primary teeth were mildly irregular. His permanent upper front teeth erupted in a 'crooked' position and have not changed since.

Medical history

Harry is fit and well.

Dental history

Harry is a regular attender at his general dental practitioner and has not required any dental treatment so far.

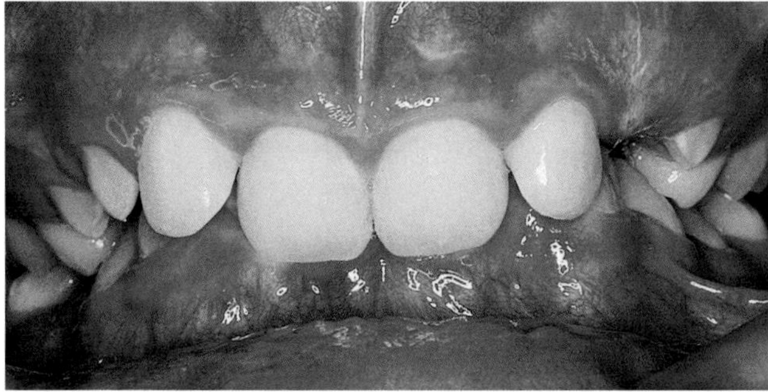

Fig. 12.1 Anterior occlusion at presentation.

Family history

Harry's father has the same arrangement of the upper anterior teeth as his son. He had four teeth removed and treatment with fixed appliances as a teenager. However, the treatment result relapsed and the upper front teeth have largely returned to their original positions. Harry's mother is keen that this does not happen to her son.

Examination

Extraoral

- ***Harry's profile view is shown in* Fig. 12.2*. What do you notice about the anteroposterior skeletal pattern and the lips?***

Harry has a Class II skeletal pattern with slightly reduced FMPA.

The lips are competent.

Intraoral

- ***The appearance of the mouth is shown in* Figs 12.1 *and* 12.3*. What do you see?***

Soft tissues appear healthy apart from mild gingival erythema related to the upper incisors.

The oral hygiene is fair with no visible carious lesions.

There are no restorations visible.

Harry is in the mixed dentition with the following teeth visible: $\frac{6E4321|124E6}{6E43|3456}$ ($\overline{21|12}$ are erupted but are covered by the upper incisors).

Mild upper labial segment crowding.

Class II division 2 malocclusion with deep complete overbite.

Buccal segment relationship is a half-unit Class II bilaterally.

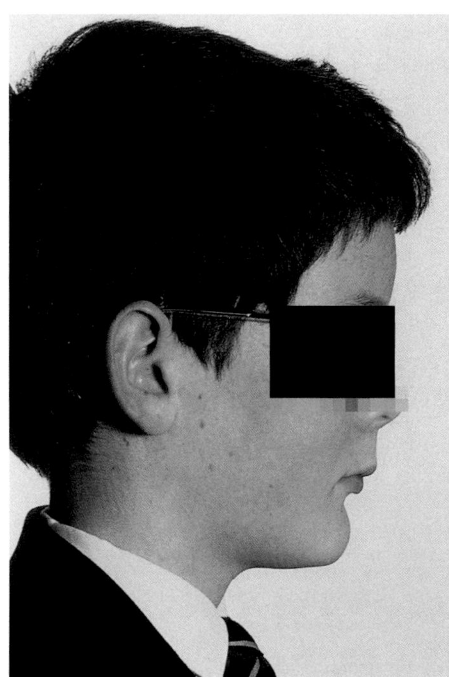

Fig. 12.2 Profile at presentation.

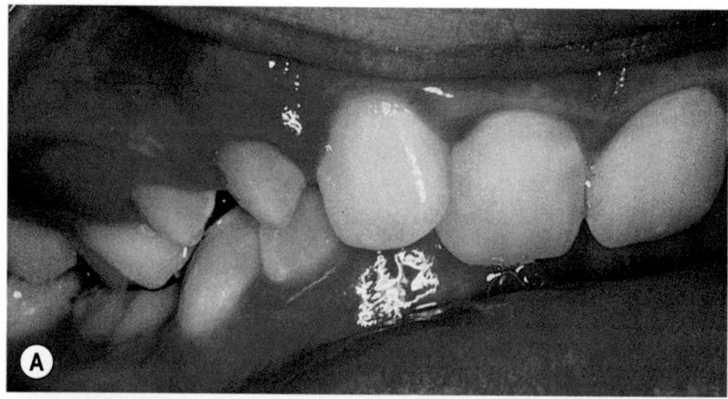

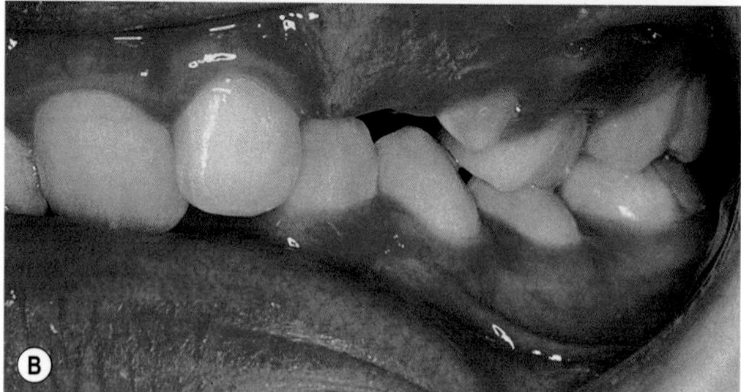

Fig. 12.3 **(A)** Right buccal occlusion. **(B)** Left buccal occlusion.

Table 12.1 Causes of increased and traumatic overbite in Class II division 2 malocclusion

Cause	Aetiology
Skeletal: anteroposterior and vertical	A Class II skeletal pattern in combination with a reduced lower facial height
Growth pattern	An anterior mandibular growth rotation tends to increase overbite
Soft tissues	Effects are via the skeletal pattern – reduced lower facial height leads to a high lower lip line that will retrocline the upper incisors, leading to overbite increase
	A hyperactive high lower lip, in association with a reduced lower facial height, leads to bimaxillary retroclination
Dental factors	Absence of a well-defined cingulum stop on the upper incisors leads to continued eruption of the lower incisors, increasing overbite

■ *What are the possible causes of the traumatic overbite?*

In a Class II division 2 malocclusion, several factors contribute to an increased overbite. These are listed in **Table 12.1**.

■ *What further investigations would you undertake?*

1. Assessment of the extent of soft tissue trauma palatal to the upper incisors and labial to the lower incisors from the increased overbite. Periodontal pocket depth should be recorded in these areas and any gingival recession should be noted. Incisor mobility should also be assessed. Although there was evidence of tooth impingement on the gingivae palatal to $\underline{1|1}$ and labial to $\overline{1|}$, periodontal probing depths did not exceed 2 mm and there was no gingival recession or incisor mobility.
2. Assessment of tooth surface wear on the upper and lower incisors – this may be on the labial aspect of the lower and/or the palatal aspect of the upper incisors as well as the incisal edges. Harry should be asked about any bruxing habit, and his mother should be asked if she is aware of him having any nocturnal bruxing habit. If wear of the incisors is observed, site and extent should be noted for future monitoring; as this is better undertaken from dental casts, impressions should be recorded of the dental arches to allow these to be constructed. There was no noticeable incisor wear, and no bruxing habit was reported.
3. Assessment of the amount of upper and lower arch crowding. Space may be obtained to relieve mild/moderate lower arch crowding and level an increased curve of Spee by some proclination of the lower labial segment and by a small amount of intercanine width expansion, which appear to be stable in this malocclusion. Therefore, in Class II division 2 malocclusion, lower arch extractions should generally only be undertaken if crowding is severe. In this case, lower arch extractions should be considered with great reservation, as this will allow the lower labial segment to drop lingually and aggravate an already traumatic overbite. There was 2 mm of lower labial segment crowding, and space analysis indicated sufficient space for the canines and premolars (21 mm present in each quadrant; 21 mm is required, on average, to accommodate $\overline{3}$, $\overline{4}$, $\overline{5}$).

> **Key point**
>
> **In Class II division 2 malocclusion:**
> - **Beware of lower arch extractions only, as a deep overbite may become traumatic.**
> - **Some proclination of $\overline{2\ 1|1\ 2}$ and mild lower intercanine expansion are often possible and stable.**

4. *Radiographic investigations.* The following views are required:
   - Dental panoramic tomogram, to account for the presence/absence, position and form of all unerupted teeth. This showed: normal alveolar bone height; a normal developing dentition with a full complement of teeth. No tooth appeared to be in an ectopic position or to be of abnormal size or shape.
   - A lateral cephalometric radiograph to assess the anteroposterior and vertical skeletal relationships and the inclination of the incisor teeth to their underlying dental bases.

■ *What is your interpretation of the following cephalometric findings (see p. 270)?*

SNA = 81°; SNB = 74°; ANB = 7°; MMPA = 22°; $\underline{1}$ to maxillary plane = 99°; $\overline{1}$ to mandibular plane = 88°; interincisal angle = 162°; facial proportion = 51%.

Relative to Caucasian norms, this indicates SNA is average; SNB is reduced; ANB is increased, indicating a Class II skeletal pattern; MMPA is reduced, which in conjunction with the Class II skeletal pattern is contributing to the increased overbite; $\underline{1}$ to maxillary plane is retroclined; $\overline{1}$ to mandibular plane is retroclined and not compensating completely for the reduced MMPA; the interincisal angle is increased; facial proportion is reduced.

Diagnosis

■ *What is your diagnosis?*

Class II division 2 malocclusion in the late mixed dentition on a Class II skeletal base with reduced FMPA.

Mild marginal gingivitis related to the upper incisors.

Traumatic overbite onto gingivae palatal to 1|1 and labial of 1|.

Mild upper and lower arch crowding.

Buccal segment relationship is half-unit Class II bilaterally.

■ *What is the IOTN (DHC) grade (see p. 264)? Explain why.*

4f – due to the traumatic overbite.

Treatment

■ *What are your aims of treatment?*

Aims of treatment are to:

Improve oral hygiene.

Relieve upper and lower arch crowding.

Reduce the overbite.

Correct the incisor relationship to Class I.

Correct the molar relationship to Class I.

Retain the corrected occlusion.

■ *How do you propose to achieve these aims?*

As Harry is growing and has Class II and deep bite skeletal problems, growth modification by a functional appliance would be the treatment of choice. A preliminary phase of upper removable appliance therapy will be required to align 1|1 by proclination and to expand the upper arch slightly, allowing the mandible to be postured forward with the arch widths coordinated for the construction bite for the functional appliance. Alternatively, a sectional fixed appliance may be used in conjunction with the upper removable appliance to align and procline 21|12 prior to functional appliance treatment. Following this, final detailing of the occlusion with full upper and lower fixed appliances is likely to be required prior to proceeding to retention.

■ *Describe the design of appliances you would use.*

The upper removable appliance to procline 1|1 would have the following design:

- *Activation:* Z springs to 1|1 (0.5 mm stainless steel wire). Midline expansion screw.
- *Retention:* Adams clasps 64|6 (0.7 mm stainless steel wire). |4 is insufficiently erupted at present to clasp.
- *Anchorage:* from baseplate.
- *Baseplate:* full palatal acrylic coverage with flat anterior biteplane, initially to half the height of 1|1. A measurement of the overjet plus 3 mm should be forwarded to the laboratory at the time of appliance construction to ensure adequate posterior extension of the biteplane.

As treatment progresses, addition of cold-cure acrylic to the flat anterior biteplane may be made at the chairside, until sufficient overbite reduction has been achieved. The upper incisor teeth should be overproclined slightly to allow for some retroclination under the influence of the functional appliance.

The patient should be instructed to turn the midline expansion screw one quarter turn per week. Arch coordination should be monitored at each recall by getting the patient to posture the mandible forward until the molars are in a Class I relationship and checking to ensure that the buccal segment teeth are not in crossbite. As the upper arch in Class II Division 2 malocclusion is usually square-shaped and the lower arch is 'u'-shaped, only a small amount of upper arch expansion is generally required to achieve coordination of the arch widths with the mandible postured forward.

An activator-type functional appliance is particularly useful in this type of malocclusion. A Herbst appliance is less recommended as it may tend to depress upper molars and inhibit correction of the deep bite problem. For this case, the construction bite for the activator appliance should be taken with the mandible postured forward edge-to-edge with the incisors 3–4 mm apart and the centrelines correct. If the centrelines had been discrepant by several millimetres initially, the bite should not compensate for this.

The design of a medium opening activator to be used here would be as follows:

- Adams clasps and occlusal rests to 6|6 (0.8 mm stainless steel wire).
- Labial bow 3| to |3 (0.8 mm stainless steel wire); palatal bow 2| to |2 (0.8 mm stainless steel wire).
- Acrylic palatal baseplate, deep acrylic capping of the lower incisors and canines with acrylic struts joining the upper to the lower part of the appliance. The acrylic should be heat-cured.

An alternative to using an upper removable appliance (with or without a sectional fixed appliance to 21|12) to procline and align the upper incisors, followed by an activator-type appliance, is to use a modified Twin-Block appliance to achieve the desired tooth movements. The design of this appliance incorporates Z springs to procline 1|1 and has no labial bow; it may also be used with or without a sectional fixed appliance to the upper incisors.

■ *What are the goals of the functional appliance treatment?*

To correct the skeletal Class II problem by differential growth of the jaws, in particular addressing the mandibular retrusion.

To increase the lower facial height and to correct the deep bite by preventing incisor eruption, controlling eruption of the upper posterior teeth while allowing eruption of the lower posterior teeth. This differential control of incisor/molar eruption aims to rotate the occlusal plane in a manner that allows Class II correction.

To convert the incisor and molar relationships to Class I.

Key point

Class II division 2 malocclusion in the mixed dentition may be amenable to functional appliance correction, taking advantage of facial growth to aid in overbite reduction.

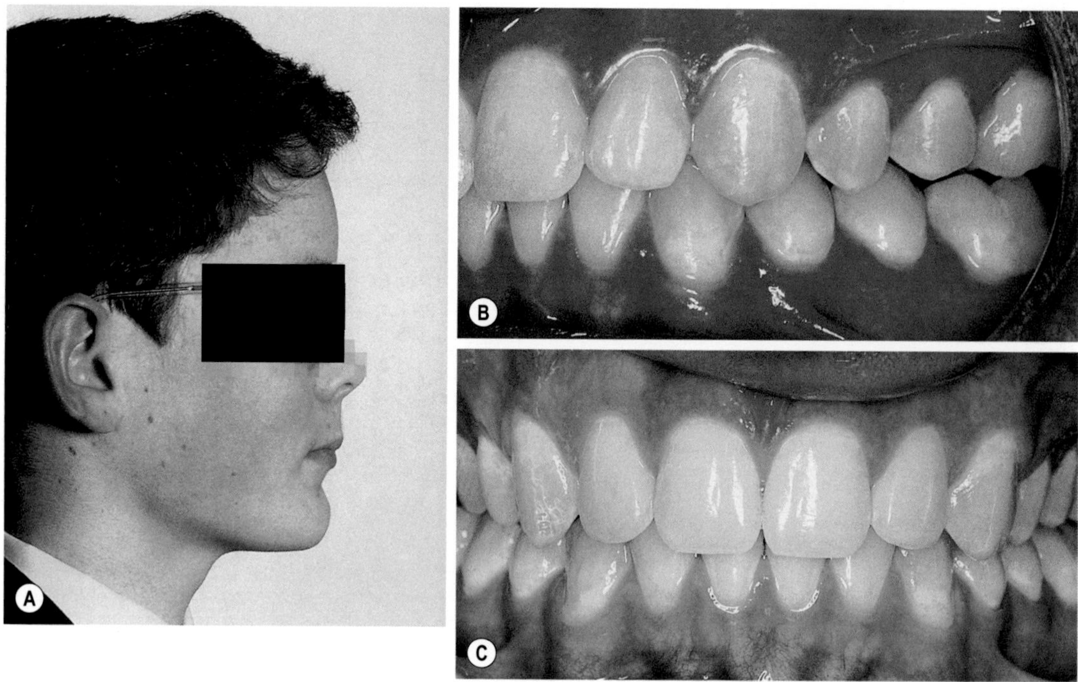

Fig. 12.4 **(A)** Post-treatment. Profile. **(B)** Post-treatment: left buccal occlusion. **(C)** Post-treatment: anterior occlusion.

■ ***Why may a later phase of fixed appliance therapy be required?***

Rotational correction, especially of 2|2, and detailing of the buccal segment occlusion require the use of fixed appliance therapy.

■ ***What aspects of the corrected occlusion are prone to relapse? How may you try to prevent/minimize relapse?***

Rotations of 2|2 – pericision (severing of the free gingival fibres) should be undertaken a few months prior to fixed appliance removal as it reduces the relapse tendency. A bonded retainer, however, will be required to maintain upper labial segment alignment in the long term.

Overbite – the tendency for anterior mandibular growth rotation to continue into late teens and beyond will encourage the overbite to increase. To combat this, a flat anterior biteplane should be incorporated on an upper Hawley retainer (designed to fit around the upper bonded retainer) to be worn at night until growth has reduced to adult levels.

Key point

The corrected aspects of Class II division 2 malocclusion most prone to relapse are:

- Rotational correction of 2|2.
- Overbite reduction.

The facial profile and the occlusion after functional appliance, followed by fixed appliance therapy, are shown in **Fig. 12.4**.

CASE 2

SUMMARY

Gillian is 14 years old and does not like the appearance of her teeth. She had |6 extracted 4 years ago due to caries. Both she and her mother would prefer to avoid any further extractions with orthodontic treatment if at all possible. What are the causes, and how may it be managed?

Examination

Extraoral

Gllian has a mild Class II skeletal pattern with slightly reduced FMPA and lower facial height. The lower lip lay at the middle to gingival third of the upper incisors. There was no facial asymmetry. There were no temporormandibular joint signs or symptoms.

■ ***What do you notice in*** *Fig. 12.5****?***

Fair oral hygiene with generalised mild marginal gingival erythema.

Apart from upper left quadrant where |6 has been extracted, 1234567 erupted in all quadrants.

6|, 6|6 and 5| restored; caries |4.

Severe lower arch crowding with |2 lingually displaced; 3| upright and |3 distally angulated; 2| mesiolingually rotated; moderate upper arch crowding with 3|3 buccally displaced; 3| upright and |3 distally angulated.

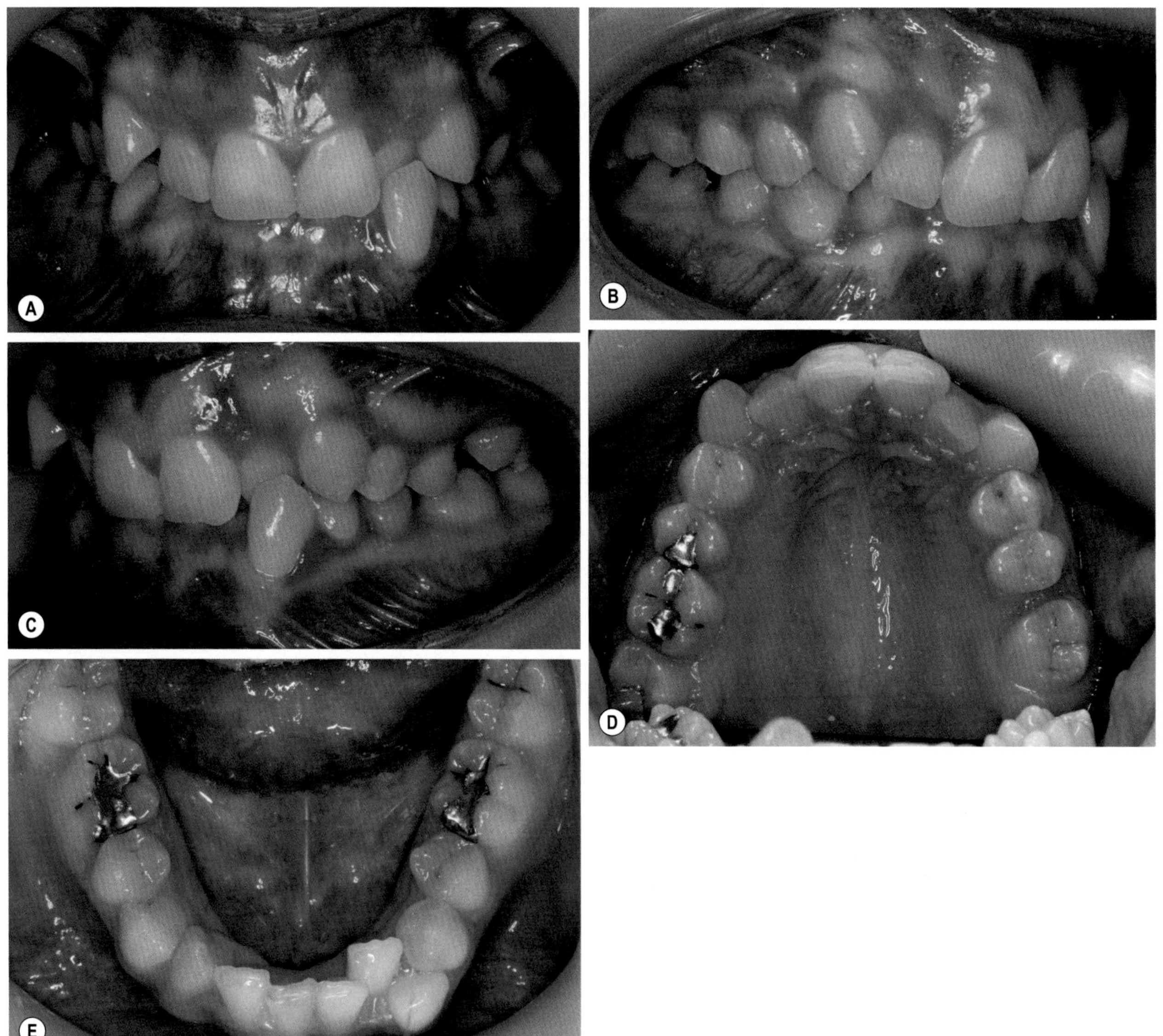

Fig. 12.5 Case 2 at presentation. **(A)** Anterior occlusion. **(B)** Right buccal occlusion. **(C)** Left buccal occlusion. **(D)** Upper occlusal view. **(E)** Lower occlusal view.

Class II division 2 incisor relationship; deep complete overbite; |2 in crossbite with ‾|3 (there was a 2.5 mm mandibular displacement between RCP and ICP).

Right molar and canine relationships, Class I; left canine relationship is Class III.

A lateral cephalometric radiograph was taken to assist with diagnosis and treatment planning.

■ ***What is your interpretation of the following cephalometric findings?***

SNA = 82°; SNB = 77°; MMPA = 23°; 1 to maxillary plane = 98°; 1 to mandibular plane = 88°; interincisal angle = 153°; facial proportion = 52%.

Relative to mean Caucasian values, SNA is slightly increased and SNB mildly reduced. The skeletal pattern (SNA-SNB) is mildly Class II (ANB 5°). The upper and lower incisors are retroclined; the lower incisor angle is not compensating for the reduced MMPA; with an MMPA of 23°, the lower incisor angle should be 97° (120° – 23°). The interincisal angle is increased, and facial proportion is slightly reduced.

Diagnosis

■ ***What is your diagnosis?***

Class II division 2 malocclusion on a mild Class II skeletal base with reduced FMPA and lower facial height.

Generalized mild marginal gingivitis.

Caries |4.

Severe lower and moderate upper arch crowding with a deep complete overbite.

Crossbite of |2 with anterior mandibular displacement on closing.

Buccal segment relationship is Class I on the right and Class III on the left.

■ ***What is the IOTN DHC grade (see Appendix A1)? Explain why.***

4c – due to the mandibular displacement.

■ ***What is the aetiology of the deep overbite?***

Several factors have contributed: mild Class II skeletal pattern, reduced MMPA and facial proportions, high lower lip line, retroclination of the upper and lower incisors producing a steep interincisal angle (**Table 12.1**).

■ ***What implications does the lower incisor inclination have on treatment planning?***

In view of the marked retroclination of the lower incisors, there is scope for these to be proclined. This will provide space for relief of the lower labial segment crowding and alignment of the lower arch; any decision regarding possible lower arch extractions should be delayed until this has been achieved.

■ ***If a non-extraction, approach is adopted for the lower arch, what impact has this for the upper arch?***

Either no further extractions are undertaken or extraction of upper first premolars is considered; in the latter case, the final molar occlusion would be a full unit Class II bilaterally. If only 4⌋ is removed, considering the previous loss of ⌊6, the molar relationship will be Class II on the right and Class I on the left.

Further upper arch extractions would be unwise as the upper incisors are already very retroclined.

■ ***What options are there to reduce the deep overbite?***

These are summarised in **Box 12.1**.

Incisor intrusion This requires fixed appliances. In reality, true incisor intrusion is difficult to achieve and 'relative' intrusion occurs. The incisors are held vertically as vertical facial growth occurs with some molar extrusion, as this occurs more readily than incisor intrusion. Placing a reverse curve of Spee in a lower rectangular archwire and/or an increased curve of Spee in an upper rectangular archwire will achieve 'relative' incisor intrusion (**Fig. 12.6A**).

Use of temporary anchorage devices (TADs) or augmenting molar anchorage, by typical addition of second molars (**Fig. 12.6B**) to the anchor unit, will increase the likelihood of incisor intrusion and limit molar extrusion. Attempts to achieve true incisor intrusion by the use of utility arches, which push the incisors against the molars, avoiding the buccal segment teeth, have achieved partial success as limited molar extrusion also takes place.

Molar eruption In a growing patient, freeing the posterior occlusion with a flat anterior bite plane on an upper removable appliance will allow the molar teeth to erupt, thereby reducing the overbite; this is accomplished by a simultaneous increase in lower facial height. The interincisal angle should also be reduced with firm incisor contact to maintain the outcome.

Molar extrusion Use of cervical headgear with a downward and backward pull will extrude the upper molars and increase lower facial height, an effect that is compensated for in a growing child. Similarly, use of mechanics listed above to attempt intrusion of incisors has in most cases the effect of also extruding the molars. Use of Class II or Class III intermaxillary elastics will extrude lower molars or upper molars, respectively, and assist with overbite reduction. Care must be taken, however, to prevent extrusion of the upper incisors with the elastics which will offset efforts to reduce the overbite.

Lower incisor proclination Moving the lower incisors labially will reduce a deep overbite but needs to be undertaken with caution as uncontrolled movement is likely to lead to relapse. In Class II division 2 malocclusion, where the lower incisors may be retroclined by the upper incisors, some lower incisor proclination may occur naturally by freeing the anterior occlusion. This may be achieved by moving the upper incisors forward, by disengaging the anterior teeth with a flat anterior bite plane on an upper removable appliance, or by placing bite turbos (see Fig. 6.9A).

Box 12.1 Options of overbite reduction

Incisor intrusion.

Molar eruption.

Molar extrusion.

Incisor proclination.

Key point

Overbite reduction by incisor intrusion is difficult to achieve.

Treatment

■ ***What are the aims of treatment?***

These are to:

- Improve oral hygiene.
- Restore ⌊4.
- Relieve upper and lower arch crowding.

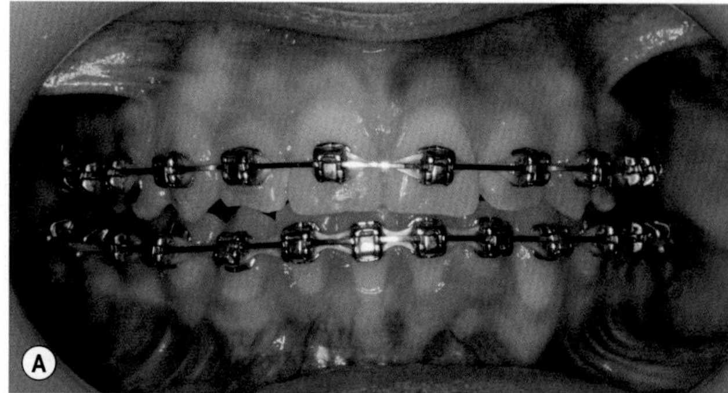

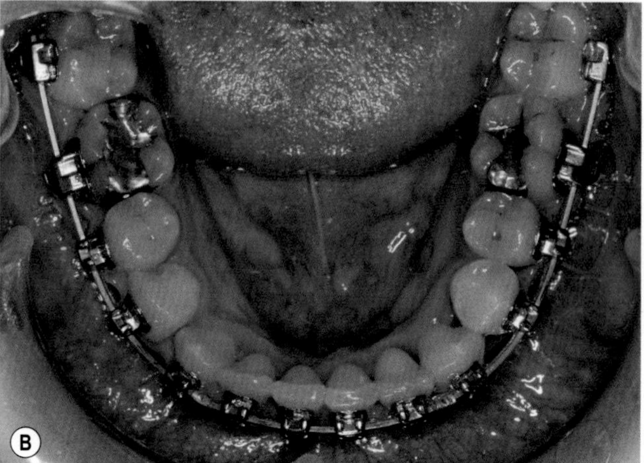

Fig. 12.6 (A) Mid-treatment: anterior occlusion. **(B)** Mid-treatment: lower occlusal view.

Reduce the overbite.

Correct the incisor relationship to Class I.

Maintain right molar relationship Class I; close ⌊6 space and establish Class I buccal segment relationship.

Retain the corrected occlusion.

How will these be achieved?

Gillian's oral hygiene and caries status will be reviewed following two visits to the dental hygienist and restoration of ⌊4. If oral hygiene is satisfactory, arrangements can be made for fixed appliance therapy to be commenced on a non-extraction basis. The upper fixed appliance can be placed initially to advance and procline the upper incisors to allow placement of the lower fixed appliance.

Why may a non-extraction approach be favoured in Class II division 2 malocclusion?

Although evidence is slim and of low quality, proposed benefits of a non-extraction approach include less or no risk of the overbite increasing, overbite reduction is favoured, there is unlikely to be any unfavourable retraction of the lips and, as there are no extraction spaces to close, treatment duration is unlikely to be protracted.

Gillian's final occlusion is shown in **Fig. 12.7A and B**.

What other non-extraction options are there for the upper arch in Class II division 2 malocclusion?

Aside from the options shown in Cases 1 and 2, other possibilities are distalization of the upper buccal segments by either:

- An upper removable appliance with 0.7 mm springs to banded $\underline{6}$'s supported by night-time (8–10 hours) headgear wear, otherwise known as a Ten Hove appliance (**Fig. 12.8**).
- TADs.

Another Class II division 2 case with increased overbite (**Figs 12.9–12.12**) is shown and was treated by using a Ten Hove appliance for distal movement of the upper buccal segments (**Fig. 12.10**), followed by fixed appliance therapy (**Figs 12.11** and **12.12**). See also Chapter 6 (Case 2).

What guidance does the best current evidence provide regarding management of Class II division 2 malocclusion?

A recent systematic review indicated that the evidence with regard to treatment and stability of this malocclusion is

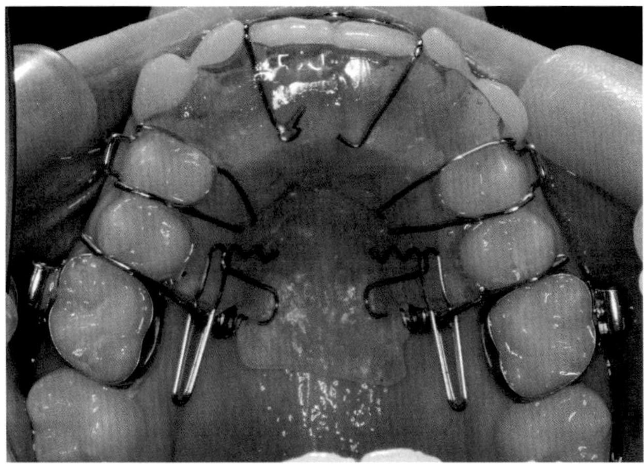

Fig. 12.8 Ten Hove appliance.

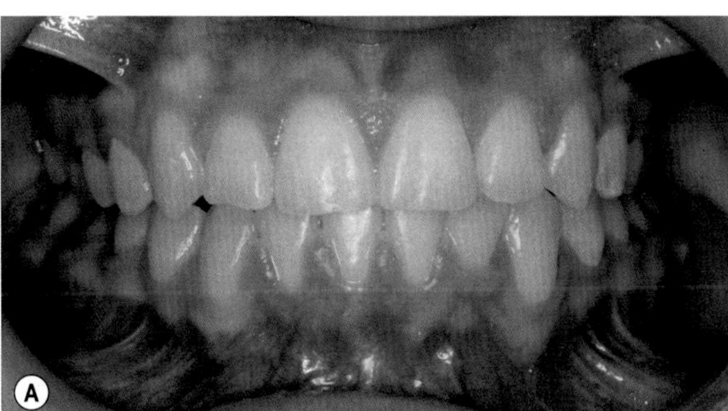

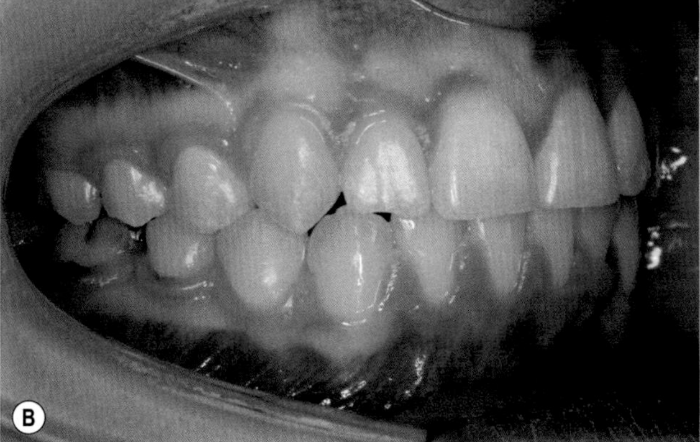

Fig. 12.7 **(A)** Post-treatment: anterior occlusion. **(B)** Post-treatment: left buccal occlusion.

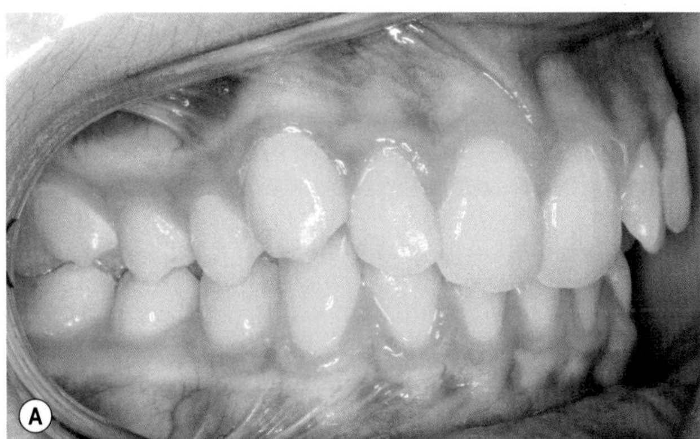

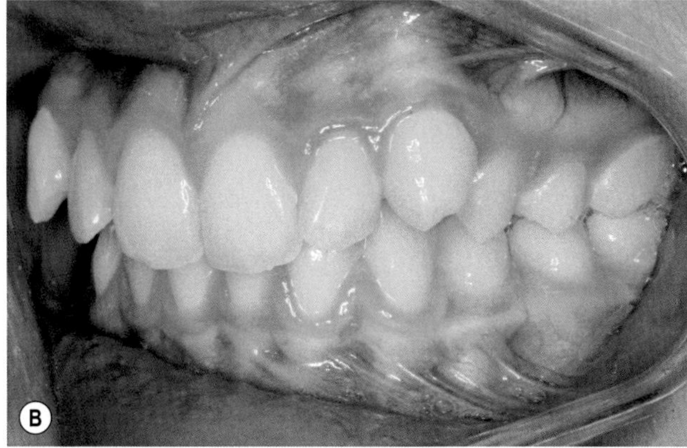

Fig. 12.9 **(A)** Pre-treatment: right buccal occlusion. **(B)** Pre-treatment: left buccal occlusion

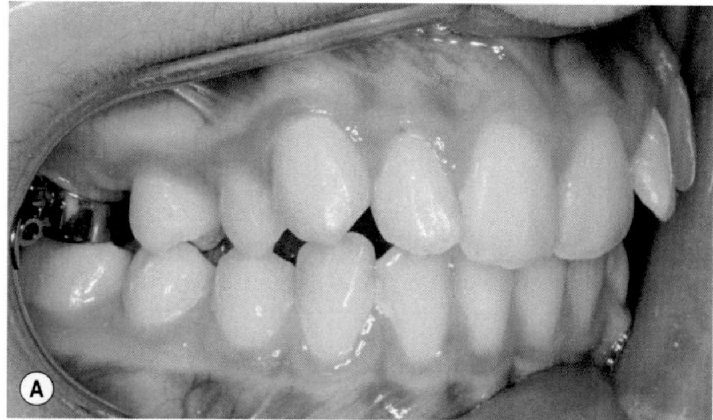

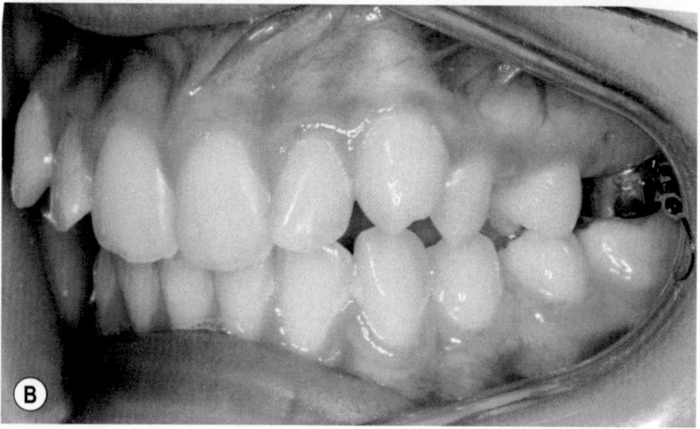

Fig. 12.10 Following retraction of 6's: **(A)** right buccal occlusion; **(B)** left buccal occlusion.

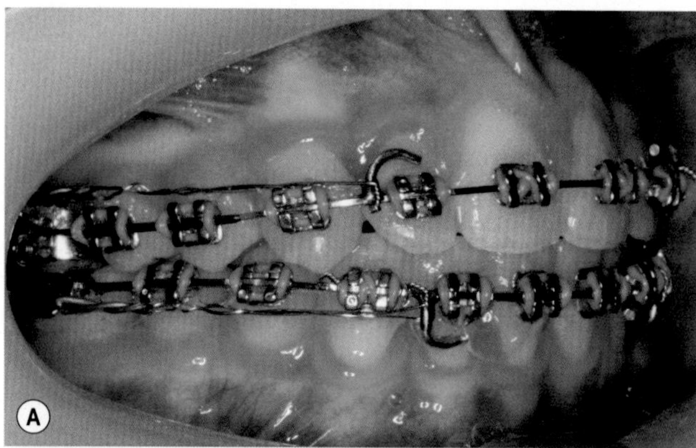

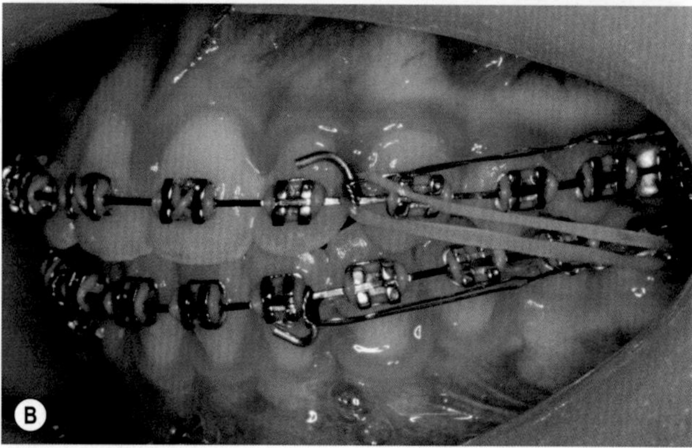

Fig. 12.11 Mid-treatment with fixed appliances. **(A)** Right buccal occlusion; note active "Berman" ligatures in place for space closure. **(B)** Left buccal occlusion with Class II elastic.

limited and highly biased. The best guidelines that were forthcoming from this review were to:

- Treat in a timely manner to maximize growth potential.
- Treat preferably non-extraction.
- Reduce the overbite and correct the interincisal angle.

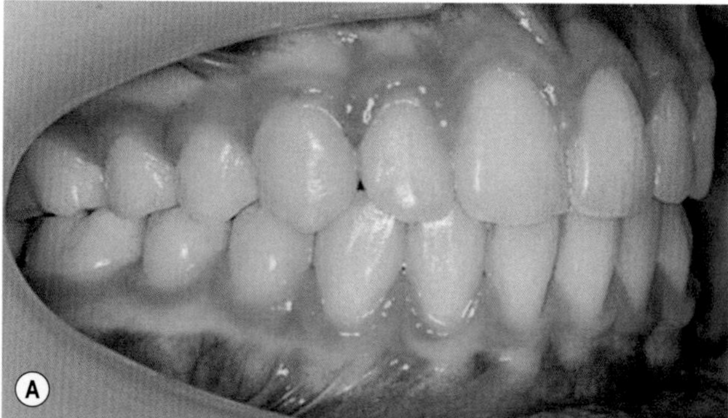

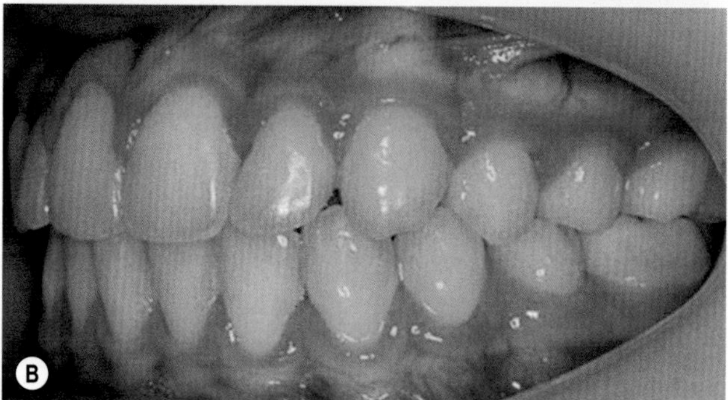

Fig. 12.12 **(A)** Post-treatment: right buccal occlusion. **(B)** Post-treatment: left buccal occlusion.

- Retain long-term with a bonded retainer with or without an upper removable appliance with flat anterior biteplane.

Key point

A non-extraction approach is favoured in management of Class II division 2 malocclusion.

Primary resources and recommended reading

Dyer FM, McKeown HF, Sandler PJ 2001 The modified twin block appliance in the treatment of Class II division 2 malocclusions. J Orthod 28:271–280.

Gianelly AA 1998 A strategy for non-extraction Class II treatment. Semin Orthod 4:26–32.

Kim TW, Little RM 1999 Postretention assessment of deep overbite correction in Class II division 2 malocclusion. Angle Orthod 69:175–186.

Lapatki BG, Mager AS, Schulte-Moenting J et al 2002 The importance of the level of the lip line and resting lip pressure in Class II division 2 malocclusion. J Dent Res 81:323–328.

Millett DT, Cunningham SJ, O'Brien KD et al 2012 Treatment and stability of Class II division 2 malocclusion in children and adolescents: a systematic review. Am J Orthod Dentofacial Orthop 142:159–169.e9.

Ng L, Major PW, Heo G et al 2005 True incisor intrusion achieved during orthodontic treatment: a systematic review and meta-analysis. Am J Orthod Dentofacial Orthop 128:212–219.

Selwyn-Barnett BJ 1996 Class II/Division 2 malocclusion: a method of planning and treatment. Br J Orthod 23:29–36.

For revision, see Mind Map 12, page 232.

13

Anterior open bite

SUMMARY

Gerald is 11 years old. He presents with no contact of his incisor teeth (*Fig. 13.1*). Identify the cause(s) and discuss the treatment options.

History

Complaint

Gerald complains that his front teeth do not meet. This embarrasses him when eating as he cannot bite into food. His parents are also concerned by this and by lisping during speech, which they attribute to the position of his front teeth. They are anxious for treatment.

History of complaint

Gerald's parents report that his primary incisors did not meet either, but the space between the upper and lower permanent incisors appears to have increased in the past year. His lisp has also become more noticeable. He has no history of thumb or digit sucking.

Medical history

Gerald is fit and well.

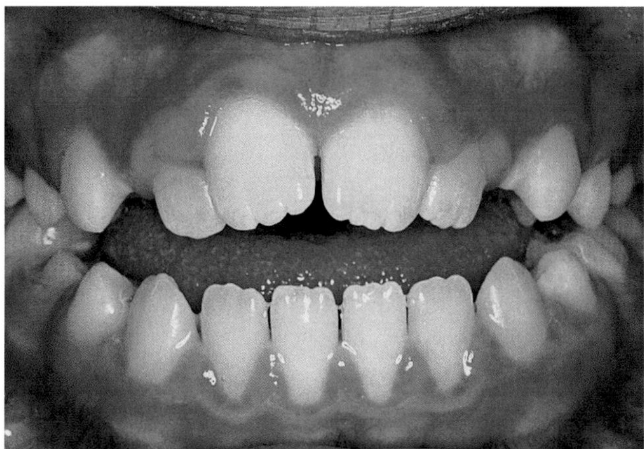

Fig. 13.1 Anterior occlusion at presentation.

Dental history

Gerald is a regular attender at his general dental practitioner and has cooperated well with previous dental treatment.

Examination

Extraoral

■ ***Gerald's facial profile is shown in* Fig. 13.2*. What do you notice?***

Gerald has a mild Class II skeletal pattern with increased FMPA and increased lower anterior facial height. The lips are competent.

There was no facial asymmetry. Mouth opening was within normal dimensions, and there was no temporomandibular joint tenderness or crepitus. No masticatory muscle tenderness was noted.

■ ***What other features should you assess? Explain why.***

1. *The swallowing pattern.* Where there is a space between the upper and lower anterior teeth, swallowing is likely to be achieved by forward positioning of the tongue between the anterior teeth to achieve an oral seal. This is particularly so where the vertical facial proportions are increased as the likelihood of lip incompetence is greater. Although such behaviour of the tongue is in most cases adaptive, in rare instances an endogenous (primary) tongue thrust exists. It has been suggested that this is associated with lisping and some proclination of the upper and lower incisors. Any attempt in these cases to close the open bite is doomed to fail as the tongue will return the incisors to their original positions.
2. *Speech.* By asking Gerald to count from 60 to 70 aloud or to say 'Mississippi', the degree of sibilance (lisping) can be detected. The tongue position during speech should also be observed.

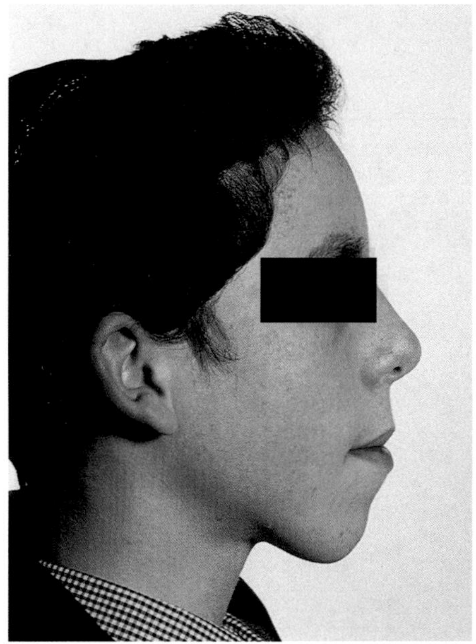

Fig. 13.2 Profile.

Gerald had a tongue to lower lip swallowing pattern, and the lisp was deemed to be mild.

■ ***What occlusal anomalies are associated with speech problems? Are the latter likely to resolve if any underlying malocclusion is treated?***

Although speech problems are associated with incisor spacing, Class II division 1 malocclusion, Class III malocclusion and anterior open bite, they do not occur in all individuals with these occlusal anomalies. Furthermore, correction of these occlusal problems is no guarantee that the associated speech problem will resolve satisfactorily. Where sibilance is judged to be marked, referral to a speech therapist would be prudent, although treatment may do little to improve matters.

Intraoral

■ ***What other features do you see (Figs 13.1 and 13.3)?***

Mild marginal gingival erythema related especially to the incisors and 4|.

No caries is visible.

Mild spacing of the upper and lower labial segments; mesiolabial rotations of 1|1.

Class I incisor relationship.

Anterior open bite (measured clinically = 6 mm from the mesioincisal aspects of |1 over |1.

Class III molar relationship bilaterally.

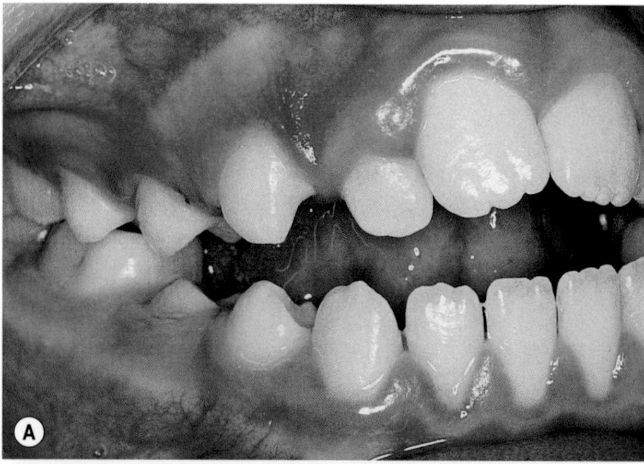

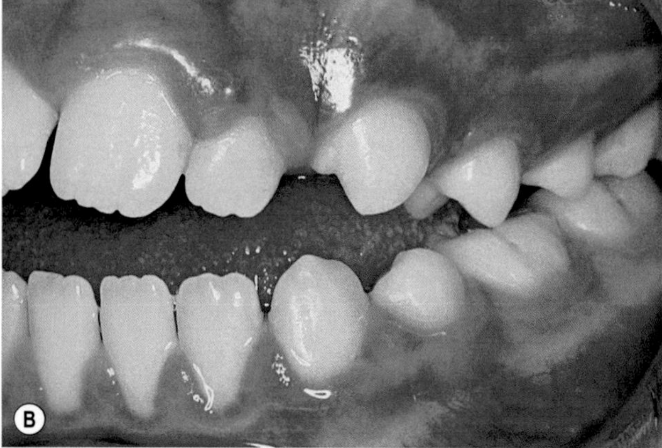

Fig. 13.3 (A) Right buccal occlusion. **(B)** Left buccal occlusion.

■ ***What are the possible causes of an anterior open bite?***

These are given in **Table 13.1**.

Key point

A persistent digit-sucking habit often produces an asymmetrical anterior open bite.

Table 13.1 Causes of anterior open bite

Cause	Aetiology
Skeletal	Increase in lower anterior facial height such that the compensatory ability of the incisors to erupt into contact is exceeded. This may be worsened by a downward and backward pattern of facial growth
Soft tissues	Rarely endogenous tongue thrust (Fig. 13.4)
Habits	Non-nutritive sucking habit (NNSH) – pacifier (dummy; Fig. 13.5), blankets, digit (Fig. 13.6) or thumb Persistent digit-sucking habit, which often leads to an asymmetrical anterior open bite (Fig. 13.7)
Localized failure of alveolar development	Occurs in cleft lip and palate, although in other cases there may be no known cause

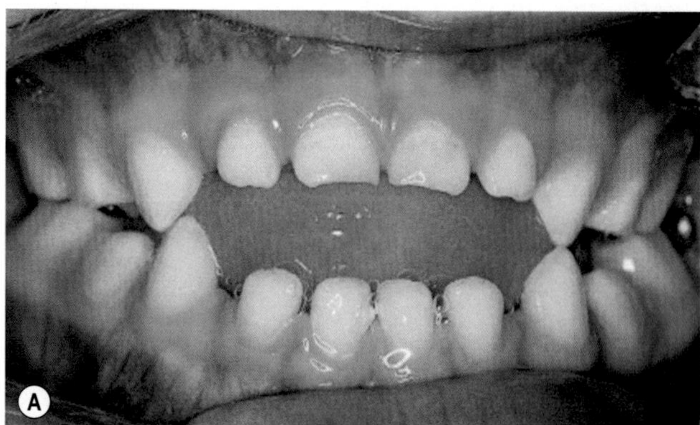

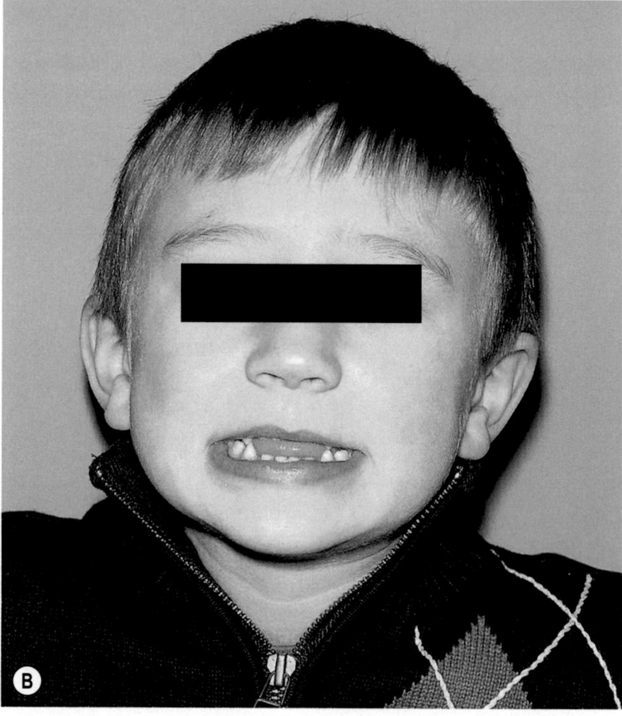

Fig. 13.4 Five-year-old boy with no history of a non-nutritive sucking habit: **(A)** anterior open bite in the primary dentition. **(B)** Suspected to be due to an endogeneous tongue thrust.

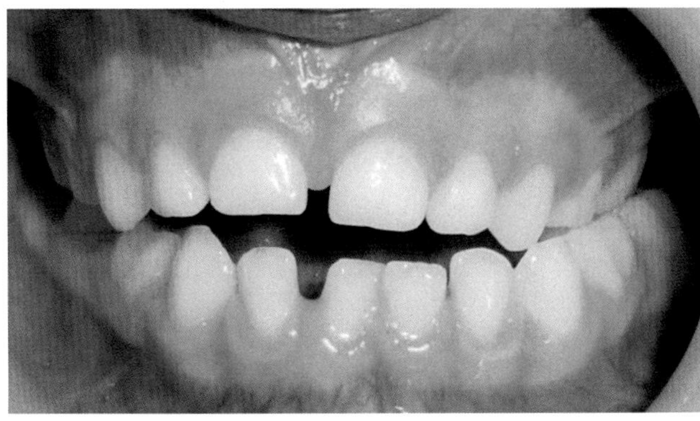

Fig. 13.5 Anterior open bite in a 3-year-old due to dummy sucking (note the buccal crossbite of $\lfloor C$ and left buccal segment).

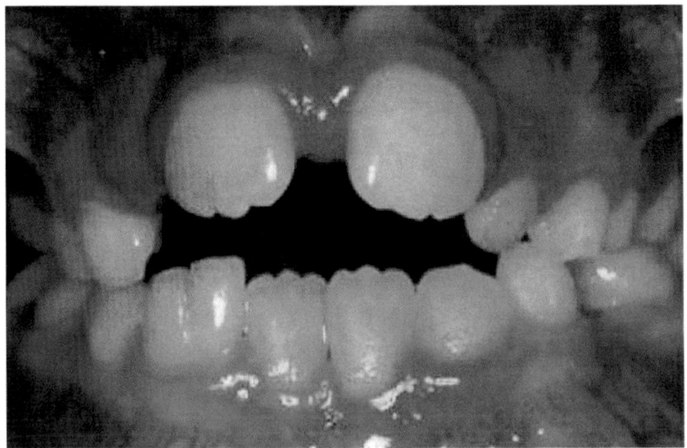

Fig. 13.6 Anterior open bite due to sucking of two digits (second and third fingers); note abnormal shape of $\overline{2\rfloor}$.

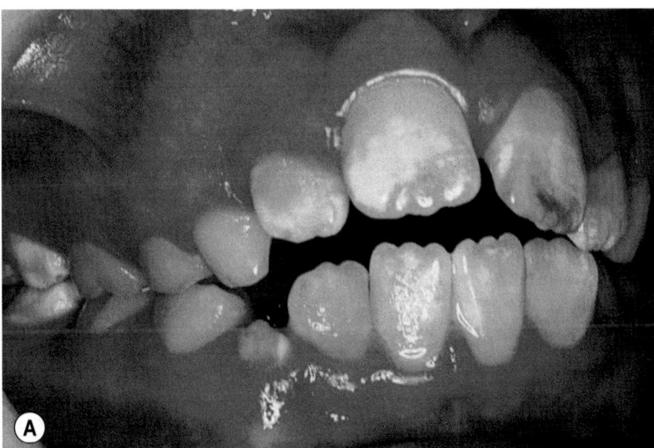

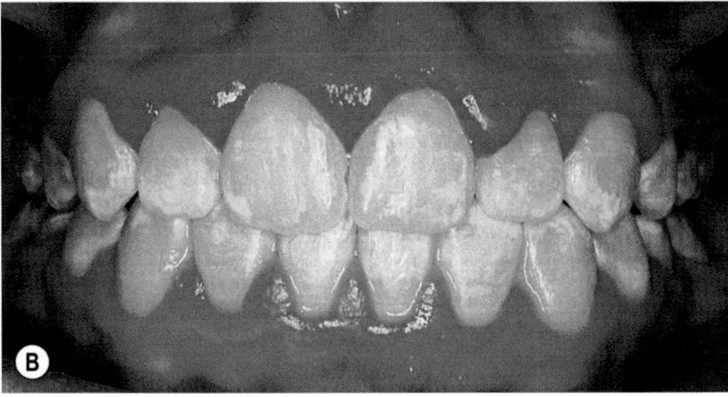

Fig. 13.7 (A) Anterior open bite due to thumb sucking. **(B)** Following cessation of the habit and fixed appliance therapy. Note that acid pumice microabrasion was used to improve the appearance of $\underline{1|1}$ (see Chapter 36).

■ ***How common are non-nutritive sucking habits (NNSHs) in children?***

The reported incidence varies depending on the age and region assessed, but NNSHs are very common in early childhood. An incidence of about 80% has been reported in the 5 months after birth in a Swedish study and of around 70% in 2–5-year-old North American children. The incidence, however, reduces with age. Almost 50% of 4-year-olds still suck a digit or pacifier, reducing to 12% past the age of 7 and to almost 2% by 12 years.

■ ***Do NNSHs always produce a malocclusion?***

Where there is a history of a NNSH, there is a greater likelihood of developing a malocclusion than without. The longer the habit continues, the greater its impact on the developing malocclusion, but it is important to realize that the effect is additive to any underlying primary skeletal cause and does not lead predictably to a malocclusion.

■ ***What are the effects of protracted pacifier use or a persistent digit-sucking habit on the occlusion other than creating an anterior open bite?***

Application of pressure from an object such as a pacifier or digit disrupts normal eruption. Development of a posterior crossbite is associated with protracted pacifier use. Persistent digit sucking may result in retroclination of the lower incisors, proclination of the upper incisors, increased overjet and a unilateral buccal segment crossbite with associated mandibular displacement (see Chapter 14).

Key point

Non-nutritive sucking habits:

- Are common in early childhood.
- Reduce with age.
- Do no predictably lead to malocclusion.

Investigations

■ ***What special investigations would you require? Explain why.***

A dental panoramic tomogram is required to indicate what other teeth have yet to erupt and to check their developmental position and form.

A lateral cephalometric radiograph is required to assess more fully the extent of the anteroposterior and vertical skeletal discrepancies, as well as the relationship of the incisors to the underlying dental bases.

The dental panoramic tomogram showed:

Normal alveolar base height.

A normal dentition. The developmental age matches Gerald's chronological age.

Third molars are present.

The cephalometric analysis revealed:

SNA = 82°; SNB = 76°; ANB = 6°; MMPA = 34°; $\underline{1}$ to maxillary plane = 111°; $\overline{1}$ to mandibular plane = 86°; interincisal angle = 126°; facial proportion = 60%.

What is your interpretation of these findings?

Relative to mean values for Caucasians, SNA is slightly increased and SNB is slightly reduced, but both are within the normal range; ANB is increased, indicating that the skeletal pattern is mildly Class II; 1 to maxillary plane shows that it is proclined relative to the mean but within the normal range; 1 to mandibular plane shows that it is retroclined relative to the mean, but it is at the correct angle to compensate for the increased MMPA (120° – 34° = 86°); relative to mean values, the interincisal angle is reduced but within the normal range and the facial proportion is increased.

Diagnosis

What is your diagnosis?

Class I malocclusion on a mild Class II skeletal base with increased FMPA.

Marginal gingivitis related to the incisors and 4|.

Mild mesiolabial rotations of 1|1 with spacing of the upper and lower labial segments. Anterior open bite.

Buccal segment relationship is Class III bilaterally.

What is the IOTN (DHC) grade (see p. 264)? Explain why.

4e – due to the anterior open bite.

Treatment

What treatment would you consider?

As the anterior open bite is not due to digit sucking, treatment is likely to be complex. Gerald has anteroposterior and vertical skeletal problems, the latter being more marked, with a downward and backward pattern of facial growth that has produced the anterior open bite. An *attempt*, therefore, to achieve incisor contact may be by growth modification aiming for effective control of maxillary vertical skeletal and dental growth.

This would require specialist care. A functional appliance with posterior bite blocks, e.g. a Twin-Block appliance, would be optimal. As the incisor relationship is Class I and the molar relationships are Class III, no forward posturing of the mandible for the registration bite is advisable. The bite, however, must be opened beyond the normal resting vertical dimension so that molar eruption is prevented. As the appliance holds the mandible in this position, a vertical intrusive force is exerted on the posterior teeth mediated by the stretch of the muscles and other soft tissues. Gerald should be instructed to wear the appliance full-time, including for meals. The anterior teeth are allowed to erupt while eruption of the posterior teeth is inhibited, thereby reducing the anterior open bite. This is supplemented by a tendency for mandibular growth to be projected anteriorly while vertical control of maxillary skeletal and dental growth is effected. In this case, high-pull headgear should not be added to the appliance. As the molar relationships are Class III, any molar distal movement is not indicated.

Currently, there is weak evidence that both the Function Regulator IV (FR IV) with lip-seal training and the palatal crib associated with high-pull chincup are able to correct anterior open bite.

Key point

Unless an anterior open bite is due to a habit, treatment is complex.

What means have been tried in an attempt to stop a digit-sucking habit?

These range from simple strategies, such as covering the digit with a plaster or painting the digit with an unpleasant-tasting substance, to attempts to modify behaviour with cognitive behavioural therapy, reward-based strategies and the use of positive reinforcement. The use of intraoral appliances has also been tried either to stop the digit being put in the habit position or to lessen the satisfaction felt in undertaking the habit.

If the anterior open bite had been due to digit sucking, what treatment would you recommend?

A recent Cochrane systematic review concluded that provision of a fixed habit breaker (palatal crib or arch; **Fig. 13.8A and B**), psychological intervention (positive or negative reinforcement) or both seem to be effective in assisting children with stopping a NNSH; this, however, was based on low-quality, highly biased evidence. If the habit ceases, the

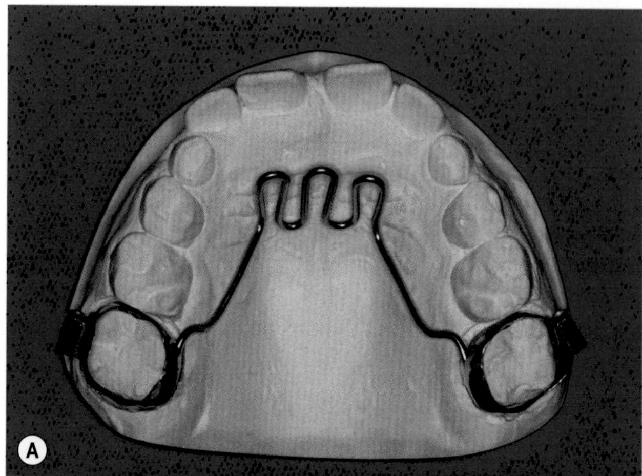

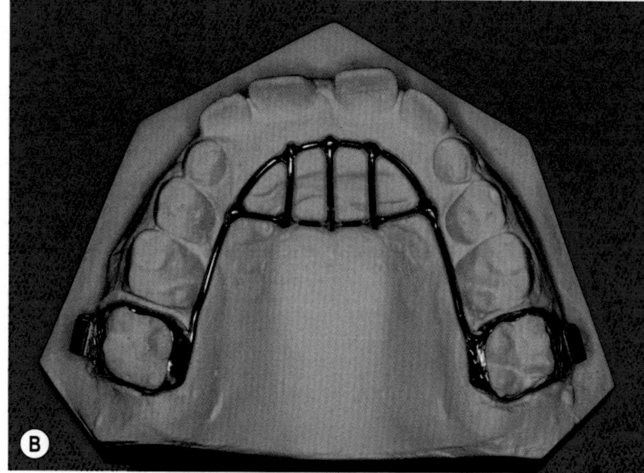

Fig. 13.8 **(A)** Palatal crib. **(B)** Modified palatal arch.

anterior open bite will usually reduce spontaneously, although this is likely to take several years.

Key point

Currently, low-quality evidence indicates that effective strategies to assist a child in stopping a digit-sucking habit include:

- Fixed habit breaker.
- Positive or negative reinforcement.
- Both.

■ *How would you manage a parent who is concerned about an anterior open bite produced by either a dummy or digit sucking habit in the primary dentition* (Figs 3.4 and 3.5)?

It would be prudent to advise the parent of the child that this is a very common issue at this stage of development and that, as the incidence of NNSHs decreases throughout the mixed dentition, a 'wait and see' approach would be beneficial. Gentle persuasion to discontinue the habit may also be considered, but as most children are likely to outgrow the habit, it would be important not to magnify the issue for the child. If either habit stops, the anterior open bite will reduce. Many changes will occur with growth of the face and the eruption of the permanent teeth, so the malocclusion can be reassessed in light of these changes at age 8 (when the incisors and first permanent molars erupt); should there be a displacement of the lower jaw due to narrowing of the upper arch by the habit, it can be assessed and corrected at that time. Any concerns regarding swallowing pattern and speech are also likely to change as the permanent teeth erupt and could be assessed by a speech therapist, also at that time, if desired.

■ *What is the likely prognosis of treatment in Gerald's case?*

As the anterior open bite is quite marked and the vertical skeletal pattern is moderately increased, the prognosis is guarded. Gerald and his parents should be made aware of this before treatment commences. Provided there is excellent cooperation with appliance wear and vertical facial growth is favourable, functional appliance treatment has a reasonable chance of success at this stage. However, a second phase of treatment with fixed appliances is likely to be required to detail the occlusion. As these appliances do not control eruption so favourably, posterior bite blocks or similar components will also be required during that phase of treatment to maintain the correction achieved in the earlier phase. Thereafter, bite blocks will also need to be incorporated in any retainer. Long-term retention will be required to avert the possible unfavourable effects of subsequent vertical facial growth.

The lisp may improve with closure of the anterior open bite, but Gerald and his parents should not have high expectations regarding this.

■ *Are there any other treatment options?*

If Gerald does not cooperate with functional appliance wear, treatment for the anterior open bite by a specific type of fixed appliance mechanics with multiloop archwires (Kim mechanics) may be considered, most likely in conjunction with the removal of the second or third molars. This approach to appliance treatment requires specialist training. The objective is to correct the cant of individual occlusal planes, uprighting the teeth in relation to the bisecting occlusal plane. As this happens, there is a reduction in posterior facial and dentoalveolar heights, which reduces the anterior open bite; anterior vertical elastics then bring the incisors into contact. Impressive and stable correction of marked anterior open bite, in adolescents and adults, has been reported using this technique. Similar results can be achieved with 'rocking horse' archwires used in combination with anterior vertical elastics.

Molar intrusion may also be achieved using temporary anchorage devices (TADs; **Fig. 13.9**) in the form of either screws or plates. To maximize molar intrusion and prevent unwanted buccal tipping of the molars, use of buccal *and*

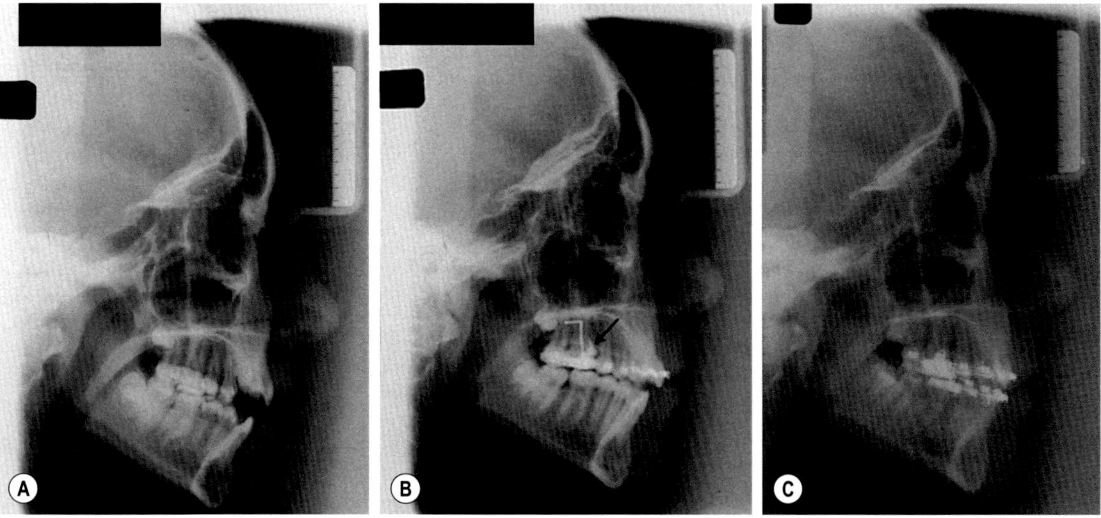

Fig. 13.9 TADs used to close anterior open bite: lateral cephalometric radiograph **(A)** pre-treatment; **(B)** following molar intrusion with TADs (arrowed) and palatal arch; **(C)** nearing the completion of fixed appliance treatment with extraction of four premolars.

palatal implants has been advised; the skeletal anchorage, however, for molar intrusion needs to be maintained during the early retention phase in an attempt to reduce relapse.

Should the anterior open bite worsen considerably, a combined orthodontic surgical approach may be sought when growth is complete.

Key point

Management options for anterior open bite may be:

- Accept.
- Habit breaker.
- Growth modification.
- Orthodontic camouflage, with or without TADs.
- Surgery.

Primary resources and recommended reading

Baek MS, Choi Y-J, Yu H-S et al 2010 Long-term stability of anterior open-bite treatment by intrusion of posterior maxillary teeth. Am J Orthod Dentofacial Orthop 138:396–398.

Borrie FBP, Bearn DR, Innes NPT et al 2015 Interventions for the cessation of non-nutritive sucking habits in children. Cochrane Database of Syst Rev Issue 3. Art No: CD008694. DOI: 10.1002/14651858.CD008694.pub2.

British Orthodontic Society 2012 Dummy and thumb sucking habits. Patient information leaflet. Available at: www.bos.org.uk.

Johnson NC, Sandy JR 1999 Tooth position and speech – is there a relationship? Angle Orthod 69:306–310.

Kim YH 1987 Anterior openbite and its treatment with multi-loop edgewise archwire. Angle Orthod 57:290–321.

Lentini-Oliveira D, Carvalho FR, Qingsong Y et al 2007 Orthodontic and orthopaedic treatment for anterior open bite in children. Cochrane Database of Syst Rev Issue 9. Art No: CD005515. DOI: 10.1002/14651858.CD005515.pub3.

Lopez-Gavito G, Wallen TR, Little RM, et al 1985 Anterior open-bite malocclusion: a longitudinal 10-year postretention evaluation of orthodontically treated patients. Am J Orthod 87:175–186.

Mizrahi E 1978 A review of anterior open bite. Br J Orthod 5:21–27.

Ngan P, Fields HW 1997 Open bite: a review of etiology and management. Pediatr Dent 19:91–98.

For revision, see Mind Map 13, page 233.

14

Posterior crossbite

SUMMARY

Kirsten is 7 years old. She presents with a crossbite of the right buccal segments *(Fig. 14.1)*. ***What will be your assessment and management options for this problem?***

History

Complaint

Kirsten's mother is concerned about the way her daughter's teeth bite together. She has noticed that Kirsten's jaw moves to one side as she closes her mouth. This makes her face appear crooked, a further cause of anxiety for her mother.

History of complaint

Kirsten used to suck her thumb until 5 months ago when $\overline{1|1}$ started to erupt. Her mother has become more aware of her daughter's 'deviated bite' in the past year and wondered if the thumb-sucking habit could have contributed to the problem.

Medical history

Kirsten is fit and well.

Family history

There is no family history of facial asymmetry.

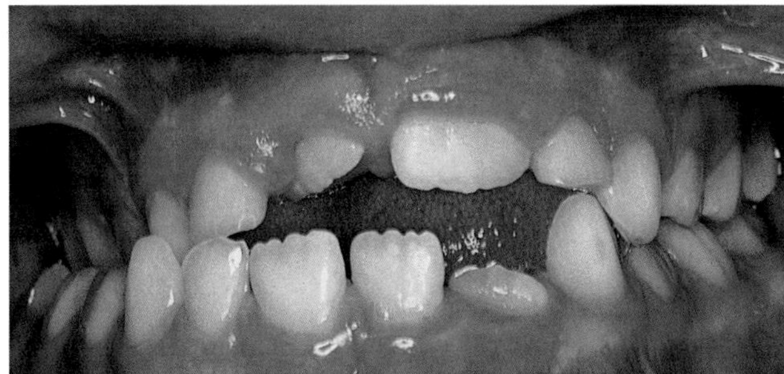

Fig. 14.1 Anterior occlusion at presentation.

Examination

Extraoral

Kirsten has a mild Class III skeletal pattern with slightly increased FMPA; the chin point is displaced slightly to the right. The lips are incompetent but habitually held together. There is a tongue to lower lip swallowing pattern. There is no masticatory muscle tenderness, temporomandibular joint tenderness or crepitus, and mouth opening is not restricted.

■ ***What other feature would you check for, bearing in mind the history? Explain why.***

It is important to check if there is mandibular displacement on closure as this would indicate that the facial asymmetry is more an apparent than a true skeletal asymmetry. For the former, orthodontic correction of an associated crossbite should be straightforward, but for the latter, further investigations would be required to determine if the asymmetry is progressive and more complex treatment would be required to address the facial and occlusal problems.

Early correction of a crossbite with a mandibular displacement is indicated to allow the occlusion to develop in an undisplaced position. It is likely also to reduce the possibility of development of temporomandibular joint dysfunction syndrome, which may occur in susceptible individuals in whom this occlusal discrepancy exists.

An anterolateral mandibular displacement on closure was detected on $\frac{C|}{C|}$ with an associated 3 mm shift between retruded contact position (RCP) and intercuspal position (ICP).

> **Key point**
>
> Early correction of a posterior crossbite with associated mandibular displacement is advisable.

Intraoral

■ ***What features are evident on the intraoral views*** *(Figs 14.1 and 14.2)*?

Mild marginal gingival erythema related to the erupting permanent incisors, but otherwise the soft tissues appear healthy. There is no caries visible.

Upper arch seems V-shaped anteriorly; lower arch is more U-shaped anteriorly.

6EDCB1 are present in both upper quadrants and in the lower right quadrant; 12CDE6 are present in the lower left quadrant.

Spacing of the upper and lower incisors with distopalatal rotation of 1|.

Class III incisor relationship.

Anterior open bite.

Lower centreline shift to the right.

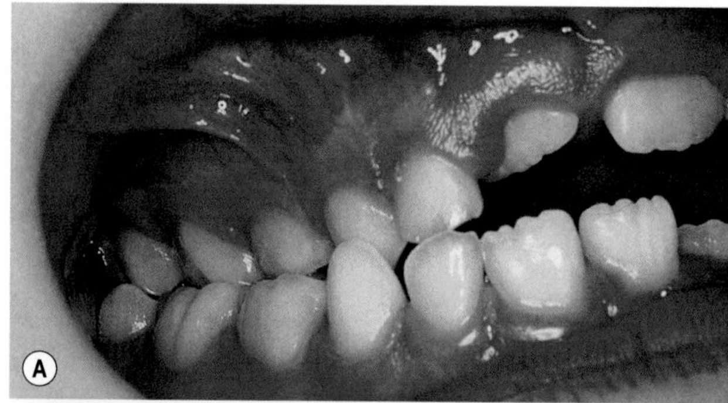

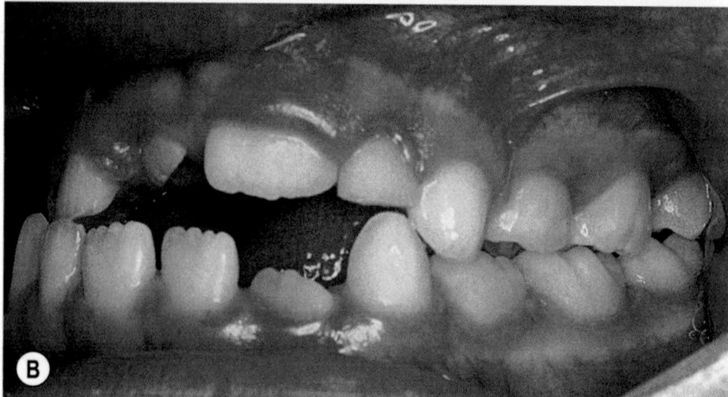

Fig. 14.2 **(A)** Right buccal occlusion. **(B)** Left buccal occlusion.

Box 14.1 Causes of a lower centreline shift

- Unbalanced loss of C, D and possibly E; the age at extraction, the degree of crowding and the tooth extracted (the more anterior, the greater the effect) influence the extent of centreline shift.
- Unilateral retained primary incisor, canine or molar.
- Hypodontia of an incisor or premolar.
- Supplemental incisor or premolar.
- Lateral mandibular displacement on closure producing unilateral buccal segment crossbite (often secondary to digit- or thumb-sucking habit).
- Early unilateral condylar fracture leading to deficient growth on the affected side.
- Hemifacial microsomia.
- Hemimandibular hypertrophy (known formerly as condylar hyperplasia). Cause is entirely unknown. Most likely in females between the ages of 15 and 20, but may occur in either sex as late as the early thirties.

Half-unit Class II right molar relationship with buccal crossbite of the right buccal segments (note palatal inclination of the teeth).

Class III left molar relationship.

■ ***How would you assess the centrelines?***

The upper and lower centrelines should be coincident with each other and with the midline of the face. Both of these aspects should be assessed, the latter by first looking at the patient anteriorly and then down on the face from above. With study models alone, it is not possible to determine the relation of the dental midlines to the facial midline.

In this case the lower centreline is displaced to the right by about half the width of a lower incisor.

■ ***What are the possible causes of a lower centreline shift?***

These are listed in **Box 14.1**. In this case it is due to the lateral aspect of the mandibular displacement on closure.

Table 14.1 Causes of buccal segment crossbite

Cause	Aetiology
Skeletal	Mismatch in the widths of the dental arches and/or an anteroposterior skeletal discrepancy – buccal and anterior crossbites are most commonly found in Class III malocclusion. Rarely, mandibular growth restriction following condylar trauma or hemimandibular hypertrophy may be implicated, both producing asymmetry
Soft tissues/habit	With a digit-sucking habit, the tongue position is lowered with the teeth apart, and cheek contraction is unopposed during sucking, narrowing the upper arch slightly

■ ***What factors may be implicated in the aetiology of the crossbite?***

These are summarized in **Table 14.1**.

■ ***What is the most likely cause of the posterior crossbite in this case?***

The thumb-sucking habit (see also Chapter 13).

Key point

A digit-sucking habit may lead to posterior crossbite with associated mandibular displacement.

■ ***What is a possible explanation for the mandibular displacement being on a primary canine rather than on the molars?***

As the corners of the mouth experience the greatest cheek pressure during thumb sucking, it seems plausible for greater narrowing to occur across the canines rather than the molars, resulting in a V-shaped upper arch (see **Fig. 14.1**); hence premature occlusal contact on one of the primary canines is the likely trigger for a lateral mandibular displacement on closure.

A narrow, V-shaped upper arch is more likely to result when the thumb is sucked intensely than when it just rests in the mouth.

Kirsten's mother reported that Kirsten used to suck her thumb for at least 12 hours per day for the past several years but gave up the habit in recent months.

Investigations

■ ***What special investigations would you undertake and why?***

A dental panoramic tomogram (**Fig. 14.3A**) is required to survey the developing dentition for any abnormalities of tooth number, size and position.

Impressions of the dental arches and a wax registration in maximum intercuspation should be taken to allow study models to be constructed. These will allow a thorough occlusal assessment to be performed and will act as a baseline record of the malocclusion.

■ ***What does the dental panoramic tomogram show?***

Normal alveolar bone height.

All permanent teeth developing apart from third molars.

No apparent caries or other pathology.

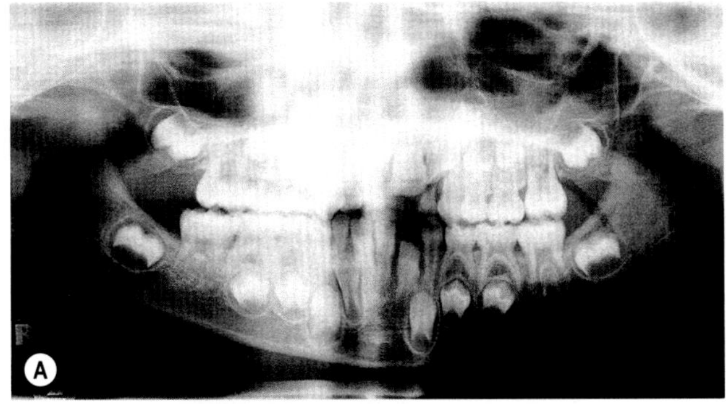

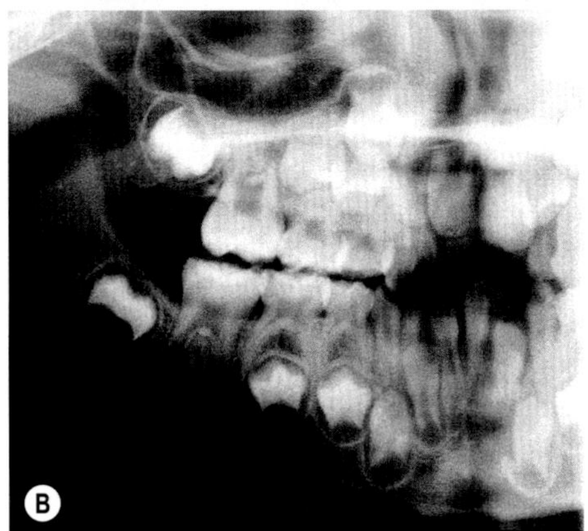

Fig. 14.3 **(A)** Dental panoramic tomogram. **(B)** Repeat of right half dental panoramic tomogram.

■ ***What is the most likely reason for the blurred image on the right half of the dental panoramic tomogram?***

Movement of the patient during image capture, most probably due to swallowing, is the likely cause.

■ ***Why was a right half, rather than a full, dental panoramic tomogram retaken*** *(Fig. 14.3B)****?***

In line with current radiology guidelines, the radiation dosage to the patient should be as low as reasonably achievable for the diagnostic purposes required. Retaking the right-half image only satisfies diagnostic needs here.

Diagnosis

■ ***What is your diagnosis?***

Class III malocclusion on a mild Class III skeletal base with slightly increased FMPA; anterolateral mandibular displacement on closure on $\frac{C|}{C|}$.

Mild marginal gingivitis related to the erupting incisors.

Spacing of the upper and lower incisors with 1| distopalatally rotated.

Anterior open bite; lower centreline shift to the right.

Buccal segment relationship half-unit Class II on the right and Class III on the left.

Buccal crossbite of the right buccal segments associated with the mandibular displacement.

■ ***What is the IOTN (DHC) grade (see p. 264)? Explain why.***

4c – due to mandibular displacement >2 mm between the RCP and the ICP.

Treatment

■ ***What treatment plan would you propose?***

Oral hygiene instruction to improve gingival health.

Correction of the right buccal segment and anterior crossbites.

Regular review of the developing occlusion.

■ ***How may the crossbites be corrected? Describe the design of any appliance you would use.***

Possible approaches to treatment are as follows:

1. As the digit-sucking habit has been abandoned and the mandibular displacement arises from premature contact on $\frac{C|}{C|}$, judicious grinding of their cusp tips may remove the occlusal interference and correct the buccal segment crossbite, although the success rate with this treatment has varied considerably, from 27–64%. Placing composite onlays to allay mandibular shift where occlusal interferences exist has also been tried but with outcomes inferior to active appliance therapy.

   The permanent incisors are erupted insufficiently, at present, to consider their proclination and which means will be best.
2. As the upper buccal segment teeth are not tilted buccally, upper arch expansion by a midline screw in an upper removable appliance may be considered. The appliance may be clasped on 6D|D6 (Adams clasps: 6|6 0.7 mm stainless steel wire; D|D 0.6 mm stainless steel wire). Buccal capping will facilitate tooth movement by disengaging the posterior occlusion. Kirsten should be encouraged to turn the screw one quarter turn twice weekly (0.25 mm of activation with each turn) until the crossbite is corrected. A small amount of overexpansion is advisable as some relapse is to be expected. Then the capping should be reduced to half its height at one visit and removed completely at the following visit to allow the buccal segment teeth to erupt into occlusion. Provided there is a well-interdigitating buccal segment occlusion, the appliance should then be worn as a retainer at night for several months; 6 months of retention will likely suffice.

   The final occlusion following crossbite correction by an upper removable appliance is shown in **Fig. 14.4**. Correction of the incisor relationship and improvement in 1| alignment occurred spontaneously.
3. Alternatively, upper arch expansion may be undertaken using a quadhelix (see **Fig. 4.11A**). This consists of bands cemented to the first permanent molars with soldered arms, which in this case should extend forward to the palatal aspects of the C's. Alternatively, a preformed quadhelix may be employed that fits into sheaths soldered to the palatal aspects of the molar bands, allowing easy removal for adjustment. Activation is usually half a tooth width on each side. To facilitate crossbite correction, it may be necessary to disengage the buccal occlusion temporarily by placing glass ionomer cement on the occlusal surfaces of the molars. Once the crossbite has been corrected, the cement may

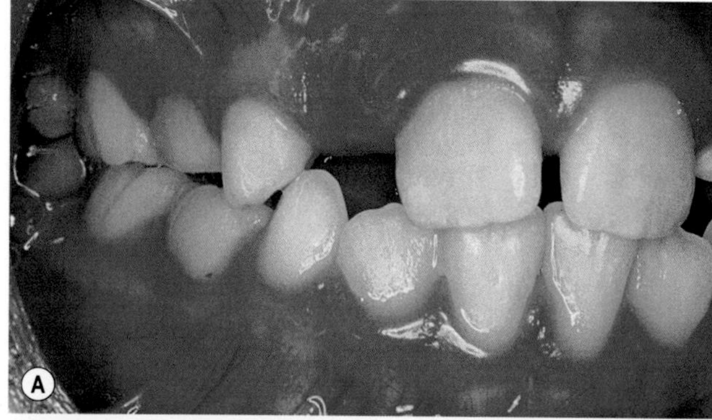

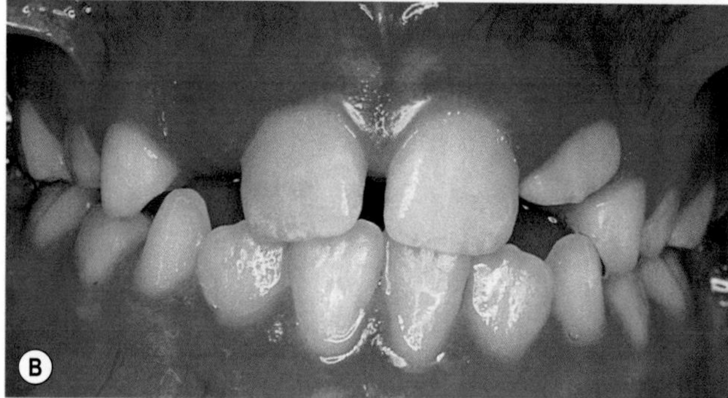

Fig. 14.4 Post-treatment **(A)** Right buccal occlusion. **(B)** Anterior occlusion.

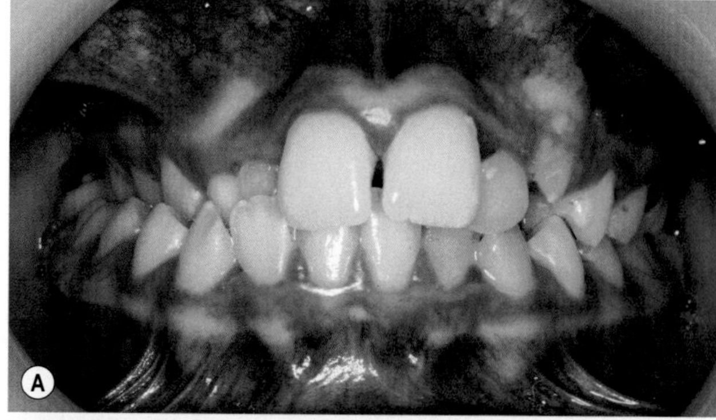

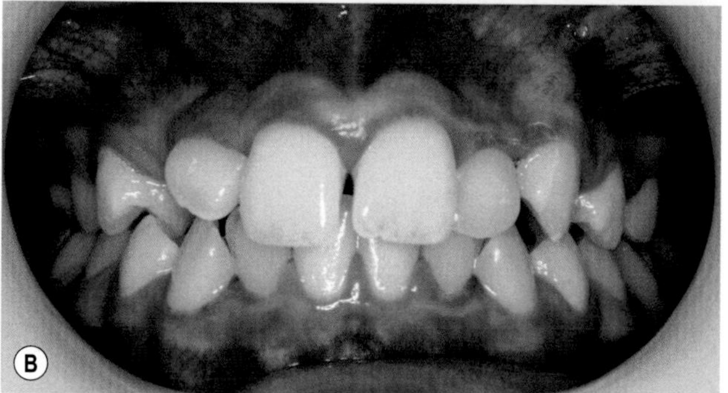

Fig. 14.5 **(A)** Pre-treatment: anterior occlusion (note C⌋ retained and mobile; 3⌋ unerupted). **(B)** Post-treatment: anterior occlusion.

be removed and the quadhelix should be rendered passive prior to cementation for 3–6 months as a retainer.

Another case treated by a quadhelix is shown in **Figs 14.5A and B.**

> **Key point**
>
> Management options for a unilateral posterior crossbite with associated mandibular displacement in the mixed dentition:
>
> - Grind C's.
> - URA with midline screw.
> - Quadhelix.

■ *Based on current evidence, what treatment modality is most effective for correction of a buccal segment crossbite in the mixed dentition?*

A recent systematic review suggests that crossbite correction and expansion of the intermolar width for children in the early mixed dentition (aged 8–10) may be more successful with a quadhelix than with an upper removable expansion appliance, although the quality of evidence was low to moderate. Compared with removable expansion plates, a quadhelix appliance may achieve 1.15 mm more molar expansion and may be 20% more likely to correct crossbites. There was insufficient evidence to favour one intervention over another with regard to the other outcomes assessed (intercanine expansion, stability of crossbite correction, signs and symptoms of temporomandibular joint dysfunction, signs and symptoms of respiratory disease and quality of life).

■ *What will determine if the corrected buccal segment crossbite is likely to be stable?*

Good buccal segment interdigitation and absence of any displacing occlusal contacts.

> **Key point**
>
> Correction of a unilateral buccal segment crossbite in the mixed dentition may be more successful with a quadhelix than with a removable expansion plate.

Primary resources and recommended reading

Agostino P, Ugolini A, Signori A et al 2014 Orthodontic treatment for posterior crossbites. Cochrane Database of Syst Rev Issue 8. Art No: CD000979. DOI: 10.1002/14651858.CD000979.pub2.

Primozic J, Ovsenik M, Richmond S et al 2009 Early crossbite correction: a three-dimensional evaluation. Eur J Orthod 31:352–356.

For revision, see Mind Map 14, page 234.

15

Bilateral crossbite

CASE 1

SUMMARY

Jean has just turned 12. She presents with bilateral buccal crossbites (*Fig. 15.1*). What are the possible causes, and how could it be managed?

History

Complaint

Jean does not like the 'narrow' appearance of her upper teeth, especially when she smiles.

History of complaint

Her mother says that Jean's 'baby' teeth had the same appearance, and she also has a similar appearance of her upper teeth to her daughter. Jean's teeth erupted in the position they are in at present. There is no history of trauma to her upper jaw, and birth was normal.

Medical history

Jean is asthmatic and uses a salbutamol (Ventolin) inhaler. She is prone to upper respiratory tract infections and is unable to breathe through her nose. Her mother reports that she snores and is prone to day-time drowsiness, which her teachers have noticed. Otherwise she is well. Her mother wonders if the narrow appearance of Jean's upper teeth is related to her mouth breathing and snoring. She is keen to know if Jean's mouth breathing and snoring could be improved by any brace treatment.

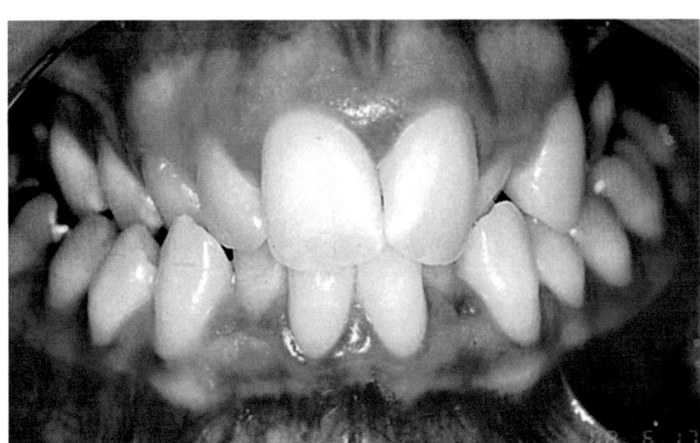

Fig. 15.1 Case 1: anterior occlusion at presentation.

■ ***What is the relevance of Jean's mode of breathing to snoring and to her complaint?***

Compulsive mouth breathing, due to inability to breathe through the nose, may contribute to an altered head posture and low tongue position; this may lead to unopposed action of buccinator musculature and bilateral narrowing of the upper arch creating bilateral buccal crossbites.

Inability to breathe through the nose is also linked with snoring, which is associated with sleep apnoea, a major cause of day-time drowsiness. Prolonged inflammation of the nasal mucosa associated with allergies (in Jean's case there is a history of asthma) or chronic infection (she is prone to upper respiratory tract infections) could produce some degree of nasal obstruction and lead to mouth breathing. The normally large pharyngeal tonsils or adenoids in children may also contribute.

Key point

- Mouth breathing may contribute to altered head posture, low tongue position and bilateral buccal crossbite, but it is not the sole or even the major cause of such crossbites.

Dental history

Jean is an irregular attender at her general dental practitioner. She has fissure sealants to several molar teeth and one filling. There is no history of digit-sucking.

■ ***How may a digit-sucking habit cause a buccal segment crossbite?***

This is given in **Table 14.1** (p. 88).

Social history

Jean has two younger sisters. Neither of them have had orthodontic treatment, and neither of them have teeth like hers.

Examination

Extraoral

Jean has a Class I skeletal pattern with slightly increased FMPA and no facial asymmetry. Lips are incompetent. There are no signs or symptoms associated with the temporomandibular joints.

Intraoral

■ ***The appearance of the teeth on presentation is shown in*** *Figs 15.1* ***and*** *15.2****. Describe what you see.***

Fair oral hygiene with generalized marginal gingival erythema.

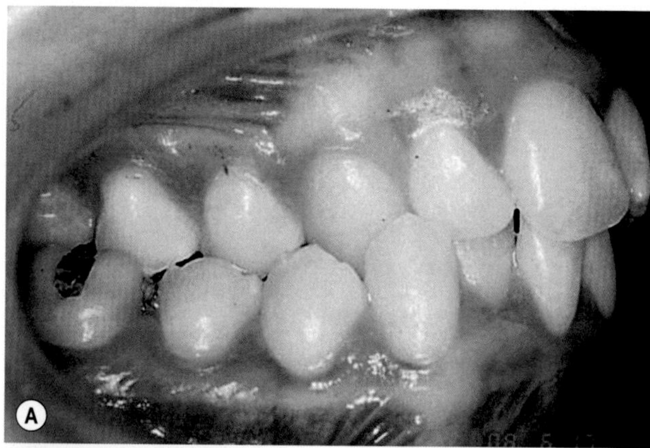

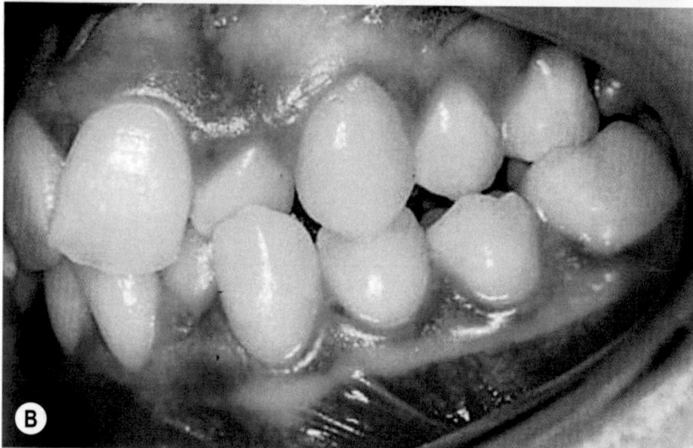

Fig. 15.2 (A) Case 1: right buccal occlusion. **(B)** Case 1: left buccal occlusion.

$\frac{654321|123456}{7654321|1234567}$ visible (please note $\underline{7|7}$ are also erupted).

All teeth visible appear caries-free; amalgam restoration in $\overline{6|}$.

Moderate lower arch crowding; $\overline{1|1}$ appear slightly small (contact point displacements were 3 mm between $\overline{|1}$ and $\overline{|2}$; also between $\overline{|2}$ and $\overline{|3}$); mild upper arch crowding.

Class I incisor relationship; average and complete overbite; upper and lower centreline shifts (upper appears to the left, lower to the right); $\underline{2|2}$ in crossbite.

Molar relationship is Class I on right and Class III on left with bilateral buccal crossbite affecting $\frac{6543|456}{6543|\ 56}$.

■ ***What are the possible causes of bilateral buccal crossbite?***

Factors implicated in the aetiology of a bilateral buccal crossbite are given in **Table 15.1**.

Investigations

■ ***What investigations would you undertake in relation to the bilateral buccal crossbite? Explain why.***

Clinical

It would be important to ascertain if there is an associated mandibular displacement, although this is rare with bilateral crossbites. It is more usual to have a mandibular displacement associated with a unilateral buccal crossbite.

No mandibular displacement was noted.

Table 15.1 Possible causes of bilateral buccal crossbite

Bilateral buccal crossbite	Possible causes
Skeletal	Mismatch in relative widths of arches or anteroposterior discrepancy (commonly associated with Class III malocclusion)
Soft tissues	Possible role of adenoids/tonsils (see text)
	Low tongue position possibly due to altered head posture associated with mouth breathing
	Scar tissue of cleft repair restraining growth in upper arch width

Radiographic

A dental panoramic tomogram would be useful to determine the presence, position and form of unerupted third molars. A lateral cephalometric radiograph will also be required to ascertain the inclination of the upper and lower incisors to their respective dental bases.

The dental panoramic tomogram indicated four third molars of good form and position to be present.

The cephalometric findings were as follows:

SNA = 81°; SNB = 79°; MMPA = 28°; $\underline{1}$ to maxillary plane = 113°; $\overline{1}$ to mandibular plane = 93°; interincisal angle = 138°; facial proportion = 56%.

■ ***What is your interpretation of these findings?***

Relative to mean values for Caucasians, SNA is normal; SNB is slightly increased; ANB (SNA − SNB) = 2°, indicating a Class I skeletal pattern; MMPA is slightly increased; $\underline{1}$ to maxillary plane is increased, so the upper incisors are slightly proclined; $\overline{1}$ to mandibular plane is normal; interincisal angle is slightly increased; facial proportion is slightly increased.

All values are within the normal range for Caucasians.

Diagnosis

■ ***What is your diagnosis?***

Class I malocclusion on a Class I skeletal pattern with slightly increased FMPA and no facial asymmetry.

Generalized marginal gingivitis.

Moderate lower labial segment crowding: mild upper labial segment crowding with $\underline{2}$'s in crossbite; upper and lower centreline shifts.

Molar relationship is Class I on the right and Class III on left with bilateral buccal crossbite affecting $\frac{6543|456}{6543|\ 56}$.

■ ***What is the IOTN (DHC) grade (see p. 264)? Explain why.***

3d – due to contact point displacement between $\overline{|1}$ and $\overline{|2}$; also between $\overline{|2}$ and $\overline{|3}$.

Treatment

■ ***What are the aims of treatment?***

To improve oral hygiene.

To correct the bilateral buccal crossbite.

To relieve upper and lower arch crowding.

Table 15.2 Management options for bilateral buccal crossbite

Management option	Indications	Comments
Accept and monitor	Patient not keen for correction.	Not an option here as Jean is keen for correction
	Part of underlying skeletal III problem which is likely to worsen with mandibular growth, especially in males	
Removable appliance with midline screw or heavy midline spring	Primary/early mixed dentition	Rate of expansion must be quite slow and force employed low: otherwise retention of appliance compromised by higher expansion forces
		Compliance with wear and activation may be problematic
		Not cost-effective as often lengthy time required to produce desired expansion
Quadhelix	Preferred approach in early mixed dentition	Made of 1 mm stainless steel wire attached to bands cemented to molar tooth on each side
	3–5 mm maxillary expansion required (mainly dental but some skeletal expansion)	Delivers few hundred grams of force
	Teeth preferably tipped palatally but molar inclination may be adjusted with fixed appliances later	Produces efficient slow expansion
		May derotate molars
		May be adjusted to give more expansion posteriorly or anteriorly
		May be custom-made or preformed types available
		Activation half a tooth width each side
Rapid maxillary expansion (RME)	Child/adolescent	Produces ~ equal amounts of dental/skeletal expansion
	Minimal/no palatal tipping of the buccal segment teeth, i.e. skeletal crossbite	May be undertaken using a banded or bonded appliance (the latter limits the amount of downward-backward rotation of the mandible)
	>5 mm transverse maxillary expansion required	
	Mild anterior maxillary crowding	The older the age at expansion, the less likely the increase in vertical facial height will be recovered by subsequent growth
Surgically assisted rapid maxillary expansion (SARPE)	Skeletally mature patient with severe skeletal crossbite in whom segmental expansion in Le Fort I osteotomy might compromise blood supply to segments	Not an attractive option if further maxillary repositioning in the anteroposterior or vertical plane is required later
	>5 mm transverse maxillary expansion required	

To align upper and lower arches with centreline correction.

To correct the left buccal segment relationship to Class I.

What treatment would you provide?

Oral hygiene instruction by a hygienist. Provided the marginal gingivitis is corrected then proceed to correction of the bilateral buccal crossbite (the need for extractions for relief of crowding and centreline correction should be reviewed following crossbite correction).

What options are there for management of the bilateral buccal crossbite? Which would you choose?

The options are given in **Table 15.2**. In view of the severity of the crossbite and the desire to simultaneously, if possible, improve nasal breathing, rapid maxillary expansion (RME) would be the preferred choice of treatment.

What factors should be checked before using this treatment? What are the chances of opening the mid-palatal suture in this patient?

It is particularly advisable to check that there is adequate buccal supporting bone and width of attached gingiva on all of the upper buccal segment teeth. Before the age of 15, the chances of successful opening of the mid-palatal suture are almost 100% but reduce after that due to greater interdigitation of the sutures.

Key point

- Mid-palatal suture opening by RME is almost 100% guaranteed before age 15.

Describe the design of the appliance you would use. What instructions would you give Jean regarding this appliance?

The mechanism of mid-palatal suture separation is expansion by a screw built into a fixed appliance that is attached rigidly to as many teeth as possible.

The appliance may only comprise metal or acrylic framework against the teeth, which does not contact the palatal mucosa or may be made with acrylic palate-covering shelves. The latter type may, in theory, produce more bodily positioning of the alveolar processes but may impinge on the palatal tissues. For that reason, appliances that are tooth-borne are preferred.

The appliance used in Jean's case was as follows (**Fig. 15.3**):

- *Activation:* mid-palatal expansion screw (Hyrax).
- *Retention:* bands on 4's and 6's.
- *Anchorage:* 4's and 6's and the joining metal struts between the bands on these teeth.
- *Baseplate:* no palatal acrylic or buccal capping.

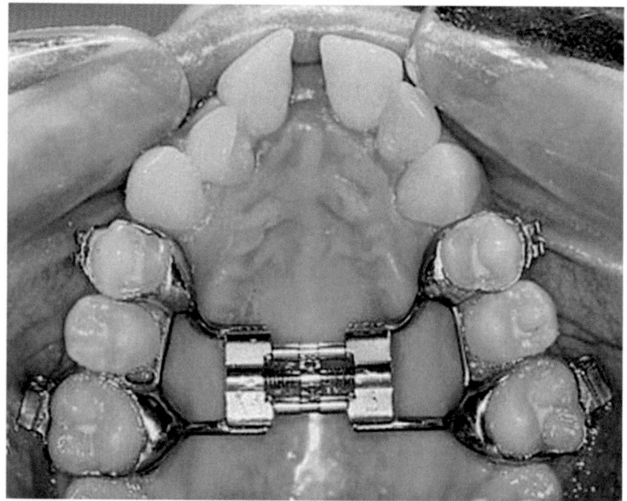

Fig. 15.3 Case 1: rapid maxillary expansion appliance with Hyrax screw.

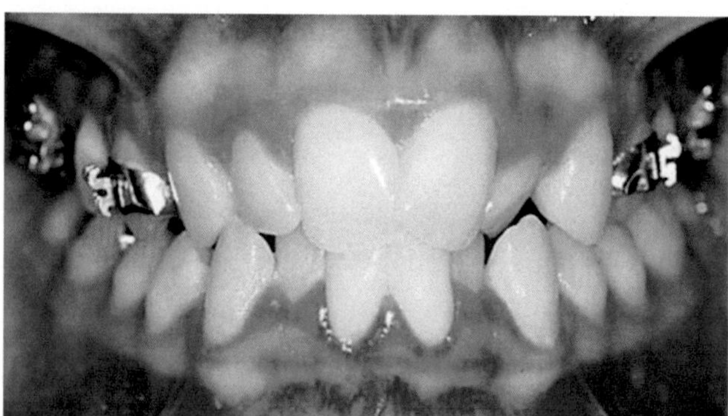

Fig. 15.4 Case 1: anterior occlusion following RME and prior to proceeding to upper/lower fixed appliance therapy.

■ *What should Jean be advised of regarding the effects of expansion?*

As the suture expands more anteriorly than posteriorly, an upper median diastema will usually develop within days of appliance activation (**Fig. 15.3**). Following correction of the bilateral crossbite and several months retention, during which time the appliance is left in place, the pull of the gingival fibres and some skeletal relapse will close the diastema (**Fig. 15.4**).

With transverse maxillary expansion, some molar extrusion is likely and cuspal interferences are created that cause the mandible to rotate downward and backward. This will reduce the overbite.

■ *Describe how the appliance works.*

It separates the mid-palatal suture as if on a hinge at the nasal base. Rapid expansion is achieved using forces of 10–20 lb (approximately 4.5–9 kg) over 2–3 weeks with the patient turning the screw twice daily (~0.5 mm movement per day). This contrasts with slow expansion (force of 2–4 lb (0.9–1.8 kg) over about 2.5 months with the screw being turned once every other day, 1 mm per week). Minimal suture disruption takes place with slow expansion.

With a screw device for rapid expansion, force is transmitted first to the teeth and then to the suture, producing microfractures of the interdigitating bone spicules. Because closure begins posteriorly in the mid-palatal suture and the other maxillary structures also exert a buttressing effect in this region, the suture opens wider and faster anteriorly, often producing a median diastema. Some overcorrection is advisable (maxillary palatal cusps in line with mandibular buccal cusps) as there is a strong relapse tendency due to palatal soft tissue elasticity.

> **Key point**
>
> Rapid mid-palatal suture expansion:
>
> - Exerts a force of 10–20 lb (approximately 4.5–9 kg) over 2–3 weeks.
> - Produces ~0.5 mm movement per day.
> - Creates a median diastema.
> - Has a strong relapse tendency, requiring overcorrection.

■ *How will you retain the crossbite correction?*

The expansion appliance should be rendered passive and remain in place for 3 months as a retainer. On its removal, a removable retainer with palatal acrylic coverage should be fitted unless further treatment is being carried out immediately, in which case a heavy expanded maxillary archwire may be placed for retention. A modified transpalatal arch with arms extending to the mesial of the 4's or a 1 mm stainless steel archwire through the headgear tubes are alternatives while light wires align the remaining teeth. On completion of treatment, an upper Hawley retainer (see p. 123) or a fitted palatal arch may be placed.

The occlusion at removal of the RME appliance and immediately prior to proceeding to further fixed appliance therapy is shown in **Fig. 15.4**.

CASE 2

SUMMARY

Aidan is 19 years old. He presents concerned about the appearance of his top teeth and his bite (*Fig. 15.5*). How may it be treated?

■ *What are the main features of note in Fig. 15.5?*

Narrow maxillary arch.

Bilateral posterior buccal crossbite, extending to include 3|.

Upper labial segment crowding with incisor rotations; very mild lower labial segment crowding.

Class III incisor relationship with 2|2 in crossbite (distal aspects of 1|1 also in crossbite).

Upper and lower centreline discrepancy (appears that lower centreline is shifted to the right).

Minimal overbite.

Lateral open bites.

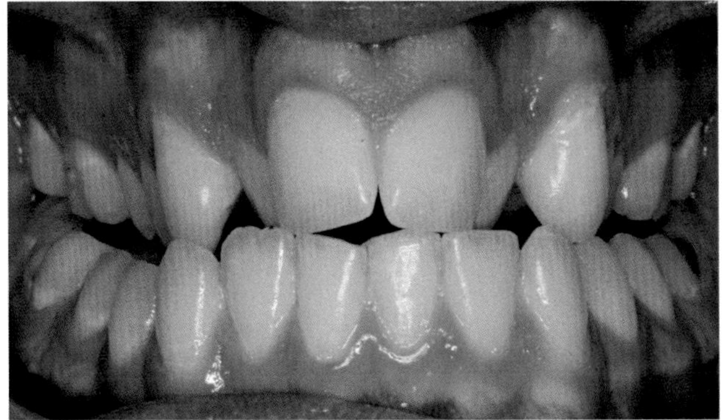

Fig. 15.5 Case 2: anterior occlusion at presentation.

History

Complaint

Aidan has been concerned for some time regarding his dental appearance. He now has a new job with a retail firm and feels embarrassed when he smiles. A previous orthodontist told him that he would need to wait until he was in his late teens before anything could be done regarding the bite of his front teeth.

■ ***What makes a smile attractive?***

On smiling, the full height of the upper incisors should be seen (usually at rest, there is 1 mm incisor show in males and 3 mm incisor show in females). Although some gingival display is acceptable, the interproximal gingivae only should be visible for optimal aesthetics. The contour of the upper incisor edges should match that of the lower lip (smile arc), with no upper incisor/lower lip contact. In the transverse dimension, the smile should include at minimum the upper first premolars. The distance between the inside of the cheek and the maxillary posterior teeth (buccal corridor), particularly the premolars, should be narrow.

Key point

An attractive smile comprises:

- Full length of the upper incisors.
- Related interproximal gingivae.
- Upper incisor edges contour matches that of the lower lip.
- Extends laterally to include no less than upper first premolars.
- Narrow buccal corridors.

Medical and dental history

Aidan is in good health. He is unable to breathe through his nose.

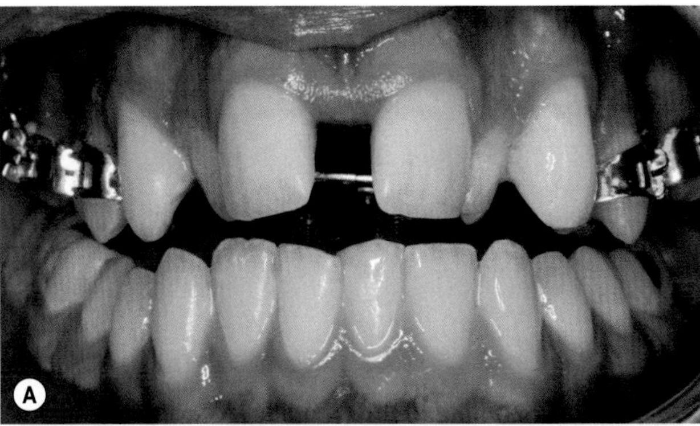

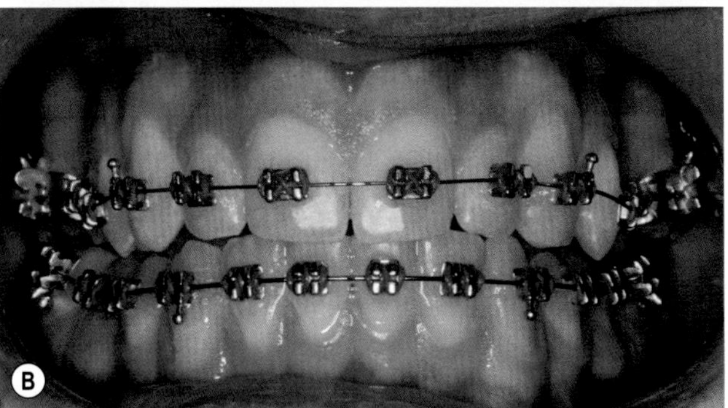

Fig. 15.6 **(A)** Case 2: expansion appliance in situ after surgery. **(B)** Case 2: completion of alignment by fixed appliances.

Treatment

■ ***Why is RME not feasible?***

In adults the mid-palatal and lateral maxillary sutures are well-interdigitated, which afford increased resistance to the orthopaedic-type palatal expansion (RME) that may be used in adolescents.

■ ***How is SARPE undertaken?***

Originally, surgically assisted rapid palatal expansion (SARPE) was undertaken using bone cuts only in the lateral maxillary buttress to decrease resistance such that in adults the mid-palatal suture could be microfractured by forced opening. Although this is commonly successful in patients under 30 years old, in older patients there is a risk of unwanted fractures in other areas. Currently, the procedure is often undertaken using cuts as for a Le Fort I osteotomy but without maxillary down-fracture. The maxilla is thus able to widen in a process akin to distraction osteogenesis (see p. 97) as resistance is provided by the soft tissues only. The RME appliance is cemented prior to surgery, and activation of the screw usually commences within 2 days at the same rate as for non-surgically assisted RME. Fixed appliances are required to complete alignment (**Fig. 15.6**).

The improved occlusion on completion of treatment is shown in **Fig. 15.7**.

■ ***How stable is SARPE?***

SARPE appears to be more stable than surgical widening of the maxilla. The latter has a high relapse tendency due to elastic rebound of the stretched palatal mucosa. Even after SARPE, wear of a palate-covering retainer for at least the first post-surgical year is recommended to control relapse.

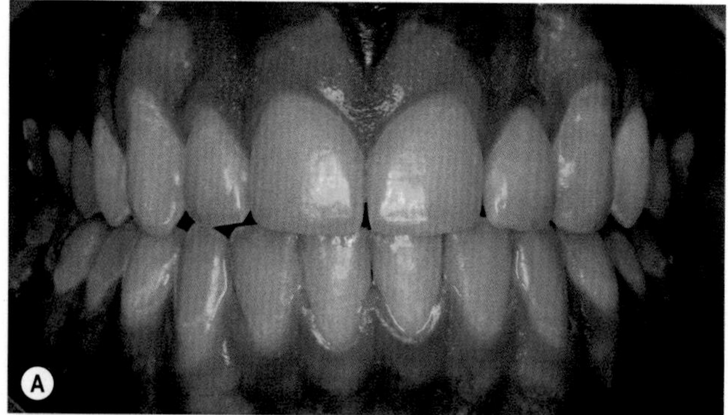

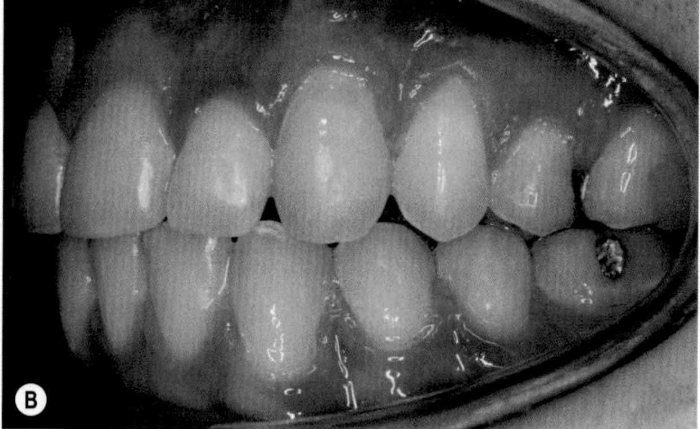

Fig. 15.7 (A) Case 2 post-treatment: anterior occlusion. **(B)** Case 2 post-treatment: left buccal occlusion.

Key point

SARPE:

- Is indicated for bilateral posterior crossbite correction in adults.
- Allows widening of the maxilla against only soft tissue resistance.
- Appears to be more stable than surgical widening of the maxilla.

CASE 3

SUMMARY

Simon is 13 years old. He presents complaining about the prominence of his top teeth and the crooked lower back teeth (Fig. 15.8). What are the causes, and what options are there for management?

■ ***What are the main features of note in Fig. 15.8?***

Enamel fracture in incisal third of ⌊1 with composite restoration (⌊1 had suffered trauma 2 years previously but was symptom-free).

Caries 5⌉ distally.

Mild upper arch crowding; moderate lower arch crowding.

Class II division 1 malocclusion; increased overjet; slightly increased overbite.

Canine relationship half-unit is Class II bilaterally.

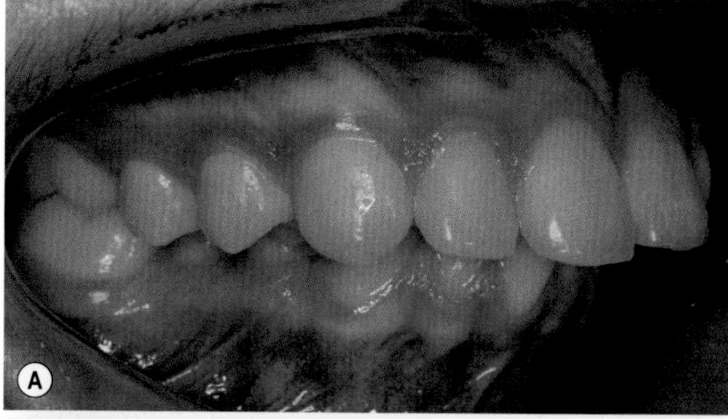

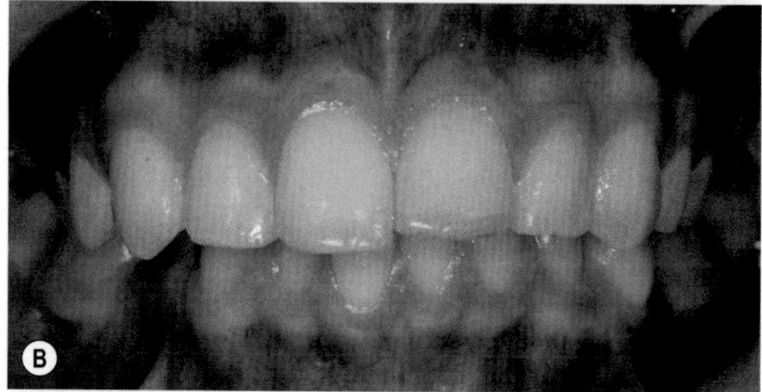

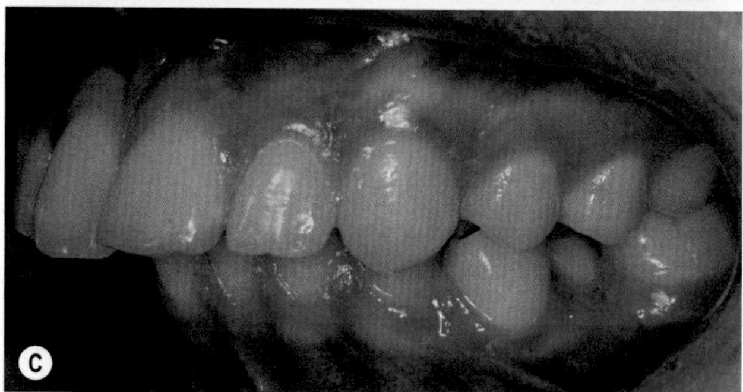

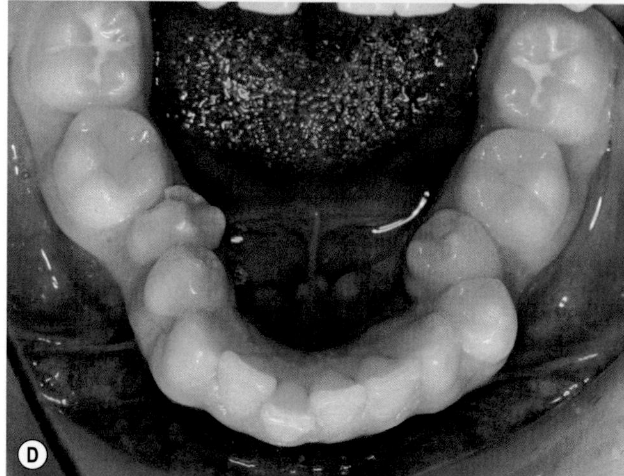

Fig. 15.8 (A) Case 3 at presentation: right buccal occlusion. **(B)** Case 3 at presentation: anterior occlusion. **(C)** Case 3 at presentation: left buccal occlusion. **(D)** Case 3 at presentation: lower occlusal view.

Bilateral lingual crossbite (also referred to as scissors bite or Brodie bite) affecting $\overline{54|5}$.

■ ***Given the position of $\overline{5|45}$, what would you enquire about?***

It would be useful to know if there had been early loss of both lower $\overline{E}$'s which would encourage mesial drift of $\overline{6}$s and lingual displacement of $\overline{5}$s.

Simon had $\overline{E|DE}$ removed when he was 7 years old.

Key point

Lingual crossbites are associated with Class II malocclusions.

Extraoral

Simon has a Class II skeletal pattern with slightly reduced FMPA; there is no facial asymmetry.

No mandibular displacement or temporomandibular joint signs or symptoms were detected.

■ ***What are the causes of bilateral lingual crossbite?***

These are given in **Table 15.3**. In Simon's case, a combination of local and skeletal causes are implicated in the bilateral lingual crossbite.

■ ***What treatment options are there for correction of bilateral lingual crossbite?***

It is important to ascertain the number of teeth affected and to check the inclination of the affected teeth. These will help to indicate the severity of any underlying skeletal component and whether reciprocal movement of the affected teeth with the opposing teeth only will suffice for correction. Management options are given in **Table 15.4**.

In view of the underlying Class II skeletal problem, Simon was treated first by growth modification with a Frankel II appliance followed by non-extraction upper and lower fixed appliance therapy (**Fig. 15.9**).

Key point

Correction of a bilateral lingual crossbite:

- Single tooth affected on each side: consider extraction of displaced teeth.
- Several teeth affected on each side: consider combination of buccal movement of affected lower teeth/palatal movement of affected upper teeth.

■ ***Simon was treated with the fixed appliances shown in*** *Fig. 15.9*. ***What type of appliance is this? What are its claimed advantages compared with conventional fixed appliance systems?***

This is a self-ligating fixed appliance (Damon). The archwire is not pressed firmly against the bracket base but is held in place by either a rigid (as with the Damon system) or spring clip (Speed) or retaining springs (Smart-Clip). These replace the stainless steel ligatures or elastomeric modules that are used (the latter mainly) to retain the archwire in the bracket slot with conventional non-self-ligating systems. Claimed advantages include faster ligation, lower friction, faster treatment, less pain and fewer appointments. Compared with conventional pre-adjusted edgewise brackets, current prospective evidence for self-ligating brackets indicates no clinically significant difference in treatment duration between the two systems; similar effects on arch form for

Table 15.3 Causes of bilateral lingual crossbite

Local	Bilateral early loss of $\overline{\text{E}}$'s may allow $\overline{5}$s to be displaced completely lingually
Skeletal	Mismatch in relative width of arches or a Class II skeletal discrepancy
Combination of local and skeletal	
Rarer causes	Pierre Robin anomaly (mandibular retrognathia, cleft palate, glossoptosis)

Table 15.4 Management options for bilateral lingual crossbite

Option	Possible indications
Extraction	Single tooth on either side affected and completely excluded lingually
Reciprocal movement of affected upper and lower teeth	Depends on inclination of teeth, number of teeth affected and presence/absence of underlying Class II skeletal discrepancy
	Fixed appliances required
Growth modification	An appliance that influences soft tissue force balance may be useful, eg, Frankel II
Orthodontic camouflage	Extraction/non-extraction therapy depending on local/skeletal components
	An appliance that facilitates lower interpremolar expansion may be helpful, eg, Damon appliance
Midline distraction osteogenesis	Severe mandibular crowding with well-aligned upper arch, v-shaped mandible and narrow mandibular arch with bilateral scissors bite affecting several teeth
Orthognathic surgery	Adult skeletal Class II with mandibular deficiency

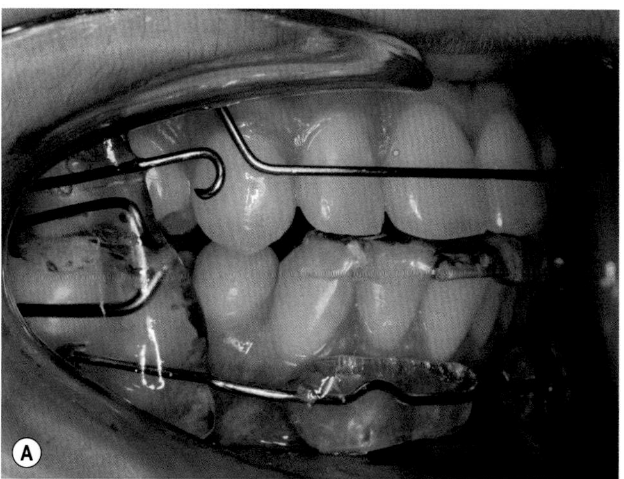

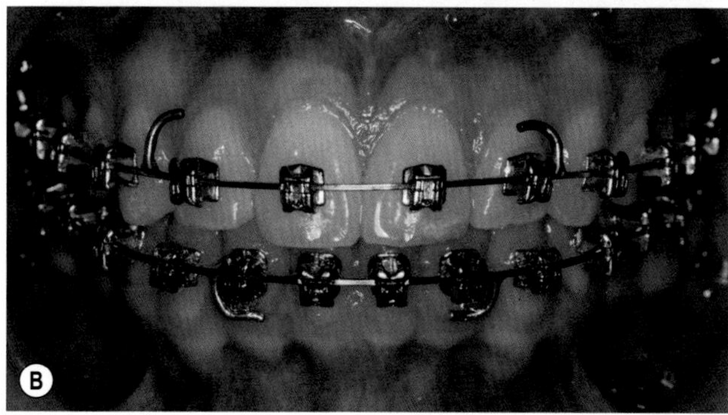

Fig. 15.9 **(A)** Case 3: mid-treatment with Frankel II. **(B)** Mid-treatment with fixed appliances.

each system; modest time-saving for tying and untying self-ligating brackets, but time saving varies with bracket design. More well-designed prospective clinical trials using identical wire sequences and mechanics are required to provide more robust data regarding self-ligating brackets.

How does distraction osteogenesis work, and what are the complication risks of mandibular midline distraction?

Based on the manipulation of a healing bone, distraction osteogenesis stretches an osteotomized site before calcification has taken place to generate formation of additional bone and investing soft tissue. As there is insufficient soft tissue in the mandibular symphyseal area to cover a bone graft necessary for widening the mandibular symphysis by orthognathic surgery, distraction affords the opportunity for formation of new bone (osteogenesis) and soft tissue (histogenesis) to create new periosteum over the distracted area. Although in concept mandibular midline distraction is basically the same as SARPE, in contrast to the maxilla no lateral surgical disjunction is performed as the mandible is not connected rigidly to the skull. Distraction of the mandible, therefore, will not be parallel but will always rotate around the condyles. Vertical cuts are made through the mandibular facial and lingual cortical plates, usually extending all the way through the symphysis. Following a 5–7-day latency period, distraction begins by turning the screw twice per day (0.5 mm) until the desired movement is achieved. The distractor may be tooth-borne or screwed to the bone; in the latter case, it is removed about 4 months post-operatively.

Complications of mandibular midline distraction, arising within 2 weeks post-operatively, are relatively rare and mainly of a mild or transient nature. Only 3% of patients experience more serious damage due to fractured incisor roots or gingival recession. Mandibular midline distraction, thus, appears a relatively safe method for expansion of the mandible.

Simon's final occlusion is shown in **Fig. 15.10**. A well-interdigitating buccal occlusion will facilitate stability of bilateral lingual crossbite correction.

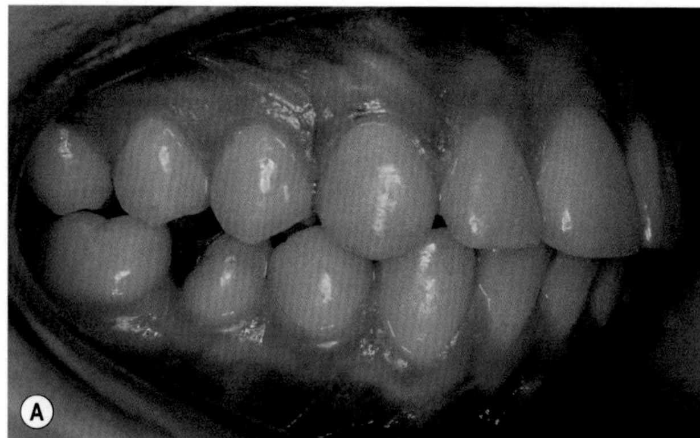
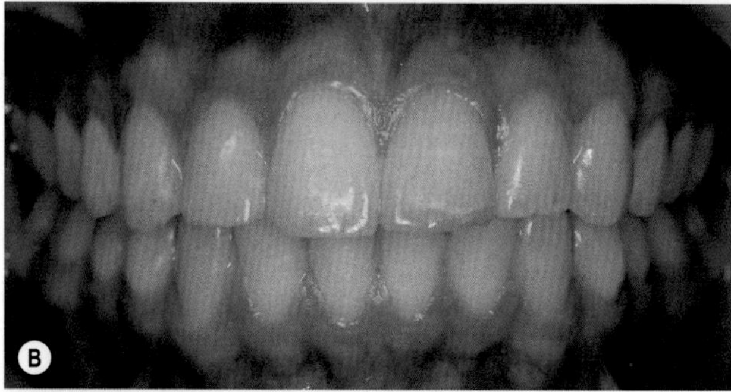
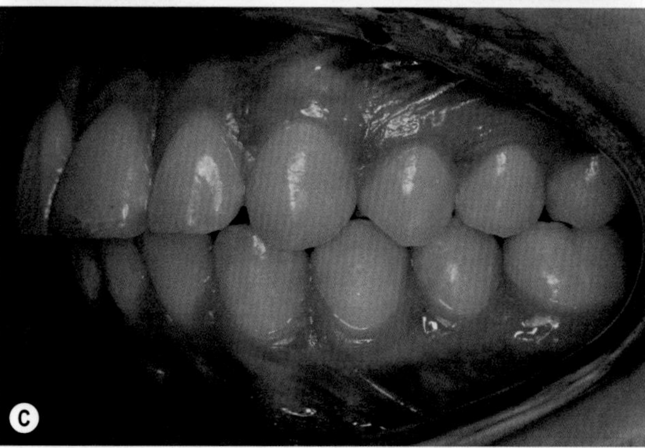

Fig. 15.10 **(A)** Case 3 post-treatment: right buccal occlusion. **(B)** Case 3 post-treatment: anterior occlusion. **(C)** Case 3 post-treatment: left buccal occlusion.

Primary resources and recommended reading

Battagel JM 1996 Obstructive sleep apnoea: fact not fiction. Br J Orthod 23:315–324.

Fleming PS, Johal A 2010 Self-ligating brackets in orthodontics: A systematic review. Angle Orthod 80:575–584.

Freeman DC, McNamara JA Jr, Baccetti T et al 2009 Long-term treatment effects of the FR-2 appliance of Frankel. Am J Orthod Dentofacial Orthop 135:570.e1–e6.

Herold JS 1989 Maxillary expansion: a retrospective study of three methods of expansion and their long-term sequelae. Br J Orthod 16:195–200.

Lagravere MO, Major PW, Flores-Mir C 2005 Long-term dental arch changes after rapid maxillary expansion treatment: a systematic review. Angle Orthod 75:155–161.

Koudstaal MJ, Poort LJ, van der Wal KG et al 2005 Surgically assisted rapid maxillary expansion (SARME): a review of the literature. Int J Oral Maxillofac Surg 34:709–714.

Magnusson A, Bjerklin K, Nilsson P et al 2009 Surgically assisted rapid maxillary expansion: long-term stability. Eur J Orthod 31:142–149.

Parekh SM, Fields HW, Beck M et al 2006 Attractiveness of variations in the smile arc and buccal corridor space as judged by orthodontists and laymen. Angle Orthod 76:557–563.

Vig KWL 1998 Nasal obstruction and facial growth: the strength of evidence for clinical assumptions. Am J Orthod Dentofacial Orthop 113:603–611.

von Bremen J, Schafer D, Kater W et al 2008 Complications of mandibular midline distraction. Angle Orthod 78:20–24.

For revision, see Mind Map 15, page 235.

16

Late lower incisor crowding

SUMMARY

Graham is almost 20 years old. He presents with crowding of his lower incisors (*Fig. 16.1*). What is the cause, and how would you treat it?

History

Complaint

Graham is concerned about the crowding of his lower front teeth and wonders if it will get worse.

History of complaint

His lower front teeth were straight until 18 months ago, when he noticed crowding developing. He now finds it more difficult to keep his lower front teeth clean. Calculus build-up also seems to occur more easily on the inside of the lower teeth, which he finds annoying. He is also aware of the two wisdom teeth erupting at the back of his lower jaw for the past 18 months. These do not cause him any problems, but he wonders if they are making his lower front teeth crooked.

Medical history

Graham is fit and well.

Dental history

Two years ago Graham had a course of fixed appliance therapy to close a large space between 1|1, followed by composite build-up of 2|2.

Examination

Extraoral examination

Graham has a Class I skeletal pattern with average FMPA and no facial asymmetry. Lips are competent. There are no signs or symptoms associated with the temporomandibular joints.

Intraoral examination

The appearance of the teeth on presentation is shown in **Figs 16.1** and **16.2**.

- ***What do you notice?***

Soft tissues appear healthy with the possible exception of mild gingival erythema related to |34 associated with slight plaque deposits; otherwise oral hygiene appears good; slight gingival recession on |4.

All lower permanent teeth present; 21|123456 visible in upper arch (note |7 was erupted).

Lower labial segment crowding with 8|8 erupting; worst incisor contact point displacement was 2.5 mm.

Upper left quadrant appears aligned.

Class I incisor relationship, although it appears to be tending towards Class III.

Left buccal segment relationship is Class III.

- ***Is development of lower incisor crowding common in the late teens?***

In modern populations, there is a strong tendency for crowding of the lower incisor teeth to develop in the late teens. This occurs even if the teeth were well aligned or spaced initially, leading usually to mild crowding, whereas

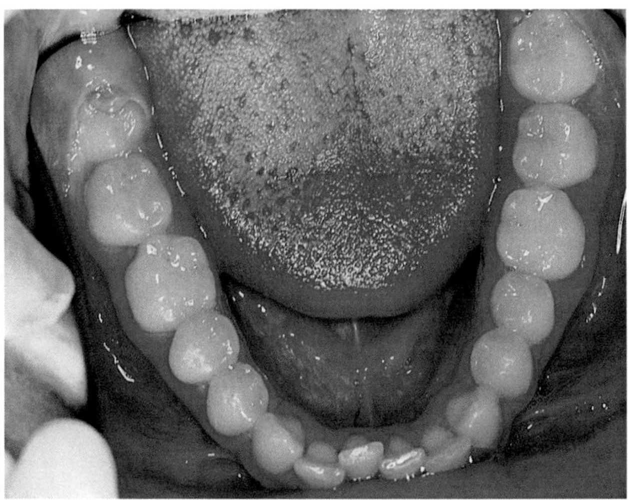

Fig. 16.1 Lower occlusal view at presentation.

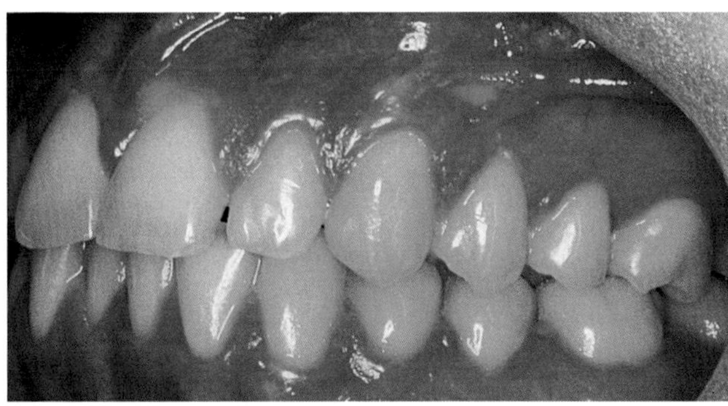

Fig. 16.2 Left buccal occlusion.

initial mild crowding tends to become worse. Lower labial segment crowding also occurs in patients in whom extractions for relief of crowding and fixed appliance therapy have been undertaken (unless a bonded lingual retainer has been placed).

■ ***What are the possible causes of late lower incisor crowding?***

The aetiology is multifactorial and the major theories proposed are as follows:

Late mandibular growth. Forward mandibular growth, especially if a growth rotation is also present, and where maxillary growth has stopped, aided by lip pressure, tends to reposition the lower incisors lingually, reducing arch length and causing anterior crowding. Currently it is thought that as the lower incisors, and perhaps the whole lower dentition, move posteriorly relative to the mandibular body late in mandibular growth, lower incisor crowding almost always develops. The greater the magnitude of late mandibular growth when other growth has essentially stopped, the greater the likelihood of developing late lower incisor crowding. On average, in a male patient, as is the case here, mandibular growth is complete by 19 years of age, but it may continue for longer.

Gingival and/or occlusal forces. Pressure from the transseptal fibres and/or the anteriorly directed component of occlusal forces lead to mesial migration of the dentition.

Lack of approximal attrition in modern diet. This was thought to explain absence of lower labial segment crowding in Australian aborigines but has not been borne out by research findings.

Reduction in intercanine width. The mandibular intercanine width reduces gradually during the teenage years, and this decrease progresses at a reduced rate into adult life. The result is an increase in lower labial segment crowding, most marked during the late teens.

The presence of third molars. Their role is controversial. Two theories abound:

- They may exert mesial pressure on the lower dentition during eruption, tending to produce lower labial segment crowding.
- They may prevent the lower teeth from moving distally in response to forces generated by mandibular growth or soft tissues.

However, late lower incisor crowding develops even when third molars are absent so their presence is not the critical factor in the aetiology of the problem. The amount of late mandibular growth is paramount.

Key point

Possible factors in the aetiology of late lower incisor crowding include:

- Late mandibular growth.
- Gingival and/or occlusal forces.
- Reduction in intercanine width.
- Third molars?

Investigations

■ ***What investigations would you undertake? Explain why.***

Radiographic

A dental panoramic tomogram would be useful to assess the position and inclination of the partially erupted lower third molars. As a radiograph was taken prior to commencing orthodontic treatment, this should be consulted first, and the need for a further radiograph should be assessed based on the clinical assessment and the radiographic findings.

Study models

Upper and lower impressions and a wax registration in centric occlusion should be taken for study models to record accurately the current malocclusion and to aid further treatment planning.

■ ***What do you notice on the dental panoramic tomogram taken pre-orthodontic treatment (Fig. 16.3)?***

Normal alveolar bone height.

All teeth present and of good quality.

$\overline{8|}$ is slightly mesioangularly impacted.

$\overline{|8}$ is upright.

Bone overlies the distal half of the crown of both lower third molars.

Diagnosis

■ ***What is your diagnosis?***

Class I malocclusion on a Class I skeletal base with average FMPA.

Lower incisor crowding.

Impacted third molars.

Left buccal segment relationship is Class III.

■ ***What is the IOTN DHC grade (see p. 264)? Explain why.***

3d – based on the 2.5 mm worst contact point displacement between the lower incisor teeth.

■ ***What are the management options for late lower incisor crowding?***

Accept and monitor. As this is a normal maturational change in the lower arch, it would be sensible in a late teenager, and

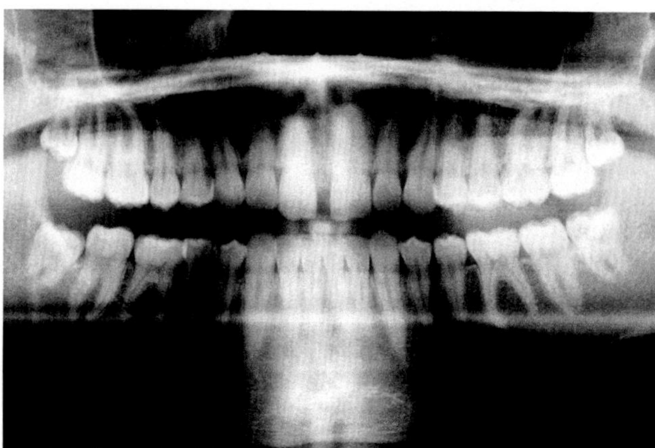

Fig. 16.3 Dental panoramic tomogram.

where the crowding is mild, to keep it under observation. Where more marked crowding is present, intervention may be considered.

Interproximal stripping. This is only acceptable in an adult with *mild* lower incisor crowding. By removing 0.25 mm at most from the mesial and distal aspects of each incisor, up to 2 mm of space can be obtained for relief of crowding. Incisor alignment may then be achieved by either a sectional fixed appliance or a removable appliance. For ultimate aesthetics, a lingual fixed appliance may be used. A removable appliance clasped on the first permanent molars, with an acrylated labial bow or Invisalign® (a clear vacuum-formed thermoplastic aligner) made to fit a duplicate study model with the incisors aligned with their mesial and distal surfaces reduced, are alternative approaches. With Invisalign®, however, several appliances will be required to achieve incremental change (~0.25–0.3 mm per aligner worn for about 20 hours per day and changed about every 2 weeks) until the final alignment has been realized. A bonded retainer will be required to maintain the result long term.

Aside from enhanced aesthetics, are there other advantages of lingual appliances?

Tooth position is easier to discern, as the labial crown is clearly visible. There is also no risk of labial enamel demineralization. There are, however, some shortcomings of lingual orthodontics and clear aligner therapy; these are given in Chapter 18, page 112.

Extraction of a lower incisor. Where the lower labial crowding is marked, removal of a lower incisor may be indicated to give sufficient space for alignment of the remaining units. It is advisable to carry out a diagnostic wax-up on a duplicate set of study models to ascertain what the final result is likely to be and to ensure the patient is happy with this before proceeding with the extraction. Unless the incisor to be extracted is completely excluded from the arch and the remaining incisors are well aligned, fixed appliance therapy is inevitably indicated to detail the position of the remaining labial segment teeth. Bonded lingual retention will then be required.

Are there any possible undesirable effects from extraction of one permanent lower incisor?

The patient should be warned of the possibility of two undesirable sequelae: the upper labial segment moving palatally, with resultant misalignment, in response to the lower labial segment being aligned slightly lingually and/or a slight increase in overjet.

Extraction of lower premolars. Where the buccal segment occlusion is well interdigitated and crowding is confined to the lower labial segment, it is preferable to avoid lower mid-arch extractions because these will disrupt the buccal occlusion. Instead removal of a lower incisor will expedite lower labial segment alignment while preserving the integrity of the buccal segments.

Would you advise removal of the lower third molars?

Lower third molars should not be removed in an attempt to prevent further increase in lower labial segment crowding, as their relation to this aspect of malocclusion is unproven.

Current guidelines advise removal of lower third molars only if they are associated with recurrent episodes of pericoronitis or other pathology. In this case, as neither of these apply at present, the lower third molars should be retained and their position reviewed if symptoms develop.

Key point

Management options for late lower incisor crowding:

- Accept and monitor.
- Interproximal stripping with appliance therapy.
- Lower incisor extraction with appliance therapy.

How would you manage the lower incisor crowding?

As the lower labial segment crowding is mild, Graham should be advised to accept it for the present. It should be kept under review, and if the crowding increases, consideration could be given to treatment.

The eruption of the lower third molars should be monitored.

Primary resources and recommended reading

Dacre JT 1985 The long-term effects of one lower incisor extraction. Eur J Orthod 7:136–144.

Ghaeminia H, Perry J, Nienhuijs MEL et al 2016 Surgical removal versus retention for the management of asymptomatic disease-free impacted wisdom teeth. Cochrane Database of Syst Rev Issue 8. Art No: CD003879. DOI:10.1002/14651858.CD003879.pub4.

Harradine NW, Pearson MH, Toth B 1998 The effect of extraction of third molars on late lower incisor crowding: a randomized controlled trial. Br J Orthod 25:117–122.

Little RM, Riedel RA, Artun J 1988 An evaluation of changes in mandibular anterior alignment from 10 to 20 years postretention. Am J Orthod Dentofacial Orthop 93:423–428.

NHS Centre for Reviews and Dissemination, York 1999 Prophylactic removal of impacted third molars: is it justified? Br J Orthod 26:149–151.

Richardson ME 2002 Late lower arch crowding: the aetiology reviewed. Dent Update 29:234–238.

For revision, see Mind Map 16, page 236.

17

Prominent chin and TMJDS

SUMMARY

Jocelyn, aged 23, is referred by her general dental practitioner because of her prominent chin (*Fig. 17.1*) and pain in her left temporomandibular joint (TMJ). What are the causes and how would you manage these problems?

History

Complaint

Jocelyn's main concern is that she does not like the prominent appearance of her chin and her upper teeth biting inside her lower teeth. She has pain in her left jaw joint and has some difficulty chewing. She is also aware that she has a lisp, which she dislikes.

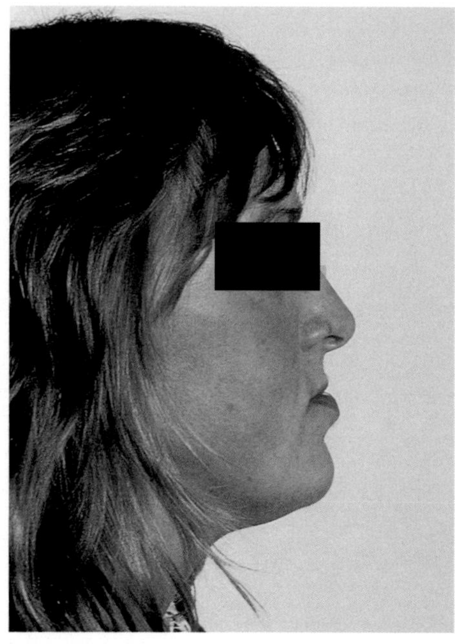

Fig. 17.1 Profile at presentation.

History of complaint

Jocelyn has been more aware of her prominent chin and her bite since she was in her last year at school. After consultation with an orthodontist at age 12, she had two upper teeth removed to provide space for the upper eye teeth (she had both lower first permanent molars extracted at age 8 because of decay.) She did not wear any braces on her teeth. She was advised to wait until she was in her late teens to have the bite of her front teeth reassessed. In the past 6 months she has become quite self-conscious about her facial appearance, although she feels that her chin does not appear to have become more prominent in the past 4 years.

■ ***What questions would you ask about the temporomandibular joint pain?***

When and how the pain started.

Type and duration of pain.

Frequency.

Is it localized? Site of radiation.

Associated symptoms, e.g. muscle pain, click, jaw locking, trismus.

Aggravating factors, e.g. stress.

Any habits, e.g. nail-biting, bruxism, pen-chewing.

Relieving factors, e.g. heat, analgesics (type and amount).

The pain started suddenly when Jocelyn was preparing for examinations in her first year at university. She has had intermittent discomfort in her left jaw joint since then, but it has been of a mild nature. The discomfort is an ache that is principally in the left jaw joint area but radiates to the jaw muscles on that side. It does not keep her awake at night, but she feels it is worse in the morning. Typically it lasts for a few hours and then disappears. It tends to return when Jocelyn is stressed by work. She is aware of grinding her teeth when stressed. She does not engage in chewing pencils or pens or nail-biting. She feels that in the past year the pain has recurred more frequently and has become worse. Chewing hard food or opening her mouth too wide makes the pain worse; one or two paracetamol tablets usually relieves the ache. Jocelyn is also aware that she has a jaw click.

Medical history

Jocelyn is fit and well.

Dental history

Jocelyn is a regular attender at her general dental practitioner and brushes twice daily.

Family history

Jocelyn's sister also has a prominent chin, but not as marked as hers, and her sister's bite was corrected with fixed braces.

Examination

Extraoral examination

■ ***What do you observe from Jocelyn's profile view (*Fig. 17.1*)?***

Class III skeletal pattern with average FMPA. Competent lips.

■ ***Based on the history, what other aspects would you assess extraorally?***

Temporomandibular joints. Opening and lateral mandibular movements should be assessed by first observing the patient from the front and second by palpation of the condylar heads while listening for the presence of crepitus or a joint click. As symptoms are present, the masticatory muscles should also be palpated. A left TMJ click and left masseteric tenderness were detected.

Mandibular path of closure. The path of closure from rest position to maximum interdigitation should be assessed, noting any anterior or lateral mandibular displacement produced by a premature contact.

In this case there is an anterior mandibular displacement on closure on contact of $\frac{7|}{8|}$ (centric relation to occlusion shift of ~3 mm).

Intraoral examination

The intraoral views are shown in **Fig. 17.2**.

■ ***What do you see?***

Gingival tissues appear healthy; gingival recession related to $\dfrac{63\,|\,356}{7\,|\quad}$.

Oral hygiene appears overall good, apart from slight plaque deposit on $\underline{|3}$ $\dfrac{765321\,|\,12356}{8754321\,|\,123457}$ are visible.

No obvious caries.

Very mild lower incisor crowding with spacing between the $\overline{4}$'s and $\overline{5}$'s.

Very mild upper arch crowding with slight mesiolabial rotations of $\underline{2|2}$.

Class III incisor relationship with reverse overjet (measured 4 mm clinically), reduced overbite and coincident dental centrelines.

Class I canine relationship bilaterally.

Buccal crossbite affecting $\frac{7|}{8|}$.

■ ***What is the most likely cause of the considerable spacing in the lower premolar areas with $\overline{5}$'s drifted into contact with $\overline{7}$'s?***

Early removal of $\overline{6E|E6}$ in an uncrowded arch is the most likely explanation for the spacing. An uncrowded lower arch is common in Class III malocclusion.

■ ***What occlusal features may predispose to temporomandibular joint dysfunction syndrome?***

Crossbites, Class III malocclusion and anterior open bite have been shown to have a significant association with temporomandibular joint dysfunction syndrome (TMJDS) in some studies while others have found no link between signs and symptoms of TMJDS and mandibular displacement. The aetiology of TMJDS is multifactorial with the implicated involvement of psychological, traumatic and occlusal elements. The most salient factor is probably stress,

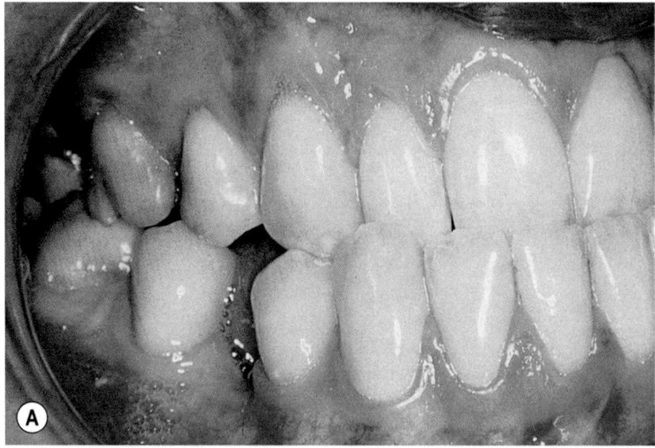

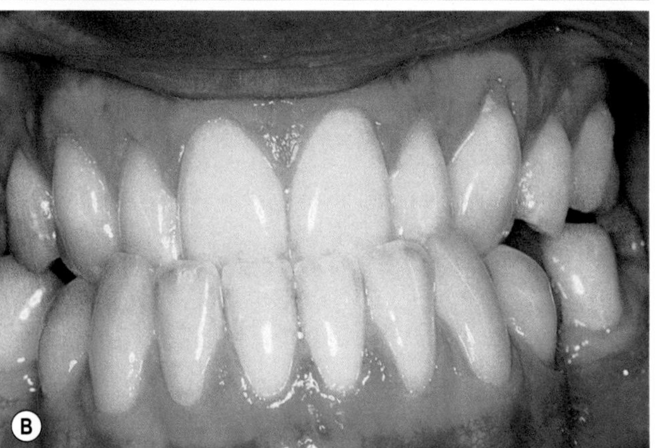

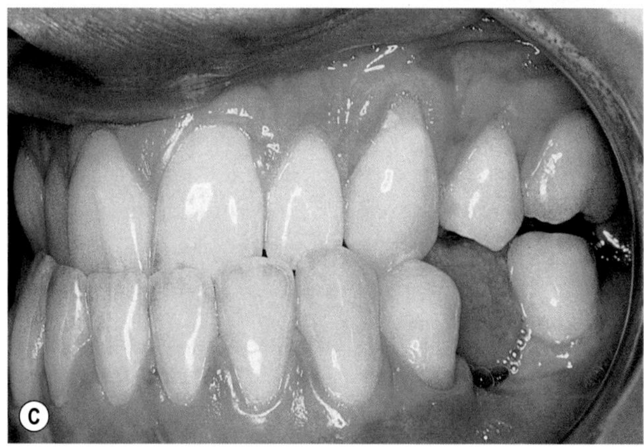

Fig. 17.2 **(A)** Right buccal occlusion. **(B)** Anterior occlusion. **(C)** Left buccal occlusion.

which may transmit its effect by a parafunctional habit, stemming from a displacing occlusal contact in susceptible individuals. In this case a displacement exists on $\frac{7|}{8|}$ on closure. There are also anterior and posterior crossbites present.

■ ***Why was Jocelyn advised to wait until her late teens for reassessment?***

In a Class III malocclusion, the amount of reverse overjet tends to increase with forward mandibular growth during teenage years. Waiting until mandibular growth is essentially completed, which is generally about 17 years of age in girls and 19 years of age in boys, has three advantages. First, it allows treatment planning to be undertaken with reasonably stable facial and occlusal characteristics. Second, if treatment is undertaken, it safeguards against relapse due to further growth. Third, the magnitude of occlusal change due to mandibular growth influences whether treatment can be undertaken by orthodontic means alone or whether a combined orthodontic-surgical approach is necessary. Orthodontic treatment involves inducing dentoalveolar compensation for the underlying skeletal pattern, but if unsuccessful due to continued adverse mandibular growth, the compensation would need to be undone as part of pre-surgical orthodontics. This may involve opening up lower premolar extraction spaces. Hence the decision to treat a Class III malocclusion in early teenage years by orthodontic camouflage that includes lower arch extractions must be made with great caution.

In this case the severity of the anteroposterior skeletal pattern, the likely pattern of mandibular growth, the amount of dentoalveolar compensation, the amount of overbite and the relative absence of crowding (following the removal of upper first premolars and lower first permanent molars) would all have been considerations in delaying any further orthodontic intervention. Whether the patient could achieve an edge-to-edge incisor relationship would also need to have been assessed.

Key point

Waiting until at least the late teens before considering an orthodontic-surgical approach is desirable, as:

- Facial and occlusal characteristics stabilize.
- It safeguards against relapse due to further growth.
- Camouflage or surgery is determined by the extent of mandibular growth.

Investigations

What investigations are required and why?

The patient's primary concern is about her facial appearance, and she has a malocclusion which is likely to be untreatable by orthodontic means alone. A combined orthodontic-surgical approach is required. The investigations required, in such cases, together with reasons for their selection, are listed in **Table 17.1**. If possible, three-dimensional (3D) facial images, at rest and smiling, should also be recorded at this stage to act as a baseline from which to monitor robustly the 3D facial changes produced by surgery and during subsequent follow-up. Similarly, if feasible, cone beam computed tomography (CBCT) may be undertaken.

- The TMJ assessment has already been undertaken for Jocelyn (p. 103).
- The dental panoramic tomogram showed no condylar pathology.

Table 17.1 Investigations required in combined orthodontic-surgical planning*

Investigation required	Reason
Thorough clinical assessment of facial form in full face and profile	To locate any cranial, maxillary, nasal, mandibular or chin deformities
	To assess the height and width proportions of the face, interalar distance, nasolabial angle, upper incisor exposure, relation of upper dental midline to other facial midlines, the form and tone of the soft tissues
Assessment of TMJ	To record signs and/or symptoms of TMJ dysfunction. Treat these conservatively if possible prior to treatment; if marked occlusal problems contributing to dysfunction, aim to correct these with treatment
Dental panoramic tomogram (DPT)	To assess the general dental status and prognosis of the dentition as well as the position of unerupted third molars (bitewing or periapical radiographs may be required depending on clinical and/or DPT findings)
Lateral cephalometric radiograph	To ascertain the aetiology of the malocclusion and to facilitate surgical planning
Facial and dental photographs	To record the facial and dental characteristics of the malocclusion
	To allow surgical planning by matching the digital profile facial image with the lateral cephalometric tracing
Study models and duplicates mounted on an articulator	To allow thorough orthodontic/occlusal assessment and model surgery

*Three-dimensional (3D) facial images, where possible, and when combined with cone beam computed tomography, allow 3D surgical planning, although further development is required to optimize this.

The cephalometric values are as follows:

SNA = 79°; SNB = 85°; ANB = –6°; $\underline{1}$ to maxillary plane = 113°; $\overline{1}$ to mandibular plane = 82°; interincisal angle = 139°; MMPA = 26.5°; SN to maxillary plane = 11°; facial proportion = 56%.

What is your interpretation of these findings (see p. 270)?

Moderately severe Class III skeletal pattern due to a combination of maxillary retrognathia and mandibular prognathism. As SNA is 2° less than the mean of 81°, application of the Eastman correction adds 1° to the ANB to give a revised ANB value of –5°.

Slightly proclined upper incisors (although inclination is within the normal range) and markedly retroclined lower incisors indicating dentoalveolar compensation for the Class III skeletal pattern. The lower incisor angle should be 120° – 26.5° = 93.5° but is 82°.

Interincisal angle is increased but within the normal range for Caucasians.

MMPA, SN to maxillary plane and facial proportion are all slightly out of the mean values but lie within the normal range for Caucasians.

Diagnosis

■ ***What is your diagnosis?***

Class III malocclusion on a Class III skeletal base with average FMPA.

TMJDS with left TMJ click.

Gingival recession on $\underline{63|356}$ and $\overline{7|}$.

Previous loss of $\overline{6}$'s and $\underline{4}$'s.

Very mild upper and lower labial segment crowding.

All of the upper arch in crossbite with the exception of $\underline{65|56}$.

Buccal crossbite on $\frac{7|}{8|}$ with associated mandibular displacement.

■ ***What is the IOTN DHC grade (see p. 264)? Explain why.***

5 m – due to reverse overjet greater than 3.5 mm with reported masticatory and speech difficulties.

Treatment

■ ***What are the aims of treatment?***

- Relief of the TMJDS.
- Control of the gingival recession.
- Correction of the underlying skeletal Class III problem.
- Establish Class I incisor and molar relationships.
- Correct the buccal segment crossbites.
- Restore the lower buccal segment spaces.

■ ***What treatment is required? Explain why.***

A combined orthodontic-surgical-restorative approach is needed due to:

The patient's concern relating to facial and dental appearance.

The severity of the underlying Class III skeletal pattern.

Despite the degree of dentoalveolar compensation, a reverse overjet of 4 mm exists.

An ANB angle of greater than –4° and lower incisor angulation to the mandibular plane of less than 83° have been found indicative of an orthodontic-surgical approach.

Pre-surgical lower arch decompensation will open up more space between the premolars and then require restorative management to optimize the final occlusion.

In addition, lower incisor decompensation may run the risk of creating gingival recession, particularly as Jocelyn already has several teeth affected by minor gingival recession. A specialist periodontal opinion should be sought before embarking on pre-surgical orthodontics.

It was decided that the spacing in the lower buccal segments would be managed by resin-retained bridgework following uprighting of the premolars. The periodontist advised Jocelyn to adjust her toothbrushing technique, and she was given appropriate oral hygiene instruction aimed to prevent any deterioration in the areas affected by gingival recession. A pre-treatment gingival graft to the lower incisors was not deemed necessary; maintenance of good oral hygiene practices during orthodontic appliance therapy was emphasized. Periodontal review was arranged 6 months into orthodontic treatment.

■ ***How will this case be managed?***

Short term A hard full coverage upper acrylic splint should be made, and Jocelyn should be instructed to wear this full-time until the TMJ symptoms subside. She should also be advised to take a soft diet and to avoid straining her jaw joints by, for example, yawning widely. Mild analgesics should also be taken as required.

Longer term A combined orthodontic-surgical-restorative approach is required to correct the facial and occlusal problems. The TMJDS symptoms may ease with orthodontic treatment. This is due to tooth movement rendering the teeth tender on biting, so parafunctional activity stops because tooth clenching/grinding does not produce the same subconscious pleasure as previously. The improvement in symptoms may be transient, even if displacing occlusal contacts (present here on $\frac{7|}{8|}$) are eliminated.

The patient should be warned about the unpredictable impact of orthognathic surgery on TMJDS to avoid unreasonable expectations of treatment.

Key point

Orthodontic treatment and/or orthognathic surgery cannot be guaranteed to eliminate TMJDS.

■ ***Explain how you would proceed with surgical planning for this case.***

1. A team approach is required involving the orthodontist and the oral and maxillofacial surgeon. The input of a restorative specialist is also required in relation to management of the lower premolar spacing. The involvement of a clinical psychologist with an interest in orthognathic surgical cases would also be helpful. Jocelyn must understand that to obtain the best facial and occlusal result possible, fixed appliance therapy is essential to the overall plan.
2. Surgical planning may be undertaken by various means. To provide information about the inter-relationships of the dentofacial complex components, namely the cranium and cranial base, nasomaxillary complex and maxillary dentition, mandible and related dentition, specialized cephalometric analyses exist. These allow comparison of individual cephalometric data with 'normal' data that should be matched for age, gender and racial background. Computer programs then allow surgical, skeletal and dental movements to be planned and displayed visually on screen before printing.
3. By linking the patient's digital profile image with the cephalometric tracing, specialized planning software can

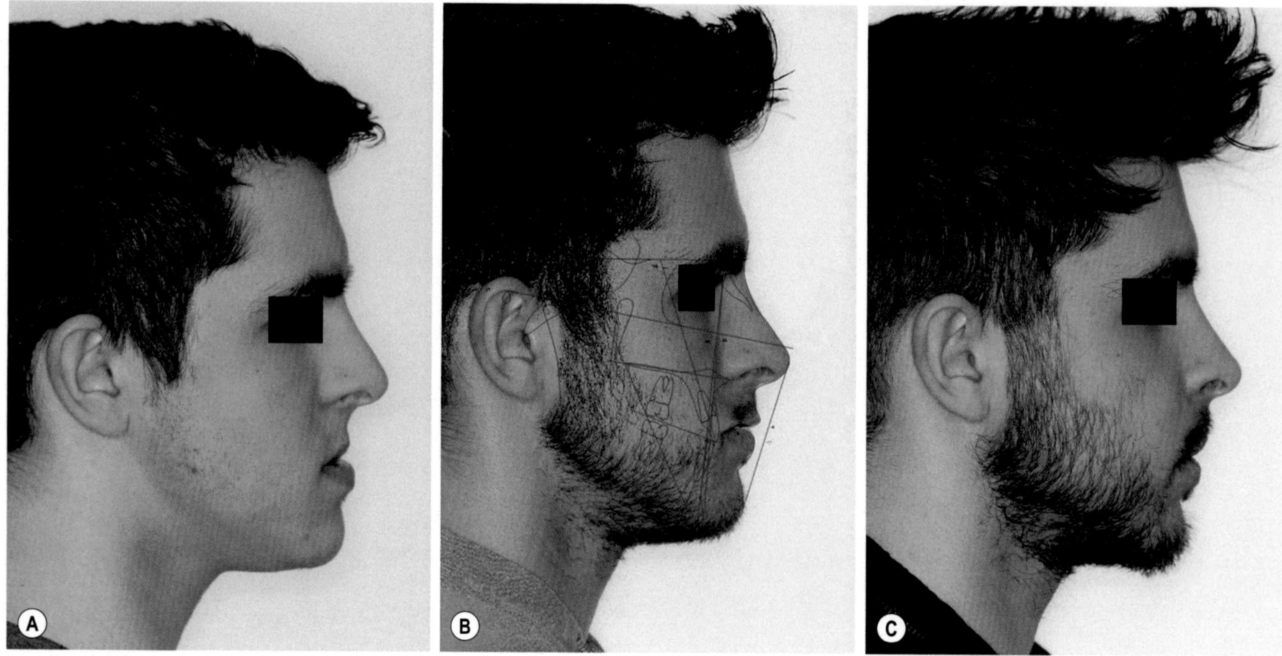

Fig. 17.3 Another case: **(A)** Pre-treatment: profile. **(B)** Super-imposition of lateral cephalometric radiograph tracing on a digital profile view and morphing using Dolphin® software to simulate the post-treatment profile. **(C)** Post-treatment: profile.

automatically morph the image in response to planned surgical and orthodontic movement undertaken virtually on the computer. The likelihood of different treatment options can thus be explored. In addition, the patient can view the final computerized prediction to appreciate more clearly the possible likely outcome on profile aesthetics, although it should be understood that this is not guaranteed (**Figs 17.3A–C**). Using reference lines to measure distances, planned surgical movements should then be transferred to a duplicate set of study models, mounted on a semi-adjustable articulator in this case as maxillary surgery is planned. The ability to plan orthognathic surgery in 3D (superimposing 3D facial images and CBCT scans) is being developed and offers exciting possibilities.

4. The final plan should be explained to Jocelyn, ensuring that she is aware that her profile will be worsened by pre-surgical orthodontics and that she realizes what her final facial appearance is likely to be. Provision of an information leaflet and DVD on orthognathic surgery will also assist in recognizing the full consequences of what treatment involves and are an important part of obtaining informed consent.

Key point

Planning orthodontic-surgical treatment:

- Requires a team approach.
- May be assisted by matching the digital facial profile image with the lateral cephalometric tracing and using computer prediction software.

Describe the phase of pre-surgical orthodontics.

This phase of fixed appliance treatment aims to allow the jaws to be moved to their desired location without interference from tooth positions. The upper and lower arches are aligned and coordinated as well as establishing the vertical and anteroposterior position of the incisors. This involves decompensating for any existing dentoalveolar compensation. For Jocelyn, this will involve primarily labial movement of the lower incisors, which will eliminate the mild crowding and slight uprighting of the upper incisors. The full extent of the skeletal discrepancy is thus revealed, maximizing the extent of possible surgical correction. Class II intermaxillary traction may be required to aid decompensation. No extractions are indicated in this case to achieve the desired tooth movements. The gingival status, labial to the lower incisors, should be monitored during decompensation to ensure that gingival recession does not ensue.

When the requisite tooth movements have been achieved, rigid rectangular stainless steel archwires should be used to passively stabilize tooth position. Final pre-surgical records – study models, photographs and a cephalometric film – will then be taken to assess the changes that have occurred and to decide if the original surgical plan will be followed or require some amendment. Hooks should be attached to the archwires just prior to surgery unless brackets with an integrated hook on each tooth have been used. The hooks facilitate intermaxillary fixation and/or elastic traction post-operatively.

What surgical procedures are likely to be required?

Le Fort I advancement.

Mandibular setback.

Key point

Pre-surgical orthodontics:

- May involve extractions.
- Usually involves decompensation for any dentoalveolar compensation.
- Aligns and coordinates arches or arch segments.
- Establishes the vertical and anteroposterior position of the incisors.
- Place rigid rectangular archwires with ball-hooks (unless brackets with integrated hooks are used) immediately pre-surgically.

What form of splint and fixation is likely to be required?

An interocclusal acrylic wafer, fabricated to fit articulator mounted casts positioned to the desired occlusal result, is recommended routinely to ensure accuracy of the post-surgical result. Following Le Fort I advancement and mandibular setback osteotomies, mini-plates and mini-plates/screws are likely to be required respectively for fixation. Intermaxillary elastics then direct the teeth into the required position and assist with jaw function.

Describe the post-surgical orthodontic phase.

With some mild jaw exercises, mouth opening is usually satisfactory within a few weeks. Lighter, round stainless steel archwires should then be placed to allow for occlusal settling, often aided by the use of posterior box elastics with a slight anterior force vector, which helps maintain the sagittal correction. When good interdigitation has been achieved, elastic wear should be discontinued. Rarely will this phase of treatment take longer than 6 months to complete. A period of retention is then required, no different from that for other adults who have completed routine orthodontic treatment. Surgical follow-up should be for a minimum of 2 years.

What factors influence post-surgical stability?

Stability will be influenced by:

- Orthodontic and surgical plans being correct, realistic, well-integrated and undertaken competently.
- Modest surgical movement – no greater than 6 mm in any direction in the maxilla or 8 mm in the mandible. This does not place the soft tissues under tension, and the condyles are not distracted at surgery.
- Absence of tongue thrust, previous surgical scarring.
- Patient compliance with all aspects of treatment, particularly post-surgical wear of elastic traction.
- Adequate fixation.
- The post-surgical profile and occlusion are shown in **Fig. 17.4**.

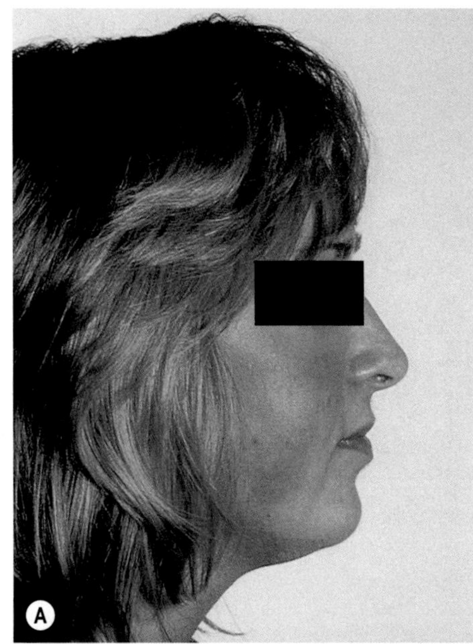

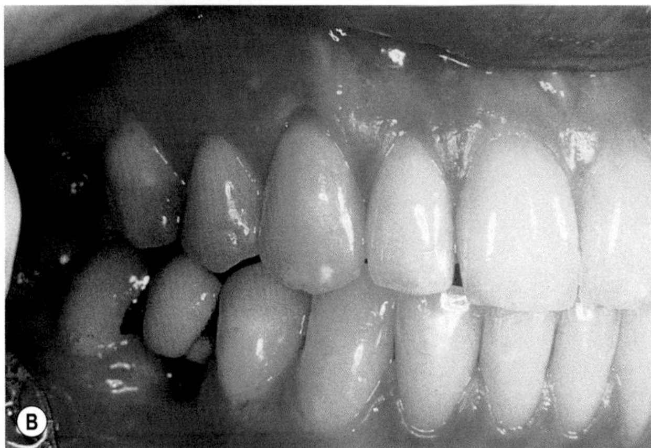

Fig. 17.4 **(A)** Post-treatment: profile. **(B)** Post-treatment: occlusion.

Key point

Stability is enhanced when surgical movement is modest and does not induce soft tissue tension.

Primary resources and recommended reading

British Orthodontic Society 2012 Temporomandibular Disorders (TMDS) and the Orthodontic Patient. Advice sheet. British Orthodontic Society, London.

Cevidanes LHC, Tucker S, Styner M et al 2010 Three-dimensional surgical simulation. Am J Orthod Dentofacial Orthop 138:36–371.

Hajeer MY, Millett DT, Ayoub AF et al 2004 Applications of 3D imaging in orthodontics: Part II. J Orthod 31:154–162.

Hunt NP, Rudge SJ 1984 Facial profile and orthognathic surgery. Br J Orthod 11:126–136.

Luther F 2007 TMD and occlusion part I. Damned if we do? Occlusion: the interface of dentistry and orthodontics; TMD and occlusion part II. Damned if we don't? Functional occlusal problems: TMD epidemiology in a wider context. Br Dent J 202:E2, Br Dent J 202:E3.

Proffit WR, White R, Sarver D 2003 Contemporary Treatment of Dentofacial Deformity. Mosby, St Louis.

Ryan F, Shute J, Cedro M et al 2011 A new style of orthognathic clinic. J Orthod 38:124–133.

For revision, see Mind Map 17, page 237.

18

Drifting incisors

SUMMARY

Iain, a 51-year-old man, presents with spacing and mobility of his upper incisors (*Fig. 18.1*). What is the cause, and what can be done?

History

Complaint

Iain complains of the spacing of his upper front teeth and looseness of all his front teeth, particularly of 2| and |2. He is self-conscious of the spacing and is worried in case his front teeth fall out.

History of complaint

He has noticed increasing mobility of his upper front teeth over the past few months. The spacing between the teeth appeared at the same time and is becoming progressively worse. There is no pain associated with the mobility of the teeth, but eating has become uncomfortable. He is also aware of mobility of his lower front teeth and of several upper and lower back teeth. Recently he has experienced an unpleasant taste in his mouth, which appears to be derived from the upper front teeth.

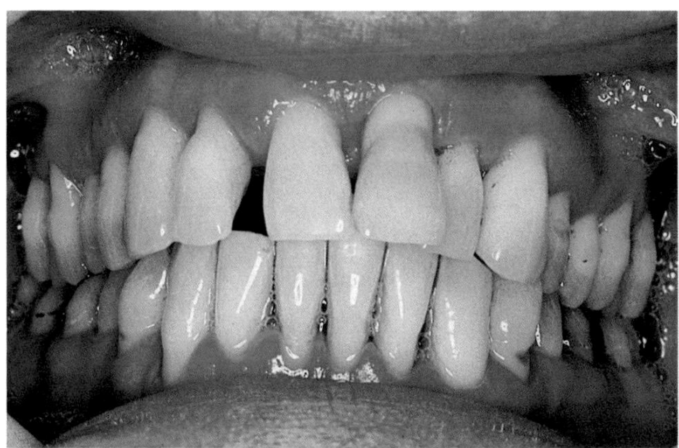

Fig. 18.1 Occlusion at presentation.

Dental history

Iain has been a regular attender at another dental practice for many years before moving to your area. He is highly motivated and does not wish any tooth to be lost. |1 was traumatized in his early twenties and has become progressively darker, but he is unconcerned by this. Iain had orthodontic treatment with fixed appliances as a teenager because his upper and lower teeth were crooked. No teeth were extracted, and he wore removable retainers for 1 year (6 months full-time and 6 months part-time) following treatment. After he stopped wearing the retainers, his bite changed and his orthodontist said it was due was due to his lower jaw growing more.

Medical history

Iain has diabetes which is well controlled by insulin. He is otherwise fit and well.

Social history

Iain smokes 10 cigarettes a day and has done so for 30 years.

Examination

Extraoral

There are no palpable submandibular or cervical lymph nodes.

Intraoral

■ ***What do you notice in* Figs 18.1 *and* 18.2*?***

Oral hygiene appears fair with generalized interproximal staining. Interdental gingivae related to the lower central and lateral incisors appears slightly oedematous.

Generalized gingival recession.

Heavily restored dentition with |1 discoloured.

7654321 present in all quadrants; 8 also in lower right quadrant.

Mild lower incisor crowding.

Uncrowded upper arch with incisor spacing.

Class III incisor relationship with minimal overbite and overjet except for 2|1; upper and lower centrelines are not coincident.

Class I molar relationship bilaterally.

■ ***Based on what you know so far, what are the possible factors implicated with respect to mobility and drifting of 21|12?***

Chronic periodontal disease is a definite possibility when the overall periodontal condition is observed.

Periapical periodontitis is another possibility, but this would also tend to lead to extrusion of these teeth, which is not markedly evident.

Root resorption. This would have to be extensive to produce such spacing and mobility.

Root fractures. This is not a possibility in view of the history.

Other pathology such as radicular cyst or bony lesions are rarer possibilities.

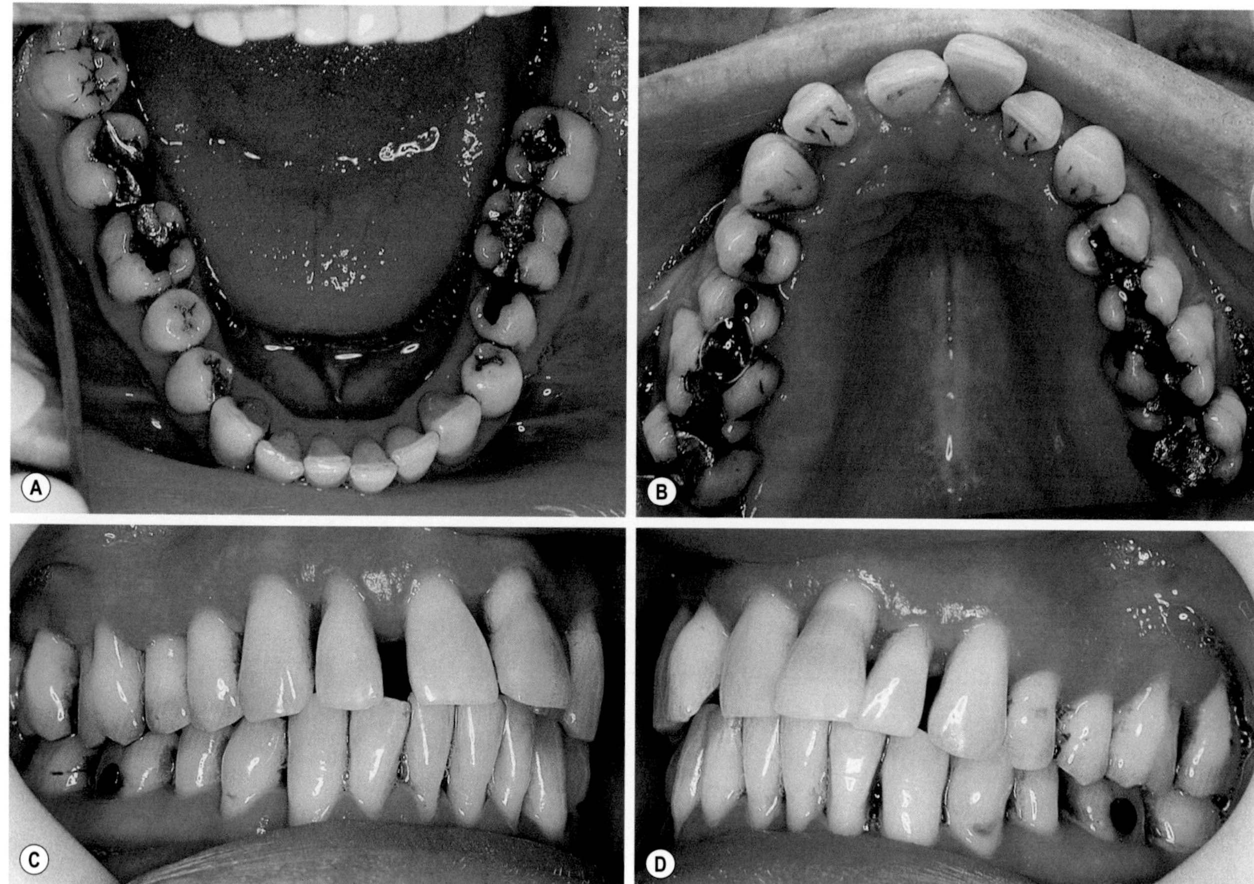

Fig. 18.2 **(A)** Lower occlusal view. **(B)** Upper occlusal view. **(C)** Right buccal occlusion. **(D)** Left buccal occlusion.

■ ***What would you check for specifically in relation to the history?***

Degree of any tooth mobility.

Presence, extent and location of plaque and/or supragingival/subgingival calculus deposits.

Presence/site of bleeding on probing.

Presence/site of periodontal purulent exudate.

Presence/site of a sinus and/or associated exudate.

Presence/site of any deep carious lesion.

Occlusal factors that may contribute to tooth mobility, e.g. displacing occlusal contacts and/or a bruxing habit.

Other habits, e.g. pen-chewing, nail-biting.

Calculus is present subgingivally on all teeth with generalized 4–6-mm pocketing and delayed bleeding on probing. There is a purulent discharge from the periodontal pocket on the mesial aspect of 2⌋. No sinuses are present. There are no carious teeth.

Upper and lower molars, premolars and canines exhibit grade I mobility buccolingually but not vertically. Upper and lower incisors have grade I mobility buccolingually but *not* vertically except for ⌈2, which exhibits grade II mobility buccolingually and vertically.

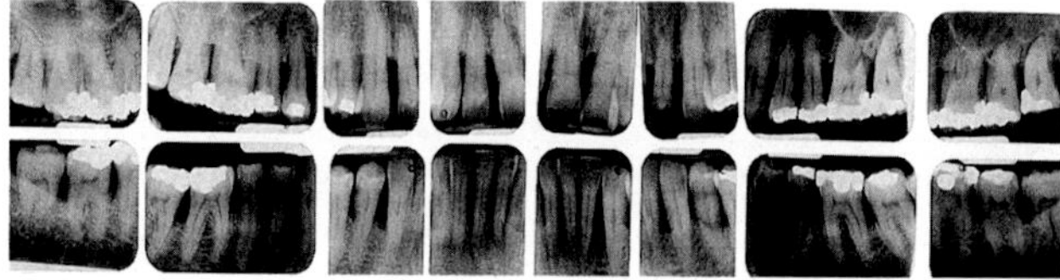

Fig. 18.3 Full-mouth periapical radiographs.

lain has right and left group function in lateral excursions. There are no occlusal interferences in protrusion. There is no bruxism, pen-chewing or nail-biting habit.

Investigations

■ ***What other investigations would you carry out? Why?***

Full-mouth periapical radiographs are required to assess accurately the periodontal status, particularly the alveolar bone height as well as the presence of any periapical pathology.

■ ***Full-mouth periapical radiographs are shown in** Fig. 18.3**. What do you see?***

Generalized horizontal bone loss of at least 50% with angular bone defects affecting $\begin{array}{c|c} 2 & 1 \\ \hline 63 & 26 \end{array}$.

70–80% alveolar bone loss affecting the lower incisor teeth.

Heavily restored dentition, but no caries visible.

Diagnosis

■ ***What is your diagnosis?***

Chronic moderate periodontitis with localized areas of advanced disease.

Class III malocclusion with mild lower incisor crowding and spacing/drifting of the upper incisors.

Upper and lower centreline shifts.

Buccal segment relationship is Class I bilaterally.

■ ***With loss of periodontal attachment, how may labial drifting of the incisors occur?***

Alveolar bone loss compromises the ability of the teeth to deal with soft tissue and occlusal forces, thereby leading to tooth movement.

A traumatic occlusion may result from extrusion as a consequence of periodontal disease. Drifting may occur where periodontal support is also reduced.

Labial shift of periodontally involved upper incisors may result also from a displacing occlusal contact on closure producing a forward mandibular slide.

Undue forces may be placed on the incisors, where posterior tooth support is lacking due to tooth loss, and these can lead to upper incisor proclination.

> **Key point**
>
> Migration of periodontally involved incisors may be exacerbated by:
>
> - A forward mandibular displacement on closure.
> - Deficient posterior occlusal support.

■ ***What is the significance of the medical history and social history to the diagnosis?***

Diabetes affects the host response to periodontal pathogens by altering polymorph chemotaxis. Although Iain's diabetes is well controlled, periodontal disease is chronic and generalized due to inadequate oral hygiene measures aggravated by the host response.

Smoking contributes significantly to periodontal disease through a variety of means. Gingival blood flow is reduced; salivary flow is slowed also, leading to poorer removal of periodontopathic bacteria and encouraging calculus build-up.

Treatment

■ ***What treatment would you advise?***

Cessation of smoking. The patient should be encouraged to stop smoking to prevent any further insult to his periodontal health imposed by this habit.

Referral for joint periodontal/orthodontic consultation. Iain's condition requires specialist care in view of the advanced nature of the periodontal disease.

■ ***What periodontal treatment do you envisage will be required?***

Oral hygiene instruction, particularly in the use of interproximal cleaning aids.

Full-mouth scaling and root planing.

Reassessment.

Consider localized surgery to those areas where response to primary phase therapy is inadequate, i.e. bleeding/purulent exudate on probing persists.

■ ***How would you describe the prognosis of Iain's dentition?***

Prognosis depends on the response to initial therapy and patient factors such as motivation towards maintenance of a very high standard of oral hygiene and cessation of the smoking habit.

Based on the amount of alveolar bone loss, the prognosis of the upper incisors is likely to be better than that of the lower incisors.

■ ***What are the treatment options for the upper labial segment spacing?***

1. Orthodontic alignment of the upper labial segment teeth with space closure. Six months after completion of periodontal therapy, the periodontist should re-evaluate the periodontal status. Provided it has not deteriorated and Iain is not averse to the prospect of wearing an orthodontic appliance, orthodontic treatment could be considered.
2. Extraction of 2| or of 21|12 and replacement on a partial upper denture or adhesive bridgework. Extraction of 1|12 may be required also with similar prosthetic replacement to the extracted upper units.

Iain opted for fixed appliance therapy to align the upper teeth (**Fig. 18.4**).

■ ***What options are there with regard to improving appliance aesthetics in an adult patient?***

Options are aesthetic brackets (polycarbonate or ceramic), clear aligner therapy (Invisalign®) and lingual orthodontics. Each, however, is not without its shortcomings (**Table 18.1**).

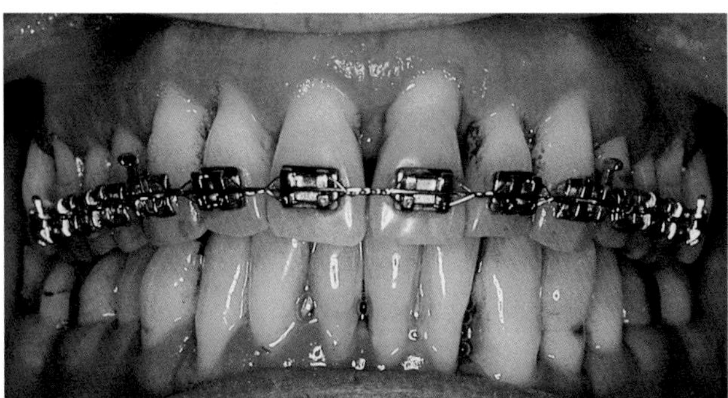

Fig. 18.4 Upper fixed appliance.

Table 18.1 Shortcomings of aesthetic orthodontic appliances

Treatment option	Shortcomings
Aesthetic brackets	
Polycarbonate brackets	Stain, deform, poor torque control (improved with metal insert)
Ceramic brackets	Cannot bond to composite unless a silane-coupling agent is used, which increases bond strength and risk of enamel damage at debond (overcome by different base designs to allow mechanical bond)
	Enamel damage at debond (problem overcome with different base design but must follow manufacturer's instructions specific for different bracket designs)
	Bracket breakage
	Wear of opposing enamel
	Increased friction compared with metal (overcome by insertion of metal slot)
Clear aligner therapy	Control of root movement and possible intermaxillary correction limited unless bonded attachments added appropriately
	Extraction site space closure difficult
Lingual appliances	Tongue discomfort
	Speech adjustment
	Difficult to place (indirect bonding required) and adjust (operator/patient time and cost implications)

What special considerations are there with orthodontic treatment in a periodontally compromised dentition?

Bands should be avoided due to the risk of further compromising periodontal support by placement of the band margin subgingivally, creating a nidus for plaque accumulation. Bonded attachments, therefore, should be placed on all teeth including molars. It is also preferable to use stainless steel ligatures rather than elastomeric modules to retain orthodontic archwires, as modules attract higher levels of plaque micro-organisms.

If several posterior teeth have been lost, anchorage for the tooth movements required may not be sufficient and reinforcement with a bonded transpalatal arch or a temporary anchorage device may be necessary.

With reduced alveolar bone support, light forces should be applied to the teeth.

When gingival recession is evident pre-treatment, the patient should be warned as to the possibility of this being aggravated by orthodontic tooth movement.

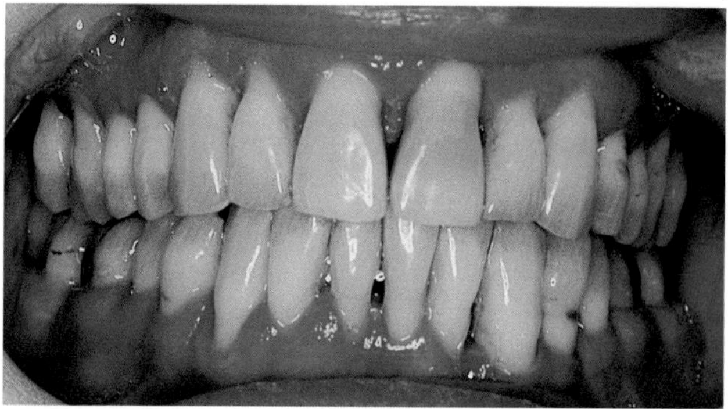

Fig. 18.5 Final occlusion (bonded palatal retainer in place).

Regular periodontal recall should be undertaken throughout orthodontic treatment.

Due to the loss of periodontal attachment and alveolar bone, permanent bonded retention will be required.

The final occlusion is shown in **Fig. 18.5**.

> **Key point**
>
> For orthodontic treatment in a periodontally involved dentition:
>
> - Avoid bands.
> - Use light forces.
> - Ensure regular periodontal recall during treatment.
> - Retain permanently.

Primary resources and recommended reading

Gustke CJ 1999 Treatment of periodontitis in the diabetic patient. A critical review. J Clin Periodontol 26:133–137.

Joffe L 2003 Invisalign®: early experiences. J Orthod 30:348–352.

Joss-Vassalli I, Grebenstein C, Topouzelis N et al 2010 Orthodontic therapy and gingival recession: a systematic review. Orthod Craniofac Res 13:287–297.

Johnson GK, Hill M, 2004 Cigarette smoking and the periodontal patient. J Periodontol 75:196–209.

Nattrass C, Sandy JR 1995 Adult orthodontics – a review. Br J Orthod 22:331–337.

For revision, see Mind Map 18, page 238.

19

Appliance-related problems

CASE 1

SUMMARY

Owen, an 8-year-old boy, presents for a routine check of his upper removable appliance. You notice a reddened palate (*Fig. 19.1A*). What is your diagnosis and how would you manage this?

History

Complaint

Owen's only complaint is that his upper removable appliance is loose. He is not aware of any problem with his palate.

History of complaint

Owen has been wearing the upper removable appliance for the past 8 weeks to correct a crossbite on |1. The current appliance has been getting progressively looser over the past month.

Medical history

Owen is asthmatic and has used a salbutamol (Ventolin) inhaler for the past 4 years. His asthma is well controlled.

Examination

Extraoral

Owen has a Class I skeletal pattern with average FMPA and no facial asymmetry. His lips are competent, with the lower lip just covering the incisal third of the upper anterior teeth. There are no temporomandibular joint signs or symptoms.

Intraoral

The soft tissues appear normal except for generalized mild marginal gingivitis and the palatal mucosa, which is shown in **Fig. 19.1A**. Oral hygiene is fair.

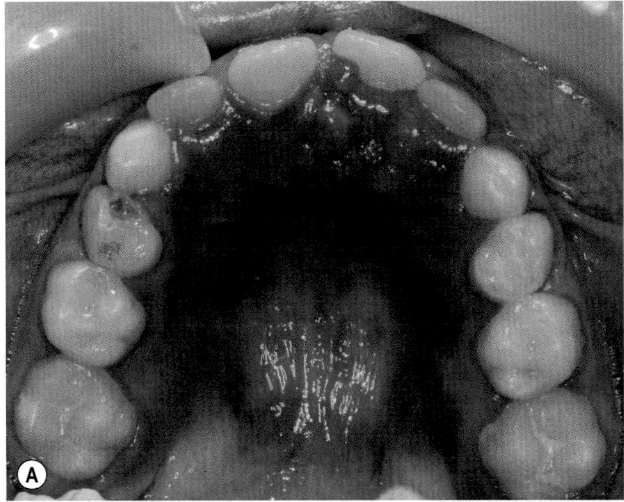

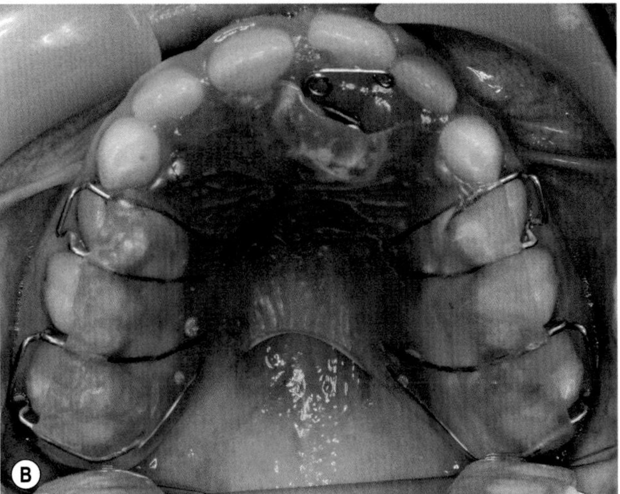

Fig. 19.1 **(A)** Appearance of the palate at presentation. **(B)** Upper removable appliance.

■ ***Describe the appearance of the palate.***

The lesion affecting the palate can be described as follows:

Site – palatal mucosa and attached gingivae.

Size – area affected relates primarily to that covered by the baseplate of the upper removable appliance (**Fig. 19.1B**).

Shape – the outline is defined by, and posteriorly extends slightly beyond, the shape of the baseplate.

Colour – uniformly reddened appearance of the palate and attached gingiva primarily underlying the baseplate.

Background – mucosa and gingivae not covered by the baseplate appear of normal colour except an area in the palatal midline beyond the baseplate.

■ ***What are your observations regarding the upper removable appliance?***

The appliance has Adams clasps on 6|6 and D|D with a Z spring to |1. The distal arrowhead on D| clasp and the mesial arrowhead on |6 clasp do not engage the undercuts optimally.

The baseplate has posterior capping over 6ED|DE6.

Appliance hygiene does not appear as it should – food debris and plaque deposits are visible, through the baseplate, on the fitting surface of the appliance.

What is the most likely diagnosis based on the information you have so far?

Palatal (denture) stomatitis, as the patient is symptom-free.

What other condition would produce a similar appearance?

Acrylic allergy. This, however, is unlikely as a 'burning' sensation of the mucosa underlying the baseplate would have been reported early after insertion of the appliance and there would be erythema of all of the soft tissues adjacent to the acrylic.

What is the aetiology of 'denture' stomatitis?

Candida is the principal cause. Although a normal oral commensal, proliferation of *Candida* is facilitated by local environmental or systemic factors, thereby allowing it to become pathogenic (**Table 19.1**).

> **Key point**
>
> *Candida* is the principal cause of palatal stomatitis related to an upper removable appliance.

What factors in this case may have predisposed Owen to 'denture' stomatitis?

The use of a steroid inhaler, poor appliance hygiene and full-time wear of the appliance are likely to be the main contributory factors. A direct relationship has been shown between the presence of an upper removable appliance, *Candida* and low salivary pH levels. In addition, upper removable appliance therapy has a positive, though transient, influence on the prevalence of *Candida* and density of oral candidal carriage, suggesting that the carrier state may be initiated by the appliance.

Investigations

How would you confirm the diagnosis?

The ideal investigation is a smear from the palatal mucosa underlying the baseplate for microbiological testing.

Table 19.1 Causes of denture stomatitis

Factor	Aetiology	
Local	Infection with *Candida* (~90% due to *Candida albicans*)	
	Poor denture/appliance hygiene	
	Night-time wear of denture/appliance	
	Possible trauma	
	Poor salivary clearance of oral commensals	
	High sugar intake providing substrate for *Candida* proliferation	
Systemic	Iron and vitamin deficiencies	predispose to *Candida* infection
	Steroids	
	Drugs that cause xerostomia	
	Endocrine abnormalities, e.g. diabetes	
	Antibiotic therapy	

Saliva sampling for *Candida* counts.

Culturing for accurate identification and sensitivity testing may also be undertaken.

What stains identify Candida?

Gram stain: *Candida* is strongly Gram positive.

Periodic acid–Schiff (PAS): the magenta stain locates carbohydrate in fungal cell walls.

Treatment

How would you treat this condition?

Owen should be advised to:

1. Leave the appliance out at night. Due to the infection, it would be wise to wear the appliance throughout the day but remove it at night until the palatal mucosa returns to health.
2. Improve appliance hygiene – brush the fitting surface and soak it in a 1% hypochlorite solution.
3. Improve oral hygiene – teeth, gingivae and palatal mucosa should be brushed thoroughly after every meal.
4. Reduce sugar intake – alter diet to low carbohydrate consumption.
5. Antifungal agents (nystatin or amphotericin suspension or miconazole oral gel) should be applied to the fitting surface of the appliance four times daily. A 0.2% chlorhexidine mouthwash may also be beneficial due to its antifungal effect.

As the asthma is well controlled, there is no need to refer Owen to his general medical practitioner.

> **Key point**
>
> Management of palatal stomatitis:
> - Leave appliance out at night.
> - Improve appliance and oral hygiene.
> - Reduce carbohydrate consumption.
> - Antifungal agents.

What is the prognosis for this condition?

Provided all the above strategies are followed, the condition should resolve completely within a few weeks.

CASES 2 AND 3

SUMMARY

Two common fixed appliance problems are shown. What is the cause of each, and what treatment would you provide?

What problem do you notice in *Fig. 19.2A***?**

A bracket has become debonded from 5⏌.

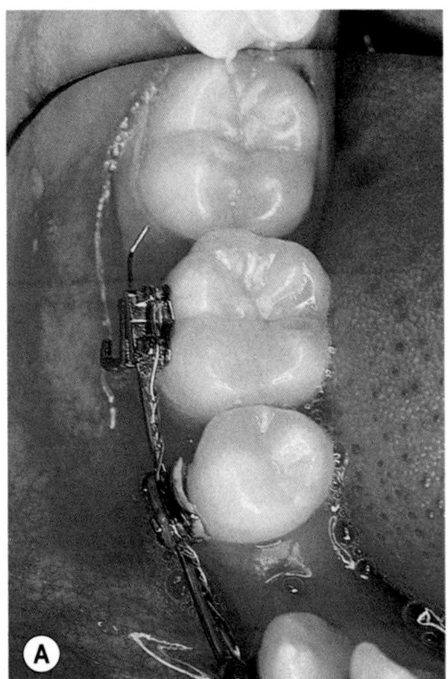

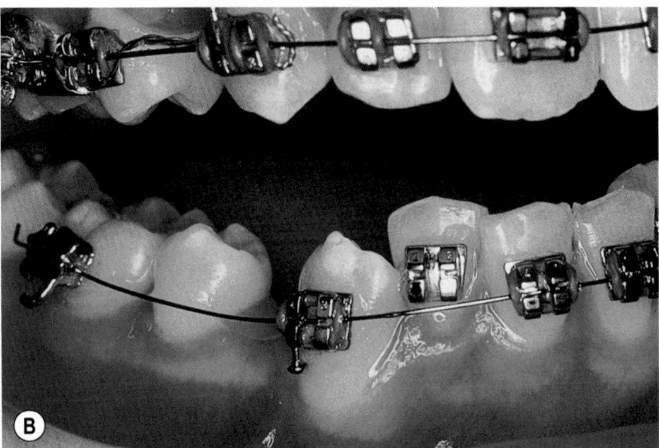

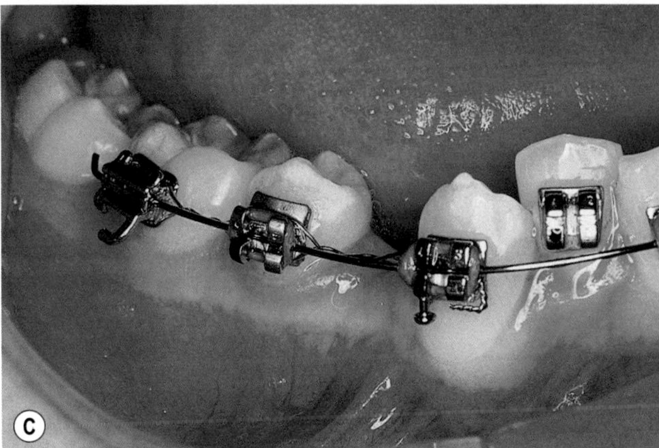

Fig. 19.2 **(A)** Lower occlusal view. **(B)** Following removal of ligature wire and $\overline{5}|$ bracket. **(C)** Following replacement of ligature wire and rebonding of a $\overline{5}|$ bracket.

Table 19.2 Causes of bracket bond failure

Factor	Aetiology
Operator	Insufficient etch time
	Poor etch pattern*
	Poor moisture control during bonding
	Non-adherence to manufacturer's instructions with the bonding adhesive chosen
	Movement of the bracket after initial placement, which interferes with bond formation within the adhesive
	Application of high force to the bracket to accomplish archwire engagement
Patient	Eating hard/sticky foods
	Possibly use of phenolic-containing mouthrinses that soften composite
	Occlusal trauma/bruxing habit
	Pen-chewing/nail-biting

*Etch pattern is poorer on premolars than on canine or incisor teeth. This contributes to the greater bond failure rate on premolars (note failure in Fig. 19.2A is on $\overline{5}|$).

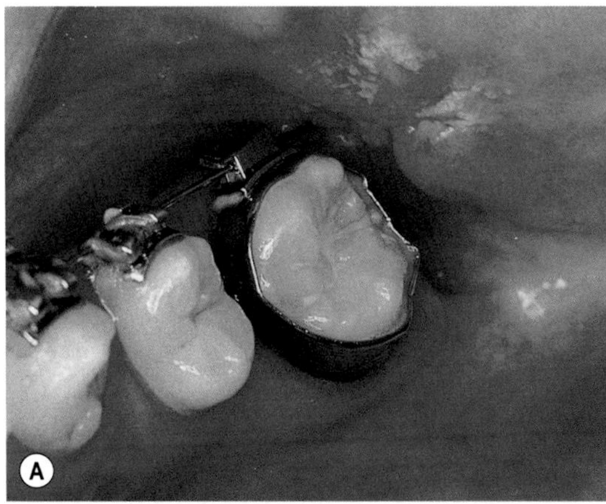

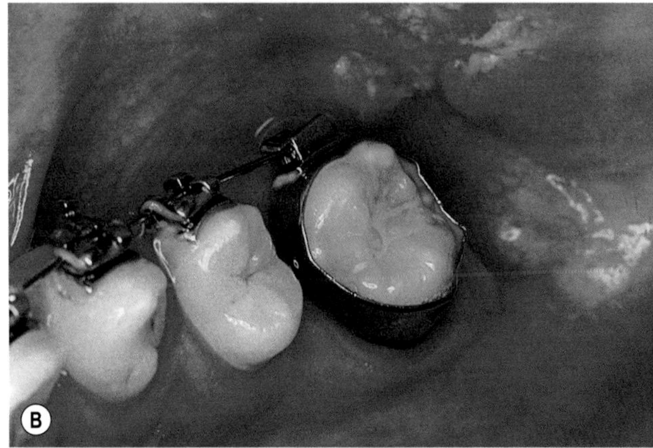

Fig. 19.3 **(A)** Upper occlusal view. **(B)** Following shortening and adjustment of upper archwire.

■ ***Why has this occurred?***

Bond failure may occur for various reasons (**Table 19.2**).

Treatment

■ ***What treatment would you provide? Explain why.***

The patient should be advised first to contact their orthodontist for repair of the appliance (**Figs 19.2B,C**).

If this is not possible and the loose bracket is at risk of being swallowed or inhaled, it should be removed. In this case, however, this risk is less likely as the bracket remains attached to a ligature wire and elastometric module.

Should the loose bracket be a source of discomfort to the patient, as a general dental practitioner, you could remove the loose bracket and the loose ligature. The patient should be appointed with their orthodontist at the earliest opportunity.

■ ***What problem do you notice in*** *Fig. 19.3A****?***

The cheek mucosa is ulcerated due to trauma from the over-extended round archwire.

How has this problem arisen?

The amount of projection of the archwire beyond the molar band may have been overlooked at the time of archwire placement, or the archwire may have moved to its current position following insertion, as the teeth aligned or due to loss/bond failure of another appliance component.

How would you manage this problem?

As a general dental practitioner (GDP), you should, first, advise the patient to contact their orthodontist to deal with this problem. If this is not possible then you should provide emergency care.

As a GDP, what emergency care would you provide?

The distal end of the archwire should be cut flush with the terminal aspect of the molar tube or the archwire end turned underneath the molar tube or angled inward away from the cheek. As a round nickel titanium wire is in place, with the terminal end heat-treated (note blackened appearance), this is easily cut to the desired length or positioned to avoid cheek trauma (**Fig. 19.3B**).

The patient should be advised to maintain a high standard of oral hygiene and to rinse with lukewarm salty water after meals until the ulceration heals. Provision of a supply of soft wax to apply over the molar tube and the adjusted wire end may also be helpful in the intervening period. The patient should also schedule an appointment in the near future with their orthodontist.

Key point

Emergency treatment for:

- Loose bracket: remove if risk of ingestion/inhalation.
- Overextended archwire: cut wire and/or turn wire end inward away from the cheek.

CASES 4 AND 5

SUMMARY

Two problems with retainers are shown. How might each of these have occurred, and what treatment would you provide?

What problem do you notice in *Fig. 19.4A*?

There is a midline fracture of a lower vacuum-formed (Essix) retainer.

How might this problem have occurred? How may it have been prevented?

This is a clean-cut fracture rather than a small crack and, as such, is unusual with a vacuum-formed retainer. Crazing of the retainer or small cracks are more typical. Extraorally, accidentally dropping the retainer while cleaning or rinsing it, followed by an impact from a sharp or heavy object, is possible; repeated flexure of the retainer would also lead to reakage. Intraorally, eating hard foods with the retainer in situ or 'biting' the retainer into place with the opposing

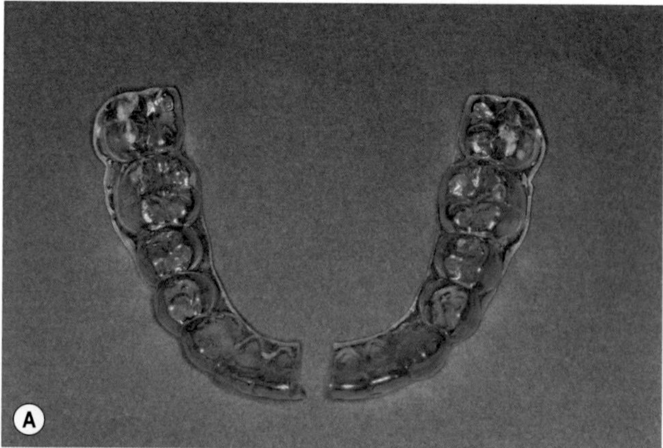

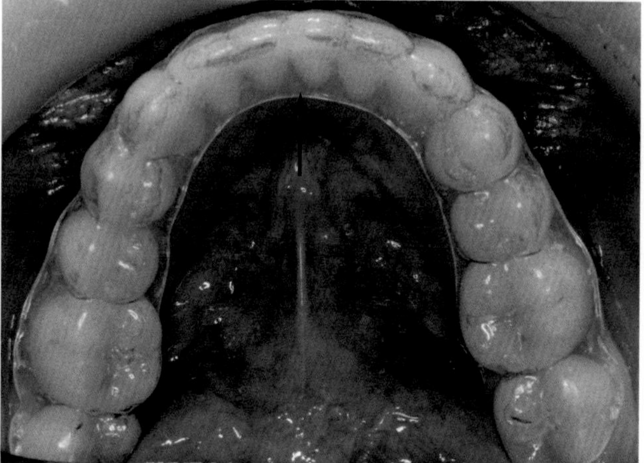

Fig. 19.4 **(A)** Lower retainer. **(B)** Lower occlusal view showing retainer halves abutted; arrow indicates fracture line.

teeth are also possibilities. A weakness in the retainer during manufacture is another option.

Accidental damage is difficult to prevent, but on issuing the retainer the patient should have been instructed to take care when rinsing or cleaning the retainer to avoid it being dropped and damaged; wear of the retainer for eating is also not required. Flexing the retainer is to be avoided; when not in use, it should be stored in the hard, plastic retainer box provided. The lower alginate impression should have been checked for any tray contact of the lower incisors or 'dragging' that could compromise the manufacturing process.

In this case the retainer had been accidently stood on after being dropped during rinsing. It had only been issued 2 weeks prior to the incident, when the lower fixed appliance was removed.

Treatment

As a GDP, what treatment would you provide? Explain why.

The patient should firstly be informed to make contact with his or her orthodontist to explain the situation and arrange to be seen as soon as possible for a replacement retainer. If this is not possible, you should check each part of the retainer to see if the pieces fit together and, if so, rinse and disinfect them before assessing the fit in the mouth. As the pieces abutted well (**Fig. 19.4B**), they could be worn as a temporary measure to prevent any relapse until a replacement retainer is issued. Until a replacement retainer is fitted, day-time wear, apart from eating and drinking, would be preferable to night-time wear, as there is a risk of one or both parts of the retainer becoming dislodged and perhaps being swallowed. If, however, the orthodontist is agreeable, an alginate impression could be taken for a replacement retainer, which you may fit with his or her guidance. A follow-up appointment with the orthodontist should be scheduled for the near future.

■ ***Could such a problem have been preempted at debond?***

At debond, it is advisable to issue the patient with two vacuum-formed retainers to allow for inadvertent breakage or loss. The spare retainer can be worn until another appointment is possible with the orthodontist, at which time a new spare vacuum-formed retainer can be made from the models constructed when the fixed appliance was removed.

■ ***What problem (arrowed) do you notice in*** *Fig. 19.5A* ***?***

The composite overlying the wire on 2⏋ has been lost exposing the wire. (Note the retainer wire had previously fractured in the midline; the wire ends had been smoothed and covered with composite.)

■ ***How has this occurred?***

Eating sticky or hard foods or chewing gum is the most likely cause.

■ ***How will you manage the problem?***

Enquire from the patient when the exposed wire on 2⏋ was first noticed, whether there are presently or have been any problems with this, how long the retainer has been in place and if the orthodontist still sees the patient for review.

The patient first noticed this 2 weeks ago after chewing a toffee; it rubs the tongue and has produced a small ulcer. The retainer fractured in the midline 2 years ago, at which time it had been in place for 1 year; the wire ends were smoothed and covered with composite. Since then there have been no problems. The patient is due for a review with the orthodontist next year. As such, the patient should contact the orthodontist to have the retainer assessed with regard to repair or replacement as soon as possible.

■ ***In the meantime, what would you do to improve patient comfort?***

As 2⏋ is still aligned with the adjacent teeth and composite remains attached to the enamel and undersurface of the wire, a small composite addition could be made to the wire on 2⏋. The wire surface should be cleaned gently with pumice, the composite roughened slightly on 2⏋ with a green stone, then resin and composite applied and light-cured. An appointment should be arranged with the orthodontist in the near future.

■ ***What further treatment do you think will be required?***

In light of the minor shifts in alignment that are now visible on several teeth (**Fig. 19.5A and B**), removal of the retainer, alignment with clear aligner therapy and replacement of the bonded retainer would be optimal.

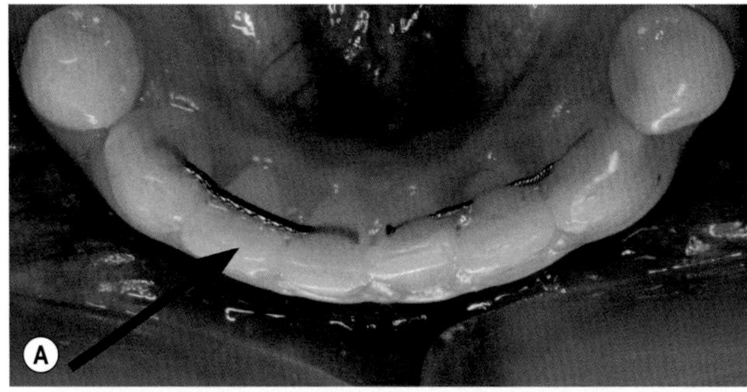

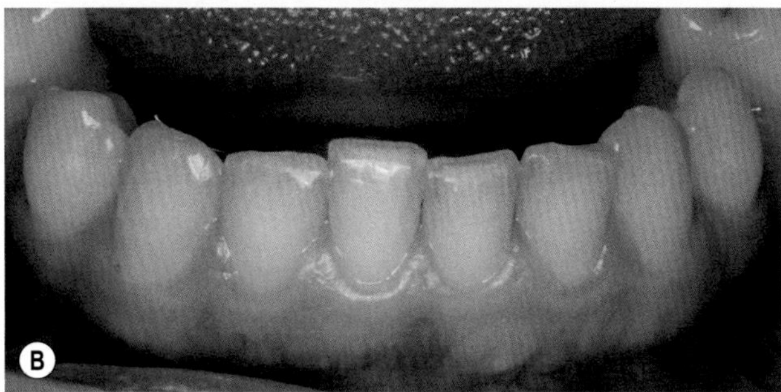

Fig. 19.5 **(A)** Lower occlusal view. **(B)** Anterior view.

Key point

Emergency treatment for:

- Broken vacuum-formed retainer: arrange replacement.
- Bonded retainer: composite repair/smooth wire end or arrange replacement.

Primary resources and recommended reading

Arendorf T, Addy M 1985 Candidal carriage and plaque distribution before, during and after removable orthodontic appliance therapy. J Clin Periodontol 12:360–368.

Hobson RS, Rugg-Gunn AJ, Booth TA 2002 Acid-etch patterns on the buccal surface of human permanent teeth. Arch Oral Biol 47:407–412.

Mandall NA, Millett DT, Mattick CR et al 2002 Orthodontic adhesives: a systematic review. J Orthod 29:205–210.

Patel A, Sandler J 2010 First aid for orthodontic retainers. Dent Update 37:627–730.

Wilson J 1998 The aetiology, diagnosis and management of denture stomatitis. Br Dent J 185:380–384.

For revision, see Mind Map 19, page 239.

20

Tooth movement and related problems

CASE 1

SUMMARY

Darren, a 13-year-old boy, has been undergoing upper removable appliance therapy for 6 months to retract and align 3|, following extraction of 4|. Tooth movement has been very slow with no movement recorded at the last two visits.

- ***What are the possible reasons for a slow rate of orthodontic tooth movement?***

These can be divided broadly into patient, appliance and operator factors.

Patient factors Non-compliance with instructions regarding wear of the appliance.

Incorrect positioning of the spring on appliance insertion or distortion of the spring.

Contact of the tooth with the buccal cortical plate or with a retained root part of 4|.

Occlusal interference from the opposing arch.

Appliance factors Acrylic and/or wire may be interfering with tooth movement.

Operator factors Design flaws, underactivation, overactivation or activation of the spring such that 3| is directly buccally into contact with the cortical plate rather than through the cancellous corridor of bone.

- ***What force range is optimal for retraction of 3| by tipping movement?***

The optimal force range is 30–50 g or 0.3–0.5 N.

- ***What cellular response is there following activation of the spring to retract 3| by tipping movement?***

The consequence of activating the spring is to set up zones of pressure and tension within the periodontal ligament. Half of the periodontal ligament is stressed with maximum pressure created at the alveolar crest in the direction of movement and at the diagonally opposite apical area (**Fig. 20.1**).

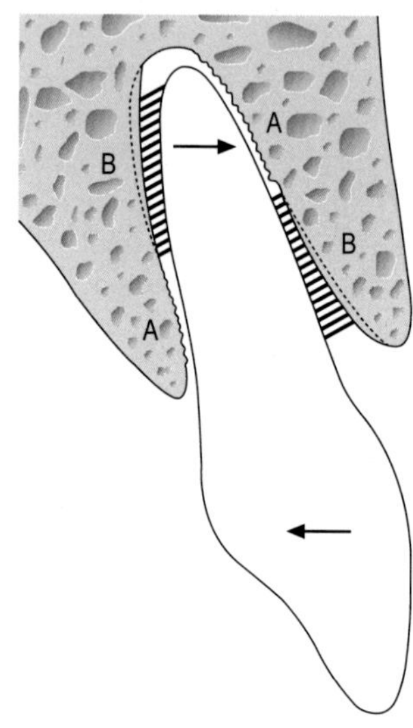

Fig. 20.1 Diagram illustrating zones of pressure **(A)** and tension **(B)** in the periodontal ligament induced by a tipping force.

> **Key point**
>
> Tipping movement, typically, requires forces of 30–50 g or 0.3–0.5 N.

Pressure zones The cellular response depends on whether a light or heavy force is applied. With a light sustained force, tooth movement occurs within a few seconds as periodontal ligament fluid is squeezed out and the vascular supply is compressed, setting off a complex biochemical response. Within 2 days, osteoclast invasion occurs and frontal resorption follows.

When a heavy sustained force is applied, the periodontal ligament is compressed to such a degree that the blood supply is cut off completely, producing an area of sterile necrosis (hyalinization). Small areas of hyalinization are inevitable, even with light forces, but the area of hyalinization is extended with forces of greater magnitude. Osteoclast differentiation is impossible within the necrotic periodontal ligament space, but after several days osteoclasts appear adjacent to and within the adjacent cancellous spaces. From there they invade the bone adjacent to the hyalinized area and tooth movement eventually occurs by undermining resorption.

Tension zones Following initial application of a light force, the blood vessels vasodilate and the periodontal ligament fibres are stretched while fibroblast and preosteoblast proliferation occurs. The stretched fibres become embedded in osteoid, which later mineralizes. The normal periodontal ligament width is eventually regained by simultaneous collagen fibre remodelling.

With heavy forces, rupture of blood vessels and severing of the periodontal ligament fibres are likely, but both are restored with the remodelling processes.

> **Key point**
>
> Application of a sustained force to a tooth creates areas of pressure and tension within the periodontal ligament which ultimately lead to bone resorption and deposition, respectively.

■ ***What is the mechanism for tooth movement?***

Although the histological response to an applied orthodontic force has been investigated extensively, the mechanism by which a mechanical stimulus is transferred to a cellular response is complex and is at present unresolved. It is likely that vascular changes in the periodontal ligament in areas of pressure and tension, electrical signals in response to alveolar bone flexing following force application, as well as prostaglandins and cytokine release interact in this process.

■ ***How would you manage the problem in this case?***

Management is specific to each cause. The action taken may be one or more of the following:

- The need for full-time wear of the appliance must be emphasized to the patient/parent. They must be made aware that treatment will stop unless full cooperation is forthcoming.
- Show the patient how to insert the appliance with the spring positioned correctly and explain the action of the spring. Ensure that the appliance is not being removed by the spring.
- Check the activation of the spring and adjust it appropriately.
- Remove any acrylic or wire obstruction to tooth movement. This may require a remake of the appliance to an improved design.
- Add to a flat anterior biteplane or buccal capping to disengage the occlusion, if this is hampering tooth movement.
- Ask the patient and check his or her case notes for any recorded problem with 4⌋ extraction. If indicated, take a periapical radiograph of 4⌋ area to check for a retained root fragment. If this is detected, seek an oral surgical opinion regarding its removal or whether it could be left in situ and its position monitored radiographically.
- Check 3⌋ is not ankylosed. This is unlikely in this case as some movement of 3⌋ has occurred since 4⌋ was extracted.
- Darren admitted to intermittent wear of the appliance and, in particular, to leaving it out at meals. He was advised accordingly.

> **Key point**
>
> Full-time wear of an upper removable appliance is required for an optimal rate of tooth movement.

■ ***What do you notice on the periapical radiograph of another case (Fig. 20.2)?***

There is a small retained apical root fragment of 4⌋.

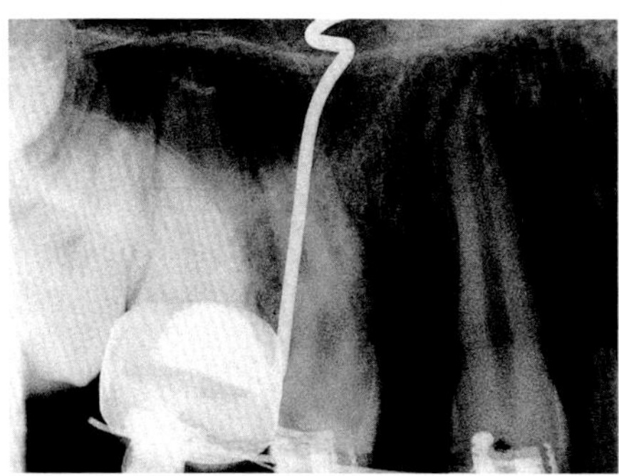

Fig. 20.2 Periapical radiograph.

■ ***What treatment would you advise?***

Complete retraction of 3⌋ is unlikely due to the presence of this root fragment. However, its removal would require a surgical procedure, which would remove a considerable amount of alveolar bone and may damage the roots of the adjacent teeth. The root fragment may resorb in time and become confluent with the alveolar bone.

In view of the surgical risks, it would be wise to leave the root fragment in situ, monitor its status radiographically and accept the limitation this poses to complete retraction and alignment of 3⌋. The patient should be advised accordingly.

CASE 2

SUMMARY

Alan is reviewed 3 months after completion of a 2-year course of upper and lower fixed appliance therapy. He is wearing upper and lower removable retainers at night only. On removal of the retainers, you detect grade 2 mobility of the upper incisors and grade 1 mobility of all other teeth anterior to and including the first permanent molars in both arches. His oral hygiene is good, and there is no bleeding on probing. You order a dental panoramic tomogram.

■ ***Why is the radiograph ordered?***

It will allow a general screen of alveolar bone height and root length of all teeth.

■ ***What do you notice on the film (Fig. 20.3A)?***

Generalized apical blunting (root resorption) of all teeth, anterior to and including the first permanent molars with the possible exception of the second premolars. The upper incisors appear to have the most root resorption.

■ ***Which teeth experience most orthodontically induced root resorption?***

The upper incisors, followed by the lower incisors and first permanent molars, have consistently more root resorption than other teeth irrespective of suggested genetic or treatment-related risk factors.

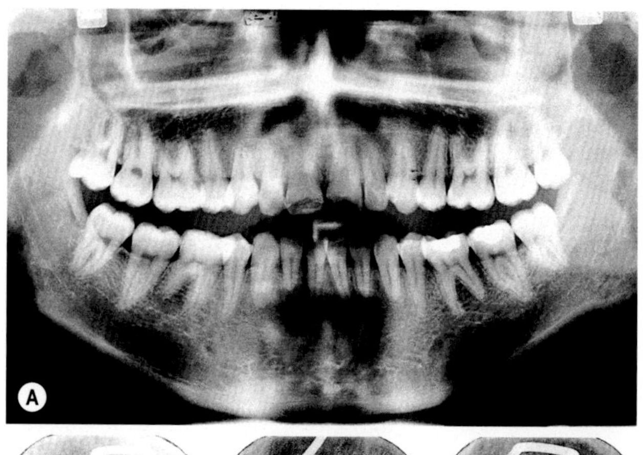

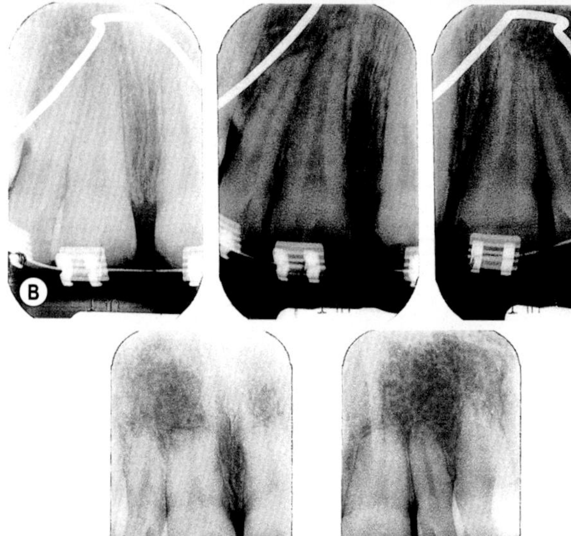

Fig. 20.3 **(A)** Dental panoramic tomogram. **(B)** Periapical radiographs of upper incisors taken 6 months into treatment. Note no apical root resorption apparent on |12, but slight apical resorption of 21| roots. **(C)** Periapical radiographs indicating marked root resorption of 21|12.

What risk factors have been suggested in relation to orthodontically induced root resorption?

Suggested patient-related risk factors include patient age and sex, root shape, history of previous trauma, teeth with short roots and previous root resorption, cortical bone proximity to the root, genetic factors and systemic factors.

Suggested treatment-related risk factors include length of treatment, force magnitude and method of application, direction of movement, appliance type, treatment mechanics and extent of apical movement.

What does current evidence suggest with regard to orthodontically induced root resorption?

Systematic reviews indicate that previous trauma and unusual root morphology are unlikely causes; root filled teeth do not appear to be more vulnerable than contralateral vital teeth. An increased incidence and severity occurs with comprehensive orthodontic treatment with total root resorption reduced by a 2–3-month pause in treatment. Bracket prescription, self-ligation and archwire sequence do not affect this. Heavy forces produce most root resorption, and evidence supports the use of light forces, especially for incisor intrusion.

Alan sustained coronal fractures to 1|1, involving enamel and dentine, 3 months before starting orthodontic treatment.

> **Key point**
>
> Root resorption:
>
> - Increases in incidence and severity with comprehensive orthodontic treatment.
> - Is promoted by the use of heavy forces.

Could root resorption have been prevented?

Root resorption is regarded as an unavoidable sequela of orthodontic tooth movement. Although, on average 1 mm of root length will typically be lost over a 24-month course of orthodontic treatment, wide individual variation exists. Determining risk factors to identify those susceptible to orthodontically induced root resorption, and the means by which its severity and prevalence may be reduced, requires further well-designed clinical research studies.

During treatment excessive force application should be avoided. Where early root resorption is detected on progress radiographs, taken 6–12 months into treatment (**Fig. 20.3B**), further root resorption may be reduced by a 2–3-month pause (with a passive archwire). Where severe root resorption is detected (>4 mm or one-third of the original root length), the treatment goals should be reconsidered with the patient and other options explored.

What must the orthodontist ensure before treatment commences?

The risk of apical root resorption as a consequence of orthodontic treatment must be explained to the patient/parents and discussed with them. In addition, an informed consent form signed by patient/parents and the orthodontist must describe, in particular, the risk of apical root resorption. Treatment should not be offered unless the anticipated benefits far outweigh the risk of minor apical resorption seen in most patients.

Appropriate radiographs should be available, and the need for progress radiographs, as required, should be explained.

> **Key point**
>
> - Root resorption is a common consequence of orthodontic treatment.
> - Explain the risk to the patient before treatment starts and obtain consent.
> - Monitor radiographically as required.

What would you do in this case?

Ask the patient if he is aware of marked mobility of any teeth and/or any other symptoms.

Clinically, the mobility of all teeth should be recorded. Alan was aware of upper incisor mobility.

Enquire about bruxism or other habits, such as nail-biting. None were reported.

Sensibility testing of the incisors and canines should be undertaken. All teeth were responsive to sensibility testing and no marked differences in recordings were detected between each tooth and its opposite number in each arch.

■ ***What treatment would you provide?***

Alan should continue with night time wear of his retainers. The retention plan may need to be re-evaluated depending on the resorption status of the incisors (see below).

Periapical radiographs should be taken of the upper incisors as these exhibit grade 2 mobility (**Fig. 20.3C**). Follow-up radiographic examinations and sensibility tests are recommended at 6 months to ascertain if the apical root resorption is progressive. This, however, should be unlikely as 'active' orthodontic treatment has been concluded. In the unlikely event that further resorption is observed at follow-up, radiographic examination is recommended until the resorption is stabilized. In the long term (10–25 years) after orthodontic treatment, teeth with root length of ≥10 mm and a healthy periodontium have been shown to remain stable.

CASE 3

SUMMARY

Lisa, an 18-year-old girl, had previous extraction of lower first premolars and fixed appliance therapy to successfully correct her Class III malocclusion. Both upper second premolars were congenitally absent. On removal of the fixed appliances 1 year ago, a palatal bonded retainer was placed from 3⌋ to ⌊3; she was also issued an upper Hawley retainer, designed to fit over the bonded retainer, and a lower vacuum-formed retainer. Both removable retainers were to be worn at night only.

■ ***What do you notice in** Figure 20.4 A and B**?***

Soft tissues appear healthy; 6⌋ seems to be restored with an amalgam restoration.

Lower arch is reasonably aligned with a small space between 5⌉ and 3⌉.

Right upper buccal segment and labial segment aligned with the possible exception of 6⌋.

Spacing between 1⌋⌊1 and ⌊1 and ⌊2 with slight mesiolabial rotation of ⌊1 and ⌊2.

Average overjet; overbite average to slightly reduced but complete; mild centreline discrepancy (lower appears shifted to the left by about 2 mm).

Molar relationship is Class I with crossbite affecting the mesiobuccal cusp of 6⌋.

■ ***What does this indicate?***

There has been relapse in the position of Lisa's teeth following treatment.

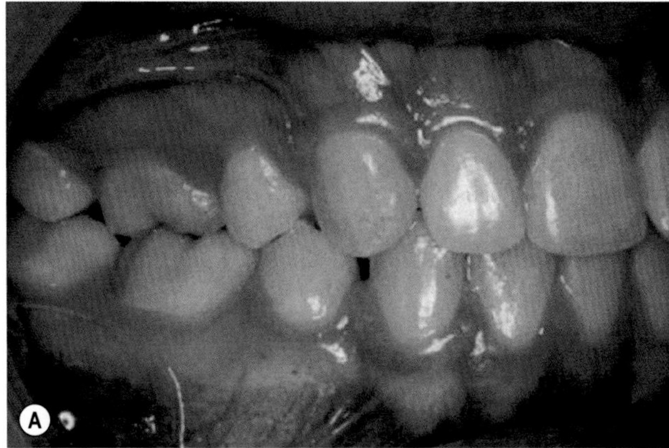

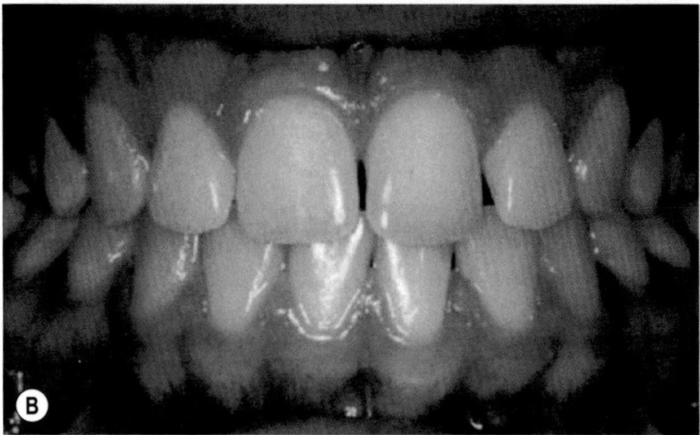

Fig. 20.4 (A) Right buccal occlusion at presentation. **(B)** Anterior occlusion at presentation

■ ***Why has this occurred?***

The following factors are likely to destabilize the final orthodontic result.

Forces from the supporting tissues Reorganization of principal periodontal ligament fibres and supporting alveolar bone occurs within 4–6 months after cessation of active tooth movement. At least 7–8 months, however, are required for the supracrestal fibres to reorganize because of the slow turnover of the free gingival fibres. Rotational correction and space closure are, therefore, liable to relapse. Pre-treatment views of Lisa's malocclusion are shown in **Figs 20.5A and B**. Note the rotated teeth and spacing of the arch.

Forces from the orofacial soft tissues Following appliance therapy, the teeth should be in a position of soft tissue balance. The original mandibular arch form should remain unchanged as marked alteration in the inclination of the lower incisors will promote relapse. Limited proclination of the lower labial segment, however, may be stable in Class II division 2 malocclusion, or if the lower incisors were retroclined by a thumb-sucking habit or by a lower lip trap.

If a thumb- or digit-sucking habit is not ceased before treatment commences, its persistence will promote overjet relapse.

One-third to half of the labial surface of the upper incisors should be covered by the lower lip to give the best chance of stable overjet correction. Where the lips are grossly incompetent post-treatment, the upper incisor position will

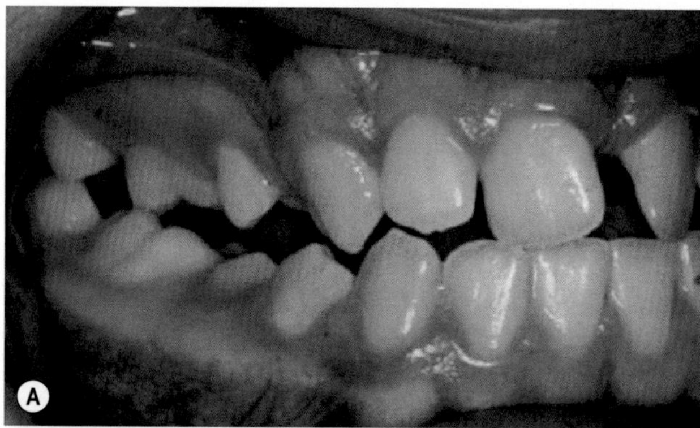

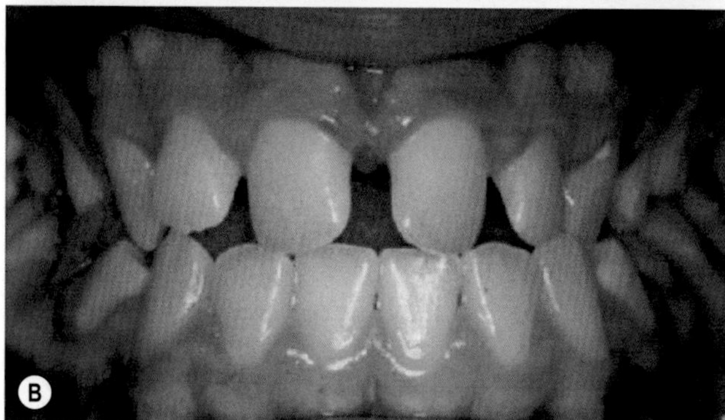

Fig. 20.5 **(A)** Right buccal occlusion (pre-treatment); note rotations of 621|1 and spacing. **(B)** Anterior occlusion (pre-treatment); note incisor spacing and rotations.

be inherently unstable, and the mechanism by which an anterior oral seal is achieved will aggravate this further.

Occlusal factors A poor buccal segment interdigitation with displacing occlusal contacts and an unfavourable interincisal angulation will encourage instability.

Post-treatment facial growth Facial growth continues into adult life and, although of lesser magnitude than that observed during childhood, it varies among individuals. On average, females tend to demonstrate a backward mandibular rotation, and this will not aid overjet stability. Late facial growth also impacts on the development of late lower incisor crowding.

Retention plan An inappropriate design of retainer, retention regimen and/or inadequate compliance by the patient with the prescribed retainer wear will facilitate relapse. Firm rules, however, do not exist for retention following active tooth movement; instead the retention plan should be decided individually for each case. How long this should be for is unknown at present and probably unlikely to be ascertained due to the multiplicity of complex factors involved in malocclusions and their treatment, as well as the inherent difficulties in undertaking clinical trials on the many likely retention strategies. It is acknowledged that the only means of guaranteeing that the post-treatment result remains unchanged long-term is to advise long-term retention. This should be explained to the patient by the orthodontist before treatment starts as a part of informed consent; importantly, the patient's responsibility in the retention process must also be emphasized.

Key point

Relapse may be due to:

- Forces from:
  - Supporting tissues.
  - Orofacial soft tissues.
  - Occlusion.
  - Facial growth.
- Inappropriate retainer design or retention regime, and/or patient compliance.

Pre-treatment:

- Discuss relapse and retention as part of informed consent.
- Highlight patient's responsibility to adhere to long-term retainer wear.

Lisa indicated that she had worn the removable retainers for a few months at night but then had discontinued wear. The upper bonded retainer had come away from |13 2 weeks ago, and the wire had fractured between 1|1. She was now concerned about the spaces that had developed and that her front teeth were 'twisting' back to the way they used to be.

What designs are there of fixed and removable retainers?

Several designs of fixed retainers exist, although in the lower arch this is most commonly either a smooth, round wire with sandblasted ends bonded to the canines only or a multistrand/spiral wire bonded to each of the incisors and canines individually (**Fig. 20.6**). In the upper arch, a multistrand wire is commonly bonded to the incisors only or to the canines and incisors. For either arch, a 020 in multistrand wire is recommended. Bonding is usually with light-cured composite. Removable retainers may either be vacuum-formed (**Fig. 20.7**) or have a wire labial bow (usually Hawley or Begg type: **Fig. 20.7**; **Fig. 20.8A**); the latter may be acrylated to improve appearance (**Fig. 20.8B**).

What does current evidence indicate with regard to post-orthodontic retention?

A recent update of a Cochrane review found that most studies on types of retainers and duration of retainer wear were of low quality. Based on a small number of participants in one well-conducted short term (6 months) study, moderate quality evidence indicates that there is no difference in stability between full-time or part-time wear of thermoplastic retainers. There is, however, insufficient high quality evidence with regard to retention protocols and procedures following orthodontic treatment to make firm recommendations.

How can relapse be prevented long-term?

Night-time wear of a removable thermoplastic retainer should continue long-term, although wear on alternate nights reduced to biweekly may be sufficient with the onus on the patient to monitor occlusal change.

Due to the unpredictability, but high likelihood, of late lower incisor crowding developing post-treatment (see Chapter 16), instead of advising long-term wear of a removable retainer, a bonded lingual retainer may be fitted to the

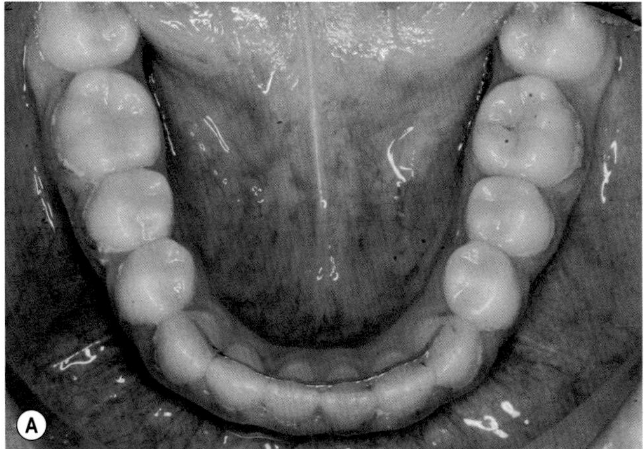

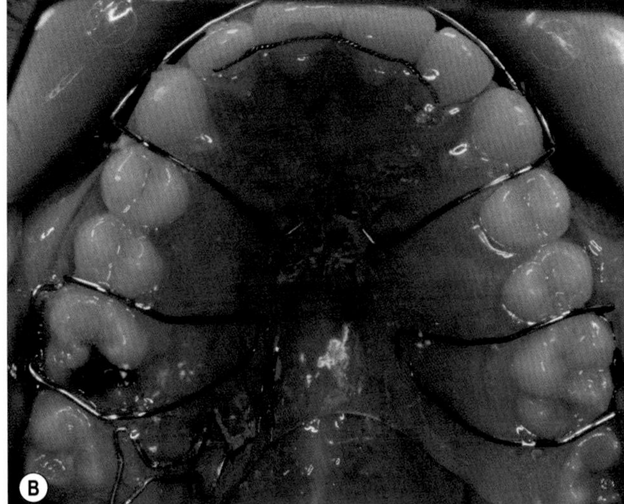

Fig. 20.6 (A) Lower bonded retainer (multistrand wire). **(B)** Upper bonded retainer (multistrand wire) with Hawley retainer.

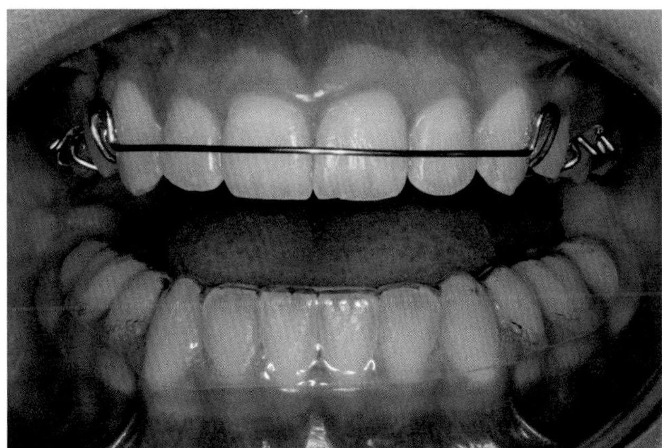

Fig. 20.7 Lower vacuum-formed retainer and upper Hawley retainer.

lower incisors and canines; increasingly this is left in place permanently to maintain lower incisor alignment.

> **Key point**
>
> In the short-term, night-time wear of a thermoplastic removable retainer seems sufficient to maintain tooth alignment after fixed appliance therapy (except in cases with high relapse potential when a bonded retainer is required).

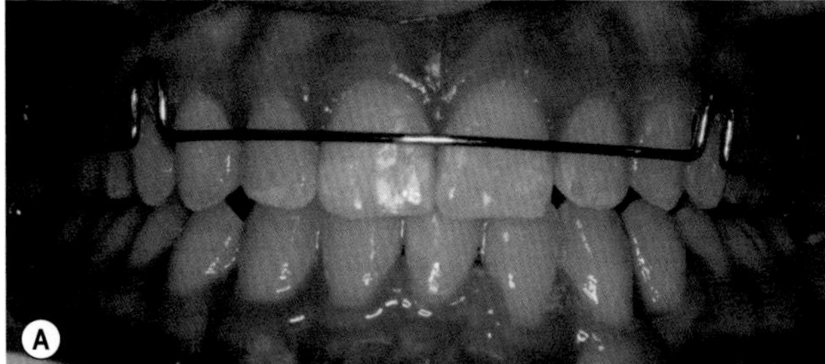

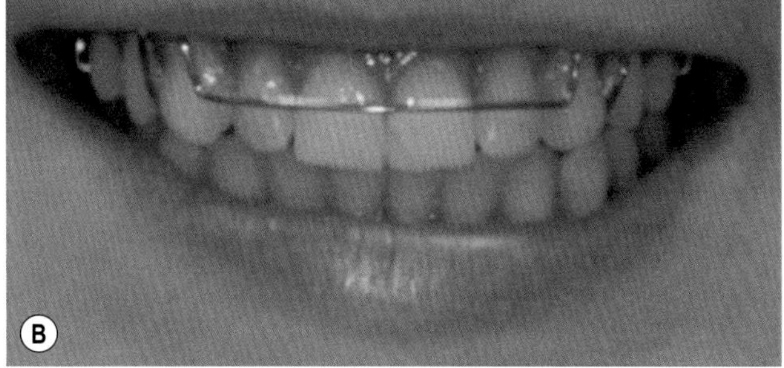

Fig. 20.8 (A) Upper Begg retainer. **(B)** Upper Hawley retainer with an acrylated labial bow.

What specific indications are there for a fixed (bonded) retainer over a removable retainer?

A fixed bonded retainer is indicated in the following circumstances: when the lips are incompetent after correction of an increased overjet; following space closure in spaced dentitions (**Figs 20.5A,B**; also includes median diastema, Chapter 1); where the anteroposterior position of the lower labial segment has been radically altered; after alignment of severely rotated teeth (**Fig. 20.5**) or of an impacted upper incisor (Chapter 2) or periodontally involved dentitions (Chapter 18); cleft lip and palate (Chapter 21) and when minimal overbite exists following incisor crossbite correction (Chapter 10). In addition, where a compromised occlusion was the treatment goal, albeit with improved appearance, fixed retention should be used.

> **Key point**
>
> A bonded retainer is indicated following correction of:
>
> - Severely rotated teeth and spaced dentitions.

Has the general dental practitioner (GDP) got a role with regard to orthodontic retention?

The GDP has a general informative and important supportive role with regard to post-orthodontic retention and retainer wear by their patients. This is summarized in **Table 20.1**

What oral hygiene measures should the patient be instructed to follow after placement of a bonded retainer?

In order to maintain optimal oral hygiene in relation to the bonded retainer, the patient should be taught how to effectively use interdental cleaning aids such as Superfloss and interdental brushes.

Instructions in relation to a removable (Essix) retainer are given in Chapter 5.

Table 20.1 Role of the general dental practitioner (GDP) in relation to post-orthodontic retention and retainer wear

When	Role	Specific aspect of retention
Referral/pre-treatment	Inform	Retention vital component of treatment
Post-treatment at review	Reinforce	Need for retainer wear and how to maintain optimal oral and retainer hygiene
Removable retainer	Confirm	Retainer wear as advised
	Ensure good fit	Adjust as required
	Repair/replace?	*Depends if still under review with orthodontist
Bonded retainer	Check	Wire/composite, integrity of bond and related oral hygiene
	Repair	*Seek advice, as required, from orthodontist regarding repair of broken/debonded retainer

*It is important when the patient is no longer under review by the orthodontist, but still wearing retainers, that the orthodontist communicates with the GDP with regard to the retainer type and retention protocol.

Key point

Following placement of a bonded retainer, instruction must be provided in relation to interdental cleaning.

■ *What management options are there for Lisa's problem?*

The following options exist:

1. Accept and monitor – study models should record the current tooth position and occlusion to allow for comparison with the pre- and post-treatment study casts and to act as a baseline from which to assess any further occlusal change. If there is further relapse, then consider options 2 or 3 below.
2. Re-treatment – full case assessment is required with study models and photographs; radiographs are not indicated. For comprehensive recorrection, fixed appliance therapy is an option, but clear aligner therapy with Invisalign is also likely to produce a satisfactory outcome due to the mild nature of the relapse; the slight centreline shift could be accepted with the latter treatment option. Long-term bonded retention will be required, thereafter, to the upper labial segment; it would also be advisable to provide a vacuum-formed retainer to fit over the bonded retainer. Although this dual retention (fixed and removable retainer) strategy was adopted formerly, it must be emphasized to Lisa that should the bonded retainer partially debond, then the vacuum-formed retainer must be worn to maintain tooth alignment prior to repair or replacement of the bonded retainer.
3. A compromise plan would be to use a sectional clear aligner to the upper labial segment teeth only. Then, prolonged retention would be required to maintain the result, as outlined in option 2 above, with the vacuum-formed retainer confined solely to the labial segment.

As Lisa is now a university student, she was not keen for further fixed appliance therapy and opted for sectional aligner therapy followed by prolonged retention.

Primary resources and recommended reading

Brezniak N, Wasserstein A 2002 Orthodontically induced inflammatory root resorption. Part I. The basic science aspects. Part II: The clinical aspects. Angle Orthod 72:180–184.

Hartsfield JK Jr, Everett ET, Al-Qawasmi RA 2004 Genetic factors in external apical root resorption and orthodontic treatment. Crit Rev Oral Biol Med 15:115–122.

Henneman S, Von den Hoff JW, Maltha JC 2008 Mechanobiology of tooth movement. Eur J Orthod 30:299–306.

Johnston CD, Littlewood SJ 2015 Retention in orthodontics. Br Dent J 218:119–122.

Jonsson A, Malmgren O, Levander E 2007 Long-term follow-up of tooth mobility in maxillary incisors with orthodontically induced apical root resorption. Eur J Orthod 29:482–487.

Kotescha S, Gale S, Khamasha–Ledezma L et al 2015 A multicenter audit of GDPs knowledge of orthodontic retention. Br Dent J 218:645–653.

Littlewood SJ, Millett DT, Doubleday B et al 2016 Retention procedures for stabilising tooth position after treatment with orthodontic braces. Cochrane Database of Syst Rev Issue 1. Art No: CD002283. DOI: 10.1002/14651858.CD002283.pub4.

Little RM 2009 Clinical implications of the University of Washington post-retention studies. J Clin Orthod 43:645–651.

Melrose C, Millett DT 1998 Toward a perspective on orthodontic retention? Am J Orthod Dentofacial Orthop 113:507–514.

Pandis N, Vlahopoulos K, Madianos P et al 2007 Long-term periodontal status of patients with mandibular lingual fixed retention. Eur J Orthod 29:471–476.

Ren Y, Maltha JC, Kuijpers-Jagtman AM 2003 Optimum force magnitude for orthodontic tooth movement: a systematic literature review. Angle Orthod 73:86–92.

Roberts-Harry D, Sandy J 2004 Orthodontics. Part II: orthodontic tooth movement. Br Dent J 196:391–394.

Walker SL, Long DT, Flores-Mir C 2013 Radiographic comparison of the extent of orthodontically induced external apical root resorption in vital and root-filled teeth: a systematic review. Eur J Orthod 35:796–802.

Weltman BJ 2011 External root resorption and orthodontic treatment—assessment of the evidence. In: Huang GJ, Richmond S, Vig KWL (eds), Evidence-based orthodontics. Wiley-Blackwell, Chichester, pp. 63–88.

For revision, see Mind Map 20, page 240.

21

Cleft lip and palate

SUMMARY

Karen, a 9-year-old girl, is unhappy about the appearance of her teeth (*Fig. 21.1*). What is the cause, and how will it be treated?

History

Complaint

Karen does not like the crookedness and spacing of her upper front teeth. Her mother is also aware that the bite of Karen's side teeth is not correct and feels that she moves her jaw to the side when she closes her teeth together.

History of complaint

Karen's baby front teeth were also crooked and spaced. Her mother has noticed the problem with her bite for several months.

Medical history

Karen was born with a cleft lip and palate (CLP), which has been repaired.

Family history

Karen's parents have no family history of cleft lip and palate. Her older brother and sister are also unaffected.

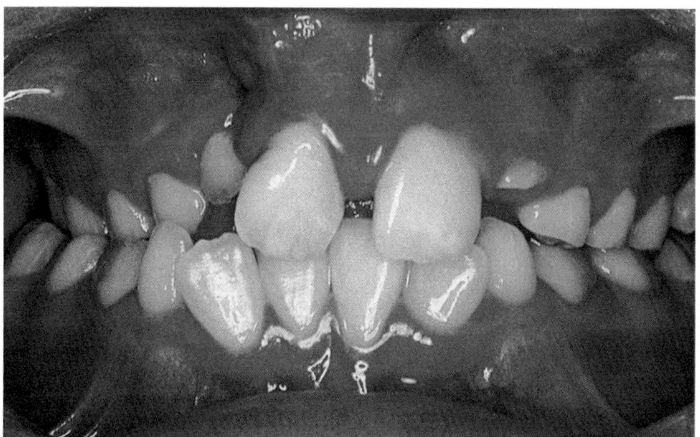

Fig. 21.1 Anterior occlusion at presentation.

■ *How common is a family history with cleft lip and palate? Is this the same for cleft palate (CP) only?*

In around 40% of cases with CLP, there is a family history. For CP alone, however, a family history is less (around 20%).

■ *What is the prevalence of cleft lip and palate?*

It affects about 1 in 700 live births among Caucasians, but the prevalence varies between racial groups as well as geographically and is increasing. Cleft lip only is found in about 9% of all clefts, whereas a cleft of the lip and alveolus comprises about 3% of all clefts. Complete unilateral CLP is the most common type of cleft and represents 50% of all clefts.

■ *Is there a sex and side variation for CLP?*

Females are affected less frequently than males, and the right side is involved less commonly than the left.

■ *How does this malformation occur?*

Failure of fusion of the median and lateral nasal processes and the maxillary process at about 4–6 weeks of intrauterine life leads to a cleft of the primary palate (the upper lip and the alveolus in the anterior region as far posteriorly as the incisive foramen). Cleft of the secondary palate (hard palate from incisive foramen back and soft palate) is due to failure of the palatal shelves to elevate and fuse at about 8 weeks in utero.

Genetic and environmental factors, e.g. steroid therapy, folic acid deficiency or anticonvulsant drugs, interact in the aetiology.

Key point

CLP:

- Prevalence of 1 in 750 live Caucasian births.
- Aetiology due to genetic and environmental factors.
- Positive family history in ~40% of cases.
- More common in males and on the left side.

■ *What genetic risk is there of CLP? How does this compare to CP alone?*

As in this case of CLP, where neither parent has a cleft and one child is affected, there is a small (4%; 1 in 25) risk that the following child will be affected; if the mother or father is affected, there is a 2% (1 in 50) likelihood of the first child having CLP. Due to the lesser genetic involvement in clefts of the secondary palate, for unaffected parents of a child with isolated CP, the risk of a subsequent cleft-affected child is 1 in 80.

Key point

There is a greater genetic risk with CLP than there is with CP.

Karen has been attending a cleft clinic at the regional dental teaching hospital since birth.

■ ***Why is this? What treatment will have been provided to date, and what role have you to play as her general dental practitioner?***

Due to the interdisciplinary care required, treatment is facilitated for the patient and family by coordinating management in a specialized centre with a team comprising an orthodontist, speech therapist, health visitor and clinical psychologist as well as plastic, ENT and maxillofacial surgeons.

Treatment until now is likely to have been as follows:

Neonatal period to 18 months

Parental counselling by a member of the Cleft Lip and Palate Association (CLAPA) and/or clinical psychologist, as well as reassurance of the future treatment by an orthodontist and member of the surgical team.

Advice and support to the parents by a specialized health visitor, particularly in relation to feeding. In this case feeding problems are likely to have been modest, as the cleft only involves the primary palate.

Planning of lip repair: this usually occurs at 3 months, although neonatal repair is being assessed. In this case closure of the alveolar defect may be undertaken at the same time. Where a palatal cleft exists, on average, this is repaired between 6 and 9 months.

Primary dentition

First formal speech and hearing assessment at around 18 months and then speech therapy as required.

Regular speech and hearing assessments should be undertaken; consider closure of any palatal fistulae to assist speech development. Consider pharyngoplasty to reduce velopharyngeal incompetence at 4–5 years, thereby attempting to improve any nasal intonation to speech.

Consider lip revision at 4–5 years only if clearly indicated.

As a general dental practitioner your role is to:

Liaise with the CP team.

Provide dietary advice and oral hygiene instruction to the parents, at regular intervals, from eruption of the primary incisors.

Consider the use of fluoride tablets if the level of fluoride in the local domestic water supply is below 1 ppm.

Attend to any dental treatment required.

Your particular aim in dental care is to promote and maintain excellent dental health for Karen, thereby avoiding the need for restorative treatment or enforced loss of primary teeth through dental caries.

> **Key point**
>
> Management of CLP requires a team approach.

■ ***What skeletal/dental/occlusal problems are commonly found with CLP?***

Skeletally, there is a tendency for the maxilla and mandible to be retrognathic, the upper facial height to be reduced and the lower facial height to be increased. A Class III skeletal pattern is common.

On the cleft side, 2 is either absent, of abnormal size and/or shape, hypoplastic or present as two conical teeth on either side of the cleft.

A supernumerary or supplemental tooth may exist on either side of the cleft.

1 is often rotated and tilted toward the cleft and may be hypoplastic.

Eruption is delayed.

Tooth size elsewhere in the mouth is small.

Class III incisor relationship is common with crossbite of one or both buccal segments and a lateral open bite on the cleft side.

> **Key point**
>
> Incisor and buccal segment crossbites are common in repaired CLP.

Examination

Extraoral

■ ***What do you notice from** Fig. 21.2**?***

Karen has a Class I skeletal pattern with average FMPA and no obvious facial asymmetry. The lips are competent with a scar on the right side of the upper lip.

No clicks, locks or crepitus of the temporomandibular joints were detected.

■ ***How is lip closure achieved?***

A Millard repair with or without its modifications is the most popular, aiming, after dissection, to place the lip muscles and alar base in their correct anatomical location. Whether subperiosteal or supraperiosteal dissection and skin-lengthening cuts are used, to obtain tissue movement, remains controversial. The extent of alar cartilage dissection or the use of a vomer flap also remains unresolved.

Intraoral

■ ***The appearance of the teeth is shown in** Figs 21.1 **and** 21.3**. What are your observations?***

Oral hygiene is fair. Plaque deposits are visible on several teeth. There is marginal gingival erythema related to most teeth.

EDCB1 | 12CDE
6EDC21 | 12CDE6 visible (6|6 were erupted but not shown).

E| restored; possible caries in E|DE; 1| slightly hypoplastic.

Mild lower labial segment crowding.

Spaced upper labial segment with 1| distolabially rotated.

The cleft repair involves the right upper lip and alveolus – a bony depression is evident in the 2| area.

Class III incisor relationship with average overbite; B| in crossbite; lower centreline shift to the right.

Right molar relationship half-unit Class II with buccal segment crossbite involving CDE|; (6| was also involved but not shown); left molar relationship is Class I.

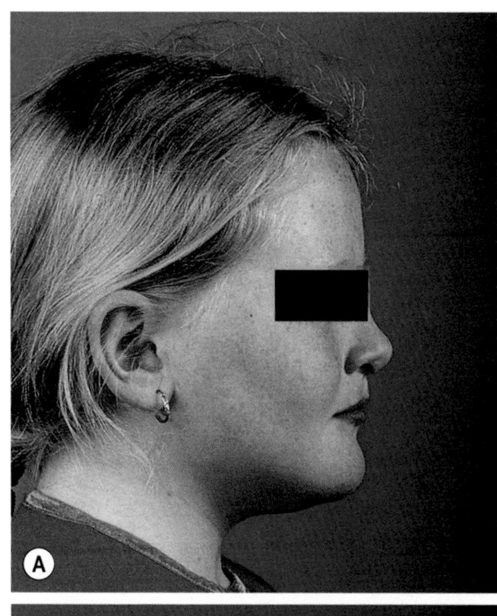

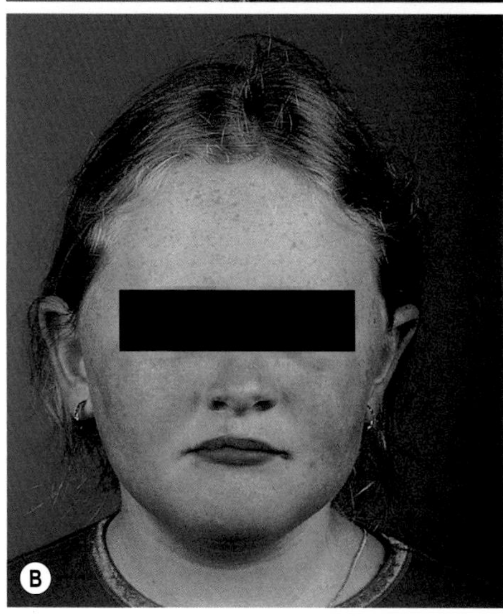

Fig. 21.2 **(A)** Profile. **(B)** Full face.

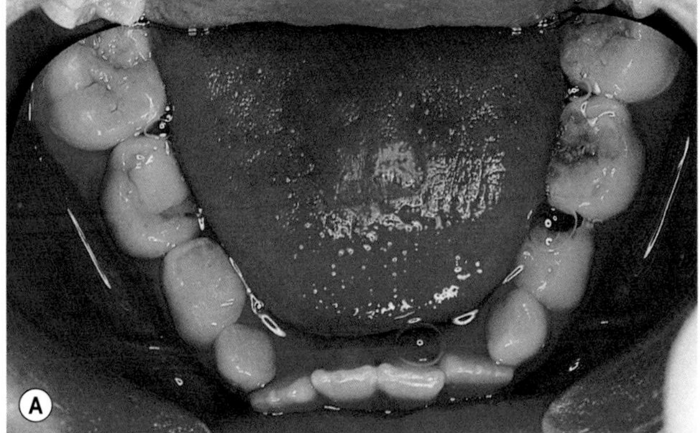

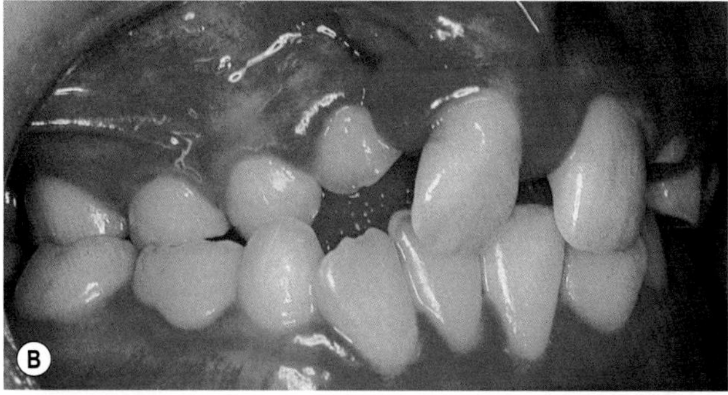

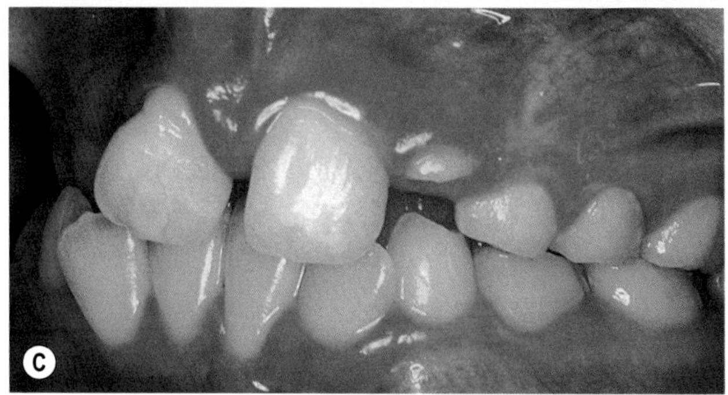

Fig. 21.3 **(A)** Lower occlusal view. **(B)** Right buccal occlusion. **(C)** Left buccal occlusion.

■ ***In view of the unilateral crossbite of the right buccal segment, what should you check for? How would you do this?***

It would be important to check if there is a mandibular displacement on the path of closure associated with the crossbite. As Karen's mother has already noticed a shift of the lower jaw on closure, a displacement is likely. To detect this, Karen should be instructed to maintain the tip of her tongue in contact with the back of her palate as she closes her teeth together. Careful observation should be made of first tooth contact on the path of closure and the extent and direction of any mandibular displacement into maximum intercuspation should be recorded.

There is a mandibular displacement to the right on closure resulting from premature contact of $\frac{C|}{C|}$.

Investigations

■ ***What investigations are required? Explain why.***

A dental panoramic tomogram should be taken to account for the presence and position of any unerupted teeth and to ascertain whether there are any permanent teeth absent.

An upper anterior occlusal radiograph is required to determine the extent of the alveolar cleft and the position of the permanent maxillary canine on the cleft side.

■ ***Karen's dental panoramic tomogram and upper anterior occlusal radiograph are shown in*** *Fig. 21.4*. ***What do you notice?***

The dental panoramic tomogram shows:

- Normal alveolar bone height except for the alveolar cleft in the $\underline{2|}$ area, which extends to involve $\underline{3|}$.
- All permanent teeth are present, except for $\underline{2|}$ and third molars; $\overline{ED|DE}$ are slightly infraoccluded.
- $\underline{1|}$ is hypoplastic; $\overline{E|E}$ appear to have secondary caries underneath the restorations with possible furcation radiolucencies.
- There is carious involvement of $\overline{D|D}$ distally.
- The upper anterior occlusal radiograph confirms the extent of the alveolar cleft, and when assessed in combination with the dental panoramic tomogram, $\underline{3|}$ appears to be lying in the line of the arch.

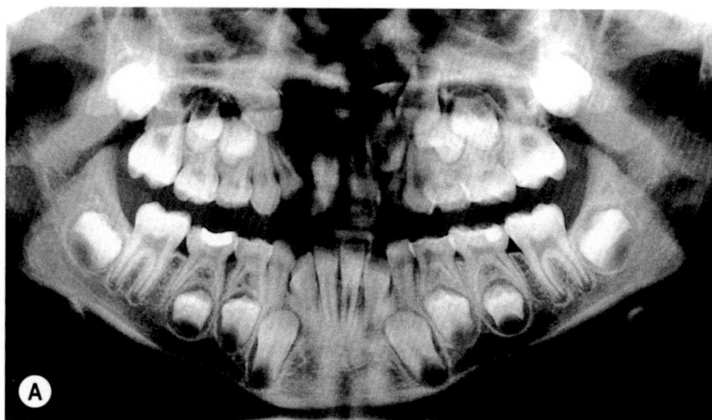

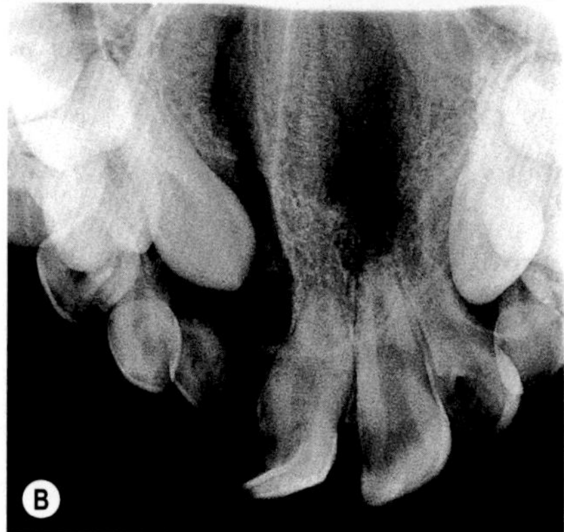

Fig. 21.4 **(A)** Dental panoramic tomogram. **(B)** Upper anterior occlusal radiograph.

Diagnosis

■ ***What is your diagnosis?***

Repaired right unilateral cleft lip and alveolus.

Class III malocclusion on a Class I skeletal base with average FMPA.

Mandibular displacement to the right on closure on $\frac{C|}{C|}$.

Generalized mild marginal gingivitis.

Caries $\overline{\text{ED|DE}}$.

Mild lower labial segment crowding.

Spaced upper labial segment with 1| distolabially rotated; absent 2|.

Lower centreline to the right.

Right molar relationship half-unit Class II with buccal crossbite of the right buccal segments; left molar relationship is Class I.

■ ***What is the IOTN DHC grade (see p. 264)? Explain why.***

5p – due to CLP.

Treatment

■ ***What are the aims of treatment at this stage?***

Caries control.

Elimination of the mandibular displacement with correction of the right buccal segment crossbite.

Elimination of the alveolar cleft defect.

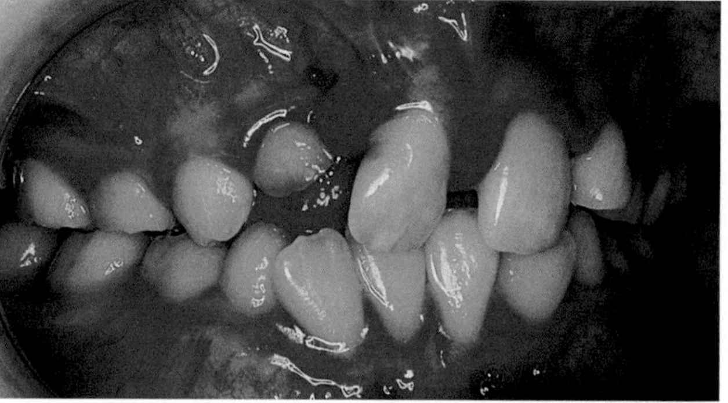

Fig. 21.5 Right buccal occlusion following crossbite correction with quadhelix.

■ ***What would you do at this stage?***

Reinforce oral hygiene practice in preparation for forthcoming orthodontic treatment.

Restore the lower primary molars.

Fissure seal the first permanent molars.

Liaise with the orthodontist on the cleft team regarding the planned orthodontic treatment.

■ ***What form do you envisage the orthodontic treatment to take?***

Upper arch expansion, by a quadhelix appliance, to correct the right buccal segment crossbite is likely to be undertaken prior to alveolar bone grafting.

■ ***When is secondary alveolar bone grafting usually undertaken and what advantages does it confer?***

Optimally, it is usually undertaken at around 9–10 years. It provides bone through which 3 can erupt, restores arch integrity, improves alar base support, aids closure of an oronasal fistula and allows orthodontic space closure.

■ ***The occlusion prior to bone grafting is shown in*** *Fig. 21.5*. ***What may you consider at this stage?***

Due to the advanced state of root resorption of C| (see also **Fig. 21.4**), it would be useful to remove this at least 3 weeks before grafting to allow time for socket healing, thereby improving the likelihood of graft success as an access route for oral infection is removed.

■ ***What treatment will be required following alveolar bone grafting?***

Once 3| erupts, consider space closure with 2| replacement by 3| as the right upper buccal segment is brought forward. This is a feasible plan and is the preferred option, as it obviates the need for any prosthetic replacement of 2|.

Consider relief of crowding in the non-cleft quadrant and in the lower arch. Delay any lower arch extractions if orthognathic surgery is planned at a later date.

Fixed appliance therapy will be necessary for the active tooth movements required.

Bonded retention will then be required to maintain upper labial segment alignment, and restorative treatment will be required to make 3| simulate an upper lateral incisor.

What restorative considerations are there when 3| replaces 2|?

Restorative considerations depend on the colour, size and shape of 3| in 2| position and an assessment of functional occlusion (see Chapter 3). Close assessment should be made of |2, so that insofar as possible, 3| is a close match to |2. Bleaching of 3| may be required to tone in with the incisors. Some reshaping of the 3| crown is also likely – in particular, reducing the prominence of the cusp tip and possible composite addition to the mesial surface so that it more closely resembles a 2|.

As 4| will then be in the position of a canine, occlusal adjustment of the palatal cusp may be necessary to remove any interference in lateral mandibular excursions. Alternatively, if 4| has been intruded orthodontically to achieve coincidence of the gingival margins of 4| and 1|, composite addition may be needed to achieve 'canine' guidance.

In the late teenage years, consideration may be given to further lip revision or orthognathic surgery with rhinoplasty later, if a marked anteroposterior and/or vertical skeletal discrepancy exists.

In Karen's case, provided facial growth is reasonably favourable, orthognathic surgery may not be required.

Key point

Secondary alveolar bone grafting:

- Provides bone for 3 eruption.
- Restores arch integrity.
- Improves alar base support.
- Aids oronasal fistula closure.
- Allows orthodontic space closure.

Primary resources and recommended reading

Bergland O, Semb G, Abyholm FE 1986 Elimination of the residual alveolar cleft by secondary bone grafting and subsequent orthodontic treatment. Cleft Palate J 23:175–205.

Guo J, Li C, Zhang Q et al 2011 Secondary bone grafting for alveolar cleft in children with cleft lip or cleft lip and palate. Cochrane Database of Syst Rev Issue 6. Art No: CD008050. DOI: 10.1002/14651858.CD008050.pub2.

Mossey P, Little J, Munger RG et al 2009 Cleft Lip and Palate. Lancet 374:1773–1785.

Rivkin CJ, Keith O, Crawford PJM et al 2000 Dental care for the patient with a cleft lip and palate. Part 1: From birth to the mixed dentition stage; Part 2: The mixed dentition stage through to adolescence and young adulthood. Br Dent J 118:78–83, 131–134.

Thom AR 1990 Modern management of the cleft lip and palate patient. Dent Update 17:402–408.

For revision, see Mind Map 21, page 241.

22

Nursing and early childhood caries

SUMMARY

Kelly-Ann is only 3 years old. She has been brought to the dentist by her mother because her upper front teeth are 'wearing away' (Fig. 22.1). What has caused this, and how may it be treated?

History

The teeth apparently never came through properly and were never white like the rest of her teeth. There has been no pain from the teeth, and Kelly-Ann is eating and drinking normally.

Medical history

Kelly-Ann is a healthy child. She has had all her vaccinations and has had no illnesses. She has never taken any medication.

Examination

Extraorally there is no swelling and no facial asymmetry. Intraorally she is in the full primary dentition with the second primary molars having just erupted. There is caries affecting the upper incisors and cavitation in all first primary molars.

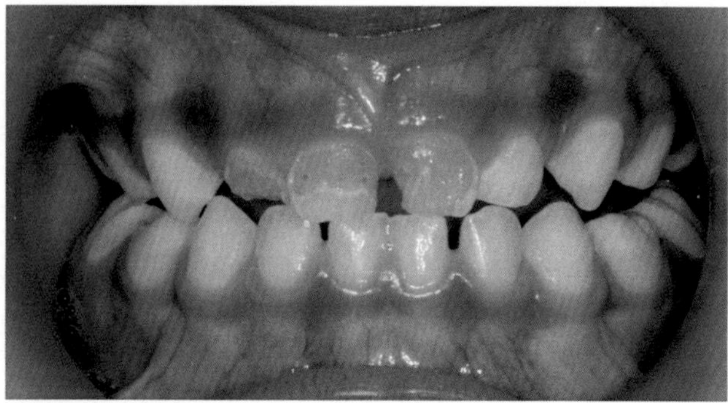

Fig. 22.1 Early cavitation in nursing caries affecting upper right lateral and central primary incisor and upper left central incisor.

■ ***What is the cause of this pattern of decay?***

'Nursing caries', or 'nursing bottle mouth' or 'bottle mouth caries'.

■ ***What can cause this?***

Consumption of a sweetened drink or fruit-flavoured drink from a bottle or dinky feeder, especially if the feeder is constantly in the mouth or the child falls asleep with it in the mouth. Care should also be taken with lactulose-free alternatives to dairy milk such as soya or rice milk.

Persistent on-demand breastfeeding at night after 12 months of age (child is allowed to sleep on the breast) may cause caries. There are many biological and social variables that confound this complex relationship.

As can be seen, the term 'nursing caries' is probably the most accurate as it encompasses both breastfeeding and bottle feeding.

■ ***Why are the teeth affected in this pattern?***

Teeth become carious in the order in which they erupt (**Fig. 22.2**), with the exception of the lower primary incisors, which are protected by two major mechanisms: the position of the submandibular ducts that open adjacent to these teeth and the position of the tongue in suckling, which covers the lower incisors.

■ ***What additional factors make the upper primary incisors more predisposed to caries?***

High bow-shaped upper lip in infants which does not cover the upper incisors and results in an increased evaporation of any saliva on these teeth.

Gravity, which keeps submandibular saliva pooled around the lower incisors and less likely to reach the upper incisors.

Any liquid with sugar that is allowed to bathe the teeth on a frequent basis will cause caries. This is especially so at night when the protective function of saliva reduces as less saliva is produced. Even breast milk, formula milk or cows' milk with their lowered natural sugars can still be cariogenic on this basis.

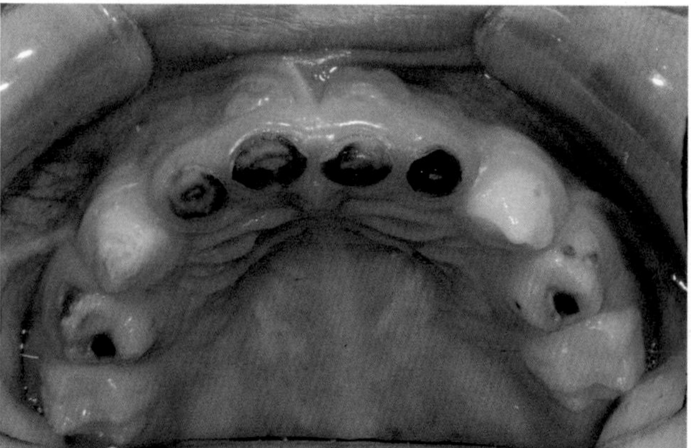

Fig. 22.2 Classical distribution of affected teeth in nursing caries in upper arch. This is a more advanced case than Kelly-Ann's, with signficant caries involving all maxillary primary incisors and upper central incisors non-vital and infected. Occlusal caries is also seen in upper first primary molars.

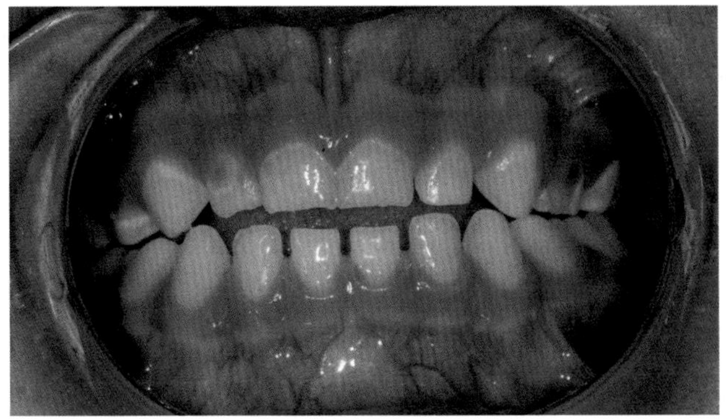

Fig. 22.3 Hypomineralization and hypoplasia are seen on the buccal surfaces of DBA|ABD.

In some situations maxillary incisors may erupt with hypoplastic or hypomineralized defects, thus making the teeth less resistant to the development of dental caries (**Fig. 22.3**).

> **Key point**
>
> Nursing caries:
>
> - Affects teeth in order of eruption.
> - Lower incisors are protected by saliva.
> - Can be caused by any sugar-containing liquid even if the sugar is naturally occurring rather than added to the liquid.

■ ***What should be your advice about night-time feeding?***

Only water should be given during the night after 12 months of age.

The term early childhood caries (ECC) is a further term used to describe caries presenting in one or more primary teeth of children under the age of 5. Some children present with extensive caries that does not follow the 'nursing caries' pattern and often present later, between 3 and 5 years old (**Fig. 22.4**).

■ ***How could you identify pre-school children in need of dental care?***

Encourage parents to bring their children for a dental check-up as soon as the first primary tooth erupts.

Develop good working relationships with local health visitors, baby clinics, mother and baby groups, nurseries and their local general medical practice to encourage wider health and nursery staff to provide appropriate oral health advice. This advice should follow the guidance of the Department of Health (DoH) Prevention Toolkit. Public health programmes in some countries encourage and train general health professionals, such as health visitors, to 'lift the lip' to identify early caries affecting the upper maxillary incisors.

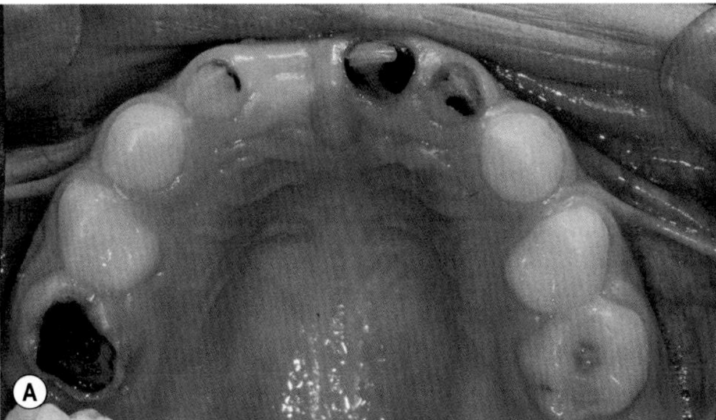

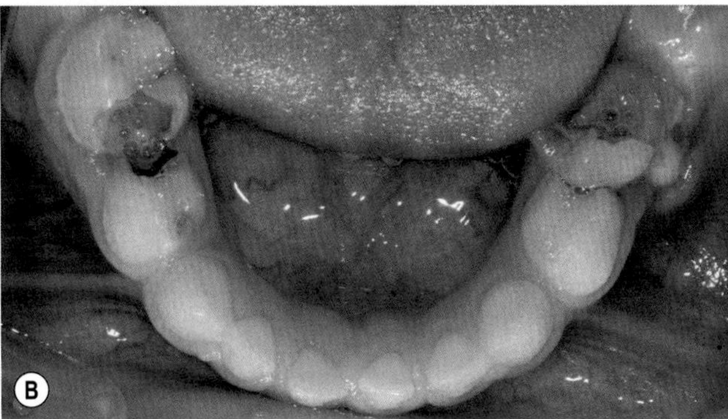

Fig. 22.4 (A & B) Upper and lower dentition of a child with extensive early childhood caries (EB|ABE over ED|DE) with a differing pattern to that of nursing caries. Please note the gross caries in the lower second primary molars with an associated sinus E| and exposure of root |E.

Treatment

Prevention

■ ***Kelly-Ann is at high risk for caries. List all the main factors you can think of for placing someone in the high risk group for dental caries.***

See **Table 22.1**.

■ ***What preventive advice would you provide for Kelly-Ann's mother?***

Preventive advice should follow the DoH Prevention Toolkit guidance. This provides advice for children of different ages (in Kelly-Ann's case, 0–3 years old) following placement in the high risk for caries category.

Home based advice Although many parents are fully aware of the causes of dental caries in their child or children, changing family behaviour to undertake healthier routines is more complex. Consequently, careful consideration is needed in how preventive advice is given and who delivers it. All members of the dental team should have a basic understanding of how they can support parents and children to undertake these changes, and those delivering these preventive messages should have a more detailed knowledge of behaviour change strategies.

Toothbrushing and fluoride toothpaste Kelly Ann's parents should undertake toothbrushing for her last thing at night

Table 22.1 'High-risk' factors for caries

Risk factor	Aetiology
Clinical evidence	New lesions
	Premature extractions
	Anterior caries or restorations
	Multiple restorations
	Fixed appliance orthodontics
	Partial dentures
Dietary habits	Frequent sugar intake
Social history	Social deprivation
	High caries in siblings
	Low knowledge of dental disease
	Irregular attendance
	Ready availability of snacks
	Low dental aspirations
Use of fluoride	Drinking water not fluoridated
	No fluoride supplements
	No fluoride toothpaste
Plaque control	Infrequent, ineffective cleaning
	Poor manual control
	Lack of parental involvement in brushing
Saliva	Low flow rate
	Low buffering capacity
	High *Streptococcus mutans* and *Lactobacillus* counts
Medical history	Medically compromised
	Physical disability
	Intellectual disability
	Xerostomia
	Long-term cariogenic medicine

and at least on one other occasion every day. On each occasion, a smear of 1350–1500 ppm toothpaste should be used.

Why is parental involvement important?

Children need help from their parents if effective oral hygiene is to be achieved. This help should extend up to at least 7 years old. Brushing needs to start as soon as the first tooth erupts. Standing or kneeling behind the child in front of a sink or mirror is often the best way to brush a young child's teeth. Other successful ways include the child lying on his or her parents' legs. Supervision of brushing is important so that an appropriate amount of paste is placed on the brush to prevent/reduce ingestion of paste. Careful questioning of parents and hands-on demonstration of how to undertake toothbrushing is important. Qualitative research has reported a number of barriers that parents describe when trying to undertake their child's toothbrushing. A number of these barriers relate to parenting skills, such as managing toddlers who want to brush themselves, or establishing and maintaining routines. Consequently advice and guidance needs to address these wider parenting issues. The use of simple serial plaque and gingivitis scores (with or without a disclosing agent) allows the dental professional to monitor parental compliance with the toothbrushing advice.

What advice should be given if Kelly-Ann does not like strong, mint-flavoured toothpaste?

Some children struggle with the strong mint flavours used in adult toothpaste. As a dental care professional, you should be able to advise on alternative child-friendly toothpastes. These should have a mild, non-minty flavour that still have the required levels of fluoride. Other children may struggle with the foaming action of the toothpaste, and again you should be able to provide advice on the availability of toothpastes without these agents (for example, sodium lauryl sulphate-free toothpastes).

Is there a role for fluoride supplements?

Fluoride supplements although still recommended are no longer considered a mainline intervention. The reason for this relates to the poor compliance with these supplements in the families with children at high risk. All fluoride products, including toothpaste, should be treated as a medicine and kept out of reach of young children to prevent excessive ingestion. The DoH Prevention Toolkit provides further reading and advice on preventing fluorosis, especially for children at low caries risk living in areas with fluoridated water supplies.

Diet advice The only way to effectively undertake dietary advice is to ask parents to complete a 4-day diet diary. From this a written analysis can be produced. It is important to try to obtain 1 day's history from a weekend, as they are invariably different from weekdays. In modern society it is common for most parents to work and the child to be looked after by a carer or nursery. It is critical to establish who is the carer on weekdays and weekends. Advice needs to be clear at all times, but if it has to be relayed from a parent in the surgery to a carer, then it needs to be clear, succinct and written. Frequent consumption of sugar-containing drinks and foods is the key aetiological feature in many pre-school children with caries. Reducing the frequency of sugar-containing snacks is an important message. If the child is a 'poor eater', there is need to build up the amount of food at mealtimes and, therefore, reduce the need for frequent snacking. Children do not need fizzy drinks or fruit-based drinks. These drinks often make up for calories missed at mealtimes. Only milk and water should be taken between meals. A small amount of fruit-based drink can more safely be taken with a meal. As previously mentioned, it is critical to stop the night-time bottle with anything other than water.

In your dietary advice you must be *practical*, *personal* and *positive*. Avoid making the parent feel excessively guilty, but concentrate on practical strategies. It is probably unreasonable to give out more than four pieces of written advice. These should concentrate on day-time drinks, night-time drinks, between-meal snacks, and making sure the child has no food or drink for 1 hour before going to bed and cleans their teeth just before bed. Furthermore, dietary advice should not be limited to sugary snacks but also briefly evaluate the diet as a whole and assess if it is in line with the eat well plate.

Medication For children on regular medication, this should, where possible, be sugar free. Often this will require liaison with their general medical practitioner. A careful medical history-taking is essential, as some parents may not perceive regular nutritional supplements or laxatives as medication.

Professional interventions For Kelly-Ann, current advice is that fluoride varnish should be applied to her teeth three to four times a year. Site-specific application of fluoride varnish can be very valuable in the management of early, smooth-surface and approximal carious lesions. The most commonly used varnish – 5% sodium fluoride – has 22 600 ppm. Before applying the varnish the child's asthma status and any history of allergy to colophony should be checked. In cases where children have been hospitalized for their asthma or have a history of an allergic reaction to sticky plasters (which can contain colophony), the use of colophony containing fluoride varnishes are contraindicated. Alternative, non-colophony-containing varnishes are available. When applying the varnish, ensure the correct dose and instructions are given.

The recall interval between dental clinic visits will reduce to 3 months. This will enable the more frequent application of fluoride varnish, more intense preventive support and the examination of Kelly-Ann's dentition for caries progression or new lesions.

Why can Kelly-Ann not have fluoride mouthwash? These are contraindicated in children less than 6 years of age because more than half the mouthwash will be swallowed, increasing the risk of flurosis. This is also the reason why parents are advised to use only a smear-sized (for 0–3-year-olds) or pea-sized (for 4–6-year-olds) amount of toothpaste and why the child is encouraged to spit out the excess residue of the toothpaste as soon as he or she is able to do so.

Treatment

Restorative care

(Please see Chapter 24, which provides greater detail of treatment options and treatment planning.)

Kelly-Ann has caries involving her upper incisors (**Fig. 22.1**) and cavitated occlusal caries in her first primary molars. Treatment can be provided in a number of ways and relates to parental expectations and willingness to comply with the home-based preventive advice, parents' expectations and wishes, child's cooperation and any history of toothache or other symptoms. Child cooperation can change rapidly as the child grows, and consequently, over a few months, different treatment options may be appropriate with improving behaviour and cooperation. In Kelly-Ann's case, with no history of pain, time was available at first to temporize and seal in the caries with glass ionomer cement (GIC) until cooperation improved.

■ ***How would you restore the upper incisors?***

There are a number of different options and materials available. These include the prevention-only approach with no caries removal or disking, temporarization with GIC or complete caries removal with definitive restoration using either a direct composite or a composite crown using a plastic strip crown. Following the temporary GIC restorations, Kelly-Ann's cooperation improved significantly to permit the placement of direct composite restorations under local anaesthetic several months later.

■ ***How would you restore the early cavitation in the first primary molars?***

Similar to the incisors, different options are available:

Prevention only – namely to modify the cavity to permit plaque removal using a toothbrush and regular application of fluoride varnish. Regular plaque scores will allow you to monitor how well parents are complying with your toothbrushing instructions.

Seal with partial or no caries removal – namely to seal the caries with composite and/or fissure seal following limited caries removal with a slow handpiece.

Complete caries removal – using local anaesthetic, rubber dam and handpieces to remove caries followed by composite restorations.

Initially a preventive approach was taken with the carious first primary molars. As Kelly-Ann's cooperation improved, a complete caries removal approach was undertaken, as both her and her mum wanted white coloured fillings rather than stainless steel crowns.

■ ***What method of caries removal, without a handpiece, may be applicable here?***

With the advent of the Hall technique (see Chapter 24) chemical caries removal has had limited use. An example of chemo-mechanical caries removal is the use of Carisolv. It consists of a pink gel that contains mainly the amino acids leucine, lysine, glutamic acid and hypochlorite. In addition, there is cellulose and a colouring agent, erythrocin. The amino acids and hypochlorite work to separate carious dentine from sound dentine, and the carious dentine is removed with the aid of special hand instruments that have different cutting edges and hand actions to excavators. They are used in a whisking, rotating or up-and-down movement. Because the sound dentine is not stimulated by the temperature or vibration of a handpiece, or the temperature changes of a three-in-one spray, it is a painless procedure. The cavity should be dried by saline-dampened cotton wool, then dry cotton wool, prior to restoring with an adhesive material. Bond strengths to adhesive materials are the same as conventionally prepared cavities. The disadvantages of the technique include the taste of Carisolv if it should leak out of the cavity, the time taken to remove caries and the noises and sensation of the hand instruments.

■ ***How is pain relief best achieved in the child with nursing caries in** Fig. 22.2**?***

This is a case where general anaesthesia for tooth removal is justified. This is covered in Chapter 26. Depending on the type of the general aneasthetic (extraction only or comprehensive care), dental care would consist of either extracting all carious teeth (DBA|ABD) or extracting irreversibly inflamed and non-vital primary teeth and restoring other teeth affected by caries together with fissure sealants of other primary molars.

Primary resources and recommended reading

American Academy of Pediatric Dentistry 2014 Guideline on caries-risk assessment and management for infants, children, and adolescents. Pediatr Dent 36 (6):127–134.

American Academy of Pediatric Dentistry 2014 Policy on early childhood caries (ECC): unique challenges and treatment options. Pediatr Dent 36 (6):53–55.

Deery C 2013 Caries detection and diagnosis, sealants and management of the possibly carious fissure. Br Dent J 214 (11):551–557.

Healthcare Improvement Scotland 2014 SIGN 138: Dental Interventions to Prevent Caries in Children. Edinburgh, SIGN. Available at: http://www.sign.ac.uk/pdf/SIGN138.pdf.

Public Health England 2014 Delivering Better Oral Health: An Evidence-Based Toolkit for Prevention, 3rd ed. London, Public Health England. Available at: https://www.gov.uk/government/uploads/system/uploads/attachment_data/file/367563/DBOHv32014OCTMainDocument_3.pdf.

Scotish Dental Clinical Effectiveness Programme (SDCEP) 2010 Prevention and Management of Dental Caries in Children: Dental Clinical Guidance. Dundee, SDCEP. Available at: http://www.sdcep.org.uk/wp-content/uploads/2013/03/SDCEP_PM_Dental_Caries_Full_Guidance1.pdf.

Marshman Z, Ahern S, McEachan R et al Parents experiences of tooth brushing with children: a qualitative study. Accepted for publication in Journal of Dentistry Clinical and Translational Research, 2016.

For revision, see Mind Map 22, page 242.

23

High caries risk adolescents

SUMMARY

Peter is 13 years old. He is concerned about the appearance of his teeth, especially the spaces between his front teeth, and would like this improved (*Fig. 23.1*). He is not very keen on the prospect of complex restorative or orthodontic treatment. On assessment he is diagnosed as high caries risk. How would you plan preventive treatment for this patient?

History

Complaint

Peter attends your surgery for the first time in a number of years. He advises you he would like the spaces between his front teeth corrected (**Fig. 23.1**).

History of complaint

Peter is a sporadic attendee. He reports no pain from any of his teeth. He is now keen on having the appearance of his front teeth improved and is eager to learn how this can be achieved.

Medical history

Peter is fit and well. He is not taking any medication.

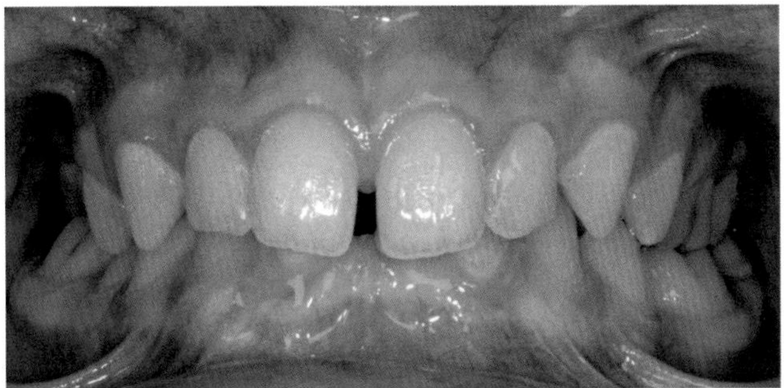

Fig. 23.1 Anterior view of teeth at presentation.

Dental history

At the age of 5 years he had a number of his primary teeth extracted under general anaesthetic.

He has subsequently required restorative care and an extraction of his upper right first permanent molar under local anaesthetic several years ago. You have not seen Peter for at least 3 years (**Fig. 23.1**).

■ ***Which aspects of his presentation and history help to determine his caries risk status so far?***

- Social history – irregular attendance and low dental aspirations to date (high caries risk).
- Fluoridated water – living in an area with no fluoride in the drinking water (high caries risk).
- Medical history – fit and well (low caries risk).
- Dental history – primary tooth extractions under general anaesthesia and subsequent permanent tooth extraction and restorations with local anaesthetic (high caries risk).

Examination

Extraoral

Nothing relevant is revealed.

Intraoral

Peter's oral hygiene is poor. Basic Periodontal Examination (BPE) scores of one in each sextant are recorded. Normal saliva levels are noted. Caries is evident in the lower left second permanent molar. He is in the permanent dentition with missing both lower central incisors and a retained lower left primary central incisor. His upper right first permanent molar was extracted previously and the upper and lower left first permanent molars and lower right first and second molars restored. No fissure sealants are present. There is evidence of mild buccal crowding in the lower arch with lower left second permanent premolar lingually placed. The upper left second permanent premolar is unerupted and palatally displaced (**Figs 23.2** and **23.3**).

■ ***Which further aspects of his clinical presentation help determine his caries risk status?***

Clinical evidence

New caries in the lower left second permanent molar, previous restorations and a missing permanent tooth which

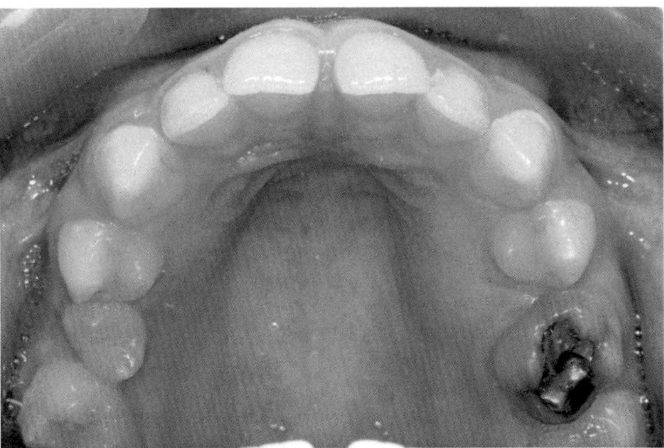

Fig. 23.2 Upper occlusal view at presentation, with upper right six previously extracted.

was extracted are all noted (high caries risk). This caries risk category will have the largest weighting in scoring overall caries risk.

Plaque control

Oral hygiene poor, BPE scores all one. His oral hygiene is especially poor in the upper anterior region (high caries risk).

Saliva

Normal saliva levels noted (low caries risk).

For a full list of caries risk factors, see Chapter 22, **Table 22.1**. This will help build up a picture of caries risk and formulate a prevention plan that is tailored to the patient's requirements.

- ***At present what caries risk status would you assign Peter to?***

High caries risk.

- ***What further information would you ask Peter to complete his caries risk assessment?***

Fluoride history

What strength/type of fluoride toothpaste does he use? If Peter is not aware of the fluoride strength of the toothpaste he uses, he should be shown how to determine this on a toothpaste tube. He should be using toothpaste strength at least 1350–1500 ppm F (children 6 and older). He is presently using a brand which is the correct strength/type for a low caries risk child of his age.

How many times a day does he brush his teeth? He presently brushes twice daily, but not effectively. Twice daily for 2 minutes should be recommended and the technique demonstrated.

Does he presently rinse with water after brushing? He rinses his teeth with water after brushing. The 'spit but don't rinse' with water guidance should be recommended.

Is he presently using any fluoride mouthwash? If so, when does he do this? At present only toothpaste is used. Fluoride mouthwash should be recommended 0.05% NaF at a separate time to brushing his teeth, for example after coming in from school or after dinner is well remembered by many high caries risk patients.

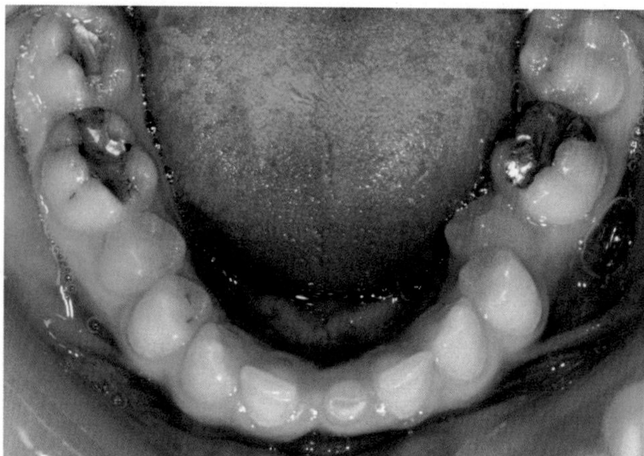

Fig. 23.3 Lower occlusal view at presentation.

Dietary history

Frequency and timing of all food and drinks including milk and water? Carbonated drinks are consumed at least four times a week with diluted juice consumed on a daily basis.

Frequency and timing of food. Peter is a grazer and likes to eat well into the evening. Peter is advised to complete a 4-day diet diary (at least 1 day should be completed over the weekend; high caries risk).

Peter's history, clinical assessment and further questioning combine to give a final caries risk assessment, which indicate a high caries risk status (**Table 23.1**).

> **Key point**
>
> Caries risk assessment:
>
> - The largest weighted caries risk assessment category is clinical evidence.
> - The completion of a caries risk assessment helps formulate an enhanced prevention plan specific to this patient.

Preventive care and treatment

Peter is presently high caries risk. Prior to restorative work being undertaken, the preventive treatment plan should ensure that his caries risk status is reduced and he remains caries free in the future.

Radiographs

- ***After the initial bitewing radiographs are taken** (Fig. 23.4), **when should Peter have radiographs taken again?***

In 6 months' time if he remains at high caries risk.

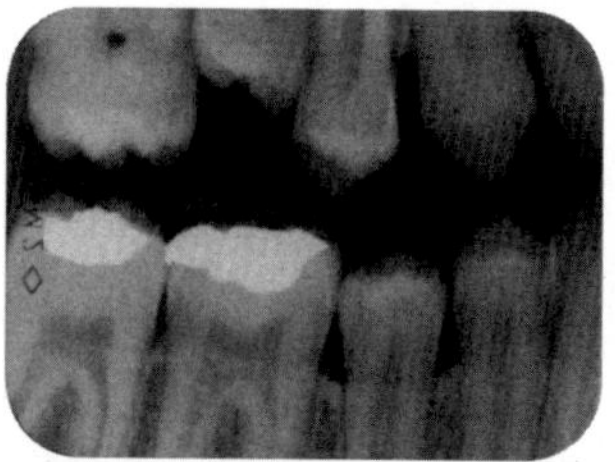

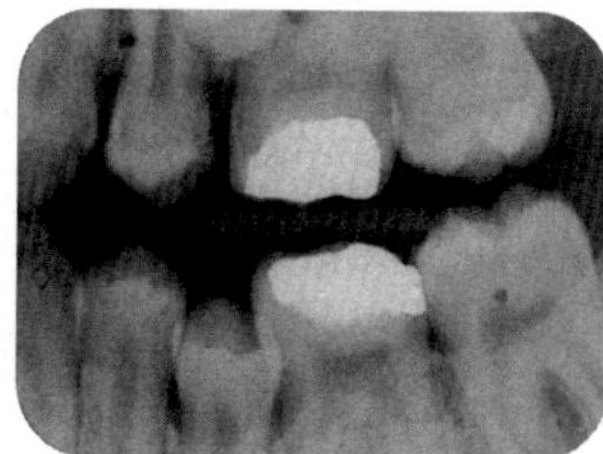

Fig. 23.4 Bitewing radiographs. These show dentinal caries in the left lower second permanent molar and enamel lesions on upper left first permanent premolar and the lower right first permanent molar.

Table 23.1 Peter's caries risk assessment

Clinical evidence	Dietary habits	Social history	Fluoride use	Plaque control	Saliva	Medical history	Caries risk
L **H**	L **H**	L **H**	L **H**	L **H**	**L** H	**L** H	L **H**

What other forms of preventive care would he benefit from?

Toothbrushing instruction Oral hygiene instruction with a toothbrushing demonstration at each recall visit for enhanced prevention.

Children of Peter's age should be shown how to brush their teeth using disclosing tablets or solutions. Disclosing tablets should be used before going to bed when time can be devoted to improving brushing techniques. Although patients or parents may ask about the benefits of a manual or powered toothbrush, clinically it is more important what he does with the toothbrush in respect to the thoroughness of the brushing and its frequency.

Does he use anything to clean in between his teeth? He was shown previously how to do this, but 'his mum forgot to buy more floss'. Explain the importance of interdental cleaning and ask Peter to demonstrate flossing in his own mouth. Give motivational feedback. This is especially important, as enamel lesions are visible on the bitewing radiographs.

Strength of fluoride toothpaste In addition to the advice on adult toothpaste strength on initial presentation, due to Peter's age and high caries risk status, he would gain additional benefit from a prescription of a higher-strength 2800 ppm F toothpaste.

Fluoride varnish application The evidence suggests an additional benefit of three to four applications annually of fluoride varnish for children at high caries risk. Even if Peter's caries risk status were to subsequently reduce to low caries risk, twice-yearly application of a fluoride varnish, termed standard prevention care (2.2% sodium fluoride 22 600 ppm F), would still be recommended.

Fluoride supplements Fluoride mouthwash at 0.05% sodium fluoride, alcohol free, is recommended for daily use at a separate time to toothbrushing. Demonstrate to the patient on a mouthwash bottle where the fluoride concentration information is written. This then allows the patient to make an informed choice regarding the many brands of mouthwash available for use on a daily basis. The mouthwash should be swished around the mouth for 60 seconds before spitting out the residue.

Diet analysis As stated in Chapter 22, a 4-day diet diary can highlight frequency and timing of foods that enable practical and patient-centred advice to be given. Advice should be given in line with the eat-well plate. Children of secondary school age can be given information that enables them to make informed choices regarding their eating and drinking practices. In many situations, simple changes can reduce their caries risk significantly.

Fissure sealants Peter required fissure sealants on all his premolars (**Figs 23.5** and **23.6**).

Table 23.2 helps highlight the complete package of preventive care that Peter should receive prior to any restorative work is undertaken.

Where more extensive caries is seen in an adolescent, stabilization of the dentition is often an appropriate first step. This can be undertaken with simple hand excavation and glass ionomer cement temporaries. This will slow down the progress of caries while the response of the child and family to the preventive advice can be evaluated. As gingival health improves, definitive caries removal and composite or other restorative options can be undertaken. Further benefits of this approach are discussed in Chapter 24.

Only on completion of this initial phase of prevention and simple restorative treatment should composite build-ups or other adhesive bridgework be considered (**Figs 23.7** and **23.8**). In Peter's case the retained lower left primary

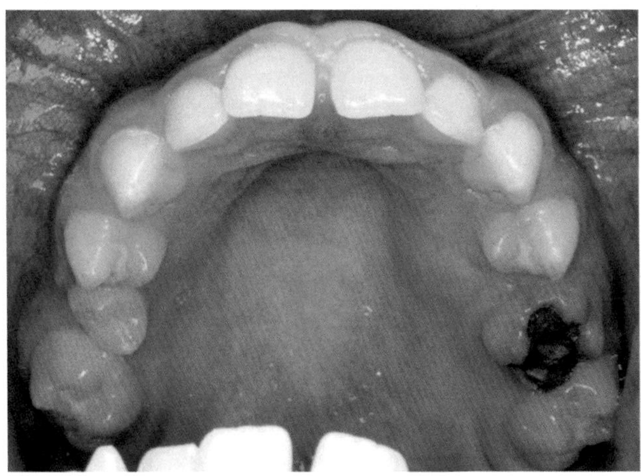

Fig. 23.5 Fissure sealants in upper premolars. The upper left second permanent premolar is unerupted and visible as a budge on the palate.

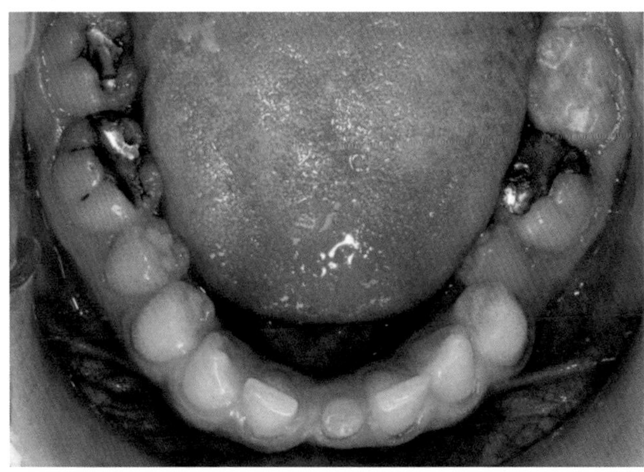

Fig. 23.6 Fissure sealants in lower premolars.

Table 23.2 Peter's prevention plan

Radiographs (Frequency)	Toothbrushing Instruction	Strength F^- toothpaste (F^- ppm)	F^- varnish (frequency)	F^- supplements (dose)	Diet analysis	Fissure sealants	Sugar-free medicines
6 months	With disclosing tablets and interdental advice and demonstration	2800 ppm F	3–4 monthly application	Daily use fluoride mouth wash 0.05% Na F	4-day food diary (in line with the eat-well plate)	Yes | Yes Yes | Yes	N/A

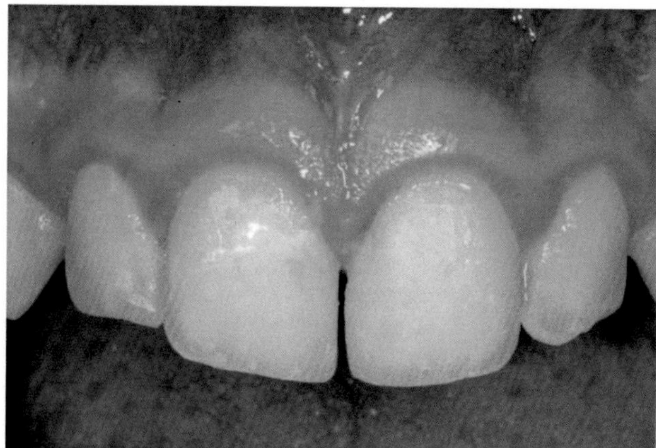

Fig. 23.7 Final restorative treatment of the upper incisors.

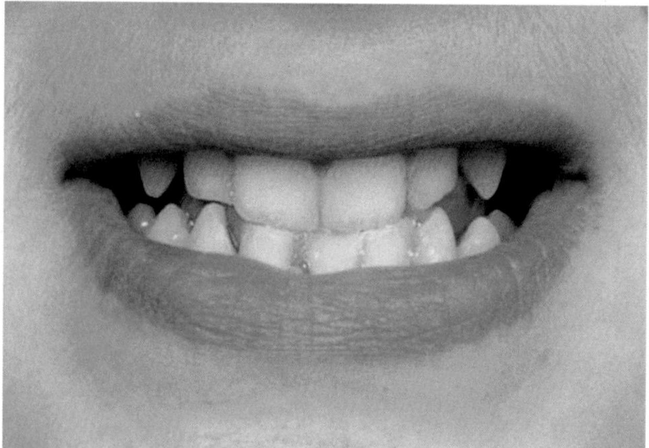

Fig. 23.8 Final restorative care of the anteriors.

central incisor was assessed and due to limited root length, he was advised of its poor long-term prognosis. The primary incisor was extracted and a one-unit Maryland bridge provided with further related oral hygiene instruction. This included the use of superfloss to clean beneath the pontic. At a later stage, should Peter decide he would like more complex treatment such as fixed orthodontics or implants, this can still be provided.

Key point

Preventive care:

- The evidence to date suggests an additional benefit from application of fluoride varnish 3–4 yearly in high caries risk children. Apply twice yearly in low caries risk children.
- Fluoride mouthwash at 0.05% sodium fluoride is recommended for daily use at a separate time to toothbrushing.
- For high caries risk children (age 10 and over) and adolescents, higher strength prescription fluoride toothpaste (2800 ppm F) is recommended.

What else might you suggest when Peter is older that could help further reduce his caries risk status for the future?

Higher strength fluoride toothpaste (5000 ppm F). The effect of fluoride toothpaste is concentration dependent. The maximal over-the-counter product is 1500 ppm fluoride. Prescription-only toothpastes containing 2800 and 5000 ppm fluoride allows the dental professional to target high caries risk adolescents. The results of a number of randomized clinical trials suggest that in the range 1000–2500 ppm fluoride, every additional 500 ppm fluoride, over and above 1000 ppm fluoride, would provide a cumulative 6% reduction in caries increment. This dose response is highest in high caries risk children and those aged over 11 years. However, this would only be prescribed after assessing suitability and compliance with instructions for the use of higher strength fluoride toothpaste. It should be emphasized that such high-strength fluoride toothpastes should be kept out of reach of younger children. Individuals for whom this toothpaste is prescribed should be encouraged to expectorate after brushing. The 5000 ppm fluoride toothpaste is used for adolescents over 16 years of age and adults.

Tooth mousse or tooth mousse plus (CPP-ACP or CPP-ACFP). Tooth mousse is a water-based cream containing Recaldent (casein phosphopeptide-amorphous calcium phosphate or CPP-ACP). Tooth mousse plus, a stronger tooth mousse, is recommended at night only for patients who either have marked salivary dysfunction or increase risk of mineral loss from dental caries or erosion of teeth. Children should be at least 6 years of age before using tooth mousse plus. The proposed anticariogenic mechanism of CPP-ACP involves the enhancement of remineralization through the localization of bioavailable calcium and phosphate ions at the tooth surface. Casein phosphopeptides (CPPs) stabilize high concentrations of calcium and phosphate ions as embryonic ACP nanoclusters together with fluoride ions at the tooth surface by binding to pellicle and plaque and act as a delivery vehicle to the tooth surface. The ions are freely bioavailable to diffuse down concentration gradients into enamel subsurface lesions, thereby effectively promoting remineralization. Tooth mousse may not be appropriate for all patients owing to its cost. This is approximately 5–10 times as expensive as a standard tube of fluoride toothpaste.

Sugar-free chewing gum. Many chewing gums are now available as sugar-free with 50% sweetened with sugar substitutes. Oral bacteria do not use these sugar substitutes to produce the acids that demineralize enamel and dentine. Furthermore, the act of chewing stimulates saliva flow, which increases buffering capacity and enhances clearance of food debris and micro-organisms from the oral cavity. Chewing gum containing xylitol, a polyol 5 carbon sweetener, reduces plaque salivary *Streptococcus mutans* levels and tooth decay, as well as enhancing remineralization.

Primary resources and recommended reading

Cochrane NJ, Saranathan S, Cai F et al 2008 Enamel subsurface lesion remineralisation with casein phosphopeptide stabilised solutions of calcium, phosphate and fluoride. Caries Res 42:88–97.

Faculty of General Dental Practice (FGDP) 2013 Selection Criteria for Dental Radiography, third ed. London, FGDP.

Healthcare Improvement Scotland, 2014. SIGN 138: Dental Interventions to Prevent Caries in Children. Edinburgh, SIGN, sections 2–8. Available at: http://www.sign.ac.uk/pdf/SIGN138.pdf.

Kiet AL, Milgrom P, Rothen M 2008 The potential of dental-protective chewing gum in oral health interventions. J Am Dent Assoc 139:553–563.

Public Health England 2014 Delivering Better Oral Health: An Evidence-Based Toolkit for Prevention, third ed. London, Public Health England, sections 2–5.

Walsh T, Worthington HV, Glenny A-M et al 2010 Fluoride toothpastes of different concentrations for preventing dental caries in children and adolescents. Cochrane Database of Systematic Reviews 2010, Issue 1. Art. No.: CD007868. DOI: 10.1002/14651858.CD007868.pub2.

For revision, see Mind Map 23, page 243.

24

Pain control and treatment planning for carious primary teeth

SUMMARY

Paul is 5 years old. He is in pain from one of his upper right back teeth. He has never had any treatment before. How would you manage Paul's problem?

■ ***What questions do you need to ask regarding the pain?***

Site – ask Paul to point to the tooth.

Severity – does the pain stop him from playing, eating or sleeping? This question you often have to ask both Paul and his parents.

Onset – what makes the pain worse? Is it in response to hot, cold or sweet stimuli, or does it occur spontaneously? Does it wake him up from sleep?

Character – is it a sharp pain or is it dull and throbbing?

Duration – how long does it last when the pain is present? How long has Paul suffered from pain? What makes the pain worse or better (e.g. painkillers)

A simple mnemonic can help you to remember the different questions, SOCRATES (Site, Onset, Character, Radiation, Association, Time course, Exacerbating and relieving factors, Severity). Young children may however find some of these questions difficult to answer, such as radiation and association. Moreover, care needs to be taken to use the most appropriate language. For example, even though children may not understand sensitivity, they or their parents are likely to report if they avoid cold drinks or ice cream.

The different characteristics of reversible and irreversible pulpitis are shown in **Table 24.1.** The initial management of a child attending in pain is often constrained by the lack of sleep on behalf of the child or time available to the dentist to treat this extra 'emergency patient'. An accurate diagnosis is essential before any treatment can be provided.

■ ***What dressings can help manage pulpitis initially?***

Reversible pulpitis – if possible, gently excavate the softest layer of coronal caries:

Place a glass ionomer cement (GIC) or other temporary restoration (Kalzinol or Intermediate Restorative Material.). If the pain settles, a more definitive restoration will be required when time permits and as part of a comprehensive treatment plan (see later).

Irreversible pulpitis – if possible, gently excavate the softest layer of coronal caries, then, place a poly-antibiotic and steroid paste (e.g. Ledermix or Odontopaste) beneath the GIC. These pastes are effective at reducing the symptoms from the tooth. Again, more definitive treatment (extraction or pulpectomy) will be required for this tooth when time permits and as part of a comprehensive treatment plan.

Acute apical periodontitis – if a tooth is abscessed, there is often significant coronal destruction. The pulp chamber of such teeth can often be accessed, and a dressing of Ledermix or Odontopaste on some cotton wool placed within the chamber and sealed with a GIC will often lead to temporary resolution of symptoms and swelling. Again, more definitive treatment (extraction or pulpectomy) will be required for this tooth when time permits and as part of a comprehensive treatment plan.

Where time and patient cooperation permit, dressing open cavities has a number of advantages (see Key Point box and Fig. 24.1):

Simple introduction to dental procedures.

Oral mutans streptococci count is reduced when excavation of gross caries is accomplished. If the cavity is then completely sealed by a GIC, there is evidence that the viability of the remaining organisms decreases and caries progression is greatly reduced. This buys the dentist time to institute preventive and behaviour management programmes before reassessing teeth with temporary restorations.

GICs act as a fluoride reservoir.

Makes toothbrushing and eating more comfortable.

Table 24.1 Pain characteristics

Reversible	Irreversible
Transient or short duration (minutes)	Long duration
Response to hot, cold, sweet	Response to pressure (chewing)
Sharp	Spontaneous
Does not stop play or sleep	Throbbing
	Stops play or sleep

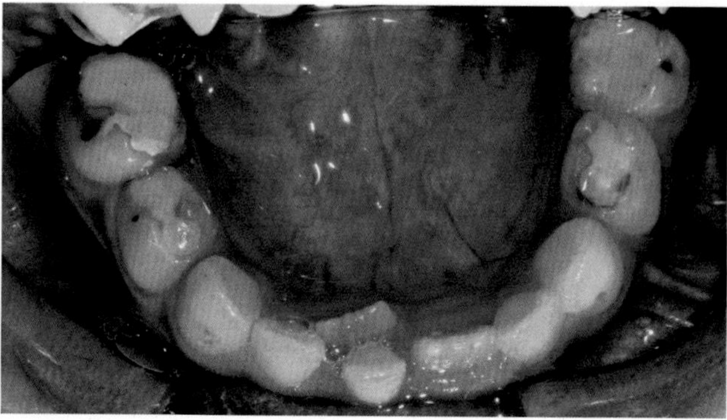

Fig. 24.1 Temporary GIC restoration placed, the benefits of which are described in the text.

Key point

Advantages of dressing (stabilization) open cavities are:

- Introduction to dental procedures and usually does not involve local analgesia or complete caries removal.
- Reduction of *Streptococcus mutans* count. The temporary restoration deprives the bacteria in the active lesion of sugar and oxygen.
- GIC acts as a fluoride reservoir.
- Eating and toothbrushing are more comfortable.

An acute and/or spreading infection or swelling may require the prescription of antibiotics. This is discussed in Chapter 25. Antibiotics should only be prescribed for pain in the absence of swelling for immunosuppressed patients.

Advice about analgesics for pain will be necessary to support the emergency treatment (**Table 24.2**).

Table 24.2 Dosages for common paediatric analgesics (for children 12 and older, refer to adult doses)

Drug	Dosage
Paracetamol	20 mg/kg initially then 10–15 mg/kg every 4–6 hours
	Maximum of four doses in a 24 hour period
	Ensure adequate hydration
Ibuprofen (non-steroidal anti-inflammatory drug (NSAID))	10 mg/kg every 8 hours
	Can be used in conjunction with paracetamol
	Best given with food and drink

History

Questioning suggested an irreversible pulpitis in the upper right quadrant.

Examination

Paul has no extraoral swelling or asymmetry. Intraorally he has all his primary teeth. There is occlusal caries of $\underline{|E}$ and mesial caries of $\underline{A|A}$. The $\underline{E|}$ is grossly carious (**Fig. 24.2A**). There is no associated soft tissue swelling.

What investigation is essential to allow you to formulate a treatment plan?

Bitewing radiographs are necessary to diagnose approximate caries in primary molars with their wide contact areas and to confirm the depth of dentine caries. Radiographs will increase the diagnosed yield of caries by 50%. Frequency of subsequent bitewing radiographs will depend on the classification of caries risk: high risk patients should have radiographs taken every 6–12 months; medium risk 12–18 months; low risk 18–24 months. In Paul's case, the lower arch (**Fig. 24.2B**) and bitewing radiographs (**Figs 24.3A and B**) show extensive caries of $\underline{E|}$ involving the pulp. There is also caries extending into the mid-dentine for $\frac{\;|E}{E|DE}$.

Treatment

Initial temporization of Paul's $\underline{E|}$ was with with Odontopaste and GIC.

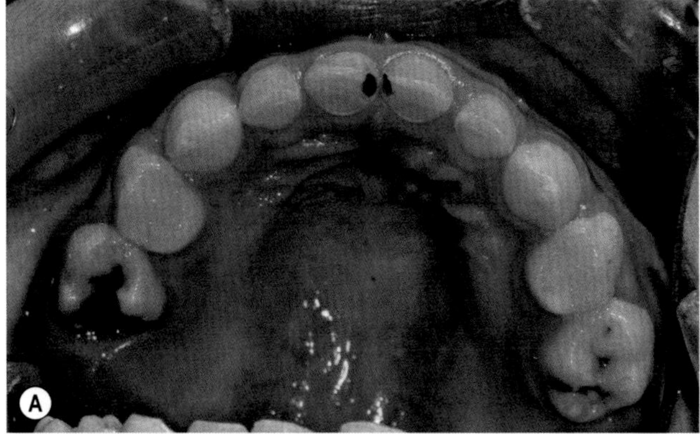

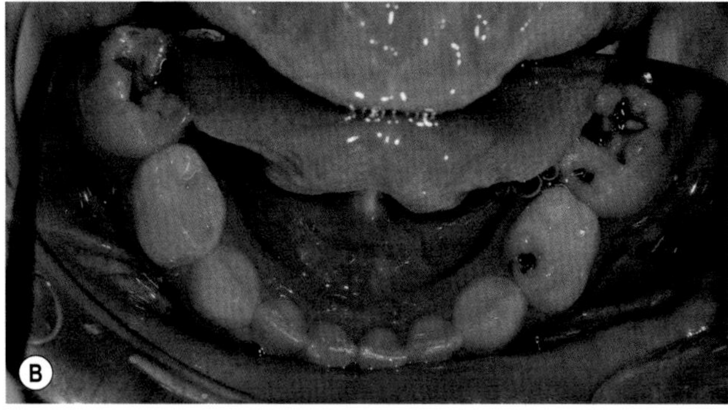

Fig. 24.2 (A & B) Paul's upper and lower arches.

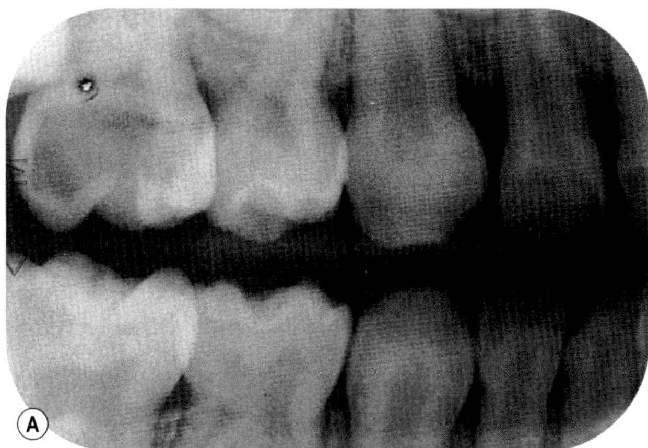

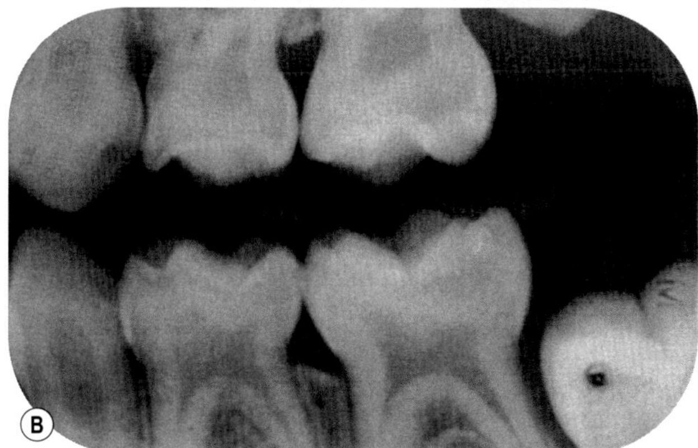

Fig. 24.3 (A & B) Paul's bitewing radiographs.

What is your definitive treatment plan for $\underline{E|}$?

The $\underline{E|}$ was unrestorable with the distal margin of the caries extending subgingivally. Therefore the only option for the $\underline{E|}$ was extraction. The temporary dressing alleviated further pain from this tooth and allowed for behaviour management and acclimatization to the dental surgery to be undertaken. Extracting primary teeth on a child's first visit to a dentist should be avoided where possible. If an extraction is undertaken on the first visit, it is likely to lead to significant dental anxiety and reluctance to attend further dental visits.

■ ***Will local anaesthetic be needed for extracting E|?***

Where the decision has been made to extract E|, *local anaesthetic is essential.* It is time consuming to give local anaesthetic in a pain free and child-friendly way and ensure the entire tooth is anaesthetized prior to the extraction. Often children and parents are surprised how quickly the tooth is extracted in comparison to the time taken for the local anaesthetic stage.

■ ***What are the consequences of extracting E|?***

Extracting the E| is likely to lead to localized space loss, with the 6| drifting mesially into this space. This especially is the case when the extraction is undertaken prior to the eruption of the first permanent molar. The drifting will exacerbate any tendency for crowding and can frequently lead to the palatal exclusion of the maxillary permanent second premolar in adolescence. Although space maintainers have been advocated to prevent space loss following premature extraction of primary molars, there is a lack of robust evidence to support their longevity and cost effectiveness in young children with extensive dental caries.

■ ***If the E| was restorable, what other treatment options would be available?***

The only other option for a tooth diagnosed with irreversible pulpitis or where it is necrotic and non-vital is a pulpectomy. A pulpectomy is similar to a root canal treatment in permanent teeth. It is made more complex by the flared and irregular shape of the root canals, as well as the need for the roots to resorb, thus allowing natural exfoliation of the primary tooth. Although hand files are used for gentle shaping, the most important stage of the procedure is disinfection of the root canal with careful use of hypochlorite. Like in the permanent dentition, a rubber dam is essential to prevent salivary ingress into the root canal and the escape of the hypochlorite into the oral cavity. Once the working length is established and the root canals disinfected, canals are filled with either zinc oxide cement or a calcium hydroxide-iodoform paste which will resorb with the root as part of the physiological root resorption.

Treatment planning

■ ***How do we undertake treatment planning and devise a plan which is appropriate for each and every patient?***

There are several important stages to treatment planning:

A. The first priority is to relieve pain. Where pain relief can be provided, even over a short time frame, this permits time to develop a holistic treatment plan described in steps B–E.

B. Identify all pathology. Bitewings (**Figs 24.3A and B**) and other radiographs are essential to support the detection of caries. A list should be drawn up of each tooth affected by caries together with the depth of caries penetration. **Table 24.3** shows such a list for Paul based on his clinical examination and bitewings.

C. Develop a robust and rigorous preventive plan as described in Chapters 22 and 23 and shown in **Table 24.4**.

D. Evaluate Paul's cooperation to treatment following the delivery of behaviour management strategies described in Chapter 26. Although several visits may be required to develop the child's cooperation, it is not acceptable to leave an infected tooth untreated for longer than 3 months.

E. There are multiple options available for treating primary teeth, and flexibility in approach is needed as treatment options may change in response to parental expectations and willingness to comply with the home-based preventive advice, the child's cooperation and the development of further toothache or other symptoms. In addition, the choice of how the treatment is undertaken, e.g. local anaesthetic, sedation or general anaesthetic, described in Chapter 26, may dictate what treatment is available and appropriate. For example, all carious teeth may be extracted even when some are restorable where an 'extraction-only general anaesthetic' is the only method available for an uncooperative child in pain.

Table 24.3 Paul's proposed treatment plan

Teeth affected by caries	Extent of caries	Restorative plan
E|	Into pulp	Extraction
A|A	Outer 1/3rd dentine	Disk
|E / E|E	Mid 1/3rd dentine	Hall crown
|D	Outer 1/3rd dentine	Partial caries removal, followed by composite restoration and fissure sealant

Table 24.4 How preventive and restorative treatment was provided for Paul on a visit by visit basis

Visit	Preventive plan	Restorative plan
1	Pain control	E| temporary
2	Bitewing radiographs	
	Toothbrushing instruction	
	Fluoride advice	
	Hand out diet diary	
	Plaque score	
	Apply fluoride varnish	
3	Collect in diet diary and give advice	Fissure seal D|D / D|D
		Disk A|A
4	Toothbrushing instruction	Plaque score
		Restore |D
		Place separators |E
5	Reinforce diet advice	Hall crown |E
		Place separators E|E
6	Toothbrushing instruction	Plaque score
		Hall crowns E|E
7	Post-extraction pain control	Extract E|

Key point

The following considerations will influence the treatment provided:

- Parental expectations and willingness to comply with home-based preventive advice.
- Child's cooperation.
- Development of further pain and symptoms.
- Dental care professional's expertise and training in different treatment procedures.

Different restorative philosophies These different approaches can be used at a patient level or at a tooth level with several employed within one patient. **Table 24.4** shows Paul's treatment plan and includes several different approaches to manage his carious teeth.

- *Prevention only.* This approach requires a high level of engagement and cooperation from the parents as treatment is predicated on their compliance with the preventive advice provided. Preventive advice as discussed in Chapters 22 and 23 is provided with regular clinic visits for fluoride varnish application. To support daily plaque removal, carious cavities can be adjusted to facilitate toothbrush access to remove plaque. For Paul, early dentinal caries was identified on the mesial aspects of A|A. The mesial aspects of these teeth were 'disked' to allow for better toothbrush access. This decision was made based on the short time these teeth had to be retained before they exfoliated, the dark appearance of the caries suggesting it was arrested, the low likelihood of caries progression or pain and parent satisfaction with this approach.
- *Sealing in caries with no or partial caries removal.* This approach is based on the biological principle that by sealing the cavity, the carious process cannot progress without nutrients and will therefore either slow down or arrest completely. Therefore ensuring a **good seal is essential**. This can be achieved using a number of different materials and with or without partial caries removal. Best examples of these techniques in the primary dentition are the Hall technique, sealing in dentinal caries and indirect pulp therapy. For Paul, his cooperation was limited and there was little likelihood of him cooperating for four separate visits of complete caries removal under local anaesthetic. Therefore Hall crowns were provided on the three other affected second primary molars (|E over E|E) and a composite restoration on |D. The |D used simple hand and slow handpiece excavation to remove only the infected dentine.
- *Complete caries removal.* This approach involves complete caries removal and necessitates the need for local anaesthetic, rubber dam and fast and slow handpieces. Consequently it requires significant levels of cooperation from the child. All infected carious dentine is removed. Only once this is completed is the tooth restored. Where caries extends into the pulp, a pulpotomy is undertaken. Paul coped with one visit of local anaesthetic where the E| was extracted. This was provided towards the end of his course of treatment. Earlier, simpler visits (**Table 24.4**) had developed his cooperation and confidence, thus permitting this more difficult procedure to be undertaken without the need to use sedation or general anaesthesia (see Chapter 26).

Key point

Advantages and disadvantages of different restorative approaches:

- Preventive

  Advantages: limited child cooperation needed, some cooperation is needed to modify carious cavities to improve toothbrushing access.

  Disadvantages: high levels of parental cooperation, as they will need to undertake a rigorous preventive plan, more frequent clinic visits, accurate diagnosis of the extent of caries to ensure these teeth are at low risk of pain or infection.
- Sealing in caries with partial or no caries removal

  Advantages: moderate child cooperation, no local anaesthetic and minimal or no drilling.

  Disadvantages: more frequent clinic visits to monitor seal, more radiographs to monitor any caries progression, accurate diagnosis of the extent of caries with a low risk of irreversible pulpitis, short term occlusal disturbance following Hall crown placement.
- Complete caries removal

  Advantages: high levels of child cooperation, can directly assess pulpal health at time of pulpotomy, permits treatment of more extensive caries, can modify crown to ensure fit of stainless steel crown, permits tooth coloured restorations for caries involving the outer and mid third of dentine.

  Disadvantages: risk of iatrogenic damage to adjacent teeth, requires high levels of clinical expertise and efficiency, local anaesthetic and rubber dam needed.

Hall crowns and indirect pulp therapy

What are Hall crowns?

Stainless steel crowns are a very effective method for restoring carious primary molars. Historically, it was only felt that these crowns could be placed using a complete caries removal approach to ensure a good fit was achieved thereby optimizing the coronal seal. Furthermore, this approach minimized any occlusal disturbance. Using this conventional approach (including occlusal reduction and mesial and distal slices) excellent long-term outcomes were achieved.

In the last ten years, an alternative (Hall crown) approach to their application has emerged. This involves no caries removal or local anaesthetic. The correct size of crown is chosen and filled with GIC. The crown is then pushed onto the tooth using the child to bite it down into place. The coronal seal generated by the crown and cement leads to the arrest of the underlying caries. Further information on the Hall technique is provided in a specific manual with the weblink provided in the Primary Resources and Recommended Reading section.

■ *When can I use Hall crowns?*

There are several important caveats to Hall crowns, and like all restorative techniques, they have advantages and disadvantages to their use. Most importantly, a careful pain history and bitewing radiographs are important stages in identifying pulpal health. Where caries is within the inner third of dentine or there is history of pain or signs and symptoms of pulpitis or pulpal necrosis, it is unwise to undertake a Hall crown. For Paul, the caries was limited to the outer half of the dentine and there were no symptoms from $\begin{array}{c|c} & E \\ \hline E & E \end{array}$.

Owing to the tight contacts seen in the primary dentition, pushing the crown through these contacts can take significant force. Where tight contacts are seen, an alternative approach is to place orthodontic separators for up to 2 weeks to provide space for placement of the crown.

■ *What will happen to the child's occlusion following the placement of a Hall crown?*

As there is no occlusal reduction as part of the Hall technique, the crown will be proud and cause occlusal interference. Research has shown that after a few weeks, there is occlusal adjustment with the crown no longer sitting proud.

A post-operative bitewing is advisory once all Hall crowns have been placed to ensure the crowns are fully seated and have sealed the carious cavity. This especially is true for proximal caries.

■ *How does indirect pulp therapy (IPT) differ from a Hall crown?*

IPT is a procedure requiring local anaesthetic and rubber dam. Infected caries is removed from the margins of the cavity. At the cavity base, careful caries removal is undertaken to remove as much soft infected dentine as possible but to ensure there is no pulpal exposure. Calcium hydroxide is then placed over the deep caries before a definitive restoration is placed. It is essential that the restoration provide an excellent coronal seal.

IPT and Hall crowns are similar in that they both require an excellent diagnosis of pulpal health. In both techniques infected caries is left, and both rely on an optimal coronal seal to prevent caries progression. The default restoration material for both techniques is a stainless steel crown. In the permanent dentition, stepwise caries removal (of which IPT is a form of) has shown very positive results in reducing the need for root canal treatment.

Pulpotomies

■ *What is a pulpotomy?*

Pulpotomy is a procedure for deep caries involving or in close approximation to the pulp. Careful pre-operative diagnosis is essential to ensure the absence of signs and symptoms suggesting irreversible pulpitis (see **Table 24.1**) or pulpal necrosis. This includes the absence of a sinus, swelling, peri-furcation radiolucency, internal resorption, tenderness to percussion or a clinical history of irreversible pulpitis.

The inflamed coronal pulp is removed under local anaesthesia (LA) and rubber dam with the healthy non-inflammed pulp stumps dressed for 15 seconds with 15.5% ferric sulphate. Following this application, bleeding from the pulp stumps should stop. The technique allows one further application of ferric sulphate if the bleeding has not stopped entirely after the first application. The chamber is then filled with zinc oxide eugenol cement or Mineral Trioxide Aggregate. The default restoration for a pulpotomised primary molar is a stainless steel crown to facilitate an excellent coronal seal. If the pulp stumps do not stop after two applications of ferric sulphate, treatment should proceed to either a vital pulpectomy (a variation of the pulpectomy technique described earlier in the chapter) or the tooth should be extracted. This continued bleeding demonstrates inflammation extending into the pulp stumps and early tooth loss is likely if a pulpotomy is undertaken (as a result of internal resorption).

Pulpotomies are an area of active research as shown by the recent Cochrane review on the subject. This identified 47 randomized controlled trials on the subject. Current areas of active research included how haemostasis is achieved and alternatives to ferric sulphate and older agents such as formocresol. Although formocresol has shown long-term success and is still used in some parts of the world, there have been international concerns over its toxicity both locally and systemically. These concerns have grown in the past 15 years with formaldehyde, one of the important components of formocresol being associated with nasopharyngeal cancer. Formocresol is no longer advocated as a front-line medicament for pulpotomies and is no longer taught in UK undergraduate curricula.

Primary resources and recommended reading

American Acedemy of Pediatric Dentistry 2014 Policy on pediatric pain management. Reference Manual 36 (6):78–79.

Pain control for children 2013 In: Cameron A, Widmer R (eds), Handbook of Pediatric Dentistry, 4th edn. Mosby, Edinburgh, pp. 25–46.

Deery C 2013 Caries detection and diagnosis, sealants and management of the possibly carious fissure. Br Dent J 214 (11):551–557.

Duggal MS, Day PF 2005 Operative treatment of dental caries in the primary dentition. In: Welbury RR, Duggal MS, Hosey MT (eds), Paediatric Dentistry, third ed. Oxford University Press, Oxford, pp. 149–174.

Evans D, Innes N 2010 The Hall Technique: A Minimal Intervention, Child Centred Approach to Managing the Carious Primary Molar. University of Dundee. Available at: https://dentistry.dundee.ac.uk/sites/dentistry.dundee.ac.uk/files/3M_93C%20HallTechGuide2191110.pdf.

Faculty of General Dental Practice (FGDP) 2013 Selection Criteria for Dental Radiography, third ed. London, FGDP.

Franzon R, Guimaraes LF, Magalhaes CE et al 2014 Outcomes of one-step incomplete and complete excavation in primary teeth:

a 24-month randomized controlled trial. Caries Res 48 (5):376–383.

Ricketts D, Lamont T, Innes NP, et al 2013 Operative caries management in adults and children. Cochrane Database of Syst Rev Issue 3. Art No: CD003808. DOI: 10.1002/14651858. CD003808.pub3.

Scottish Dental Clinical Effectiveness Programme (SDCEP) 2010 Prevention and Management of Dental Caries in Children: Dental Clinical Guidance. Dundee, SDCEP. Available at: http://www.sdcep.org.uk/wp-content/uploads/2013/03/SDCEP_PM_Dental_Caries_Full_Guidance1.pdf.

Smail-Faugeron V, Courson F, Durieux P et al 2014 Pulp treatment for extensive decay in primary teeth. Cochrane Database of Syst Rev Issue 8. Art No: CD003220. DOI: 10.1002/14651858. CD003220.pub2.

For revision, see Mind Map 24, page 244.

25

Facial swelling and dental abscess

SUMMARY

Danny is 12 years old. He attended with a large facial swelling after an episode of trauma 3 weeks previously. He feels unwell, and his right eye is closing *(Fig. 25.1)****.***

The presentation of* acute *infection, as demonstrated by Danny, is very different from* chronic *infection.

■ ***List four symptoms and signs specific to each type of infection***

Acute:

- Sick, upset child.
- Raised temperature.
- Red, swollen face.
- Reduced intake of food and drink

Chronic:

- Buccal sinus may be present.
- Mobile tooth.
- Halitosis.
- Discoloured tooth.

Other signs and symptoms can be seen in both acute and chronic infection, including pain and lymphadenopathy.

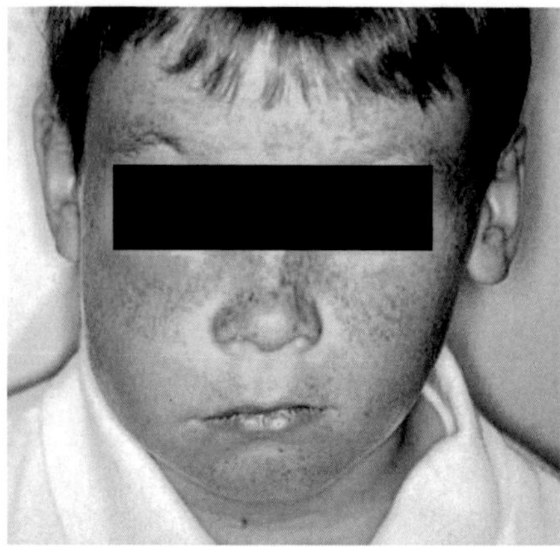

Fig. 25.1 Severe infection of canine fossa.

Acute infections tend to present with facial cellulitis rather than a facial abscess with pus. Danny was febrile, although he was not in any significant pain, because the infection had perforated the cortical plate. The mainstay of treatment is removal of the cause – either pulpal extirpation or extraction of the tooth.

History

Danny traumatized his upper right lateral incisor 3 weeks ago, sustaining a deep enamel dentine fracture. The dentine was dressed with calcium hydroxide and a glass ionomer cement was placed over the exposed dentine and enamel. He had a review appointment with his dentist the following week.

On Saturday morning his mother noticed that his cheek was swollen and the tissues around his right eye were 'puffy and red'. He attended the accident and emergency department of the local hospital, where he was prescribed Amoxicillin 250 mg tablets to be taken three times daily for 5 days. Unfortunately, by Sunday evening Danny had become listless and his swelling had increased. He felt hot.

Examination

Extraorally there was facial asymmetry with a swelling of the right maxillary canine fossa. The overlying skin was red and hot. The right eye fissure was partially closed. Danny's temperature was 39°C. Maxillary canine fossa infections can spread via emissary veins, which have no valves, to the intracranial venous system causing either a cavernous sinus thrombosis or a brain abscess. The pathways of the IIIrd and VIth cranial nerves lie in the walls of the cavernous sinus. Thrombosis in the cavernous sinus can present with a squint due to involvement of the IIIrd and VIth cranial nerves, which are involved in control of the extraocular muscles.

■ ***What is the major problem with mandibular infections?***

Spread alongside the fascial planes that surround the airway with subsequent narrowing of the airway and stridor.

Spread via the fascial planes to the mediastinum to cause a mediastinitis.

■ ***What is the basic management of any infection?***

Removal of the cause – extraction or root canal therapy.

Local drainage and debridement – via root canal or incision and drainage.

Oral antibiotics if systemic involvement (see Table 25.1) – Amoxicillin or Penicillin V are usually the drugs of first choice. Amoxicillin has the advantage that it is given with food and only needs to be taken three times per day. Metronidazole, which is active against anaerobes, can be added to either Amoxicillin or Penicillin if the infection is severe. Often the extraction of the abscessed tooth alone will bring about resolution without antibiotic therapy. It is important that antibiotics alone should not be considered as a first line of treatment unless there is systemic involvement. In a child a temperature of 39°C or higher can be considered significant (normal ≅ 37°C). Immunosuppressed patients and those with

Table 25.1 Common antibiotics used in paediatric dentistry

Drug	Route	Dose	Frequency	Notes
Antibiotics				
Amoxicillin	PO	25–50 mg/kg/day	tds	Syrup or chewable tablets for young children
	IV	100–400 mg/kg/day	tds	
Amoxicillin plus clavulanic acid	PO	20–40 mg/kg/day	tds	For beta-lactam-resistant organisms only
Ampicillin	IV	50–100 mg/kg/day	qds	
	IV	50 mg/kg	stat	
Benzyl penicillin	IV	15–350 mg/kg/day		
		20 000–500 000 U/kg/day	qds	First IV drug of choice for odontogenic infections
Penicillin V	PO	< 5 years 500 mg/day		
		> 5 years 1–2 g/day	qds	Give 1 hour before meals
Cephalexin	PO	25–50 mg/kg/day	qds	
Cephazolin	IV	25–50 mg/kg/day		
Erythromycin	PO	25–40 mg/kg/day	qds	Ethylsuccinate is readily absorbed
Metronidazole	IV	22.5 mg/kg/day	tds	Not in pregnancy
Gentamicin	PO	10–15 mg/kg/day	tds	
Clindamycin	PO, IV	15–40 mg/kg/day	qds	Risk of pseudomembranous colitis

Analgesics see Chapter 24, Table 24.2

PO, per oral; *IV*, intravenous; *IM*, intramuscular; *PR*, per rectum; *tds*; three times daily; *qds*, four times daily; *stat*, at once

(Frontline antibiotics used for facial swellings and dental abcesses are Amoxycillin, Penicillin V and Metronidazol)

cardiac disease should receive antibiotics immediately if any infection is suspected.

What are the criteria for hospital admission with orofacial infection?

Dehydration. Ask whether the child has had a decreased frequency of micturition (urine output) in previous 12 hours.

Significant infection or temperature greater than 39°C.

Floor of mouth swelling.

What will the hospital management of a severe infection involve?

Extraction of involved teeth. It is impossible to drain a significant infection solely through the root canals of a tooth. Drainage of any pus. In addition to extractions, there may be a need to incise and drain pus, often leaving a drain in situ for a few days to enhance drainage. With severe mandibular swellings or where the floor of the mouth is raised, it may be necessary to have an extraoral drain through a skin incision or a 'through and through' drain, which passes completely through the area of infection. Extraoral incisions are to be avoided if at all possible due to post-operative scarring. Swabs of pus for laboratory culture to establish accurate sensitivities of the organisms concerned to common antibiotics.

Intravenous antibiotics. Benzyl penicillin is the drug of first choice, or Amoxicillin. Cephalosporins are effective if there is a penicillin allergy, but there is some cross-reactivity in those patients allergic to penicillin and so cephalosporins should be used with care, especially when there was a severe reaction to penicillin. In severe infections, metronidazole should be added as anaerobic organisms play a significant role.

Maintenance fluids will be given until the child is drinking normally again.

Warm saline mouthwashes.

Adequate pain control commonly with paracetamol or ibuprofen (Table 24.2).

If the eye is shut due to a swelling in the canine fossa, it may be necessary to give chloramphenicol eye drops 0.5% or chloramphenicol ointment 1.0% to prevent conjunctivitis.

Key point

Hospital admission in orofacial infection is necessary with:

- Dehydration.
- Temperature >39°C.
- Floor of mouth swelling.
- Trismus or significant swelling around the eye leading to complete closure.
- Breathing and swallowing difficulties.

Treatment

Danny was treated by the following regimen:

1. Extirpation of 2|. The tooth was immature and good drainage of pus was achieved through the root canal.
2. Open drainage of the tooth for 2 days.

3. Amoxicillin 250 mg three times daily, metronidazole 200 mg twice daily for 5 days each.
4. Hot saline mouthwashes.

After 2 days Danny was reviewed. The swelling was reduced around his right cheek, and his right eye was normal. The 2| was cleaned and filed and non-setting calcium hydroxide placed into the canal. The access cavity was sealed with cotton wool and glass ionomer cement. The non-setting calcium hydroxide was replaced once after a month. Once the root canal was free from any signs or symptoms of infection, the tooth was oburated with a Mineral Trioxide Aggregate plug and warm gutta percha.

Primary resources and recommended reading

Cameron A, Widmer R (eds), 2013 Paediatric oral medicine and pathology. In: Handbook of Pediatric Dentistry, 4th edn. Mosby, Edinburgh, pp. 209–268.

American Academy of Pediatric Dentists 2015 Guideline on use of antibiotic therapy for pediatric dental patients. Ref Man 36 (6):284–286.

For revision, see Mind Map 25, page 245.

26

The uncooperative child and adolescent

CASE 1

SUMMARY

Liam is 5 years old. He is shaking and tearful as he is brought into the surgery. His mother says he has been in pain from his teeth for a long time. How would you manage Liam and his dental treatment?

■ ***What do you understand by the term behaviour management?***

Behaviour management includes a number of skills: empathy, communication, coaching and listening. These skills need to be combined with an understanding of child development and psychology.

The goals are to establish communication, alleviate fear and anxiety, deliver quality dental care, build a trusting relationship between dentist and child and promote the child's positive attitude towards oral/dental health.

All decisions must be based on a benefit versus risk evaluation. Parents/legal guardians share in the decision-making process regarding treatment of their children. They are also responsible for dental attendance, Liam's oral health regime (including purchase of toothpaste and undertaking toothbrushing) and control what Liam eats and drinks. It is therefore essential to establish a good relationship with parents to ensure they are supportive and comply with the preventive advice provided.

■ ***What history is important in Liam's case?***

Liam's dental history. It is crucial to identify any previous episodes at the dentist, doctor or hospital, usually involving needles, that may have frightened him. If there are no previous precipitating factors he may have been frightened by stories or comments from his peers or family.

Family dental history. Parental fear, and a negative attitude toward dental and oral health, can significantly affect the cooperation of a child.

Liam's development. Delayed development and poor cognition can affect the ability of a child to understand what you are trying to do to help. Children with a negative image of themselves who have never succeeded at anything will be more difficult to treat. They often give up because they 'never succeed' and are often called 'failures' by their parents or peers.

Communicative management. This is the most fundamental form of behaviour management. It is the basis for establishing a relationship with a child that will allow you to successfully complete dental procedures and help the child develop a positive attitude toward dental health.

■ ***What main forms of communicative management are there?***

Non-verbal communication.

Tell-show-do.

Positive reinforcement.

Distraction.

Voice control.

Parental presence/absence.

Non-verbal communication is the reinforcement and guidance of behaviour through appropriate contact, posture and facial expression.

Objectives:

To enhance the effectiveness of other communicative management techniques.

To gain or maintain the patient's attention and compliance.

Indications:

May be used with any patient.

Contraindications:

None.

Tell-show-do is a technique of behaviour shaping used by many paediatric professionals. The technique involves verbal explanations of procedures in phrases appropriate to the developmental level of the patient (tell); demonstrations for the patient of the visual, auditory, olfactory and tactile aspects of the procedure in a carefully defined, non-threatening setting (show); and then, without deviating from the explanation and demonstration, completion of the procedure (do). The tell-show-do technique is used with communication skills (verbal and non-verbal) and positive reinforcement. The language chosen must be appropriate to the child's level of understanding and experience.

Objectives:

To teach the patient important aspects of the dental visit and familiarize the patient with the dental setting.

To shape the patient's response to procedures through desensitization and well-described expectations.

Indications:

May be used with any patient.

Contraindications:

None.

Positive reinforcement In the process of establishing desirable patient behaviour, it is essential to give appropriate feedback. Positive reinforcement is an effective technique to reward desired behaviours and thus strengthen the recurrence of those behaviours. Social reinforcers include positive voice modulation, facial expression, verbal praise and appropriate physical demonstrations of affection by all members of the dental team. Non-social reinforcers include tokens and toys.

The delivery of positive reinforcement should follow these principles. When the desired behaviour is shown it should be *immediately* rewarded. Each time the behaviour is shown, *consistency* is needed in rewarding this behaviour. It should be *clear* what behaviour is desired. The positive reinforcer is only used *contingent* on that behaviour being displayed.

Objective:

To reinforce desired behaviour.

Indications:

May be useful for any patient.

Contraindications:

None.

Distraction is the technique of diverting the patient's attention from what may be perceived as an unpleasant procedure.

Objectives:

To decrease the perception of unpleasantness.

To avert negative or avoidance behaviour.

Indications:

May be used with any patient.

Contraindications:

None.

Voice control is a controlled alteration of voice volume, tone or pace to influence and direct the patient's behaviour.

Objectives:

To gain the patient's attention and compliance.

To avert negative or avoidance behaviour.

To establish appropriate adult-child roles.

Indications:

May be used with any patient.

Contraindications:

None.

Parental presence/absence This technique involves using the presence or absence of the parent to gain cooperation for treatment. A wide diversity exists in practitioner philosophy and parental attitude regarding parents' presence or absence during paediatric dental treatment. Practitioners are united in the fact that communication between dentist and child is paramount and that this communication demands focus on the part of both parties. Children's responses to their parents' presence or absence can range from very beneficial to very detrimental. It is the responsibility of practitioners to determine the communication methods that best optimize the treatment setting; recognizing their own skills, the abilities of the particular child and the desires of the specific parent involved.

Objectives:

To gain the patient's attention and compliance.

To avert negative or avoidance behaviours.

To establish appropriate adult-child roles.

To enhance the communication environment.

Indications:

May be used with any patient.

Contraindications:

None.

All these communication techniques may be needed to enhance the evolution of a compliant and relaxed patient. It is an ongoing subjective process rather than a singular technique and is often the extension of the personality of the dentist.

Key point

Positive reinforcement should be:

- Immediate.
- Clear.
- Consistent.
- Contingent.

Examination

After spending some time talking to Liam and showing him that you are genuine in wanting to help, he allows you to look at his teeth. Both lower first primary molars are carious. All the other teeth are sound. Liam has been frightened by stories from his friends. His family are very supportive and are regular attenders.

Liam responds well to communicative management, but although he wants to have his treatment carried out, he just cannot override his fear of the unknown.

■ ***What additional help might you consider giving Liam?***

Inhalational sedation has been an effective and safe method of reducing anxiety and enhancing effective communication for the past 30 years. Its onset of action is rapid, the depth of sedation is easily titrated and reversible and recovery is rapid and complete. Additionally, nitrous oxide mediates a variable degree of analgesia, amnesia and gag reflex reduction.

The need to diagnose and treat, as well as the safety of the patient and practitioner, should be considered before the use of nitrous oxide. The decision to use nitrous oxide must take into consideration the following points:

Alternative behaviour management modalities. (Although nitrous oxide sedation is effective for mild to moderately anxious patients, it is not effective for children who cannot or will not breath through their nose – some young children have not developed the level of maturity and understanding to be able to follow this requirement.)

Dental needs of the patient.

The effect on the quality of dental care.

The patient's emotional development.

The patient's physical considerations.

Written informed consent must be obtained from a legal guardian and documented in the patient's record prior to use of nitrous oxide.

The patient's record should include:

Informed consent.

Indication for use.

Nitrous oxide dosage:

- Percent nitrous oxide/oxygen and/or flow rate.
- Duration of the procedure.
- Post-treatment oxygenation procedure.

Objectives:

To reduce or eliminate anxiety.

To reduce untoward movement and reaction to dental treatment.

To enhance communication and patient cooperation.

To raise the pain reaction threshold.

To increase tolerance for longer or more difficult treatment.

To aid in treatment of the mentally/physically disabled or medically compromised patient.

To reduce gagging.

Indications:

A mild to moderately fearful, anxious or obstreperous patient.

Certain mentally, physically or medically compromised patients.

A patient whose gag reflex interferes with dental care.

A patient in whom profound local anaesthesia cannot be obtained.

Contraindications:

May be contraindicated in some chronic obstructive pulmonary diseases.

Where the child has a blocked nose, common cold or tonsillitis, their appointment should be postponed until they have recovered.

May be contraindicated in certain patients with severe emotional disturbances or drug-related dependencies.

Patients in the first trimester of pregnancy.

May be contraindicated in patients with sickle cell disease.

Patients treated with bleomycin sulphate.

Neuromuscular disease, e.g. myasthenia gravis, multiple sclerosis.

Liam had inhalational sedation, which enabled completion of his treatment and helped him overcome his fear of local anaesthesia.

Key point

The patient's record in inhalational sedation should include:

- Informed consent.
- Indications for use.
- Nitrous oxide dosage.

CASE 2

SUMMARY

Maria is a 12-year-old girl with early caries in her mandibular first permanent molars. She has an increased overjet, and the orthodontic plan includes four premolar extractions, provided her caries risk is reduced and the dental disease is treated.

■ ***How would you motivate Maria to reduce her caries risk and assess and treat her dental anxiety?***

History

Complaint

Maria says she does not like to smile and is getting teased at school.

History of complaint

Maria went to her local dentist recently and received preventive advice but did not mange to accept local analgesia. Further questioning revealed that she remembered being 'forced' to have a primary tooth extracted at age 6 years and has been fearful of dental treatment since then.

Medical history

There is no relevant medical history.

Family history

Maria's mother says she is also afraid of going to the dentist.

Examination

Extraoral examination

Maria has a slightly prominent increased overjet, but a Class I skeletal base and normal face height with no asymmetry.

Intraoral examination

Maria has good oral hygiene. She has stained fissures on the mandibular molars. Bitewing radiographs suggest that the caries is into the enamel only.

■ ***What recommendations are used regarding diet, toothbrushing and fluoride for adolescents?***

Ideally, we would all hope that by adolescence a child is disease free and therefore will need little operative treatment. However, there are adolescents who have caries or other dental problems, such as non-caries tooth tissue loss; perhaps due to acid erosion, or periodontal disease; or who have aesthetic needs that require orthodontic treatment, which perhaps include premolar extractions as part of the treatment plan. Adolescents who need orthodontic extractions, in particular, may not have had very much dental treatment in the past, especially if they are low caries risk. On the other hand the adolescent who has high caries risk (approximately 14% of the adolescent population,

Child Dental Health Survey 2013) often has a heavy burden of disease requiring many visits to complete their restorative treatment.

To overcome the burden of disease, preventive action is needed. This is a two-pronged approach that involves good, clear, evidence-based preventive advice from the dentist and the active agreement to implement the advised behaviour changes from the adolescent. The Department of Health (DoH) Oral Health Preventive Toolkit contains evidence-based prevention advice including twice daily toothbrushing with 1450 ppm fluoride toothpaste, the need for regular dental check-ups and reducing sugar frequency.

In Maria's case, 2800 ppm fluoride toothpaste should be recommended. This is suitable for children over 10 years of age who may be at risk for tooth decay, including patients with active tooth decay or a history of tooth decay, exposed root surfaces, high-sugar diets, orthodontic appliances or dry mouth.

Advice given should be evidence based and given in a knowledgeable context of adolescent mind-set and behaviour change psychological theory, such as using motivational interviewing and cognitive behaviour therapy. These theories are generally based on adolescents understanding their own dental needs and the challenges that they face in implementing recommendations and then taking action, and 'rewarding' themselves for doing so.

This approach to prevention will also help in Maria's anxiety management because she will feel that she has a role and a say in her own dental management. In this way, the dentist and Maria will already be working together; 'on the same side' against the dental disease.

Key point

- Prevention of further dental caries is essential, provided the caries that is already present is managed.
- Adherence to preventive advice is key to progression to orthodontic treatment afterwards.
- The DoH toolkit gives clear, evidence-based preventive recommendations.

What is the aetiology of dental anxiety?

There are two reasons behind adolescent anxiety. The first is dental anxiety that is learnt over the preceding years and caused by real or perceived trauma of previous dental or medical treatment. The second is dental anxiety that is part of a deeper psychological disturbance that is beginning to emerge.

Why should an adolescent be managed differently form a younger child?

There are some further details that a dentist cannot overlook when managing an anxious adolescent. These relate to the mind-set and to the emerging character of the adolescent themselves. Adolescents have a rather fragile self-esteem yet want to be able to determine and make their own choices in life. They have concerns about their looks, especially dental aesthetics, and want to fit in with their peers. A detailed history, perhaps based on some subtle questioning, should also include habits such as smoking, experimental drug and alcohol frequency; e.g. 'alco-pops' and also 'recreational' drugs that cause thirst leading to increased acidic/sugary drink consumption.

Key point

- Adolescents are self-conscious and can have a fragile self-esteem.
- They want to be able to determine and make their own choices in life.
- They have concerns about their looks.
- They want to fit in with their peers.
- Question for habits such as smoking, experimental drugs and alcohol.
- Be alert to bullying and safeguarding issues.

Can anxiety be measured, and what questions should be asked?

There are various anxiety scales that help alert a dentist to dental anxieties. Though these are not sensitive enough to tease out the differences between these two possible aetiologies, they may be of value. The common ones are the Modified Child Dental Anxiety Scale (MCDAS) and the Child Fear Survey Schedule (CFSS). A simpler measure, which can also be valuable in younger children, is the Facial Image Scale (FIS); this is sometimes combined with the MCDAS to assist younger children's comprehension. An example is shown in **Fig. 26.1**.

However, these also need to be augmented by careful and thoughtful questioning, especially relating to past dental history and possible perceived traumatic events. Those who report that they have a needle phobia should be asked if they managed to accept their vaccinations at school; e.g. the tetanus/polio booster is usually given at around 13 years of age in the UK.

Treatment

What are the anxiety management options?

Non-pharmacological behaviour management is just as effective with adolescents as it is with younger children, so positive reinforcement, tell-show-do and enabling a hand signal to 'stop' to enhance Maria's sense of control should all be used. Giving information about what will happen, what it will feel like and how to cope beforehand and during the procedure are all important. Psychological interventions such as cognitive behavioural therapy can also play a key role. The idea behind this technique is to help Maria reconsider her belief that a future dental extraction will be as traumatic as that remembered from her childhood.

Maria has already undergone a dental extraction at an earlier age, and in her memory this was traumatic. It is not uncommon for a child to perceive a past experience as 'traumatic', even if in reality it was not. The fact is that in Maria's own mind the event was damaging to her, so this has to be taken into account. In Maria's case, she will need to undergo extractions as part of her orthodontic treatment plan. It is

Modified Child Dental Anxiety Scale – MCDAS

For the next eight questions I would like you to show me how relaxed or worried you get about the dentist and what happens at the dentist. To show me how relaxed or worried you feel, please use the simple scale below. The scale is just like a ruler going from 1, which would show that you are relaxed, to 5, which would show that you are very worried.

1 would mean: relaxed/not worried
2 would mean: very slightly worried
3 would mean: fairly worried
4 would mean: worried a lot
5 would mean: very worried.

How do you feel about ...					
... going to the dentist generally?	1	2	3	4	5
... having your teeth looked at?	1	2	3	4	5
... having your teeth scraped and polished?	1	2	3	4	5
... having an injection in the gum?	1	2	3	4	5
... having a filling?	1	2	3	4	5
... having a tooth taken out?	1	2	3	4	5
... being put to sleep to have treatment?	1	2	3	4	5
... having a mixture of 'gas and air' which will help you feel comfortable for treatment but cannot put you to sleep?	1	2	3	4	5

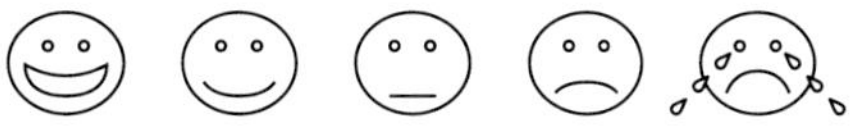

Fig. 26.1 MCDAS with FIS images.
(From Wong (1998), with permission.)

likely that discussing Maria's fears with her and putting them into a different context, in line with a cognitive behavioural therapy approach, and using excellent behavioural management skills, giving her a locus of control, and ensuring adequate analgesia will enable her to proceed to accept her planned orthodontic extractions. Resources and further guidance on the use of cognitive behavioural therapy are listed in the further reading section.

What is the commonest conscious sedative in children and adolescents?

For moderately anxious children, nitrous oxide inhalation sedation is the most commonly used sedative and is effective in adolescents who require premolar extractions. Maria may need this in addition to the behavioural techniques already described. The key is to carry out a thorough assessment based on a frank discussion with her and her parent(s) before the treatment plan is developed, to include inhalation sedation from the start if it is needed, rather than have a 'failed' behavioural management visit before considering conscious sedation as an option. It is also wise to build in a reassessment of the agreed plan after the first or second visit to assess treatment progression and to evaluate whither the plan is likely to succeed.

What treatment plan would you propose?

The treatment plan:

VISIT 1

1. Preventive advice (this is discussed in greater detail in Chapter 23) following the DoH toolkit, so including:
   a. Prescription of twice daily brushing with 2800 ppm fluoride toothpaste.
   b. Handing out a 4-day diet diary.
2. Ask Maria to sign a contract to:
   a. Reduce dietary sugar intake frequency based on tailored advice derived from her diet diary.
   b. Implement twice daily toothbrushing with a 2800 ppm fluoride toothpaste.
   c. Attend pre-agreed and booked dental appointments.
   d. Conduct a discussion between dentist, parent(s) and patient that leads to written parental consent and

adolescent assent of sedative choice and operative treatment.

e. Document the consent and assent process and document written informed consent.
f. Disclose dental plaque and modify toothbrushing technique and choice of toothpaste regarding fluoride dose; consider 2800 ppm fluoride toothpaste.
g. Introduce her to the inhalation sedation nasal mask and technique.
h. Fissure seal a maxillary first permanent molar and introduce topical analgesia.

VISIT 2 (preventive advice will continue and expand on 2a, 2b, 2f)

3. Use inhalation sedation for the first time:
   a. Fissure seal the remaining first permanent molars.
   b. Introduce topical analgesia.
   c. Reassess Maria's caries risk by checking compliance with dietary changes and toothbrushing, and confirm premolar extraction plan with the orthodontist. Reassess the use of nitrous oxide inhalation sedation. Does Maria still need it?

VISIT 3 AND 4 (preventive advice will continue and expand on 2a, 2b, 2f)

4. Begin orthodontic premolar extractions – perhaps in two quadrants per visit. Often an extraction in maxillary and mandibular quadrant is undertaken rather than extracting both mandibular premolars on the same visit. For mandibular extractions, infiltrations using Articaine local anaesthetic rather than inferior dental blocks with Lidocaine is an effective but less invasive method.

What follow-up does Maria need now?

Maria has successfully undergone the premolar extractions and has reduced her sugar frequency and is toothbrushing with 2800 ppm fluoride tooth paste. Therefore she is proceeding to have orthodontic fixed appliance treatment. As such, her caries risk is still high and she will need regular, four-monthly follow-ups during her orthodontic treatment. She will also need further bitewings to assess for new dental caries once yearly (once her orthodontic appliance is removed, until no further caries is seen and she is deemed to be at low caries risk).

Maria feels happy and proud to have undergone the extractions. She now enjoys visiting the dentist for check-ups and is excited about her new smile.

CASE 3

SUMMARY

Unfortunately, there are some children and adolescents for whom inhalational sedation is unable to overcome their anxiety, and alternative sedation agents or general anaesthesia is the only option that will allow relief of pain and completion of dental treatment.

What other sedation techniques are available?

Other sedation techniques such as oral or intravenous midazolam are effective. Dental sedationists who offer this type of treatment have to show that they have undergone further training in the technique, as well as continued competency and experience in line with contemporary national guidelines and recommendations.

For young children oral sedation is a viable option using midazolam. A number of recent studies have shown that its use in a dose of 0.3–0.5 mg/kg, depending on age, has been therapeutically effective in producing sedation that has allowed subsequent dental treatment.

For adolescents who require more invasive procedures or who are more severely phobic, midazolam intravenous sedation is an option because it has the added benefit of causing amnesia. Amnesia also occurs with oral midazolam. The patient cannot remember undergoing the procedure. They may remember the start of the dental visit and the beginning of the sedation, but nothing until after the sedative effect has begun to wear off.

What are the indications for general anaesthesia?

Patients who are unable to cooperate due to a lack of psychological or emotional maturity and/or mental, physical or medical disability.

Patients for whom local anaesthesia is ineffective because of acute infection, anatomical variations or allergy.

The extremely uncooperative, fearful, anxious or uncommunicative child or adolescent.

Extensive dental caries involving dental treatment in multiple quadrants.

Patients requiring significant surgical procedures (for example, the extraction of all first permanent molars or a severely infraoccluded primary molar).

Patients for whom the use of general anaesthesia (GA) may protect the developing psyche and/or reduce medical risks.

Patients requiring immediate, comprehensive oral/dental care.

What are the contraindications for general anaesthesia?

A healthy, cooperative patient with minimal dental need.

Predisposing medical conditions that would make GA inadvisable.

General anaesthesia is a controlled state of unconsciousness accompanied by a loss of protective reflexes, including the ability to maintain an airway independently and respond purposefully to physical stimulation or verbal command. It should only be provided in premises with resuscitation capability and intensive care back-up (e.g. an acute hospital setting). All equipment must follow current guidelines (please see reference section).

Parental or legal guardian informed consent must be obtained and documented prior to the use of general anaesthesia. The patient's record should include:

- Informed consent.
- Indications for the use of GA.

Informed consent

Regardless of the behaviour management techniques utilized by the individual practitioner, all management decisions must be based on a subjective evaluation weighing benefit and risk to the child. Considerations regarding need of treatment, consequences of deferred treatment and potential physical/emotional trauma must be entered into the decision-making equation.

Delivery of dental treatment is often a complex decision. Decisions regarding the use of behaviour management techniques other than communicative management cannot be made solely by the dentist. Decisions must involve a legal guardian and, if appropriate, the child. The dentist serves as the expert about dental care, i.e. the need for treatment and the techniques by which treatment can be delivered. The legal guardian shares with the practitioner the decision whether to treat or not to treat and must be consulted regarding treatment strategies and potential risks. Therefore the successful completion of diagnostic and therapeutic services is viewed as a partnership of dentist, legal guardian and child.

Although the behaviour management techniques included in this chapter are used frequently, parents may not be entirely familiar with them. It is important that the dentist inform the legal guardian about the nature of the technique to be used, its risks, benefits and any alternative techniques. All questions must be answered. This is the essence of informed consent.

Who can consent for a child?

Mother – all mothers automatically have parental responsibility.

Fathers – if married at the time of the child's conception, birth or sometime after this, this responsibility is not lost if the mother and father divorce.

Unmarried fathers – only have parental responsibility if either given parental responsibility by a court order or in agreement with the mother that is registered with the High Court or the child was born after 1/12/03 (for England and Wales) and is named on the birth certificate.

Step parents – only have parental responsibility if given by a court order.

Grandparents, relatives, friends – other people may be given responsibility by a court order or by being appointed guardian upon the death of the parents.

Social services – social care may have, or share, parental responsibility if a child is under a care order or is a ward of court. (Reproduced with kind permission of Bradford District Care NHS Trust.)

Can an adolescent consent for themselves?

Adolescents want to be in charge of their destiny and feel that they are competent to make their own decisions. Legally, written consent for treatment, such as sedation, does still require written parental agreement, but the discussions that lead up to this should include the adolescent's wishes and incorporate their assent.

Therefore agreeing to a contract with an adolescent patient, where they sign-up to agree to dietary behaviour changes and regular toothbrushing with the correct dosage of fluoride toothpaste, not only provides them with a sense of self determination and esteem but also tailors and clarifies the preventive practices that underpin the dental treatment plan.

It is always prudent to involve both the adolescent and the adult with parental responsibility. Children under 16 years of age can consent for treatment if they understand what is proposed. 'It is up to the dentist to decide whether the child has the maturity and intelligence to fully understand the nature of the treatment, the options, the risks involved and the benefits. A child who has such understanding is considered Gillick competent.

Key point

- It is good practice to gain consent from the adult with parental responsibility and assent from the child up to 16 years of age.
- Where a child is considered Gillick competent, they can consent for their own dental treatment.
- Different ages and rules apply in different parts of the UK.

Primary resources and recommended reading

American Academy of Pediatric Dentistry 2015 Guideline on behavior guidance for the pediatric dental patient. Reference Manual 37 (6):180–193.

American Academy of Pediatric Dentistry 2015 Guideline on use of local anesthesia for pediatric dental patients. Reference Manual 37 (6):199–205.

American Academy of Pediatric Dentistry 2015 Guideline on use of nitrous oxide for pediatric dental patients. Reference Manual 37 (6):206–210.

Campbell C, Soldani F, Busuttil-Naudi A et al 2011 Non-Pharmacological Behaviour Management Guideline. Available at: http://bspd.co.uk/Portals/0/Public/Files/Guidelines/Non-pharmacological%20behaviour%20management%20.pdf.

Davies C, Harrison M, Roberts G 2008 Guideline for the Use of General Anaesthesia (GA) in Paediatric Dentistry. London: Royal College of Surgeons of England. Available at: http://www.rcseng.ac.uk/fds/publications-clinical-guidelines/clinical_guidelines/documents/Guideline%20for%20the%20use%20of%20GA%20in%20Paediatric%20Dentistry%20May%202008%20Final.pdf.

Hosey MT 2002 Managing anxious children: the use of conscious sedation in paediatric dentistry. UK National Clinical Guideline. Int J Paediatr Dent 12:359–372.

Intercollegiate Advisory Committee for Sedation in Dentistry 2015 Standards for Conscious Sedation in the Provision of Dental Care. London: Royal College of Surgeons of England. Available at: https://www.rcseng.ac.uk/fds/Documents/dental-sedation-report-2015-web-v2.pdf.

Marshman Z, Baker S, Creswell C et al 2016 Cognitive behaviour therapy for dental anxiety. Resources are available for the dental team, children and their parents. Available at: http://dental.llttf.com.

Medical Protection Society 2014 Consent – children and young people. Available at: http://www.medicalprotection.org.

Nunn J, Foster M, Master S et al 2008 Consent and the Use of Physical Intervention in the Dental Care of Children. London: Royal College of Surgeons of England. Available at: https://www.rcseng.ac.uk/fds/publications-clinical-guidelines/clinical_guidelines/documents/paed_dent_intervention.pdf.

Public Health England 2014 Delivering Better Oral Health: An Evidence-Based Toolkit for Prevention, third ed. Public Health England, London. Available at: https://www.gov.uk/government/uploads/system/uploads/attachment_data/file/367563/DBOHv32014OCTMainDocument_3.pdf.

Wong HM, Humphris GM, Lee GTR 1998 Preliminary validation and reliability of the modified child dental anxiety scale. Psychol Rep 83:1179–1186.

For revision, see Mind Map 26, pages 246–247.

27

Children with disabilities and learning difficulties

SUMMARY

Sanjeev is an 8-year-old boy with Asperger's syndrome. You receive a letter from a community dentist who has undertaken a routine school inspection. The letter reports that Sanjeev has caries in his first and second primary molars. On entering the clinic, Sanjeev's mother gives the receptionist a communication passport (http://www.autism.org.uk/living-with-autism/out-and-about/my-hospital-passport.aspx). She asks the dentist to read the passport before seeing her son (Fig. 27.1).

■ ***How will you manage him?***

History

Complaint

Sanjeev's mother reports that she does not think he is in pain. He has been eating and sleeping normally. Sanjeev says, but only when he is prompted, that he has occasional pain when he eats sweets.

History of complaint

There is no relevant history.

Medical history

Sanjeev is fit and well. He was diagnosed with Asperger's syndrome last year. He does not take any medication. Asperger's syndrome is a type of high-functioning autism.

Social history

Sanjeev is in a mainstream school and receives additional support during his lessons from a teaching assistant. His mother reports that she had to fight very hard for this support and went through numerous education assessments – especially before the Asperger's syndrome diagnosis was finally made. Sanjeev's mother has only recently returned to part-time work, now that he seems more settled in school.

■ ***What challenges has Sanjeev's family faced?***

The family may have faced genuine difficulties relating to access to medical and dental care. A key focus for Sanjeev's parents was to get a thorough assessment of his medical condition. They also had to work with his school and with social services to have his educational and social needs assessed. As a result of these assessments, Sanjeev now has better access to health care, social and educational support, and his parents have been in touch with other parents who have children with Asperger's syndrome.

Sanjeev has two healthy brothers who also need support and attention in their own right. Sanjeev's mother gave up her part-time job to look after him. Although she is pleased that she has achieved stability, support and medical care for her child, she is worried about his teeth. She has previously prioritized the many educational and school assessments, which led to Sanjeev's irregular dental attendance.

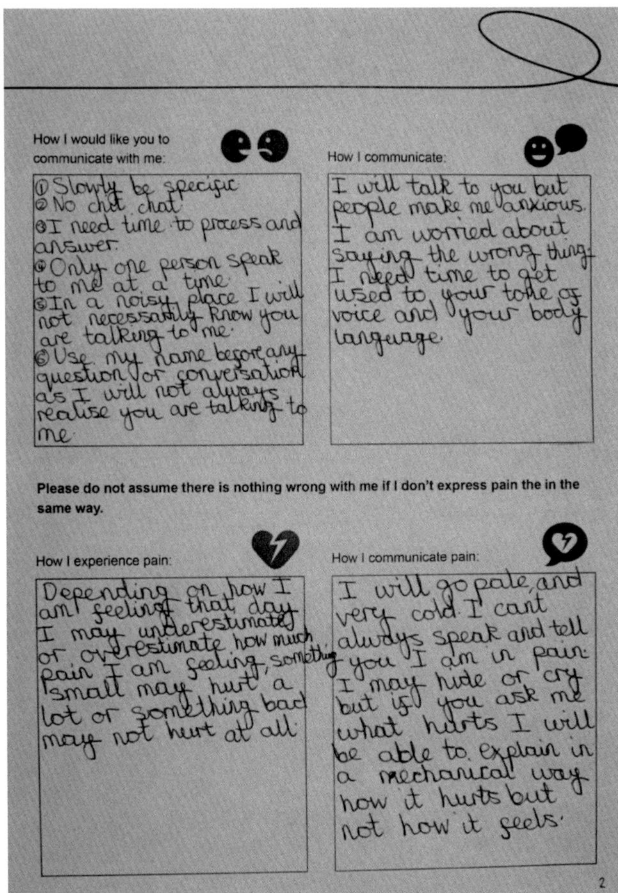

How I would like you to communicate with me:

① Slowly be specific
② No chit chat
③ I need time to process and answer.
④ Only one person speak to me at a time.
⑤ In a noisy place I will not necessarily know you are talking to me.
⑥ Use my name before any question or conversation as I will not always realise you are talking to me.

How I communicate:

I will talk to you but people make me anxious. I am worried about saying the wrong thing. I need time to get used to your tone of voice and your body language.

Please do not assume there is nothing wrong with me if I don't express pain the in the same way.

How I experience pain:

Depending on how I am feeling that day I may underestimate or overestimate how much pain I am feeling, something small may hurt a lot or something bad may not hurt at all.

How I communicate pain:

I will go pale, and very cold. I cant always speak and tell you I am in pain. I may hide or cry but if you ask me what hurts I will be able to explain in a mechanical way how it hurts but not how it feels.

2

Fig. 27.1 Sanjeev's communication passport where he describes how best to manage his dental visit. Passport originated by National Autism Society. See http://www.autism.org.uk/about/health/hospital-passport.aspx.

Key point

Key features of Autism, Asperger's syndrome and Attention Deficit Hyperactivity Disorder (ADHD):

- Please see http://www.autism.org.uk for further information.

Autism is a spectrum of disorders with children showing varying levels of severity in three key categories:

- Communication – children show delayed language development and limited comprehension of non-verbal communication. Severely affected children may have rudimentary or no speech.
- Social interaction – children often live in their own world and have limited interest and interaction with other children and adults.
- Social imagination – children may struggle to interpret other people's feelings and actions.

Asperger's syndrome, as already described, is at the high-functioning end of the autistic spectrum. It is characterized by normal spoken language development, and the child can have average or above average intelligence. He or she often does not have learning delay but can have specific learning difficulties. There are three key features of the diagnosis:

- Love of routines.
- Intense interests.
- Sensory impairment which can be either under or over functioning, for example taste, sound, sensation, hearing or sight.

ADHD is a diagnosis made before the age of 7 with children demonstrating a triad of symptoms, which can be treated with medication or therapeutic interventions.

- Inattention.
- Impulsivity.
- Hyperactivity.

Although many children are diagnosed with high-functioning autism and ADHD, they are two separate conditions.

■ ***What can dentists do to assist the family and help them overcome barriers of access to dental care?***

Managing children with disabilities and learning difficulties can sometimes seem to be a challenge, but it is always rewarding. For many of these families, being able to access dental care in a primary setting is a welcome respite from the other specialist services that they attend. Many dentists who begin to treat a child with a disability often continue to deliver care for the whole family and provide a continued source of support. For many children with Asperger's syndrome, routine is very important and being seen by the same dentist in the same surgery helps with familiarization and their cooperation.

From a dental point of view, it is not uncommon to have a 'warrior-mum' who has become conditioned to fight for her child's care and so can appear overly demanding or impatient. However, being aware of these other challenges that the family is facing can help develop a strong affinity and level of trust. Parents will be grateful for appointments and treatments that minimize the amount of time out of school and away from work.

Examination

■ ***How will you examine Sanjeev?***

Sanjeev has provided considerable help and guidance on how best he can cope with the dental examination. Following his advice will only help with the appointment. Many children with disabilities and learning difficulties can readily accept a dental examination. However, some can have more challenging behaviour and even a dental examination can be difficult to perform. Some of these difficulties can be overcome by a sequence of short introductory visits, each one set up in exactly the same way as the previous but just building on the examination; this can work well with a child with autistic spectrum disorder. Other distractions around the surgery should be minimized, e.g. noise or interruption.

Keeping instruction simple and direct helped Sanjeev sit in the dental chair and allowed for a quick dental examination.

Extraoral

There were no relevant findings.

Intraoral

Caries was identified in the occlusal surfaces of all four second primary molars. There were distal cavities on both mandibular first primary molars.

Radiographic investigation

■ ***What is the best radiographic investigation?***

With careful and simple explanation, Sanjeev tolerated bitewing radiographs.

If this was not possible, a 'teeth-only dental panoramic tomogram (DPT)' or a standard DPT (depending on what settings are available) is an alternative. A trial run to familiarize Sanjeev with the equipment and what is expected is a very helpful halfway step. This will increase the likelihood of Sanjeev staying still for the DPT. Although the radiation exposure is higher for a DPT, where a radiograph of the carious primary teeth will influence the treatment provided, this DPT radiograph is still justified if bitewings are not possible.

The bitewings showed that the:

- First permanent molars have no caries.
- Occlusal caries in the second primary molars was into the inner half of the dentine.
- Caries in the mandibular first primary molars appears close to the pulp with the roots almost completely resorbed by the permanent successors.

■ ***What is Sanjeev's dental diagnosis?***

Sanjeev appears to have reversible pulpitis from his carious and restorable second primary molars.

The mandibular first primary molars may also be causing him some annoyance, especially as they become more mobile. In common with other children his age, he may be fixated by his exfoliating teeth.

Key point

- Parents of a child with a learning disability will have many competing demands on their time.
- Routine is key and therefore it is important that the child sees the same staff, in the same surgery to develop familiarity.
- Keep instructions simple and direct.
- Children may not always sit in the dental chair and therefore take whatever opportunity arises to examine their teeth (e.g. sitting on their parents' lap, in the waiting room, on the surgery floor).
- Clear communication with a parent is essential to identify how much support and/or restraint they are happy to provide to permit a dental examination. Any restraint must be proportionate with the history and the need for a dental examination.

What are the treatment options for Sanjeev?

The management of the dental disease is the same as described in Chapter 24. but it is the method of delivery than can be different. *Prevention is the key.* The DoH Prevention Toolkit is a valuable source of guidance. Every visit presents an opportunity to prevent caries: whether this is advice to reduce sugar frequency, to use 1450 ppm fluoride toothpaste or to apply topical fluoride. There are a number of ways parents can be supported to ensure they are undertaking toothbrushing for their child. This includes modified toothbrushes (three-sided toothbrush), finger-guards or using a two toothbrush technique. The second toothbrush can be used to keep the teeth apart, thus permitting the other to brush the occlusal surfaces of the teeth.

Can Sanjeev be managed in a primary care setting?

The answer to this question depends on the definitive treatment plan and the patient's level of cooperation. Referral to a specialist (community) or hospital-based paediatric dentistry unit may be required, especially if general anaesthesia is needed.

What are the dental management options?

Sanjeev might manage to have the carious second primary molars restored with complete caries removal, but he will need to accept local analgesia owing to the depth of caries in all four of these teeth and their symptomatic history. Conventional caries removal is likely to take at least a further five visits. Therefore, in the first instance, stabilizing the caries using glass ionomer cement (GIC) temporary restorations is the best option. It also provides Sanjeev with further acclimation to the dental surgery and gives an indication of how he will cope with more invasive treatment. In these earlier visits, addressing the causes of caries is essential as described in Chapters 22 and 23. Many autistic children can struggle with some of the sensations of dentistry such as the tastes, smells, noises and textures.

Would Hall crowns be an appropriate treatment option?

The extent of the caries and the history of pain would reduce the chances that the Hall approach would be effective. Guidance for the use of Hall crowns (see Chapter 24) would advocate their use at an earlier stage of the caries process, before symptoms develop. However, in some situations, and after careful discussion with the parents, treatment may be undertaken if there is a clear understanding of the poor prognosis and the need for one or more teeth to be extracted if further signs and symptoms show irreversible pulpitis or apical periodontitis (e.g. non-vital).

For some children with disabilities, especially where there are signs of bruxism and tooth wear, great thought should be taken before applying Hall crowns. The propping open of the occlusion may exacerbate their grinding and increase the risk of a perforated crown.

When will these primary teeth exfoliate?

This is an important consideration when treatment planning. For Sanjeev, the mandibular primary first molars are likely to exfoliate very shortly and therefore, unless symptomatic, can be left to exfoliate. For the second primary molars, these teeth exfoliate around the age of 12. Therefore any restorative plan will require materials with good evidence of longevity over this 4-year time period. Such materials include composite, amalgam or stainless steel crowns. The longer the restoration needs to survive the more likely a stainless steel crown will be the restorative option as these have the greatest longevity.

Does behaviour management work with children with Asperger's syndrome?

Non-pharmacological behaviour management can work well in children with Asperger's syndrome. However, this may need to be augmented with voice control to gain Sanjeev's attention if he becomes distracted, so positive reinforcement, tell-show-do and enabling a hand signal to 'stop' should all be used. Giving simple information about what will happen, what it will feel like and how to cope beforehand and during the procedure are all important. The language used should be appropriate for his level of understanding and experience. A constant simple and repetitious dialogue needs to be maintained, otherwise Sanjeev will get distracted.

Key point

- Behaviour management techniques should be used.
- A constant dialogue should be maintained to keep the child engaged and focused on the dentist.
- Voice control may sometimes be required to focus the child's attention.

Does nitrous oxide inhalation sedation work for children with Asperger's syndrome?

Nitrous oxide inhalation sedation is the most commonly used sedative in children. The key is to carry out a thorough assessment based on a frank discussion with Sanjeev and his mother. The success of the technique is dependent on Sanjeev's ability and willingness to breathe in and out through his nose. Many children with Asperger's syndrome enjoy the active engagement of this activity. It is also wise to assess progress after the first or second visit and to evaluate whether Sanjeev will manage to accept local analgesia.

Does Sanjeev need a general anaesthetic?

This decision is a balance as there are a number of disadvantages of this approach. The whole general anaesthetic event can be traumatic for the child, and research has shown that children are more dentally anxious afterwards. However, for some parents the ability to treat the dental caries efficiently (e.g. all dental care is provided in one go) and their child's limited ability to report any pain and suffering can make a general anaesthetic an attractive option. Other considerations which influence the decision include the likelihood of the child cooperating during treatment, the pain history and the waiting time for this treatment.

Sanjeev does not need urgent treatment, and he is not in severe pain. Therefore a general anaesthetic is not currently justified especially as in Sanjeev's case there is time to stablise his caries and see how he and his symptoms respond to this initial treatment.

What treatment plan would you propose?

Using the principles discussed in Chapter 24, a treatment plan should be drawn up together with a visit-by-visit plan. As for all children, it is essential to ensure a rigorous preventive plan. Sanjeev may always need extra support when attending the dentist and therefore keeping him caries free is a key priority.

By following Sanjeev's instructions, he coped with the temporary restorations and both his mum and he engaged in the preventive regime (discussed in Chapters 22 and 23). Sanjeev's cooperation was good but limited. However, he responded well to nitrous oxide sedation. Conventional caries removal was undertaken under local anaesthetic and nitrous oxide sedation. This was very effective, and Sanjeev completed treatment. While the mandibular second primary molars were anaesthetized, the almost exfoliated mandibular primary molars were extracted.

Common disabilities

What are the common disabilities?

There are many other physical disabilities and learning difficulties. These can be grouped into sensory, physical, mental and medical disabilities. The commonest of these are shown in **Table 27.1**. Sometimes these can be intertwined. The impact of medical conditions on dental care is discussed in Chapter 28.

How would this plan be altered if Sanjeev's disability had been more severe?

Sanjeev coped well with a dental plan that was based on prevention, stabilization and then definitive care. As such, it did not challenge him too much and it also incorporated very good behavioural management. However, for some children, their physical and learning disability is more severe and their dental needs more urgent. A typical example is a child with epilepsy and cerebral palsy who is unable to control his or her movements. This child may have had a seizure and fallen, thus traumatizing a tooth. In such a case, the child may be unable to cope with treatment for a non-vital central incisor and a general anaesthetic might be required to manage the traumatized tooth. While asleep, any other dental care would also be carried out, such as fissure sealants, extractions or restorations.

Are there more complications to general anaesthesia for children with a disability?

Many children with a disability or learning difficulty are otherwise physically healthy and can undergo daycase general anaesthesia without further concern. Nevertheless, the whole general anaesthesia event can be anxiety provoking, and so preparing the child and family can help reduce the psychological anxiety that surrounds the event. Psychological support information may help; one such online and freely available package that has increased family satisfaction can be found at www.scottga.org.

Some may not have the coping skills to cooperate with the anaesthetic induction and may need pre-medication beforehand. The commonest pre-medication is midazolam 0.5 mg/kg given approximately 30 minutes before the general anaesthetic induction.

What medical comorbidities can children with a disability commonly present with?

Apart from his Asperger's syndrome, Sanjeev is otherwise healthy. However, sometimes disabilities are linked with a medical comorbidity. An example of this is a child with Down syndrome, who might not only have a cardiac defect but also be prone to acute lymphoblastic leukaemia, especially if the Philadelphia chromosome is carried together with trisomy 21.

The management of these children with complex conditions needs liaison with paediatricians and is best referred to a hospital paediatric dentistry team.

Key point

- Learning disabilities can be linked to epilepsy, cardiac defects and other medical problems.
- There needs to be liaison with the child's paediatrician.
- Referral to a community or hospital based paediatric dentistry specialist team may be needed, especially if general anaesthesia treatment is required and their medical comorbidity will complicate the general anaesthesia.

How does a dentist communicate with children with a disability?

Communication with children with complex needs includes a mixture of methods and technologies that can supplement the spoken and written word and gesture. For some, gestures, facial expressions, body postures, eye gaze and mime is needed. For others, sign language, e.g. British sign language, or other hand signals and pictures and symbols or other media such as a soundboard may be used. The best-known technique is MAKATON, developed in the 1970s to help people with learning disabilities to communicate. It uses some British sign language signs combined with speech, facial expression, eye contact and body language along with gestures and symbols. Nowadays, MAKATON

Table 27.1 Types of disability

Type	Example(s)	Dental implications	Solutions
Physical	Cerebral palsy Varying degrees of paralysis/muscular dysfunction Epilepsy Behavioural problems Visual and/or hearing impairments Compromised speech and learning skills	Bruxism Reduced vertical dimension Anterior open bite Drooling Inability to perform adequate oral hygiene Phenytoin-induced gingival hyperplasia Wheel-chair access	Oral hygiene support Modified brushes Teaching carers how to brush 2800 ppm fluoride toothpaste for children aged 10 and over Regular check-ups and scaling Corsodyl gel applied via a toothbrush daily, separate from fluoride toothbrushing Reduce sugar frequency Wherever possible consider referral to interdisciplinary team for assessment of drooling to avoid surgery to relocate submandibular salivary gland outlet, as this will significantly increase caries risk especially lower anterior teeth Augmentive and alternative communication skills
Learning	Down syndrome	Class III occlusion Macroglossia Hypodontia Microdontia Delayed exfoliation of primary teeth Predisposition to periodontal disease Medical problems: Cardiac defect Leukaemia Recurrent chest infection	Oral hygiene support Modified brushes Teaching carers how to brush 2800 ppm fluoride toothpaste for children aged 10 and over Regular check-ups and scaling Corsodyl gel applied via a toothbrush daily, separate from fluoride toothbrushing Reduce sugar frequency
	Severe developmental delay	Difficult to examine or to provide dental care	Consider gentle holding to prevent harm – known as 'clinical holding' Mouth props (thimble) Towels Pillows Safety belts Pharmacological restraint Pre-medication General anaesthesia
Sensory disabilities	Hearing	Difficulty giving a history Difficulty following instructions while in the dental chair, especially if the dentist is behind Hearing aids and cochlear implants may distort sounds and enhance the volume of dental drills and scalers so much that it is painful and distressing Uses other means of communication Sign language Lip-reading Other communcation aids or media such as VOCA	Lip-reading Do not over emphasize mouth and lips when speaking – it causes difficulties with lip-reading Find out the best means of communication Take time to ask them to show it to you and agree how you will use it to collaborate together to communicate Give child a hand mirror so that they can see you Warn to switch off hearing aid or turn down volume before drilling or scaling Agree on hand signals or gestures to allow continued communication while hearing aids are off Cochlear implants Avoid monopolar electrosurgery
	Vision	Needs toothbrushing instruction that is not based on visual cues such as disclosing Bright lights can hurt No visualization of surroundings or gestures of dentists or staff Access challenges Stairs Guide dog Directional signage	Use sunglasses and avoid shining light into eyes Give verbal cues Use and allow touch-shake-hands/touch hands and shoulder Use Braille in lifts and in signage Think about where the guide dog can be during treatment

has been augmented by new technologies and media (for example http://widgit-health.com/easy-read-sheets/pdfs/Healthy%20teeth.pdf). Speech and language therapists use all of these techniques and tailor them to each child's needs so that every child can achieve some level of communication. As can be seen from Sanjeev's case, the communication passport can work very well. The full passport contains other helpful sections such as 'things I can't cope with and make me distressed' and 'how to avoid distressing me'. Other leaflets and storybooks can help children prepare for their dental visit and what to expect.

Key Point

- Children with disabilities communicate by gestures, symbols, signing and multimedia.
- Many have their own 'communication passport'.

Primary resources and recommended reading

Faculty of Dental Surgery 2012 Clinical Guidelines and Integrated Care Pathways for the Oral Health Care of People with Learning Disabilities. London: Faculty of Dental Surgery, The Royal College of Surgeons of England.

Makaton®. Available at: www.makaton.org.

Mencap. Available at: https://www.mencap.org.uk/cqcreports.

The National Autistic Society. Available at: http://www.autism.org.uk.

Nunn J, Foster M, Master S et al 2008 Consent and the Use of Physical Intervention in the Dental Care of Children. London: Royal College of Surgeons of England. Available at: https://www.rcseng.ac.uk/fds/publications-clinical-guidelines/clinical_guidelines/documents/paed_dent_intervention.pdf.

Peninsula Cerebra Research Unit 2013 Dentistry for children and young people with learning disabilities and challenging behaviour. Available at: http://www.pencru.org/evidence/dentistry/.

Public Health England 2014 Delivering Better Oral Health: An Evidence-Based Toolkit for Prevention, 3rd edn. London: Public Health England. Available at: https://www.gov.uk/government/uploads/system/uploads/attachment_data/file/367563/DBOHv32014OCTMainDocument_3.pdf.

Research Autism. Available at: http://researchautism.net

RNIB Knowledge and Research Hub. Available at: http://www.rnib.org.uk/knowledge-and-research-hub.

Scott's Hospital Dental Visit. Available at: www.scottga.org.

For revision, see Mind Map 27, page 248.

28

Common medical problems in children

CASE 1

SUMMARY

Hannah is 9 years old. She was diagnosed with acute lymphoblastic leukaemia (ALL) 3 months ago. She has toothache, and her medical team has asked you to see her.

History

Hannah has been suffering from toothache for the last 3 days. She reports that the pain is coming from the upper left quadrant and feels her gum is swollen (**Fig. 28.1**).

Medical history

Over the 6-month period prior to her ALL diagnosis, Hannah started to feel tired and lethargic. A blood test at her general medical practitioner identified an excessive number of immature and poorly differentiated lymphocytes. A bone marrow aspiration confirmed the diagnosis of ALL. She was admitted to hospital and started on a standard chemotherapy regime. For girls, treatment involves several stages of chemotherapy over a 2 year period with the aim of eliminating the leukaemic cells and preventing their recurrence.

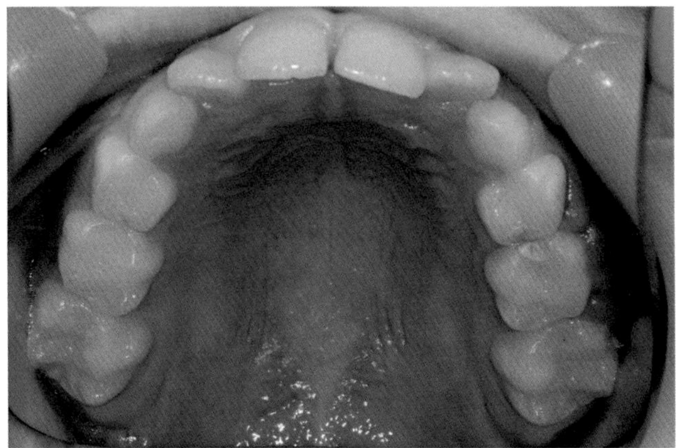

Fig. 28.1 |E with a temporary restoration, |D distal caries with buccal swelling.

Dental history

She had a previous filling in the |E with no local anaesthetic about a year ago. No bitewing radiographs were taken.

Examination

Extraorally there is no swelling and no facial asymmetry. There is left-sided submandibular lymphadopathy. Intraorally she is in the mixed dentition. Intraorally there is a fluctuant swelling associated with |DE.

■ ***Why are you concerned with this dental history?***

At the time of the filling, no bitewing radiographs were taken to identify the depth of the caries, the proximity of the caries to the pulp and the pulpal response to the caries. Moreover, the lack of local anaesthetic when undertaking conventional caries removal often results in incomplete removal, as the child finds the drilling uncomfortable. The temporary cement in the medium term will deteriorate, leading to microleakage and caries progression.

■ ***What are the effects of chemotherapy on cells with a rapid turnover?***

Chemotherapy targets different stages of cell mitosis and is toxic to all differentiating cells. Therefore hair, skin, mucosal cells lining the gastro-intestinal tract, red blood cells, white blood cells and platelets will be affected in addition to the cancer cells. This results in loss of hair, dry and fragile skin, mucositis, anaemia, leukopenia and thrombocytopenia. **Fig. 28.2** illustrates how chemotherapy works. Rapidly replicating cells (e.g. hair, mucosa, skin, red blood cells, white blood cells and platelets) are able to repair and recover quicker following chemotherapy than the cancerous cells. Each tumour will have a different chemotherapy regimen and timeline. This schematic is for a solid tumour with the bone marrow recovery taking about 3 weeks before the next dose of chemotherapy. Providing care for children on chemotherapy requires liaison with their oncologist. Acute dental care is often provided once the bone marrow counts have recovered and shortly before their next dose of chemotherapy.

■ ***What further information do you need?***

Dental information A full oral assessment is needed. At different stages of the chemotherapy cycle, patients will have very low white cell counts (in particular, low neutrophil counts), which will limit their ability to fight infections. A lack of facial swelling or lymphadenopathy does not necessarily mean there is no infection related to a necrotic tooth, especially if a patient is pyrexic. Therefore

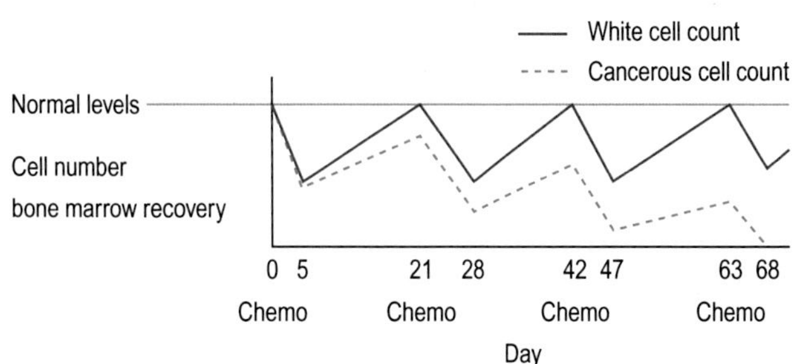

Fig. 28.2 A schematic and simple diagram to explain the effect of chemotherapy on bone marrow and cancer cell numbers.

taking Hannah's temperature is essential. Her temperature is 38.5°C.

The oral assessment should include bitewings and a dental panoramic tomogram, when the patient can tolerate these radiographs (**Fig. 28.3**). Following the clinical and radiographic examination, a complete problem list and treatment plan (see Chapter 24, Table 24.3) should be drawn up. Any primary teeth with a poor prognosis, including those with deep caries, should be extracted rather than restored. For necrotic and infected permanent teeth, either they should be extracted or first stage endodontics should be undertaken where there is confidence that the infection can be eliminated.

Medical information Close collaboration is required with the medical team coordinating Hannah's chemotherapy. There are only a few short windows in which invasive dental treatment can be provided as a result of the anaemia, leukopenia and thrombocytopenia associated with her treatment. Therefore it is essential to find out the current full blood count (red cell count, white cell count, neutrophil count and platelet count) and whether the count will improve or get worse in the immediate future. Moreover, at different points of ALL chemotherapy regimens, children will undergo a lumbar puncture and bone marrow aspiration. These are invariably carried out under general anaesthetic and may therefore provide an opportunity to undertake any acute extractions.

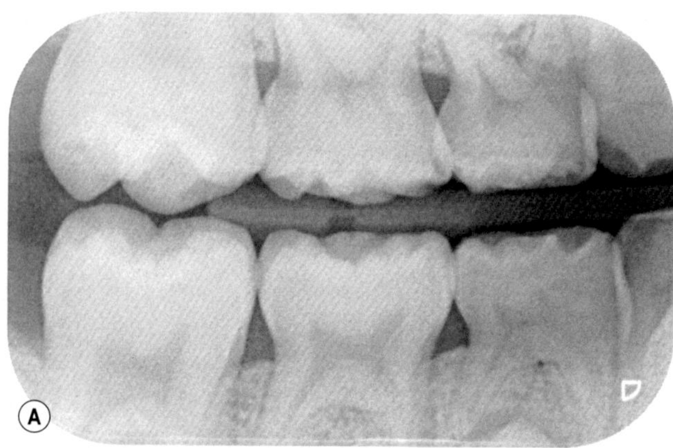

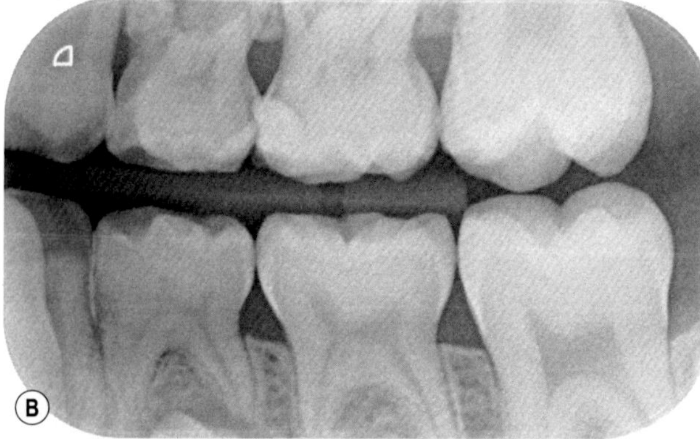

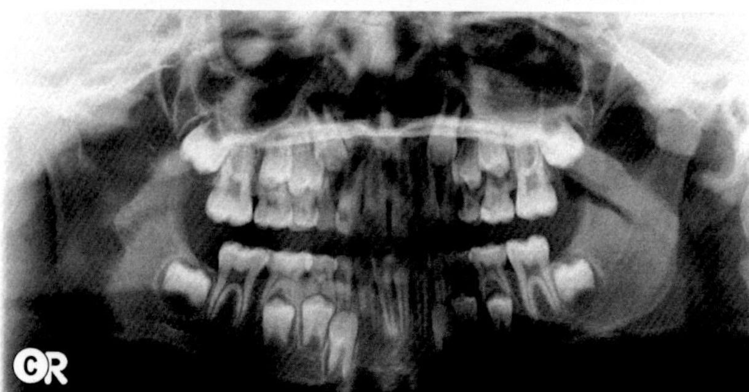

Fig. 28.3 Hannah's bitewings (A, B) and dental panoramic tomogram (C).

Treatment

What acute treatment does Hannah need?

The presence of a temperature, together with the buccal swelling associated with the |E and/or |D, needs to be discussed with the medical team immediately. Treatment will include the use of appropriate antibiotics (for example, amoxicillin and metronidazole or similar antibiotics given intravenously or orally depending on the severity of the infection) and painkillers (these are frequently paracetamol and opioids, as non-steroidal anti-inflammatories such as ibuprofen are avoided owing to the low platelet count and the risk of bleeding). Hannah was admitted to the oncology ward and started on intravenous antibiotics.

At the most appropriate time, in relation to the chemotherapy regime and full blood count, the |DE will need to be extracted. Although swelling is most likely to arise from the |E, for Hannah the safest option would be to extract both |DE to eliminate all potential sources of infection. In identifying the most appropriate time for this treatment, consideration should be given to how long it will take the socket to heal post-extraction because her counts will start to drop again with the next course of chemotherapy.

What other dental care does Hannah require?

Hannah requires an intense preventative regime against any further oral disease. For some children undergoing chemotherapy, their diet will change significantly during treatment. This is further exacerbated by the side effects of chemotherapy, such as mucositis and the need to maintain adequate calorific oral intake. On occasions where children are failing to eat sufficient calories, they may be fed via a nasogastric tube, gastrostomy or intravenously.

What are the oral implications of childhood cancer treatment?

Treatment for leukaemia and solid childhood cancers can include chemotherapy, radiotherapy and surgery. **Boxes 28.1** and **28.2** list the short- and long-term oral complications of chemotherapy and radiotherapy.

Box 28.1 Short and long-term oral side effects of chemotherapy

Short-term oral side effects – chemotherapy

At risk of peri- and intra-oral infections – bacterial, viral and fungal, especially as chemotherapy and associated medication will lead to changes in oral flora

Ulcers and mucositis

Bleeding and gingivitis

Xerostomia and dysgeusia

Dysphasia

Trismus

Phantom pain in jaw – often associated with vincristine or from leukemic infiltration into the jaw or dental pulp

Long-term oral side effects – chemotherapy

Anomalies of dental development – e.g. aplasia, hypoplasia or hypomineralized crowns, diminutive or rudimentary roots and or crown, delayed eruption and exfoliation

Box 28.2 Short and long-term oral side effects of radiotherapy involving the oral cavity

Short-term oral side effects – radiotherapy

Trismus

Osteomyelitis

Sialadenitis

Infections

Erythema

Pulp pain or hypersensitivity

Dry mouth, impaired salivary function

Long-term oral side effects – radiotherapy

Increase risk of caries

Dry mouth, xerostomia

Change in taste

Anomalies of dental development

At risk of osteoradionecrosis

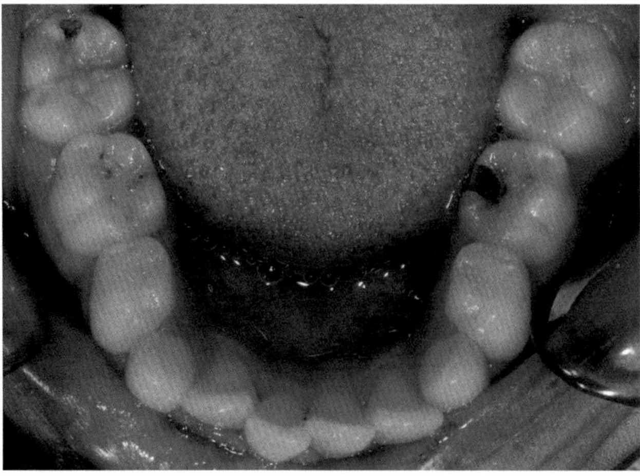

Fig. 28.4 6|E caries.

CASE 2

SUMMARY

Hugo is 8 years old and presents for a routine check-up. He has Haemophilia A. Clinical and radiographic examination reveal mid-dentine caries in |E and 6| (Fig. 28.4). A dental panoramic tomogram identifies both mandibular second permanent premolars to be missing (5|5).

History

Hugo complains of no pain or problems from his teeth.

Medical history

Hugo has severe Haemophili A and is under the care of the paediatric haematologist. He requires alternate day injections of factor VIII, which are administered at home by his mother.

What is Haemophilia A?

Haemophilia is an X-linked recessive deficiency of factor VIII. The defective gene is passed down through his mother, who is a carrier for this condition, which only affects boys. Factor VIII is an essential part of the clotting cascade and enables the platelet plug to be stabilized with fibrin. Primary haemostasis is not affected. The condition is classified by the percentage of factor VIII activity, with severe classified as less than 1%, moderate 1–5% and mild less than 5%.

What dental treatment does Hugo require?

A full clinical and radiographic examination identified mid-dentine caries in 6|E. The absence of the 5|5 will influence the treatment options available. Treatment planning for poor prognosis first permanent molars is discussed in more detail in Chapter 34. Following an orthodontic consultation, it is felt that restoration of both teeth is the most appropriate option. Conventional caries removal is the treatment choice for both 6|E.

Hugo is cooperative and happy to have the treatment provided under local anaesthetic. The quantity of treatment and the number of visits this will take may influence whether treatment is provided under local or general anaesthetic. For |E the most appropriate restoration would be a stainless steel crown, owing to its enhanced longevity in comparison to other restoration materials. Long-term outcomes for the Hall technique are only available for 5 years. Realistically the |E may survive for 15–30 years, and therefore, when the child is cooperative, conventional caries would be the most appropriate option. For the 6| a single surface restoration with either an amalgam or composite with fissure sealants of the remaining occlusal surfaces would be the most appropriate option. If a composite is chosen, treatment under rubber dam is essential to optimize moisture control and hence longevity.

As important as the restorative plan is the preventative plan to minimize further dental caries. Hugo will require enhanced prevention as discussed in Chapters 22 and 23.

What are the oral implications of Haemophilia A on Hugo's restorative treatment?

Careful liaison with the haematology team is required to discuss the treatment needed and a plan to systemically minimize any bleeding. For Hugo, the following medical plan is drawn up: Firstly, transexamic acid mouthwash is prescribed at least one dose prior to his treatment and then continued three times a day for 3–7 days depending on the dental treatment required. Hugo needs to gargle the mouthwash and then swallow it to optimize its effectiveness. Transexamic acid is an antifibrinolytic and helps prevent clot breakdown. Secondly, he is advised to take his factor VIII on the morning of his dental treatment and to take a further dose the next morning if there are any signs of post-operative bleeding from the gingivae or submucosal haematoma. If not, he should continue with his regular alternate day pattern for taking factor VIII.

What local measures can you take to minimize bleeding?

There are a number of surgical principles to minimize bleeding. These include taking great care when manipulating the soft tissues, for example, when placing rubber dam clamps and matrix band and when using high-volume suction. Where teeth have been extracted, the use of sutures, Surgicel and pressure is commonly used. On rarer occasions bone wax, Coe-Pak dressings and bipolar diathermy may be needed depending on the oral surgery being undertaken.

Care should be taken to carefully explain the post-operative instructions to prevent disturbance or loss of the blood clot, for example, avoiding poking the clot, eating hard foods, drinking hot drinks or exercise. Non-steroidal anti-inflammatory painkillers should be avoided in all patients with a bleeding diathesis.

■ *Infiltrations versus inferior alveolar block injection*

Although the factor VIII prophylaxis will cover inferior alveolar block injection, when infiltration injections will achieve similar pain control, they should be used instead. Therefore, for both the |E and 6| infiltration injections, using Articaine would be the most appropriate option. The adrenaline contained within both Articaine and Lignocaine will again help achieve haemostasis.

CASE 3

SUMMARY

Harriet is 3 years old. Her mum is concerned with the appearance of the E|. She reports that the tooth erupted with brown staining and that it appears to be getting worse (Fig. 28.5).

History

Harriet sometimes complains of pain from the E| when eating ice cream.

Medical history

Harriet has had a surgical correction for a tetralogy of Fallot at the age of 4 months. The heart condition was diagnosed in pregnancy at the 20-week scan. Her first months of life were spent in and out of hospital prior to her cardiac surgery. Currently there are no plans for further surgery, although she is still seen on a regular basis by the cardiologists.

■ *What are the oral implications of Harriet's cardiac history?*

Harriet's congenital heart defect puts her at an increased risk of infective endocarditis. Infective endocarditis is a bacterial infection in which there is potential for bacterial vegetation to become established, owing to impaired blood flow in the heart. These colonies will then cause pyrexia, new or changing heart murmurs and embolic events. Infective endocarditis carries with it significant morbidity and mortality, and consequently its prevention is a high priority for at risk children and adults. Bacteraemias from the oral cavity are common following dental extractions or other treatments involving gingival manipulation. However, bacteraemia is also seen when children brush their teeth or chew, especially if there is marked gingivitis and poor oral hygiene. Consequently, good oral hygiene is a key preventative behaviour in minimizing the risk of infective endocarditis.

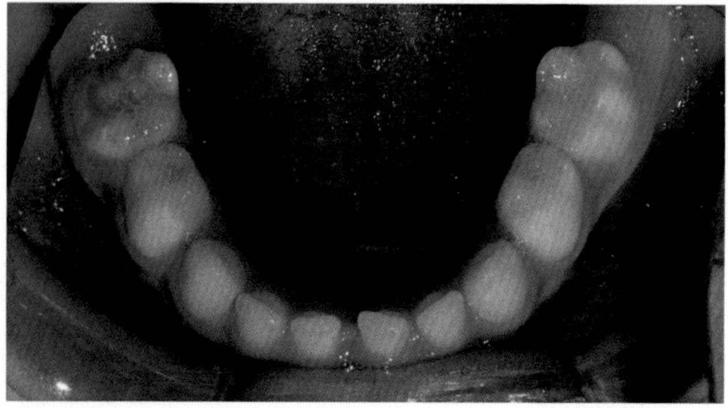

Fig. 28.5 E| hypomineralized with post-eruptive breakdown.

■ *Is antibiotic prophylaxis required for dental procedures?*

In the UK, National Institute of Clinical Excellence (NICE) guidelines advocate that no antibiotic cover is required for dental procedures. This is different in other countries, such as Australia and the USA, where antibiotics are still advocated for dental procedures that cause bacteria. The logic behind the NICE guidances was that since no antibiotic cover was advised for the frequent oral bacteraemia associated with everyday behaviours (such as chewing and brushing) it therefore did not make sense for antibiotics to be used to cover infrequent dental procedures. However, a recent article has identified an increase in infective endocarditis since this guidance was published with the consequent fall in prescribing of antibiotic prophylaxis in the UK. In light of these findings, NICE has reviewed their guidelines but has concluded that this evidence is not sufficient to change their advice.

■ *What treatment is appropriate for Harriet?*

Preventive plan It is essential that a robust preventive plan be drawn up for Harriet. Owing to her cardiac condition, Harriet should be placed on an enhanced preventative plan, as the consequences of dental caries are potentially significant. Furthermore, very careful attention should be paid to her oral hygiene. Her parents should be encouraged to actively undertake her tooth brushing and ensure that both the teeth and gingivae are brushed to minimize gingivitis and hence bacteraemias of oral origin.

Restorative care A careful clinical examination and bitewings are essential. The examination identifies that the E| is hypomineralized with post-eruptive breakdown and is sensitive to cold air. There are no signs or symptoms that the E| is non-vital and infected. The rest of the dentition is caries free. Bitewing radiographs show no radiographic signs of a non-vital E|. In discussion with Harriet's parents, they feel she would struggle to cooperate for a conventional stainless steel crown (e.g. complete caries and hypomineralized enamel removal) but may cope with a stainless steel crown placed using the Hall crown technique (e.g. no caries or hypomineralized enamel removed). Therefore a difficult choice exists because a conventional stainless steel crown would require a general anaesthetic and would involve risks of morbidity and mortality. A careful discussion with Harriet's parents is required to discuss the different treatment options. Certainly if a Hall crown was chosen, very careful follow-up, both clinically and radiographically, is

Table 28.1 Common medical problems and their impact on the provision of dental care

Type	Example(s)	Dental implications	Solutions
Medical	Cardiac – cyanotic	*Increased risk of bleeding* *Complicated and potentially high risk general anaesthetic* *Avoid stress at the dental visit* *Some cyanotic patients are on warfarin and therefore at increased risk of bleeding*	Close liaison with cardiologist; treat in a specialist cardiac centre
	Bleeding	*AV – malformation – vascular anomaly seen on perioral skin or intra mucosa* *Inherited bleeding disorder*	Close liaison with surgeon/radiologist to identify the extent of the lesion and involvement of the maxilla or mandible – risk of profuse bleeding Close liaison with haematologist – identify severity of disorder and medical management; local surgical management as described is essential
	Diabetes	*Discussed in Chapter 41*	
	Transplants	*Depends on the type of transplant they have had, however, all will be on immunosuppressants to prevent organ rejection*	At increased risk of bacterial, viral or fungal infections; some anti-rejection drugs associated with gingival enlargement (e.g. cyclosporine); liaise with paediatrician if oral infections (bacterial, fungal, or viral) are identified, as these need to be aggressively managed; careful vigilance as long-term immunosuppression is associated with development of cancers including oral cancers
	Asthma	*Identify severity of asthma, how it is managed, what triggers it, what medication they are taking and last hospital admission*	Salbutamol and inhaled steroids each have direct effects on the oral cavity (e.g. reduced salivary flow, increase risk of oral candidiasis) Ensure salbutamol is available in emergency drug box Care with some topical fluorides, as they can very rarely cause breathlessness
	Epilepsy	*Identify the type/s of seizures and their duration, when was the last seizure, how was it managed and did it require rescue medication or hospitalisation to stop the seizure*	Some epileptic medication can increase the risk of gingival overgrowth (phenytoin); risk of trauma to the dentition during seizure; parents are normally very aware and perceptive of an impending seizure; ensure anti-epileptic medication has been taken prior to attendance
	Cystic fibrosis	*Multi system disorder predominantly affecting lungs and digestive system; need to identify current respiratory status, have they been admitted for intravenous antibiotics to clear chest infections or have they been colonized by pseudomonas*	Studies show that children with cystic fibrosis have a lower risk of developing dental caries; however, if caries develops, treatment is complicated by high risk for general anaesthetic; may have nutrition supplemented by gastrostomy feeding; long-term treatment options may include lung transplant
	Metabolic	*Multiple different disorders affecting different biochemical pathways; treatment often involves strict diets that avoid amino acids, which cannot be broken down, or medication to circumvent these pathways*	A careful history is needed to identify their diet restrictions and feeding; for some children they are exclusively or predominantly gastrostomy fed; infections (including systemic infections of oral origin) can lead to decompensation and hospital admission; admission for general anaesthetic requires careful liaison to identify how best to manage pre-operative starving

required to monitor any signs of infection as a result of the tooth becoming non-vital. Avoidance of non-vital and infected teeth is essential to minimize the increased risk of infective endocarditis. Harriet's parents, following this discussion, opted for the Hall crown and very careful follow-up. They felt that if she did have a general anaesthetic, they would elect to have E| extracted.

Where a general anaesthetic is required for dental care, children with complex congenital heart defects (repaired or unrepaired) or with rhythmic disorders (for example Wolf Parkinson White syndrome) should be referred to specialized cardiac hospitals.

Examples of other common medical problems and how they impact dental care is provided in **Table 28.1**.

Key point

With all medical conditions:

- Enhanced prevention is essential to prevent or minimize caries
- Careful liaison with the medical team leading the patient's care

Primary resources and recommended reading

RCS Guideline for Oral Management of Oncology Patients Requiring Radiotherapy, Chemotherapy and/or Bone Marrow Transplantation 2012 Available at: https://www.rcseng.ac.uk/fds/publications-clinical-guidelines/clinical_guidelines/documents/clinical-guidelines-for-the-oral-management-of-oncology-patients-requiring-radiotherapy-chemotherapy-and-or-bone-marrow-transplantation.

Dayer MJ, Jones S, Prendergast B et al 2015 Incidence of infective endocarditis in England, 2000–13: a secular trend, interrupted time-series analysis. Lancet 385 (9974):1219–1228.

NICE Guideline (CG 64) 2008 Prophylaxis against Infective Endocarditis: Antimicrobial Prophylaxis against Infective Endocarditis in Adults and Children Undergoing Interventional Procedures. Available at: https://www.nice.org.uk/guidance/cg64.

AAPD guidelines 2015 Guideline on dental management of pediatric patients receiving chemotherapy, hematopoietic cell transplantation, and/or radiation therapy. Pediatr Dent 37 (6): 298–306.

For revision, see Mind Map 28, page 249.

29

The displaced primary incisor

SUMMARY

James, who is 3 years old, tripped over while playing outside. He hit his front teeth on the ground. How do you manage the immediate problem, and what do you advise his parents about potential damage to the permanent teeth?

History

Complaint

James has been brought to your surgery straight from home by his mother. She says his upper front tooth has been pushed back (**Fig. 29.1**).

History of complaint

James tripped and fell forward hitting his teeth on the ground. One tooth is 'pushed backwards'.

Medical history

James is a healthy boy who has had no significant childhood illnesses and who is up to date with all his vaccinations.

Dental history

James has been a regular attender at his dentist since the age of 2 years. He has had his teeth polished and has no caries.

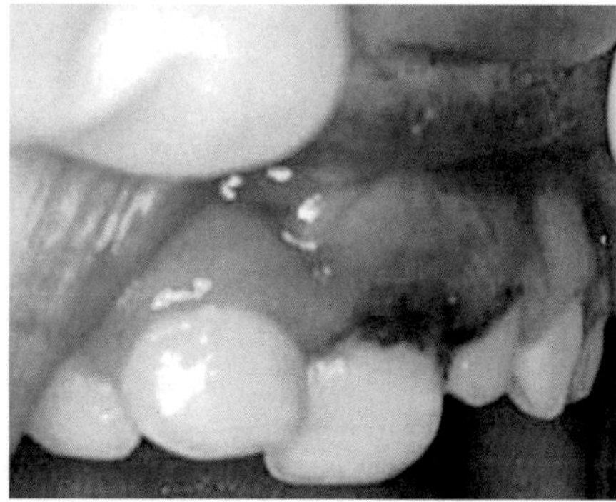

Fig. 29.1 Palatal luxation of |A.

■ ***What specific questions would you ask and why?***

Was there any loss of consciousness? If so how long? If there was, then this signifies intracranial trauma and the child should be referred to an accident and emergency department. The duration of loss of consciousness can provide an indication to the severity of the head injury.

When did the accident occur? Delay in seeking help might arouse suspicions of a non-accidental injury.

Where did the accident occur? An accident outside raises the additional problem of potential wound contamination. Any child brought up in the UK should be immunized against tetanus. If a child has not been immunized, seek the advice of a local general practitioner or accident and emergency department.

What was the surface on which the accident occurred? Newly constructed playgrounds have to conform to British Standards and should be either of an energy-absorbing polymer or bark chippings. Older playgrounds and normal pathways will have non-yielding surfaces and are likely to produce greater damage and potentially greater risk of more underlying injuries. Dirt or gravel can contaminate extra- and intra-oral wounds, and these foreign bodies will need to be carefully removed to prevent infection and reduce scarring.

How did the accident occur? This gives an indication of the force that produced the injury. The clinician needs to be highly suspicious of the high-impact injury that looks simple. Always suspect a deeper underlying injury until proven otherwise.

Fragments, where are they? Where a tooth or teeth have been fractured, these fragments need to be identified. Although in many cases they will have been spat out, there is a risk of these being swallowed, inhaled or incorporated into oral soft tissues (e.g. lacerated lips or tongue). Suspicion of inhalation of fragments is increased if there was any history of loss of consciousness, where the accident was not witnessed by an adult or if there was coughing or choking following the injury. If in any doubt, referral to an accident and emergency department to investigate this further is needed and may necessitate a chest x-ray.

What other parts of the body were injured? Frequently other parts of the body will also be injured such as abrasions to hands, elbows or knees. If visible they should be briefly examined to establish the extent of these injuries. Again, concerns of more significant injury, for example bony fractures, should be assessed at an accident and emergency department.

Examination

Extraoral

James is distressed, but there is no obvious extraoral swelling or facial asymmetry.

Intraoral

■ ***The appearance of the upper anterior teeth is shown in*** *Fig. 29.1*. ***What can you see?***

Palatal displacement of |A and associated gingival trauma.

What specific signs will you look for in your examination?

The mobility of the teeth. Are they a danger to the airway?

The occlusion. Do the injured teeth prevent normal occlusion?

Mobility of a segment of teeth, e.g. the injured teeth move together rather than individually. This indicates a dentoalveolar fracture.

What question should dentists keep at the back of their minds when examining children?

Are the injuries consistent with the history, and if you feel they are, is this normal behaviour?

Child physical abuse presents with orofacial signs of bruising, abrasions and lacerations, burns, bites and fractures in approximately 65% of cases.

Dentists should have a copy of their local area Child Protection Committee guidelines. This will tell them who they should contact for advice.

What features in the history and examination would lead to suspicions of child physical abuse?

There are 10 items to consider. Five are questions to ask yourself, and five are observations about the behaviour of the child and the parent(s):

Could the injury have been caused accidentally and if so, how?

Does the explanation for the injury fit the age and the clinical findings?

If the explanation of the cause is consistent with the injury, is this itself within the normally acceptable limits of behaviour?

If there has been delay in seeking advice, are there good reasons for this?

Does the story of the accident vary?

The nature of the relationship between parent and child.

The child's reactions to other people.

The child's reactions to any medical or dental examinations.

The general demeanour of the child.

Any comments made by the child and/or parent that give concern about the child's upbringing or lifestyle. For example, lack of parental supervision or a history of repeated trauma.

Investigations

What investigations would you perform for James? Explain why for each.

Radiographs are required to visualize the traumatized area and assess whether there are any root fractures to either the traumatized or adjacent teeth. In addition, is a dentoalveolar fracture evident? Are permanent successor teeth present?

In an intrusive injury a child may have been referred as an 'avulsed' incisor. It is imperative always to check in these circumstances that the tooth is not intruded. Re-eruption of an intruded tooth may occur, and close review is necessary. If re-eruption has not occurred within 4–6 months, an intruded primary incisor should be removed to minimize eruptive problems in the permanent dentition.

An adult periapical film used as an anterior occlusal is the easiest way to obtain a periapical view of the upper anterior region in a young child. James's radiograph did not reveal any root fractures or dentoalveolar fractures.

Vitality testing of primary teeth is not indicated, as young children are often unreliable in reporting any sensation felt.

Direction of displacement provides important information on the likelihood of any damage to the underlying permanent successor. Displacement of the crown labial indicates the root has moved palatally towards the permanent successor and vice versa.

Radiographic assessment with periapical and/or occlusal films is essential: a palatal intrusion of the root toward the successor moves away from the x-ray source and yields an elongated image.

A labial intrusion of the root away from the successor moves near the x-ray source, yielding a foreshortened image and a gap between the apex of the primary incisor and crown of its successor. Extraoral lateral radiographs have been shown to have a limited value in showing labial positioning, especially in cases of intruded lateral incisors or multiple intrusions.

Diagnosis

What is your diagnosis?

James has a palatal luxation injury to his upper left primary central incisor.

Treatment

What are the three key components of the history and examination in primary tooth trauma that will dictate if active treatment is required?

Pain. Either spontaneous or on eating suggests pathosis.

Mobility. Is the tooth a danger to the airway?

Occlusal interference. A luxation injury that has prevented normal intercuspal occlusion will prevent normal eating.

What treatments are usually required for displaced primary incisors?

Concussion and subluxation: observation.

Lateral luxation: if no occlusal interference, the tooth is allowed to reposition spontaneously; if occlusal interference, extract.

Intrusion: if the apex is displaced toward the labial bone plate, then leave for spontaneous repositioning. If no movement within 4–6 months, extract. In addition, if the root has perforated the buccal plate of bone, as identified by palpating the area, extract. If the apex is displaced into the developing tooth germ, extract.

Extrusion: extract or reposition if only a minor extrusion.

Avulsion: replantation is not indicated.

Key point

Traumatized primary teeth may need to be extracted if:

- Pain interrupts eating or sleeping.
- Excessive mobility causes a danger to the airway.
- There is occlusal interference.
- Tooth becomes non-vital and child is uncooperative for a pulpectomy. If the tooth is left in situ, further damage to the developing permanent successor can result.

■ ***What radiographs would you take for these displacement injuries?***

A periapical and/or occlusal view is indicated for all periodontal injuries including concussion, subluxation, lateral luxation, intrusion, extrusion and avulsion. Even in avulsion cases a radiograph is indicated to ensure the tooth has not been intruded, unless the parent attends with the avulsed tooth.

■ ***What are you going to tell James's mother about the risk to the permanent teeth?***

The reported incidence of damage to the developing permanent teeth as a result of trauma to primary incisors ranges from 17–64%. An easily remembered figure to tell all parents at the time of the initial presentation would be 50%. It is better to be pessimistic and then be pleasantly surprised on eruption of the permanent teeth rather than the opposite. The younger the child at the time of injury the greater the risk of damage to the permanent tooth. Other factors increasing the risk of damage include the type of injury (with avulsion and intrusion most likely to cause damage), the severity of displacement (greater displacement leads to an increased likelihood) and pulp necrosis.

■ ***What are the possible effects on the permanent successor teeth?***

White or yellow-brown discoloration of enamel (hypomineralization).

Enamel hypoplasia.

Crown dilaceration.

Crown-root dilaceration.

Root dilaceration.

Odontome formation.

Partial/complete arrest of root formation.

Sequestration of permanent tooth germ.

Disturbance in eruption.

■ ***Can you tell all of these sequelae on a periapical radiograph?***

No. Only structural abnormalities and abnormal root growth will be visible. White and brown areas of hypomineralization will only be evident on eruption of the permanent teeth.

■ ***If you retain a luxated primary tooth how often would you review it?***

One week after the injury, 1 month, then 3-monthly.

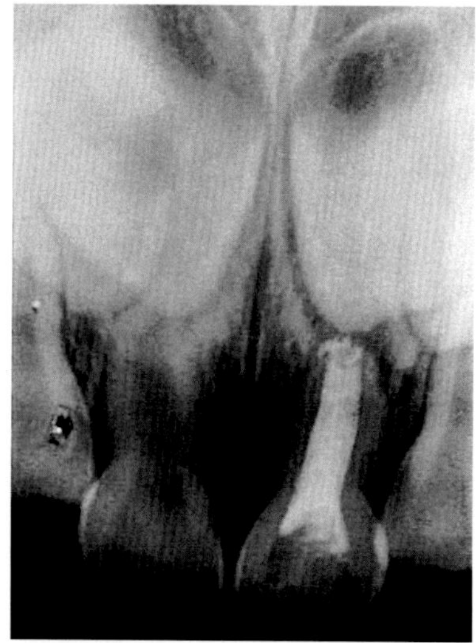

Fig. 29.2 Endodontically treated primary incisor.

■ ***How would you review it?***

Historically: symptoms.

Clinically: colour, sinus, tenderness, swelling, mobility.

Radiographically: 6-monthly for 1 year and then when clinically indicated.

Key point

After primary tooth trauma:

- Damage to permanent teeth may occur in 50% of cases.
- Intrusive and avulsion injuries cause most permanent tooth damage.

■ ***Does a discoloured primary incisor always need treatment?***

When there is progressive or persistent (greater than 3 months) greying of the injured tooth, it is highly likely to be non-vital. When there is initial grey discoloration that improves then vitality is likely to be maintained. In the absence of infection a discoloured primary incisor can be reviewed. In the presence of infection, extraction or root canal therapy with zinc oxide cement or a calcium hydroxide-iodoform paste is indicated (**Fig. 29.2**).

Primary resources and recommended reading

Andreasen JO, Lauridsen E, Bakland L et al 2014 Dental Trauma Guide. Available at: http://www.dentaltraumaguide.org.

Day P, Bussel R, Clough S 2011 Management of dental trauma in the primary dentition. e-Den. http://www.e-lfh.org.uk/programmes/dentistry/.

Malmgren B, Andreasen JO, Flores MT et al 2012 International Association of Dental Traumatology guidelines for the management of traumatic dental injuries: 3. Injuries in the primary dentition. Dent Traumatol 28 (3):174–182.

UK Committee of Postgraduate Dental Deans and Directors 2013 Child protection for the dental team. Available at: http://www.cpdt.org.uk.

For revision, see Mind Map 29, page 250.

30

The fractured immature permanent incisor crown

SUMMARY

Shay is 8 years old. While saving a penalty for his school team, he collided with the goalpost and sustained enamel-dentine-pulp and enamel-dentine fractures to his upper central incisors. How would you manage the injuries? Outline a follow-up treatment plan.

History

Complaint

The upper right and left permanent central incisors are fractured (**Fig. 30.1**).

History of complaint

The injury was sustained during a game of soccer. There were no other injuries.

Medical history

Shay is a healthy boy with no history of illness. He has had all his vaccinations, including a pre-school booster for tetanus.

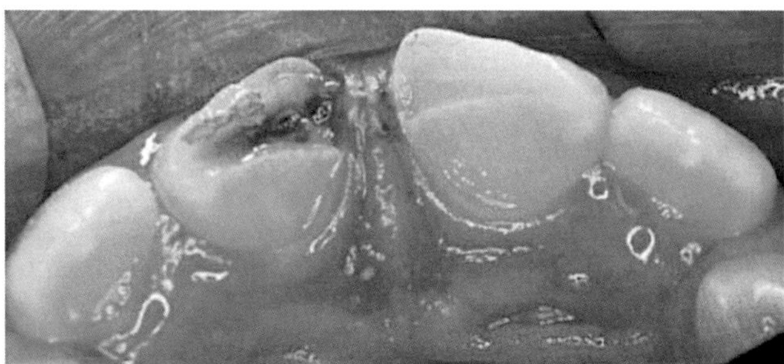

Fig. 30.1 Trauma to the central incisors. Pulp exposure can be seen affecting 1|.

Dental history

Shay is a regular attender at his dentist and has had local anaesthetic for a restoration.

■ ***What specific questions would you ask and why?***

Was there any loss of consciousness? When unconscious, patients lose their protective reflexes. Moreover, the duration of loss of consciousness together with the length of post-traumatic amnesia are key indicators for the severity of the head injury.

Was the fractured piece of tooth located?

A history of loss of consciousness together with a missing tooth fragment is an indication for a chest radiograph to check that the tooth fragment has not been inhaled.

When, where and how did the injury occur? A clear and detailed description of the injury is essential.

What other injuries were sustained at the time of the injury?

The time from the injury to presentation may affect the treatment options.

Did Shay cope well with his previous experience of local anaesthetic? The answer to this will dictate what behaviour management techniques (see Chapter 26) may be required to facilitate treatment.

Examination

Extraoral

■ ***Why is the presence of lip swelling together with a mucosal laceration important?***

This could indicate that the missing tooth fragment is retained in the lip.

■ ***How would you demonstrate there was a fragment of tooth in the lip?***

Take soft tissue radiography using two views at right angles to each other. A simple anteroposterior view using a periapical film placed behind the lip and in front of the teeth, followed by a lateral soft tissue view using a lateral occlusal film (**Fig. 30.2**). Unless experienced and trained in finding these fragments, it is sensible to refer to a surgical colleague to retrieve them.

Key point

Missing tooth fragments could:

- Be within the soft tissues if there is a laceration.
- Have been inhaled if there was loss of consciousness.
- Have been spat out at the site of the accident.
- Have been swallowed.

Intraoral

■ ***What injuries are visible in** Fig. 30.1**?***

There is an enamel-dentine fracture of |1 and an enamel-dentine-pulp fracture of 1| of greater than 1 mm in diameter.

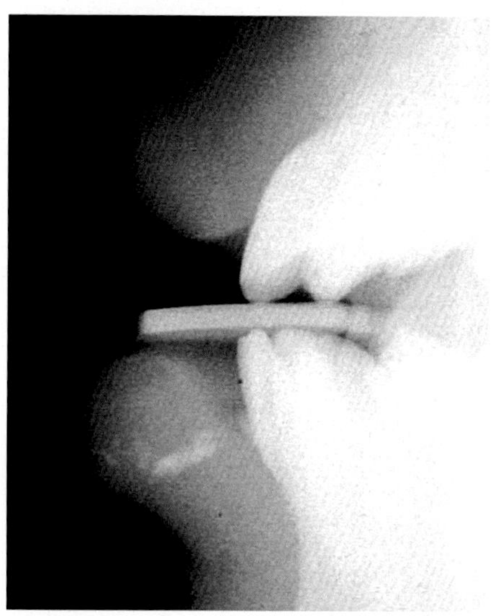

Fig. 30.2 Fragments of tooth in lower lip (different case).

It is essential that periodontal injuries are also diagnosed. Unless special tests such as mobility or tenderness to percussion are undertaken, diagnoses such as concussion or subluxation will be missed. Crown fractures combined with a periodontal injury have poorer pulp survival outcomes than those with no associated periodontal injury.

■ ***Are the roots of 1| and |1 likely to have open or closed apices?***

Open. Apices are not usually closed on upper permanent central incisors before the age of 11 years.

■ ***How would you confirm apical status?***

Periapical radiograph.

■ ***What other injuries must you exclude on the periapical radiograph?***

Root fractures.

■ ***What other features of the anterior teeth are important at examination?***

Mobility. In a buccopalatal direction. Excessive mobility suggests either a periodontal ligament injury or a root fracture.

Colour. This will indicate whether any direct pulpal damage causing haemorrhage into the dentinal tubules has occurred.

Percussion. Tenderness suggests periapical damage and oedema. A dull note may suggest a clinically undiagnosed vertical crown fracture or root fracture.

Vitality. Following trauma there may be a period of apparent loss of vitality on testing with hot and cold stimuli or the electric pulp tester even in teeth without obvious crown fractures. Nevertheless, the readings serve as a baseline against which subsequent tests can be compared. Teeth, which respond to vitality testing at the time of injury, have an excellent chance of maintaining pulp vitality. For teeth that do not respond at this time point, the pulp may be still be vital and respond at subsequent clinic visits.

■ ***What teeth should be examined after trauma affecting only the upper centrals?***

All upper and lower incisors should be included in an examination after any trauma to the anterior region. It is also appropriate to briefly check the posterior teeth as they can on rare occasions be injured as well.

Investigations

- *Radiographs* (previously mentioned) for:
  - Foreign body in soft tissues if applicable.
  - Root maturity and apical status of teeth.
  - Presence or absence of root or alveolar fractures.
- *Vitality testing* of all upper and lower incisors.

Treatment

■ ***What is the prime consideration for both the upper central incisors?***

To maintain a vital pulp within the root, which will allow ongoing physiological dentine deposition. This will result in full root growth with normal dentinal wall thickness, which will reduce the chance of late stage crown root fracture.

■ ***What is the appropriate immediate treatment for |1 (that has an enamel-dentine fracture)?***

Reattachment of the fragment.

or

A bonded restoration/'bandage', which will produce a hermetic seal. Glass ionomer cement is not an adequate material for a 'bandage' and will be lost shortly after placement resulting in bacterial ingress and thermal damage to the pulp from hot and cold stimuli. A layer of setting calcium hydroxide cement should be placed over dentine where a pulpal shadow is visible prior to placement of an adhesive (composite) bandage.

■ ***What are the treatment options for 1| (that has a pulpal exposure)?***

- Direct pulp capping.
- Pulpotomy – Cvek, coronal or radicular (depth determined by level of inflammation).

Direct pulp capping, the placement of wound dressings on an exposed pulp, is considered less unpredictable by many authors. Partial pulpotomy (Cvek) is the removal of only the outer layer of damaged and hyperaemic tissue in the exposed pulps. This will leave healthy pulp, which will permit continued full root growth. Partial pulpotomy is a highly successful technique. Where damage to the pulp has been more extensive (e.g. size of exposure or increased duration between injury and treatment), further inflamed pulpal tissue will have to be removed. Where this extends to the root canal orifice, this is called a cervical pulpotomy or a radicular pulpotomy when extending down the root canal. The important aspect of this treatment is to ensure that all inflamed pulp is removed leaving healthy (uninflammed) tissue behind.

■ ***What are the indications for permanent tooth pulpotomy?***

No history of spontaneous pain.

Acute minor pain that subsides with analgesics.

No discomfort to percussion, no sulcus swelling, no mobility.

Radiographic examination shows normal periodontal ligament.

Tissue appears vital.

Bleeding from the pulp excision site stops within 2–5 minutes.

■ *How would you carry out a pulpotomy?*

Local analgesia and rubber dam. Flush exposed pulp tissue initially with isotonic saline. Then excise a 2 mm superficial layer of exposed pulp and surrounding dentine with a high speed diamond bur using a light touch under water spray cooling (partial pulpotomy). Irrigate the surface of remaining pulp with isotonic saline. If bleeding ceases with pressure applied to the pulp stump using a damp (isotonic saline soaked) cotton wool ball for 2–5 minutes, apply a pulpal medicament with biologically available calcium hydroxide and seal coronal cavity with a bonded restoration. However, if the bleeding does not cease, further pulp tissue should be removed. Apply a cotton wool ball for a further 2–5 minutes and reassess. If bleeding has stopped, then cover with a medicament as previously stated. However, if after removing the pulp to a coronal level (a coronal pulpotomy) there is still bleeding, continue deeper into the root canal with care (radicular pulpotomy). If bleeding persists deep into the root canal, then the remaining pulp tissue should be removed and root canal treatment instigated (pulpectomy). If on accessing the pulp chamber there is no bleeding or there is an empty infected canal, then a pulpectomy is indicated. The time from injury to presentation, contamination and the size of pulp exposure will all influence the depth of inflammation and necessitate greater amounts of inflamed pulp tissue to be removed.

■ *How should the crown of 1| be restored?*

If the crown fragment has been retrieved, then this can be stored in normal saline while the pulpotomy is completed. The fragment can then be reattached.

If the crown fragment is not available or the fracture extends significantly subgingivally, a bonded composite restoration should be provided. The careful use of retraction cord or electrosurgery will ensure good bonding of the composite to the fracture margins.

Figs 30.3 and **30.4** show the crown fragments before and after reattachment in Shay's case. 1| had a partial pulpotomy as described.

■ *How should the upper centrals be reviewed and how often?*

Definitive crown morphology should be restored as soon as possible after emergency treatment to re-establish normal sagittal relations with the lower incisors.

One-, two-, and then six-monthly clinical and radiographic examinations should be carried out to check for continued vitality and normal root growth. If there is evidence of non-vitality, then the immature tooth must be extirpated and non-setting calcium hydroxide used to disinfect the root canal. Root end closure can then be achieved using Mineral Trioxide Aggregate prior to obturation with warm gutta percha.

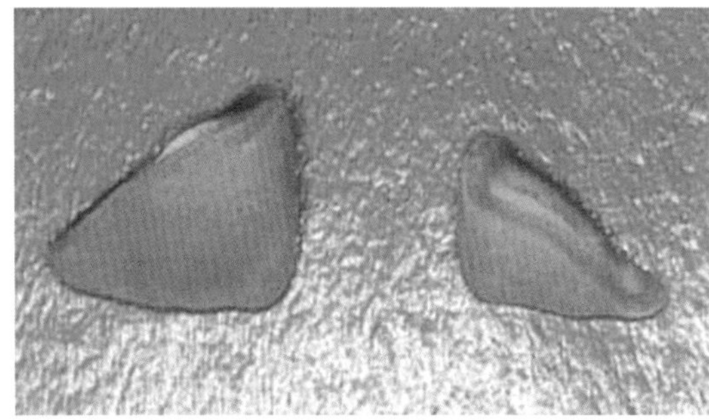

Fig. 30.3 Fragments found at scene of incident.

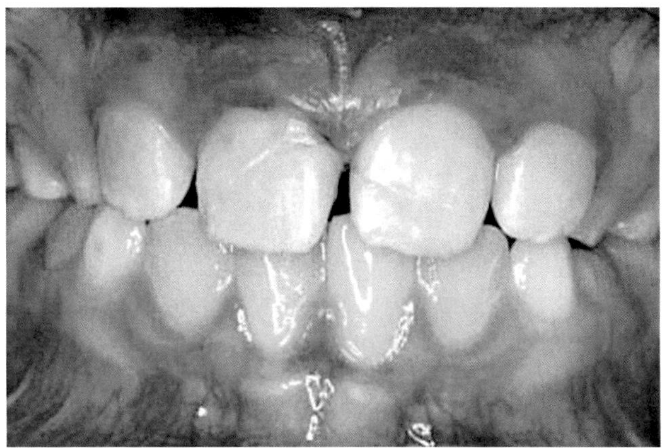

Fig. 30.4 Fragments reattached.

> **Key point**
>
> Partial or complete pulpotomy:
>
> - Has a high success rate.
> - Size of exposure and length of time between injury and treatment will influence the extent of the pulpal inflammation that will need to be removed during the pulpotomy procedure.
> - Allows full root growth with a vital radicular pulp. This will reduce the risk of long-term crown root fractures which is a common occurrence if an immature tooth was to become non-vital.

Primary resources and recommended reading

Andreasen JO, Lauridsen E, Bakland L et al 2014 Dental Trauma Guide. Available at: http://www.dentaltraumaguide.org.

Diangelis AJ, Andreasen JO, Ebeleseder KA et al 2012 International Association of Dental Traumatology guidelines for the management of traumatic dental injuries: 1. Fractures and luxations of permanent teeth. Dent Traumatol 28 (1): 2–12.

Lauridsen E, Hermann NV, Gerds TA et al 2012 Combination injuries 1. The risk of pulp necrosis in permanent teeth with concussion injuries and concomitant crown fractures. Dent Traumatol 28 (5):364–370.

Lauridsen E, Hermann NV, Gerds TA et al 2012 Combination injuries 2. The risk of pulp necrosis in permanent teeth with subluxation injuries and concomitant crown fractures. Dent Traumatol 28:371–378.

Diangelis AJ, Andreasen JO, Ebeleseder KA et al 2012 International Association of Dental Traumatology guidelines for the management of traumatic dental injuries: 1. Fractures and luxations of permanent teeth. Dent Traumatol 28 (1):2–12.

For revision, see Mind Map 30, page 251.

31

The root fractured permanent incisor

SUMMARY

Andrea is 12 years old. She was trampolining at school when she fell and sustained middle third root fractures of 1| and |1. How do you manage this type of injury, and what do you advise her about the long-term prognosis for these teeth?

History

Complaint

Andrea is brought to your surgery by a schoolteacher. She is complaining that her upper permanent central incisors are loose and feel 'funny' when she bites together.

History of complaint

Andrea fell forward while on the trampoline at school and hit her teeth. Her mother arrives at the surgery soon after Andrea and her teacher. It appears Andrea was not being supervised on the trampoline and the foam protection was not in the correct position on the metal frame of the trampoline. Her mother is not happy with the explanation by the teacher.

■ ***What does this alert you to?***

The possibility of legal action against the school. It is especially important to make drawings of any external injuries on the face and keep accurate records of intraoral injuries and subsequent treatment. A photographic record will be an advantage. A structured history form (Appendix 6) can help clinicians ensure that they undertake a comprehensive history and examination by prompting them to record different pieces of information.

Medical history

Andrea is under regular care with her dentist and has had local anaesthetic without problem.

■ ***What specific questions would you ask and why?***

Was there any loss of consciousness? If there was, then Andrea should be referred to an accident and emergency department.

Is there any pain or discomfort while opening and closing the jaw? Absence of symptoms should rule out any condylar injury/fracture. When the force that produces an injury is significant, it should raise suspicion of a deeper underlying bony injury.

Examination

Extraoral

There is some swelling of the upper lip and some bruising and swelling under the right eye.

■ ***What questions and examination would you complete regarding the swelling and bruising under the right eye?***

Is there any double vision? Palpate the infraorbital margin for 'stepping' and then check for altered sensation over the distribution of the infraorbital (V2) nerve. Check that there is a full range of eye movements – especially upward gaze. Fracture of the infraorbital margin and infraorbital floor could lead to entrapment of the inferior oblique extraocular muscle preventing upward and outward movement of the globe of the eye.

Is there any altered sensation on the cheek? Oedema surrounding the infraorbital nerve or entrapment of the nerve in a fracture can result in paraesthesia.

If there is any doubt about a fracture, then posteroanterior and occipitomental views will detect displacement of the infraorbital margin and tomograms will detect orbital floor 'blow-out' fractures.

Intraoral

There is downward and palatal displacement of the crowns of 1| and |1, which are mobile. Centric occlusion is not possible because of the slightly palatal position of 1| and |1.

■ ***What would be the diagnosis based on the clinical findings alone?***

It is important to differentiate between lateral luxations and an extrusion. On examination both diagnoses can have a similar appearance in the position the tooth or teeth are displaced to. The important difference is that the tooth will be mobile for an extrusion and immobile for a lateral luxation. With a lateral luxation there is fracture within the bony socket with the tooth locked into position.

■ ***What tests would you do prior to repositioning the teeth?***

Radiographs. Intraoral periapicals (**Fig. 31.1**) or an anterior occlusal view are needed to diagnose root fractures compared with luxation injuries. The upper lateral incisors should also be checked for injury. Consideration should also be given to taking radiographs of the lower incisors, which may also have received either direct or indirect trauma. Where there is no significant displacement of the coronal portion of a tooth with a root fracture, then an anterior occlusal radiograph will often detect root fractures that may not be so evident on periapical views. These radiographs will serve as baseline views before repositioning.

Vitality tests of all upper and lower incisors.

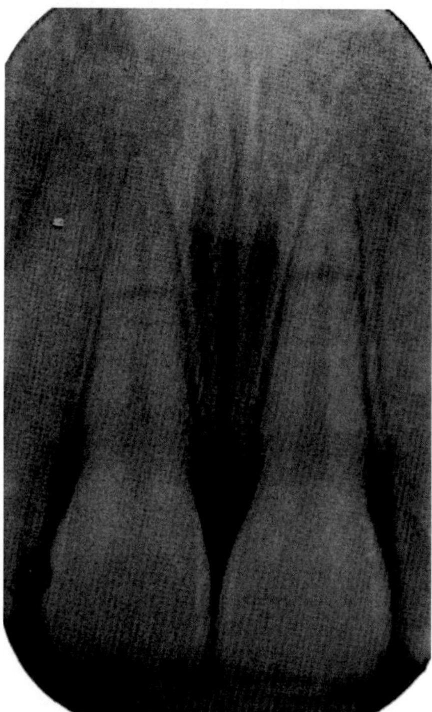

Fig. 31.1 Middle third root fractures.

■ ***What is the diagnosis based on the clinical and radiographic findings?***

For both **1|** and **|1** a diagnosis of a mid third root fracture with an extrusion of the coronal fragment.

Treatment

■ ***What design of splint would you use for 1| and |1? You have confirmed on radiography that they have middle third root fractures** (Fig. 31.1)**.***

The splint should be flexible/functional and designed to have one sound (uninjured) abutment tooth on either side of the root-fractured teeth.

■ ***How long should the splint be in place in root fractures?***

For 4 weeks in apical and middle third fractures until the majority of periodontal ligament fibres have healed. This time can be extended to 4 months in coronal third fractures. The old regimen of rigid splinting for root fractures has been shown to have no benefit. Rigid splinting was meant to give the fracture its best chance of a hard tissue union. Research has shown that hard tissue union is most likely to occur if there was little displacement at the time of the original injury rather than being a function of the type of splint employed. In other words, the larger the displacement at the fracture line at the time of the injury, the smaller the chance of a hard tissue union between the fracture ends after reduction and splinting.

■ ***Do any forms of dentoalveolar injury need to be rigidly splinted?***

No. Historically, rigid splinting was used for dentoalveolar fractures. A rigid splint involved two sound abutment teeth on either side of the injury and a stiffer arch wire. It was proposed that this style of splinting would ensure no movement between bony fragments, thereby allowing healing. Current guidance advises a flexible/functional splint for all displacement injuries including root and alveolar fractures. The only difference between injuries is the duration of splinting proposed.

> **Key point**
>
> Splinting in dentoalveolar trauma:
>
> - Flexible 2 weeks for avulsions.
> - Flexible 4 weeks for luxations, dentoalveolar fractures and apical and middle third root fractures.
> - Flexible 4 months for coronal third root fractures.

■ ***Describe step by step your procedure for reduction and splinting Andrea's 1| and |1.***

1. Give topical and local anaesthesia labially and palatally. Good and widespread anaesthesia is important to enable pain-free manual reposition.
2. While the local anaesthetic is taking effect, bend your splint so that it will sit passively on the upper labial segment of all four incisor teeth. When splinting teeth, if the splint is not passive, active orthodontic movement will be seen in the splinted teeth.
3. Gently reposition 1| and |1 and hold these in approximate position. The repositioned tooth/teeth are unstable and will need to be held in their new position. Although it is enticing to use fingers to hold the repositioned teeth, this makes the rest of the splinting procedure more complex, as both hands are needed. Some red wax palatally, which extends over the incisal edges of 1| and |1, or cotton wool rolls between the upper and lower incisors are appropriate methods to hold the repositioned teeth in the correct position. Etch the labial surfaces of 2| and |2; wash, dry and place bonding resin and a spot of composite in the centre of the labial surface. Place the splint into position on 2| and |2. Use a bonding brush to mould the composite already on the teeth over the wire. Add extra composite if required. Cure the composite.
4. Remove the wax or cotton wool rolls, and with a nonworking hand, bring 1| and |1 into an accurate position against the wire splint. Hold them in this position while etching, washing, bonding and adding composite with the working hand. Cure the composite.
5. Smooth any rough areas with sandpaper discs.

■ ***What materials could be used for splinting?***

An ideal splint should be simple and quick to place and remove, easy to bend to ensure it is passive, biologically compatible and relatively cheap. The splint must allow for functional movement of the teeth while holding the teeth in their new position and allowing thorough cleaning around the gingival margins. The most common materials used are pieces of orthodontic wire, for example 0.014-in or 0.016-in stainless steel or twistflex (which is three pieces of 0.010-in wire twisted around each other). Each of these wires requires moderate skills in wire bending to achieve a passive splint. New materials such as titanium are now available for splinting, and these have the benefit of being much easier and therefore quicker to passively adapt to teeth (Chapter 32, Fig. 32.1B).

■ ***On removal of the splint how often would you review Andrea?***

After 1 month, 3 months, 6 months and then yearly.

■ ***What tests would you complete at each of these reviews?***

For all traumatized teeth, a standard regimen should be followed. If this is carried out in every case, then omissions are less likely to be made.

- Clinical:
  - Colour (palatal surface best).
  - Buccal sulcus sensitivity to digital pressure.
  - Sinus or swelling presence.
  - Tenderness to percussion.
  - Percussion sound.
  - Mobility.
  - Sensibility testing.
- Radiography: long cone periapicals.

■ ***Is sensibility testing accurate?***

No form of sensibility testing on its own is accurate. Electric pulp testing (EPT) is probably the most accurate, but its real value lies in successive numerical readings with the same type of EPT. Numerical values can then be compared.

At each visit, responses (both positive and negative) should be compared against uninjured teeth and also if each tooth is consistent in its response and the duration before any positive sensation is acknowledged. Current sensibility testing relies on sensation of stimuli, whereas true pulpal vitality is more appropriately tested by the presence of blood flow. In the future, the widespread use of Doppler in detecting blood flow in a traumatized tooth will inform all decisions regarding pulpal necrosis and the necessity for extirpation.

Key point

What types of healing occur in root fractures?

- Hard tissue.
- Connective tissue (see **Fig. 31.2**). This type of healing is often combined with osseous healing. As the two fragments grow apart over time, bone will fill in the gap that was originally only filled with connective tissue.
- Granulation tissue. Technically this is not a type of healing but is seen when the coronal fragment is infected. Once the infection is treated, healing will take place by connective tissue.

■ ***What is the likely radiographic appearance at the fracture line if the coronal tooth portion becomes non-vital?***

There will be increasing widening and translucency surrounding and between the fractured ends of the root.

■ ***If the coronal portion of an apical or middle third root fractured tooth became non-vital, how would you root treat the tooth?***

Extirpation to the fracture line only.

Establish working length to fracture line.

Place non-setting calcium hydroxide 1 mm short of fracture line with aim of inducing barrier formation.

Change non-setting calcium hydroxide 3-monthly until barrier forms, or alternatively use MTA to generate a 4–5-mm barrier.

Obturate with gutta percha to barrier.

Annual radiographic review.

■ ***What happens to the apical fragment?***

In nearly all cases this will undergo pulp canal obliteration and will not need treatment. If there is infection of the apical fragment, it may require surgical removal. Root canal therapy across a root fracture is fraught with difficulty because of problems keeping the distal canal dry.

■ ***Is the prognosis good in coronal or gingival third root fractures?***

No. Decisions need to be made early regarding options. Long-term stability and long-term retention of the whole tooth in these injuries are uncommon. Research shows a survival rate of one-third at 10 years post-trauma, with many of these teeth being lost as a result of further trauma or excessive mobility. These consequences relate to the unfavourable crown root ratio.

■ ***What are the treatment options in coronal or gingival third root fractures?***

Retain crown temporarily with an endodontic post across the fracture line.

Remove coronal fragment. Root treat apical fragment and orthodontically extrude prior to post, core and crown placement.

Remove coronal fragment. Cover, 'bury', the apical fragment with a mucoperiosteal flap. The width and height of the alveolus are thus retained for future implant placement. Prosthetic replacement required.

Remove all portions of tooth. Prosthetic replacement required. Future implant placement.

■ ***Can root fractured teeth maintain vitality?***

Yes. The majority do so (literature reports between 72% and 90% maintain their vitality). **Figs 31.2** and **31.3** show Andrea's teeth 3 years after the original injury. The teeth maintained vitality and underwent progressive pulp canal obliteration. In addition, the distal fragments are resorbing. Importantly, there has been no infection.

■ ***Can root fractured teeth be moved orthodontically?***

Yes, but with caution. If there is not a hard tissue union between the fracture ends, then the apical portion will remain static and only the coronal portion will move. Regular radiographic review will be necessary during any orthodontic treatment. Orthodontic movement may cause further root resorption, which when combined with an already compromised crown root ratio can lead to long-term mobility of the coronal fragment at the end of orthodontic treatment. Consequently, great care is needed with the orthodontic treatment to minimize the risk of further root resorption.

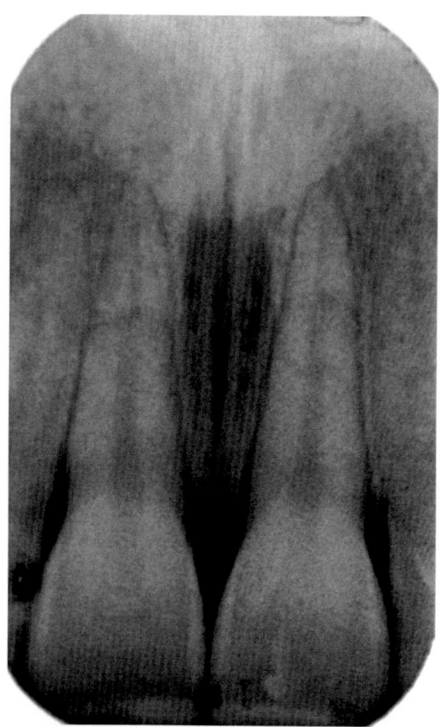

Fig. 31.2 Radiographic appearance after 3 years.

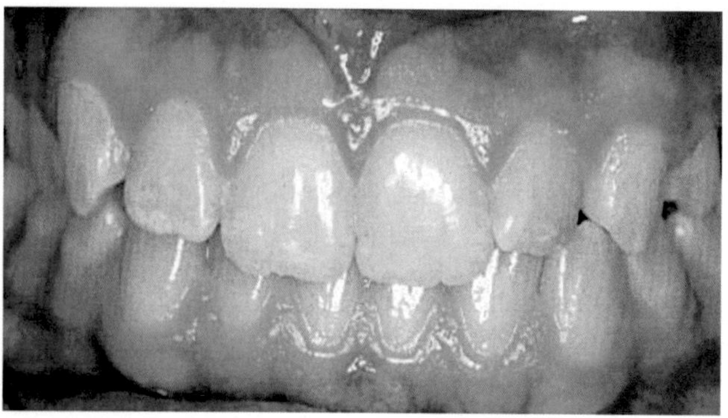

Fig. 31.3 Clinical appearance after 3 years.

Primary resources and recommended reading

Andreasen JO, Ahrensburg SS, Tsilingaridis G 2012 Root fractures: the influence of type of healing and location of fracture on tooth survival rates – an analysis of 492 cases. Dent Traumatol 28 (5):404–409.

Andreasen JO, Andreasen FM, Mejare I et al 2004 Healing of 400 intra-alveolar root fractures. 1. Effect of pre-injury and injury factors such as sex, age, stage of root development, fracture type, location of fracture and severity of dislocation. Dent Traumatol 20 (4):192–202.

Andreasen JO, Lauridsen E, Bakland L et al 2014 Dental Trauma Guide. Available at: http://www.dentaltraumaguide.org.

Diangelis AJ, Andreasen JO, Ebeleseder KA et al 2012 International Association of Dental Traumatology guidelines for the management of traumatic dental injuries: 1. Fractures and luxations of permanent teeth. Dent Traumatol 28 (1):2–12.

For revision, see Mind Map 31, page 252.

32

The avulsed incisor

CASE 1

SUMMARY

Kathryn is 9 years old. She was playing with her friends at a brownie camp with a skipping rope, when the rope caught behind one of her upper central incisors and avulsed it. Her teacher has got the tooth. How would you manage this problem?

- ***Kathryn's teacher phones your surgery for advice. She has the tooth in a handkerchief. The accident occurred 10 minutes ago. What is your advice?***

Check that Kathryn has no other injuries, i.e. head injuries that require referral to an accident and emergency department.

Check for any known medical history.

Hold tooth by crown and wash gently under cold water to remove any debris for 10 seconds.

Replant in socket ideally.

Hold tooth in socket by biting on a handkerchief. Come to surgery.

If replantation is not possible, place the tooth in either milk or normal saline (first aid box) and bring it to surgery with Kathryn as quickly as possible.

- ***The tooth is brought to the surgery in milk. How would you proceed?***

1. Check medical history for any reason not to replant. For children who are immunosuppressed (e.g. mid-chemotherapy, organ transplant or primary immune deficiency) or at risk of infective endocarditis, a discussion with their medical consultant would be prudent before replantation.
2. Gently shake the pot containing the tooth and milk to remove any foreign bodies. Check state of root development.
3. Undertake a brief history and examination to ensure there are no other injuries (see structure history form shown in Appendix 6). Examine the patient and check for other injuries. Examination shows a small intraoral laceration to the upper lip as well as an avulsion of 1⌋ and subluxation of ⌊1 (**Fig. 32.1A**)
4. Give labial and palatal local anaesthesia.
5. Irrigate socket with normal saline to remove the blood clot.
6. Recontour labial plate with flat plastic instrument, if required.
7. Gently reposition the avulsed tooth.
8. Bend a titanium trauma splint (or alternative splinting material as discussed in Chapter 31) to include one uninjured tooth on either side of the avulsed tooth (C|C) and follow guidance described in this chapter for splint placement. **Fig. 32.1B** shows the splint in situ.
9. Prescribe chlorhexidine mouthwash. Antibiotics (such as Amoxicillin or Penicillin V for 5–7 days) can be prescribed at the clinician's discretion. Chlorhexidine 0.2% should be used twice daily to enhance oral hygiene.
10. Arrange a review appointment for 14 days.

- ***What factors are important when deciding whether root canal treatment is necessary in Kathryn's case?***

Root development.

How long the tooth was out of the mouth (extra-alveolar time).

A tooth that has completed root development will not undergo revascularization. The only tooth that has a chance

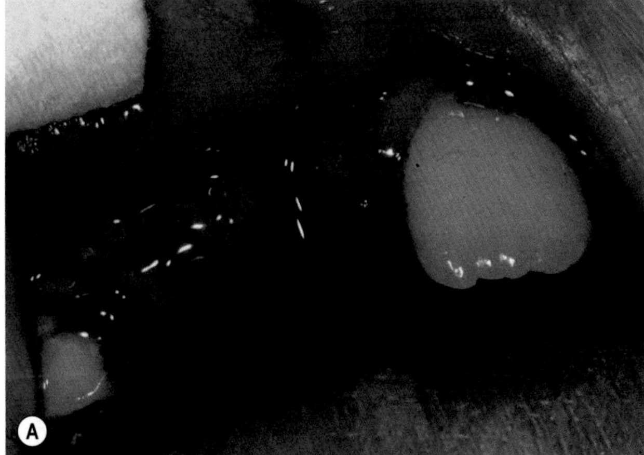

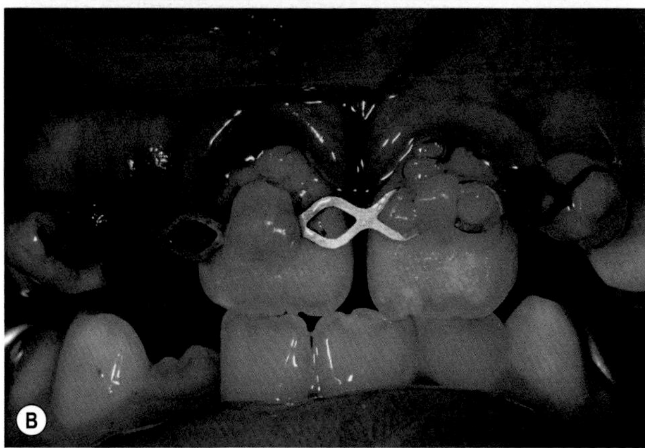

Fig. 32.1 (A) 1⌋ avulsed and ⌊1 subluxed. **(B)** 1⌋ replanted and splinted with a titanium trauma splint.

of revascularization is the immature tooth with an open apex that is replanted within 30–45 minutes. All other teeth should be extirpated prior to splint removal at 7–10 days. Different guidelines argue for different lengths of total and dry time where revascularisation is unlikely (for example, British Society of Paediatric Dentistry (BSPD) – less than 30 minutes dry time and/or 90 minutes total time; International Association of Dental Traumatology (IADT) – less than 60 minutes dry time). The reason for giving the tooth time to revascularize is only reserved for teeth where if the pulp is extirpated it would leave a non-vital immature tooth with increased risk of late stage crown root fracture. However, if revascularization does not occur, there is a strong chance of infection-related resorption, which can lead to rapid destruction of the tooth. Therefore in situations where an immature tooth is given a chance to revascularize, very careful follow-up is required to ensure any complications are identified and treatment instigated as soon as possible.

Kathryn was seen for splint removal at 14 days after the injury. The radiograph showed an immature root form. The tooth was replanted within 30 minutes, with 10 minutes stored dry and the remainder of the time kept in milk. The decision was therefore taken to see if the tooth would revascularize.

What factors are important in predicting root resorption?

Extra-alveolar dry time (EADT).

Extra-alveolar time (EAT).

Storage medium prior to replantation.

Contamination.

Root maturity.

Research has shown that teeth with a dry time of greater than 5 minutes have a significantly increased risk of resorption. The two preferred storage media, milk and normal saline, are iso-osmolar, and that is why they are the recommended storage media. Even in these appropriate media, periodontal ligament vitality is not maintained for long.

Key point

Critical information to ask about in avulsion cases:

- EADT.
- EAT.
- Storage medium and duration in it.
- Contamination of the root surface.

What types of resorption are there?

Repair-related resorption (previously called surface resorption): most commonly seen as blunting of tooth apices after application of excessive orthodontic forces or on the roots of upper lateral incisors as a result of canine tooth impaction. The vitality of the tooth is not related to this type of healing, e.g. the tooth may be vital or non-vital.

Following trauma this can be present on any part of the root surface but is only visible on conventional 2D radiographs as saucer shaped cavities along the mesial and distal surfaces of the root. Following the avulsion injury and extraoral storage there is damage to the periodontal ligament and cementum. Following replantation these areas of damage are removed including areas of adjacent root surface giving these saucer shaped cavities. Adjacent cementum and periodontal healing then grows over these cavities, and the periodontal and cemental architecture is restored.

Infection-related resorption (previously called external inflammatory resorption): this type of resorption is only seen where there is damage to the periodontal and cemental architecture (for example following trauma) combined with a non-vital and infected root canal. The immunological response (destructive phase) removes the necrotic and infected material on the root surface, thus opening up the dentinal tubules. This opens up a pathway through which the bacteria toxins are transmitted, thus exacerbating the immunological response and stimulating further the root resorption. Radiographically, the surfaces of the roots have punched-out craters with radiolucency seen in the adjacent bone. Only when the necrotic pulp is extirpated and the root canal disinfected will this resorption stop. The root surface is then able to repair (healing phase) with the type of healing dictated by the amount of damage. Either the cementum and periodontal ligament will re-establish themselves (repair-related resorption) or the adjacent bone will fuse to the root (ankylosis-related resorption).

Ankylosis-related resorption (previously called replacement resorption): this is characterized by the absence of the periodontal ligament with bone fused to the cementum and dentine. The tooth becomes part of the bone and is constantly remodelled, resulting in progressive resorption of the root until the entire root is resorbed and the crown fractures off. In growing children, ankylosis-related resorption causes the local cessation of growth with the appearance of the affected tooth or teeth staying still (infraoccluding) while the adjacent teeth continue to erupt.

Key point

Types of root resorption following trauma:

- Repair-related.
- Infection-related.
- Ankylosis-related.

What is the treatment for infection-related resorption following trauma?

The only medicament that is proven to arrest infection-related resorption is non-setting calcium hydroxide. Its antibacterial properties relate to its alkalinity (pH 11–12). It should be placed within the root canal at least twice with a month gap between applications. Applications continue until radiographs show the lack of radiolucency in the bone adjacent to the affected tooth. Once this is detected, the root can be obturated with gutta percha.

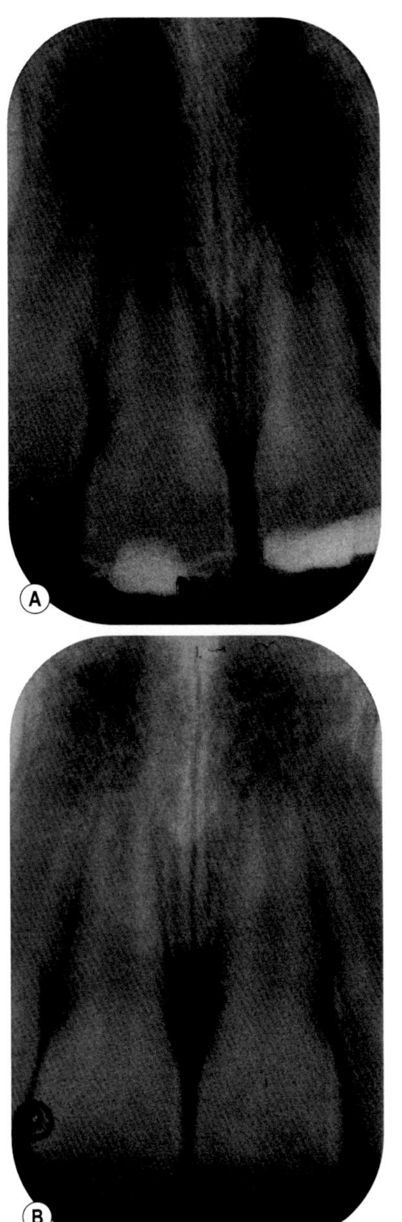

Fig. 32.2 **(A)** A post-replantation radiograph taken at 14-day review, 1⌋ showing an immature root form. **(B)** 1⌋ radiograph taken at 6-month review showing continued root development.

Following splint removal, Kathryn's 1⌋ was carefully reviewed at 6 weeks, 3 months, 6 months and 12 months. At each visit, special tests (described in Chapter 31) and radiographs were taken. This was to ascertain the type of periodontal healing and to look for signs of pulpal necrosis and or infection-related resorption. As can be seen in **Fig. 32.2**, continued root formation was seen demonstrating pulp revascularization. At 12 months (**Figs 32.3A and B**) there was clear clinical and radiographic signs of periodontal healing (re-establishment of a normal periodontal ligament with a few small areas of repair-related resorption) and continued root growth and apical closure (signs of revascularization). Kathryn was therefore discharged back to her general dental practitioner with the prognosis that the 1⌋ will be retained as a functional tooth for the rest of her life.

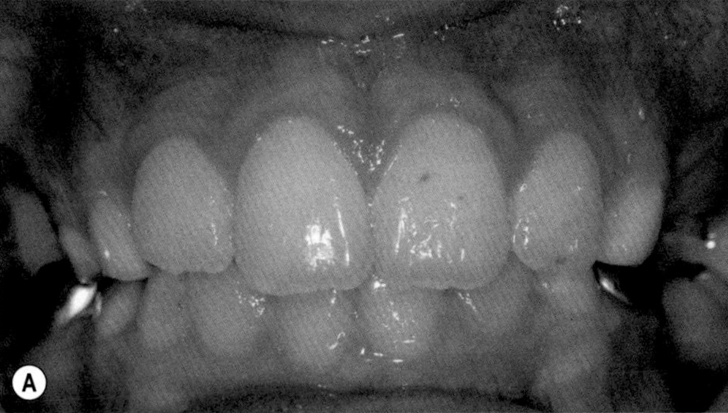

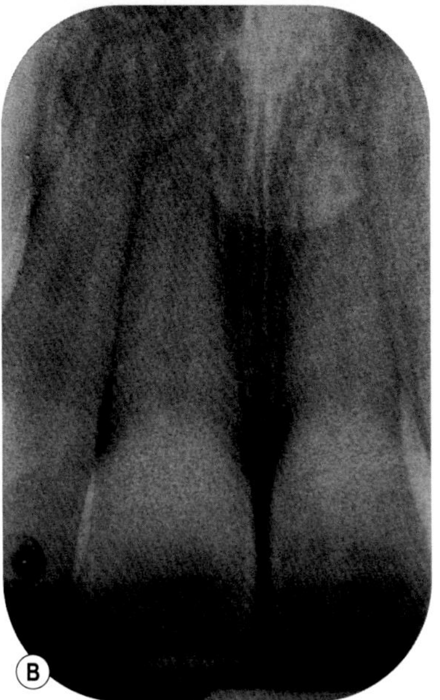

Fig. 32.3 **(A)** Clinical appearance of 1⌋ 12 months following avulsion injury. **(B)** Radiographic appearance of 1⌋ 12 months following avulsion injury, showing further root development.

CASE 2

SUMMARY

Justin is 11 years old. He fell off his scooter, avulsing his 1⌋. His friends at the park ran home to get his parents, who arrived within 15 minutes. They took Justin and his tooth to an accident and emergency department. At hospital his tooth was placed in milk. Three hours later his tooth was replanted and splinted. The EAT was 4 hours, and the EADT 1 hour.

- ***Justin's parents book an emergency appointment so see you the following day, what will you do?***

Fig. 32.4 shows a suture splint. This type of splint is inappropriate, as the patient will find it very difficult to maintain good oral hygiene. Moreover, this type of splint is unable to hold the tooth in the replanted position with the 1⌋ slightly extruded on presentation. The splint was replaced for a more conventional splint (discussed in Chapter 31); however, Justin would not tolerate further repositioning of the tooth to improve its position. Advice described earlier in this chapter is reiterated, and Justin was booked for a review appointment 8 days after his accident.

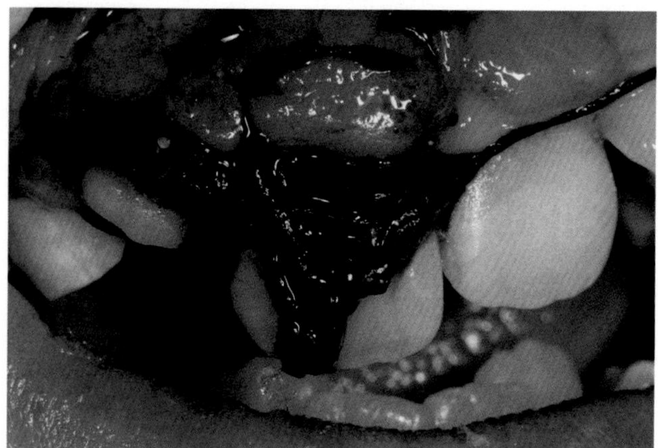

Fig. 32.4 Showing 1⌋ replanted with an inappropriate suture splint. *Reproduced with permission from the RCS EDen project, Royal College of Surgeons of England.*

What is the chance of pulp survival?

Radiographs show 1⌋ has complete root development. Therefore there is no chance of pulpal revascularization. In order to prevent infection-related resorption, root canal treatment is commenced at this visit. It is good practice to extirpate the necrotic pulp and disinfect the root canal before removing the splint. Justin was booked for a further review and disinfection of the root canal 1 month later.

What intracanal medicament should be placed in the extirpated tooth?

There has been some animal-based research that has shown that when non-setting calcium hydroxide is placed too early after replantation (within the first 7 days) in a tooth with a damaged periodontal ligament, this can aggravate favourable periodontal healing and lead to ankylosis-related resorption. With this in mind some authorities advocate that a steriod/polyantibiotic paste should be the first dressing placed in root canals of avulsed teeth as soon after the injury as possible. They argued that the steroid/antibiotic paste will dampen the immune response promoting favourable healing. Currently there is no definitive research supporting one approach over another. Therefore guidelines advocate either approach. For Justin's tooth, a non-setting calcium hydroxide dressing was placed at his day-8 review appointment.

What are the chances of periodontal healing?

There is very little chance of periodontal healing with the tooth almost guaranteed to heal by ankylosis-related resorption. Therefore early referral to an interdisciplinary team is essential. At this interdisciplinary clinic they will discuss the different treatment options with Justin and his parents.

BSPD and IADT guidelines differ slightly with their cut off points of when ankylosis-related resorption is highly likely. Beyond EADT of 30 minutes and EAT of 90 minutes, BSPD guidelines report that there is less than a 10% chance of periodontal healing. For IADT, beyond EADT of 60 minutes there is less than a 1% chance of periodontal healing. Justin is beyond both of these cut off points, and therefore ankylosis-related resorption is almost guaranteed. However, maintaining a tooth which will ultimately fail is very important over the short to medium term. The tooth will help maintain good aesthetics for the patient as well as the height and width of the alveolus. Careful follow-up is essential to diagnose infraocclusion as soon as it becomes apparent.

What long-term treatment options are available?

There are a number of different options which were assessed for Justin. These included decorontation, orthodontic space closure and camouflage of the lateral incisor, denture, resin retained bridge and premolar transplant. In a growing patient (e.g. a child or adolescent) an osseointregrated implant is contraindicated as they have not completed their facial growth.

The different options were discussed with Justin and his parents at the interdisciplinary clinic. Justin had crowding in his upper and lower arches and was keen on undergoing orthodontics to improve his appearance. As part of the treatment plan a premolar was to be extracted in each quadrant. The best prognosis for premolar transplant is when the root formation is between three-quarter and complete root length development but with an open apex. Justin fitted the criteria for a premolar transplant and both he and his parents were keen to pursue this option (see **Figs 32.5 A-D**).

Justin had a tooth extracted in each quadrant including the ⌊5 which was used for the premolar transplants. This was built up initially during the healing phase of the transplant before the orthodontic treatment was undertaken. On the completion of his orthodontic treatment, a final composite build up was provided. The transplant demonstrated both pulpal and periodontal healing. The prognosis for the transplant is that it will be retained as a functional unit for the rest of Justin's life.

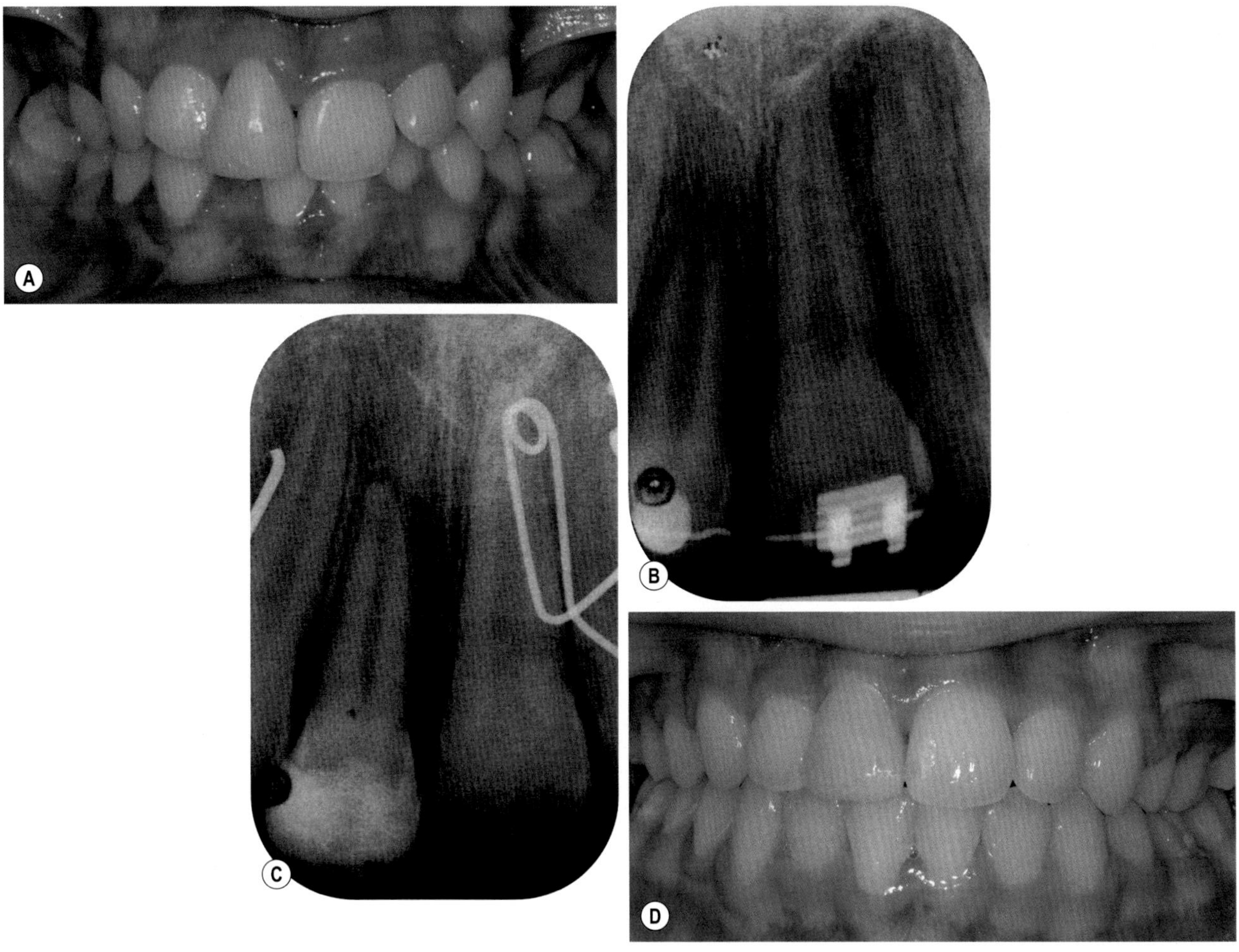

Fig. 32.5 **(A)** 1 week after the premolar transplant procedure with initial composite build up. **(B)** Radiograph of the premolar transplant taken 1 week after the premolar transplant procedure. *Reproduced with permission from the RCS EDen project, Royal College of Surgeons of England.* **(C)** Radiograph of premolar transplant taken 6 months after the premolar transplant, showing periodontal and pulpal healing (continue root growth). *Reproduced with permission from the RCS EDen project, Royal College of Surgeons of England.* **(D)** Premolar transplant (1|) after orthodontic treatment and final composite build up. *Reproduced with permission from the RCS EDen project, Royal College of Surgeons of England.*

Primary resources and recommended reading

Andersson L, Andreasen JO Day P et al 2012 International Association of Dental Traumatology guidelines for the management of traumatic dental injuries: 2. Avulsion of permanent teeth. Dent Traumatol 28 (2):88–96.

Andreasen JO, Lauridsen E, Bakland L et al 2014 Dental trauma guide. Available at: http://www.dentaltraumaguide.org/Examination.aspx.

Day P, Gregg T 2012 Treatment of avulsed permanent teeth in children. British Society of Paediatric Dentistry. Available at: http://bspd.co.uk/Resources/BSPD-Guidelines.

Day PF, Kindelan SA, Spencer J et al 2008 Dental trauma: part 2. Managing poor prognosis anterior teeth - treatment options for the subsequent space in a growing patient. J of Orthod 35:143–155.

Trope M 2011 Avulsion of permanent teeth: theory to practice. Dent Traumatol 27 (4):281–294.

For revision, see Mind Map 32, page 253.

33

Disorders of eruption and exfoliation

CASE 1

SUMMARY

***Beth was only 20 days old when it was noticed she had two teeth at the front of her lower jaw** (Fig. 33.1).*

■ ***What is the correct terminology for these early erupting teeth?***

If the teeth are present at birth, 'natal' is the correct term. If they are not present at birth but erupt within the first month of life, 'neonatal' is correct.

The prevalence rates for both natal and neonatal teeth are reported as 1 in 2000–3000 live births. The most commonly presenting tooth is the lower central incisor. More rarely, maxillary incisors or first molars have been reported. The early eruption is thought to be caused by the ectopic position of the tooth germ during fetal life. Natal and neonatal teeth may follow a sporadic pattern, or they may be familial. However, they can be associated with specific syndromes:

Pachyonychia congenita.

Ellis–van Creveld.

Hallermann–Streiff.

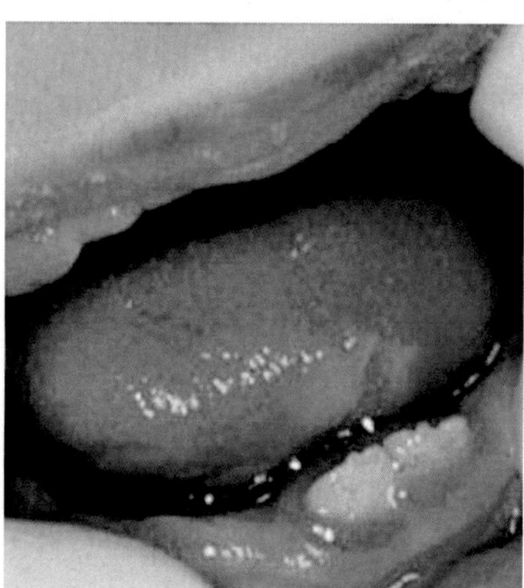

Fig. 33.1 Natal teeth.

■ ***What are the main problems associated with natal and neonatal teeth?***

Mobility.

Ulceration of ventral surface of tongue.

Nipple soreness (breastfeeding mothers).

The teeth are mobile because the development of the tooth is consistent with age. Only about five-sixths of the crown, and usually no root, is formed. Additionally, the crown is occasionally dilacerated and the enamel hypoplastic or hypomineralized.

Excessive mobility is a danger to the airway from aspiration, and the tooth should be removed. Care should be taken to ensure that the entire tooth including the pulpal tissue is removed, otherwise dentine and a root will form, which will require eventual removal. If teeth can be left, then continued root development will occur. Nipple soreness may occasionally necessitate tooth removal.

Ulceration on the ventral surface of the tongue may respond to carmellose sodium oral paste. Smoothing of the incisal edges with sandpaper discs may also help.

If the decision is made to remove the tooth, do remember the local anaesthetic doses, as these young babies are likely to weigh between 2–4 kg. Newborns are given vitamin K in the first week of life. Check that they have received this as either an injection or an oral dose in hospital or from their midwife.

Key point

Natal and neonatal teeth may need to be removed if:

- Mobility causes concern about inhalation.
- Ulceration under the ventral surface of the tongue persists.
- Nipple soreness is significant.

■ ***What factors can cause generalized premature eruption but still be considered as 'normal'?***

Familial – a family history is a common finding.

Children with high birth weights.

Maternal smoking during pregnancy.

Lower socioeconomic status.

Reduced maternal physical activity.

Race – generally Negroids tend to erupt their permanent teeth earlier than Mongoloids, who are in turn in advance of Caucasians and finally Asian children. Racial group can affect eruption times and eruption patterns of the primary dentition.

Sex – females tend to erupt permanent teeth several months ahead of males.

The opposite of premature eruption is delayed eruption.

■ ***When is generalized delay in eruption of primary teeth expected?***

Preterm infants.

Very low birth weight infants.

■ ***What conditions may lead to a generalized delayed eruption of teeth in both primary and permanent dentitions?***

Chromosomal abnormalities – Down syndrome and Turner syndrome.

Gross nutritional deficiency.

Hypothyroidism/hypopituitarism.

Hereditary gingival fibromatosis (HGF).

Acquired gingival overgrowth (drug-induced – phenytonin, cyclosporin, sodium channel blockers).

Acquired reduction in bone turnover (drug-induced – bisphosphonates).

■ ***What specific condition is associated with grossly delayed or failed eruption of teeth in the permanent dentition?***

Cleidocranial dysplasia – this is an autosomal dominantly inherited condition where, in addition to multiple supernumerary teeth causing delayed exfoliation of primary teeth and delayed eruption of permanent teeth, there is aplasia of the distal end or total absence of the clavicles.

■ ***What local factors can account for delayed eruption of permanent teeth?***

Supernumerary teeth or odontomes.

Ectopic crypt positions of permanent teeth.

Cystic change in the follicle of permanent teeth.

Crowding.

Thickened mucosa due to early primary tooth removal.

Exfoliation of teeth (like eruption) can be either premature or delayed.

CASE 2

SUMMARY

George was 3 years of age when his mother first noticed that his lower primary incisors were loose.

History

George was born after a normal pregnancy and delivery but had problems after birth with recurrent coughs and colds, upper and lower respiratory tract infections, and oral ulceration. He was extensively investigated and was confirmed as having a cyclic neutropenia.

Dental history

George and his mother had regular toothbrush instruction, and his oral hygiene was excellent. He also used 0.2% chlorhexidine gel at night instead of fluoridated toothpaste. Despite these efforts his lower primary incisors exfoliated between age 4 and 5 years, and by his sixth birthday he had erupted his lower permanent central incisors and first permanent molars (**Figs 33.2A and B**).

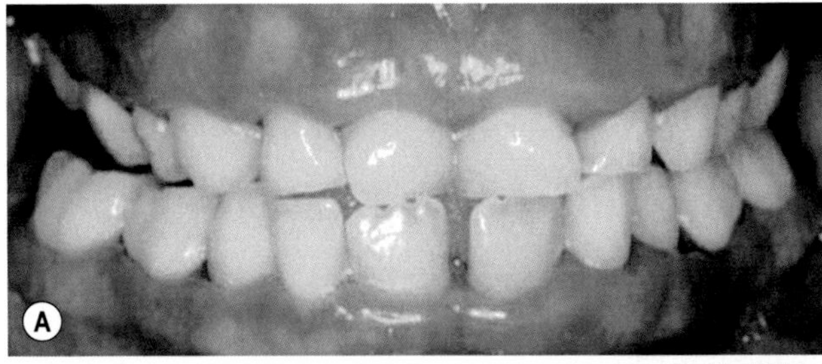

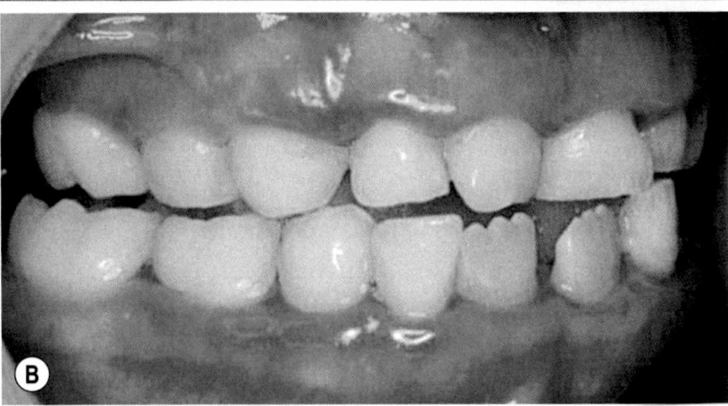

Fig. 33.2 **(A)** Cyclic neutropenia. **(B)** Cyclic neutropenia.

Box 33.1 Differential diagnosis of causes of premature exfoliation of primary and permanent teeth

- Neutropenias and qualitative neutrophil defects:
  - Cyclic neutropenia.
  - Congenital neutropenia (Kostmann disease).
  - Prepubertal periodontitis.
  - Juvenile periodontitis.
  - Leucocyte adhesion defect.
  - Papillon–Lefèvre syndrome.
  - Chediak–Higashi disease.
- Langerhans cell histiocytosis – leading to bony destruction.
- Hypophosphatasia with aplasia or hypoplasia of cementum.
- Self-injury in either a psychotic disorder or the congenital insensitivity to pain syndrome.
- Ehlers–Danlos syndrome (type VIII) – disorder of collagen formation causing progressive periodontal destruction.
- Scurvy – loss of tooth due to failure of proline hydroxylation and collagen synthesis.

Premature loss of primary teeth is an important diagnostic event, as most conditions causing it are potentially serious and warrant immediate investigation (**Box 33.1**).

Generally teeth may be lost early because of:

Metabolic disturbances.

Severe periodontal disease.

Loss of alveolar bone support.

Self-injury or non-accidental injury.

George will continue to have regular dental care and supervision of brushing. Even in the presence of immaculate plaque control we can expect that his neutrophil defect will predispose him to periodontal disease and premature loss of some if not all his permanent teeth.

The opposite of premature exfoliation is delayed exfoliation.

What causes delayed exfoliation of primary teeth?

Double primary teeth.

Hypodontia affecting permanent successors.

Ectopically placed permanent successors.

Trauma or periradicular infection of primary teeth causing interruption of physiological resorption.

Infraocclusion or ankylosis.

In 40% of cases, double primary teeth are associated with an abnormality in the permanent dentition number. Parents should be advised of this and a dental panoramic tomogram should be taken around the age of 6. Further information on double teeth is provided in Chapter 37.

Infraocclusion is the preferred term for either 'submerged teeth' or 'ankylosis' when describing teeth that have failed to achieve or maintain their occlusal relationship to adjacent or opposing teeth. Most commonly, primary teeth have reached a normal occlusal level before becoming infraoccluded.

The tooth most commonly affected is the mandibular first primary molar. Males and females are affected equally. Infraoccluded primary teeth are associated with a higher incidence of absent permanent successors. Further details of their management is discussed in Chapter 8.

Key point

Infraocclusion:

- Mandibular first primary molar is most commonly affected, with mandibular primary molars more commonly affected than maxillary primary molars.
- More common in primary teeth than in permanent teeth.
- Equal sex ratio.
- Higher incidence of absent permanent successors.
- Prevalence of 2–8%.

How is infraocclusion graded?

- Grade I – occlusal level above contact point of adjacent tooth.
- Grade II – occlusal level at contact point of adjacent tooth.
- Grade III – occlusal level below contact point of adjacent tooth.

Grade III infraocclusions, if progressive, may be completely submerged by the surrounding hard and soft tissues. Radiographs of infraoccluded teeth show blurring or absence of the periodontal space.

Primary resources and recommended reading

Aldred M, Cameron A, Georgiou, A 2013 Paediatric oral medicine, oral pathology and radiology. In: Cameron A, Widmer R (eds), Handbook of Pediatric Dentistry, 4th ed. Mosby Wolfe, St Louis.

Crawford PJM, Aldred MJ 2012 Anomalies of tooth formation and eruption. In: Welbury RR, Duggal MS, Hosey MT (eds), Paediatric Dentistry, 4th ed. Oxford: Oxford University Press.

Management of unerupted maxillary incisors 2010. London: Royal College of Surgeons of England, Faculty of Dental Surgery. Available at: https://www.rcseng.ac.uk/fds/publications-clinical-guidelines/clinical_guidelines/documents/ManMaxIncisors2010.pdf.

Ntani G, Day PF, Baird J et al 2015 Maternal and early life factors of tooth emergence patterns and number of teeth at 1 and 2 years of age. J Dev Orig Health Dis 6:299–307.

For revision, see Mind Map 33, page 254.

34

Poor quality first permanent molars

SUMMARY

Lisa is 9 years old. Her mother has brought her to your surgery because her recently erupted permanent teeth at the back of her mouth are brown and there are creamy patches on her adult incisors. What has caused these discolorations? How may they be treated?

History

Lisa has complained that for the past few months these teeth have been painful on eating hot and cold foods. The pain is of 1–2 minutes' duration. Toothbrushing also has caused sensitivity at the back of the mouth. There has been no pain on biting and eating foods. Very recently Lisa felt that one of the back teeth has started to crumble. Her mother has also noticed this when she has helped with brushing. Lisa has not required any analgesics for the discomfort caused by her teeth.

Medical history

Lisa is a healthy child who has never been in hospital.

Dental history

Lisa and her family are regular dental attenders. The family members all have a low caries risk. Lisa has had no restorations in her primary dentition. She used a children's toothpaste (1050 ppm) until recently and is now using the same adult toothpaste as her parents (1450 ppm).

Examination

Intraoral examination revealed that all four first permanent molars (FPMs) were hypomineralized with areas of brown enamel. In addition, there were areas of post-eruptive breakdown (hypoplasia) where the enamel had chipped away, exposing the underlying dentine. The maxillary molars were the worst affected by post-eruptive breakdown. 6| had a large atypical amalgam restoration. In addition, some creamy hypomineralized areas were visible on the labial surfaces of the newly erupted upper and lower permanent central incisors (**Figs 34.1** and **34.2**).

Upper and lower arches were uncrowded. Space assessed from the distal of 2's to mesial of 6's in each quadrant was 21.5 mm in the lower arch and 22 mm in each upper arch quadrant. On average, 21 mm and 22 mm are required for these distances in the lower and upper arches, to provide sufficient space for the premolars and canines to align within the arch. The incisor relationship was Class I on 1|1; the molar relationship was Class I bilaterally.

> **Key point**
>
> - **Hypoplasia** is the name given when there is a reduced thickness of enamel but the enamel is well mineralized (e.g. there is reduced quantity but normal quality of enamel).
> - **Hypomineralization** is the name given when there is reduced mineral content of enamel but a normal amount of enamel has been laid down (e.g. there is reduced quality of enamel but normal quantity).
> - **Post-eruptive breakdown** is where the tooth erupts with hypomineralized enamel. Shortly after eruption this area of enamel fractures off exposing underlying dentine.
> - **Atypical restorations** is where the classical appearance of the restoration for dental caries (following Black's cavity design) is not seen.

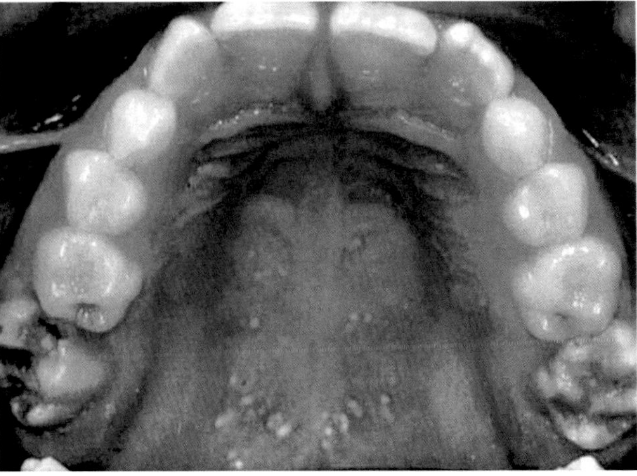

Fig. 34.1 Hypomineralized and hypoplastic upper first permanent molars.

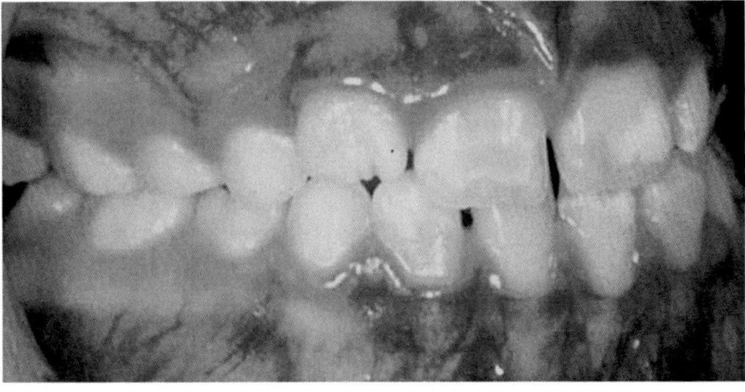

Fig. 34.2 Hypomineralized upper and lower permanent incisors.

■ ***Do you think that the enamel hypomineralization and hypoplasia noted on the first permanent molars and the permanent incisors follows a chronological pattern? If so, at what time was the affected enamel formed?***

Yes, it is possible that there is a chronological pattern. The cusp tips of the first permanent molars begin mineralizing from the eighth month of pregnancy, and the cusp tips of the incisors and cuspids (canines) from about 3 months of age (the upper lateral incisor slightly later at 10–12 months). Mineralization dates for the permanent dentition are given in **Table 34.1**.

■ ***What specific questions would you like to ask Lisa's mother?***

Pre-natal. Mother's health during pregnancy. Were there any concerns such as high blood pressure, proteinuria or preeclampsia?

Peri-natal. Difficult birth. Was the delivery prolonged? Was there a need for assisted delivery by forceps, ventouse or caesarean? All of these can be associated with fetal distress.

Post-natal. Did Lisa spend any time in the special care baby unit (SCBU)?

Illnesses in the first 2 years of life, e.g. meningitis, measles, respiratory infections, chickenpox. These disturbances may manifest as enamel defects distributed in the enamel that was forming around birth and in the first 2 years of life.

Further questioning revealed that Lisa was born after a normal pregnancy and delivery but had a significant number of respiratory infections during the first year of life. This confirms your diagnosis of chronological hypoplasia. The correct name for this condition is molar incisor hypomineralization (MIH). Post-eruptive breakdown and atypical restorations are consistent with this diagnosis.

Table 34.1 Mineralization times for the permanent dentition

Tooth	Mineralization begins (months)
Upper	
Central incisor	3–4
Lateral incisor	10–12
Canine	4–5
First premolar	18–21
Second premolar	24–27
First molar	At birth
Second molar	30–36
Third molar	84–108
Lower	
Central incisor	3–4
Lateral incisor	3–4
Canine	4–5
First premolar	21–24
Second premolar	27–30
First molar	At birth
Second molar	30–36
Third molar	96–120

■ ***What other differential diagnoses might you consider?***

- *Caries.* Newly erupted teeth are particularly prone to dental caries until their enamel maturation is complete. However, it seems very unlikely, even in the presence of particularly deep fissures, that Lisa, who has no caries in her primary teeth, should develop such caries in her permanent teeth. In addition, the overall colour of the permanent molars is not consistent with caries in a tooth of normal morphology. The exposed dentine is slightly softened and does have caries, but the overall pattern of destruction of the tooth suggests that caries is secondary to some other predisposing factor, such as hypomineralization/hypoplasia. Another factor to consider that is against a diagnosis of caries is the creamy hypomineralized areas on the incisors. They are neither the shape nor the distribution of white spot or precarious lesions that one would expect with poor oral hygiene.
- *Amelogenesis imperfecta.* Although the presenting features could be a hypomature form of amelogenesis imperfecta, there are several factors that suggest this is not the case: there is no family history; the primary dentition is not affected; the pattern of the defects is chronological. All of these combined make an inherited abnormality unlikely.
- *Fluorosis.* The severe enamel defects on the molar teeth could only occur if there was a history of very high endemic fluoride levels, probably in excess of 6 ppm. Such levels do not occur in the UK. Mild fluorosis is seen where children have swallowed toothpaste or have been given supplementation in addition to swallowing toothpaste. However, in such cases there are usually fine, opaque, white lines following the perikymata and small irregular enamel opacities or flecks that merge into the background enamel colour. Fluorosis does not produce well-demarcated opacities like those seen on the incisors.

Key point

In patients with MIH, your questioning should include:

- Pre-natal period.
- Natal period.
- Post-natal period.
- Systemic illnesses in first 2 years of life.

■ ***Is pain from such molar teeth common?***

Yes. There is evidence that these teeth have 5–10 times greater treatment need than normal teeth and are more difficult to anaesthetize. A palatal as well as a buccal infiltration is essential. There is also evidence that children with hypomineralized first permanent molars (HFPMs) have more behaviour management problems than other children, necessitating adjuncts to treatment such as sedation. In recent years, the prevalence of HFPMs varies across different populations in the world. The average prevalence is 16% with a range between 3% and 44%.

The histology of extracted HFPMs shows that the yellow/brown areas are more porous and occupy the entire enamel layer. The white/creamy areas occupy the inner parts of enamel. The affected areas have a higher carbon and lower calcium and phosphate content (e.g. less mineral and more protein).

Investigations

What investigations are indicated and why?

Intraoral radiographs are indicated in order to assess the proximity of the coronal defects to the dental pulp. These can be difficult to interpret, as MIH-affected teeth have a different radiographic appearance to dental caries. A *panoramic tomogram* is necessary to ascertain the presence and stage of development of the remaining permanent dentition in view of the poor long-term prognosis of the first permanent molars.

A panoramic tomogram revealed all permanent teeth, including third molars, to be present. The furcation of 7's was calcifying. Secondary caries was evident in all first permanent molars but was most pronounced in $\frac{6|6}{\;|6}$.

Treatment

What are the main clinical problems in this case?

Loss of tooth substance: breakdown of enamel tooth wear secondary caries.

Sensitivity.

Appearance.

> **Key point**
>
> Children with MIH:
> - Have a higher treatment need.
> - Have significantly higher behaviour management problems.
>
> Achieving good local anaesthetic of the entire tooth is essential, as frequently these teeth can be very sensitive (histology of affected MIH teeth shows significant pulpal inflammation).
>
> Treatment under rubber dam is frequently needed to prevent sensitivity from affected adjacent teeth.

What are the treatment options for the HFPMs in this case?

Sensitivity.

Composite.

Stainless steel crowns.

Adhesively retained copings.

Extraction.

Sensitivity This can be managed in a number of different ways. Advising patients to use antisensitivity toothpaste and/or toothmousse (see Chapter 23) can be affective. For children over the age of 10, use of a high-fluoride toothpaste (e.g. 2800 ppm) can also work. For localized areas that are sensitive to toothbrushing or cold drinks and food, temporary glass ionomer cements (GICs) are often used to reduce the sensitivity symptoms. This is often used to maintain symptomatic molars until the ideal age for their extraction.

Composite These can be definitive restorations when there are small areas of hypomineralization. It is important when restoring these teeth that all the hypomineralized area is removed. This is achieved with gently running a slow handpiece with a large rose bur over the discoloured enamel. The soft enamel will give way, leaving hard, less affected enamel behind.

Stainless steel crowns These are the most durable restoration and can maintain a tooth until a permanent crown can be placed in the teenage years, or until a planned extraction.

Adhesively retained copings These may be suitable for teeth that are not significantly affected by hypomineralization. When the defect has been removed and replaced by GIC, a coping can be placed on top of the restoration and cover the remainder of the occlusal and cuspal surface.

Extraction For moderate to severely affected HFPM this is the preferred treatment option because:

- HFPMs are of poor long-term prognosis. Although full coverage coronal restorations could be undertaken to retain them, this is an ambitious plan in a 9-year-old child. The restorations undoubtedly would require replacement at some future date due to possible microleakage at the margins and caries. This would incur additional inconvenience, expense and life-long treatment for the patient.
- It is the optimal developmental stage to remove $\overline{6}$'s as the furcation of $\overline{7}$'s is calcifying and predictable bodily movement of $\overline{7}$ forward is most likely. Timing of $\overline{6}$ removal is more critical than that of $\underline{6}$ as the mesial drift tendency is greater in the upper arch.
- Third molars are also developing and should erupt eventually if the 7's migrate forward to occupy the position of the 6's (**Fig. 34.3**).

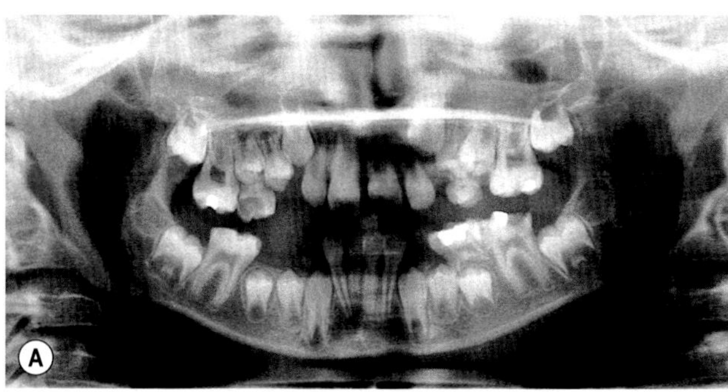

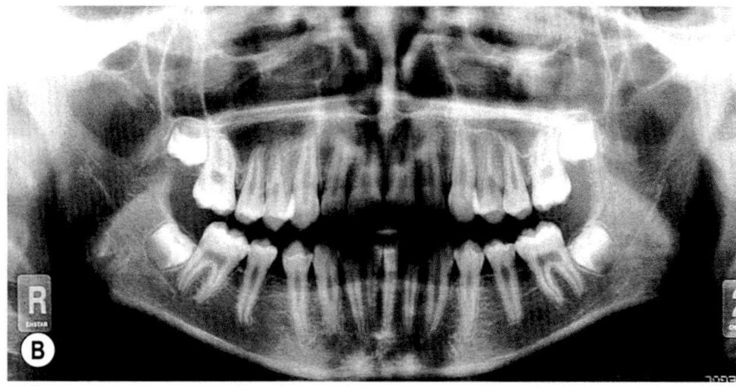

Fig. 34.3 **(A)** Dental panoramic tomogram before removal of all first permanent molars. **(B)** Dental panoramic tomogram following removal of all first permanent molars.

- As the molar relationship is Class I bilaterally, removal of $\overline{6}$'s necessitates the removal of $\underline{6}$'s to encourage maintenance of the buccal segment relationship. This is known as compensating (removal of the equivalent opposing tooth) extractions and preventing over-eruption of the $\underline{6}$'s.

Key point

- Ensure all permanent teeth, especially 5's and 8's, are present radiographically before considering FPM extraction. In some situations the FPM may be extracted even if the 8's are absent.
- An orthodontic assessment of the patient is essential to establish their malocclusion. A consultation with an orthodontist is prudent in Class II and III cases.
- Timing of the extraction of $\overline{6}$ is more critical than that of $\underline{6}$. Ideal timing for a $\overline{6}$ is between the ages of 8.5–9.5 (when there is calcification of the bifurcation of the $\overline{7}$). The timing for the extraction of a $\underline{6}$ is before the $\underline{7}$ erupts.
- Consider compensating extractions of upper FPM where there is moderate to severe MIH in lower FPM.

What are the treatment options for the incisors in this case?

Bleaching.

Microabrasion.

Localized composite restoration.

Full composite veneer.

Bleaching is controversial in these cases. Firstly, there are legal issues around bleaching children's teeth (see Chapter 36). Secondly, the bleaching can cause sensitivity, and therefore patients may struggle to comply with instructions for use when their teeth are already sensitive. Finally, the impact of the bleach is more likely to lighten the adjacent tooth around the defect, thereby reducing the contrast between the two. Importantly this is the least invasive treatment with no removal of enamel.

Controlled enamel microabrasion may produce a more acceptable result without removing the white areas. This is because the surface enamel layer after microabrasion is relatively prismless and well compacted. The optical properties are changed and a white area may become less perceptible. The technique should not be used if there is a reduced thickness of enamel.

Localized composites can give very acceptable results but are destructive of enamel and may weaken the tooth structure if large areas are removed.

Full composite veneers with a thin layer of a relatively opaque composite may produce an acceptable result without any, or very little, enamel reduction. This will, however, make the tooth bulkier.

Primary resources and recommended reading

D3 Group 2016 Development Dental Defects website. Available at: http://www.thed3group.org.

Jalevik B 2010 Prevalence and diagnosis of molar-incisor-hypomineralisation (MIH): a systematic review. Eur Arch Paediatr Dent 11:59–64.

Jalevik B, Klingberg GA 2002 Dental treatment, dental fear and behaviour management problems in children with severe enamel hypomineralisation of their permanent first molars. Int J Paediatr Dent 12:24–32.

Lygidakis NA, Wong F, Jalevik B et al 2010 Best clinical practice guidance for clinicians dealing with children presenting with molar-incisor-hypomineralisation (MIH): an EAPD policy document. Eur Arch Paediatr Dent 11:75–81.

Royal College of Surgeons A Guideline for the Extraction of First Permanent Molars in Children 2009. Available at: http://www.rcseng.ac.uk/fds/publications-clinical-guidelines/clinical_guidelines/documents/A%20Guideline%20for%20the%20Enforced%20Extraction%20of%20First%20Permanent%20Molars%20in%20Children%20rev%20March%202009.pdf.

For revision, see Mind Map 34, page 255.

35

Tooth discoloration, hypomineralization and hypoplasia

CASE 1

SUMMARY

Simon is 8 years old. He has been brought to your surgery by his mother because his teeth are very dark and he is being teased at school. How would you determine the origin of the discoloration?

History

Simon says that the colour of his permanent teeth has remained the same since they erupted (**Fig. 35.1**).

■ ***What other questions do you need to ask about the teeth?***

Do they chip or wear?

Are all the teeth affected?

Was the primary dentition affected?

Has anyone else in the family got, or had, similar teeth?

Positive answers to the last three questions may suggest an inherited abnormality of the teeth such as amelogenesis or dentinogenesis imperfecta.

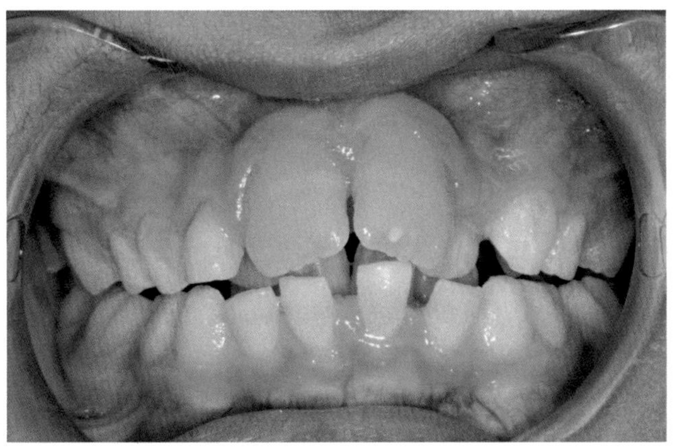

Fig. 35.1 Intrinsic discoloration.

Medical history

■ ***What specific questions do you need to ask his mother with regard to potential causes of discoloration?***

The pregnancy. The health of Simon's mother during her pregnancy and Simon's health during the birth and delivery are important when considering the condition of the first permanent molars (FPMs). The FPMs were the only permanent teeth that had started to mineralize before birth (around the eighth month of pregnancy). Conditions that may suggest some fetal distress and dysmineralization may be raised maternal blood pressure; early admission to hospital; premature delivery; prolonged delivery; assisted delivery, e.g. forceps or ventouse, emergency caesarean section; or admission to the special care baby unit (SCBU).

Childhood illnesses. These may result in a 'chronological hypoplasia' affecting those parts of the teeth that were mineralizing at the time of the illness. Although 'chronological hypoplasia' usually involves some failure of development of enamel matrix giving obvious lines or ridges on the teeth, there may be milder forms that can only be felt with a probe and that present for care because they attract extrinsic stain.

Tablets or medications taken during childhood. Tetracycline staining should not occur now in children who have been brought up in developed countries. It is still common in children from developing countries where tetracycline is still used because it is a very effective, cheap, broad-spectrum antibiotic. The only children who may still be affected in developed countries are those with cystic fibrosis who have developed multiple drug resistances as a result of recurrent respiratory infection.

Simon was born with primary biliary atresia. This resulted in progressive liver failure, increasing levels of circulating bilirubin and eventually a liver transplant at the age of 2.5 years. All the permanent teeth developing prior to the transplantation will have intrinsic discoloration as a result of the high circulating bilirubin. The primary dentition will be affected to a lesser extent as a result of staining in secondary dentine. Although not seen with Simon, some children can have gingival overgrowth as a result of immunosuppressive treatment with cyclosporine.

The colour of the second permanent molars is likely to be entirely normal as these teeth started mineralizing around the age of 3 when there was a functioning new liver and normal levels of bilirubin.

Dental history

■ ***What other lines of questioning do we need to explore if we are considering all the possible causes of intrinsic discoloration?***

Was there a history of infection and/or extraction for decay of any of the primary teeth?

Localized infection on primary teeth can cause localized abnormalities of enamel formation and mineralization of permanent teeth (Turner's tooth).

Was there ever any trauma to the primary teeth?

There is a 50% chance of enamel anomalies of permanent successor teeth after primary trauma (see Chapter 29). These will be localized anomalies.

Fluoride history.

A full history from birth, including areas that the child has lived in, fluoride supplementation and brushing habits is required. Fluorosis will produce a systemic or chronological distribution affecting the teeth that were forming when excess fluoride was taken.

The important categories and questions for a history into intrinsic tooth discoloration and hypoplasia are shown in **Box 35.1**.

Examination

The important features to note about any intrinsic discoloration or hypoplasia are:

Is it generalized or localized?

Does it affect the primary and permanent dentitions?

■ ***In the major categories for questioning shown in*** *Box 35.1*, ***which are likely to cause generalized discoloration and which are likely to cause localized discoloration?***

Generalized: medical; family; fluorosis.

Localized: pregnancy; dental; trauma.

Simon has generalized intrinsic discoloration as a result of biliary atresia causing increased levels of bilirubin.

Box 35.1 Intrinsic tooth discoloration and hypoplasia

Maternal and neonatal history

- History of pregnancy – maternal problems.
- History of birth – caesarean, forceps, fetal distress.

Family history

- Is anyone in the family similarly affected.

Medical history

- Dates of prolonged illnesses, e.g. childhood infections, haematological disorders, nutritional diseases etc.
- Medications taken (such as topical or systematic tetracyclins).

Dental history

- Does the discoloration affect all the teeth or just a few.
- Does the discoloration affect both primary and permanent dentitions.
- Has the colour got worse or did the teeth erupt with this appearance.
- History of abscesses of the primary dentition.
- Any pain or sensitivity from teeth.
- Are the teeth chipping or wearing away.

Trauma history

- Has the child any history of an accident to primary or permanent teeth.

Fluoride history

- Where has the child lived.
- History of fluoride supplements.
- Age at commencement of brushing.
- Amount and type of toothpaste.
- Toothpaste eating habits.

■ ***What is the only method of treatment that will help Simon's appearance?***

Veneering. Composite veneers should be provided until the age of 16 years when they can be replaced with porcelain veneers. Composite veneers may not mask the severe green stain unless opaquing agents are used. Porcelain veneers may be the only realistic alternative; however, they are not appropriate until the gingival margin has matured and stabilized in late teens or early twenties. The method of placement of composite veneers is covered in Chapter 36.

An alternative, less destructive approach is the use of vital nightguard bleaching (see Chapter 36, together with discussions about the current legality of bleaching for children under 18 years old). This requires no irreversible destruction of enamel, and although it may not fully correct the discolouration, it may be sufficient for the patient. For severe discolouration several months of night-time bleaching may be required. At 3 years there is reported colour relapse in a third of all cases. However, top up bleaching is feasible and an acceptable outcome for some patients and their parents.

Key point

Lines of questioning in discoloration, hypomineralization and hypoplasia:

- Maternal.
- Trauma.
- Medical.
- Fluoride.
- Dental.
- Family.

■ ***If a patient came to you with a single discoloured root-filled incisor, what form of treatment should you consider first?***

Non-vital bleaching: this technique has certain advantages, especially in the younger and adolescent patient:

Non-destructive of tooth tissue (already root filled).

No irritation to gingival health that can occur with veneers.

No change in contour of tooth that may make oral hygiene more difficult.

Patient has some control over the amount of colour change achieved, as they are responsible for the frequency and duration of application, although as the dentist, you control how many tubes of bleach (10% carbamide peroxide) are used.

The only contraindications to non-vital bleaching would be teeth that are poorly obturated as they would need retreatment.

Patients with teeth that have composites need to be warned that these may need to be replaced once bleaching has finished.

Although there are other methods, such as sealing in sodium perborate, these have very much been superseded by inside outside technique and the difficulty in obtaining sodium perborate.

Technique

Visit 1

1. Make a diagnosis for the discolouration. Take pre-operative periapical radiographs; these are essential to check if there is an adequate root filling and no symptoms or signs of apical pathology.
2. Clean the teeth with pumice and make a note of the shade of the discoloured tooth. It is prudent to take clinical photographs of the anterior teeth with and without the shade guide visible.
3. Take an upper alginate impression of the entire arch. Ask the technician to cast up the impression and to block out a well on both the buccal and palatal aspects of the affected tooth. Then to construct a soft vacuum formed tray made of thermoplastic material. The tray should be cut back and scalloped around the gingival margin.

Visit 2

4. Check that the bleaching tray fits and trim back any rough edges that may irritate the gingival margin.
5. Place rubber dam, isolating the affected tooth. Ensure adequate eye protection for the patient, operator and dental nurse.
6. Remove the palatal restoration to permit access to the root canal.
7. Remove root filling to 1–2 mm below the dentogingival junction – you may need to use adult burs in a miniature contra-angle head.
8. Place 1 mm of glass ionomer cement over the gutta percha.
9. Use an ultrasonic to remove debris blocking the dentinal tubules on the labial surface. Alternatively, very lightly use a slow hand piece with a round bur. Do not remove excessive dentine.
10. Show the patient (or parent) how to fill up the access with 10% carbamide peroxide and then seat the bleaching tray. A small amount can also be placed in the well of the bleaching tray around the discoloured tooth.
11. Provide written and verbal instructions. In summary advise the patient to remove the bleaching tray and replace the bleach 3–5 times a day. This should continue for several days up to 2 weeks until the patient is happy with the colour. It is sensible to provide the patient with a maximum of two tubes of bleach so that they are forced to return for a review appointment after a week. The bleaching tray should be worn at all times except for tooth brushing. Phoning the patient a couple of days after their visit is sensible to check how they are getting on. Often at this point they will not have seen any change in colour.

Visit 3

12. Check that the patient is happy with the colour. Wash out the access cavity and place a cotton wool ball and a temporary restoration (glass ionomer cement). Ideally the definitive composite should be avoided for several days as the bleaching may interfere with composite bonding.

Visit 4

13. Remove the glass ionomer cement and cotton wool ball and provide a definitive composite.

Slight overbleaching is desirable, as there is likely to be some relapse. Although bleaching has been associated with later occurrence of external cervical resorption, resorption has never been reported with 10% carbamide peroxide.

Key point

Restorative techniques in discoloration:

- Bleaching.
- Microabrasion.
- Localized composite.
- Composite veneers.

CASE 2

SUMMARY

Tony is 14 years old. He has come to your surgery because he is concerned by the colour of his teeth and his bad breath (*Fig. 35.2*).

History

He has noticed his teeth changing colour over the past year. His friends have also commented on his bad breath over this period of time.

The colour of the teeth in **Fig. 35.2** is a result of extrinsic staining from chromogenic bacteria due to inadequate oral hygiene. The staining is classically in the gingival and cervical areas of the teeth.

■ ***Are there any other causes of extrinsic staining?***

Food and drink. Tea, coffee and dishes such as curry can cause staining of the teeth. Most commonly this occurs in the gingival or cervical areas initially, but if oral hygiene is poor, then it can affect a significant part of the whole tooth surface (**Fig. 35.3**).

Arrested caries. This produces a brown stain as a result of chromogenic bacteria.

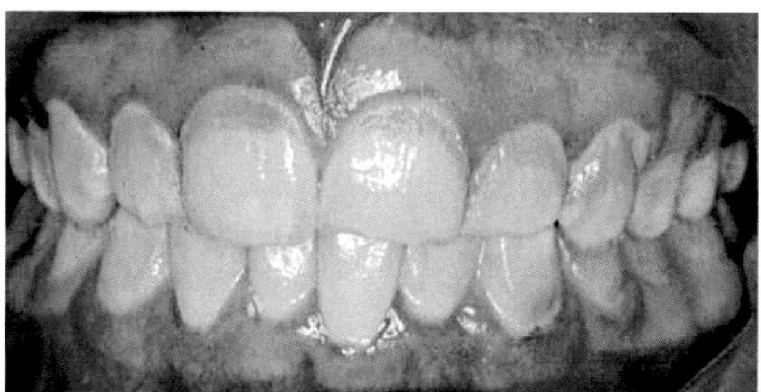

Fig. 35.2 Extrinsic chromogenic staining.

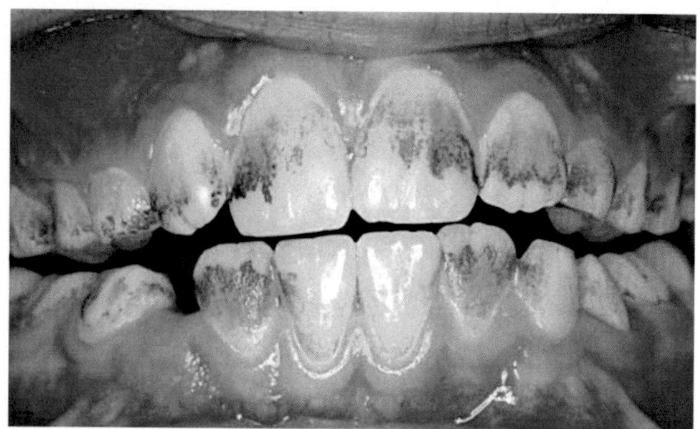

Fig. 35.3 Extrinsic food staining.

Medical condition. In biliary atresia and jaundice it is possible for bile pigments in the gingival crevicular fluid to cause extrinsic staining. This is yellow/green in colour.

Drugs. Ferrous sulphate in liquid iron preparations can result in black staining. Rifabutin, an antituberculous drug, is excreted in the crevicular fluid. This results in an orange-red staining.

Chlorhexidine mouthwash, when used frequently, can cause a brown-black staining.

All these extrinsic stains originate initially around the gingival or cervical area of the tooth but can progress to involve a significant amount of the tooth surface.

- ***How can you confirm your diagnosis of extrinsic discoloration?***

Extrinsic stains can be polished off. Carry out a prophylaxis.

- ***What additional clinical signs are there in** Fig. 35.2 **to back up your diagnosis of chromogenic staining secondary to poor oral hygiene?***

Marginal gingivitis.

'White spot' demineralization lesions in the gingival third of the labial enamel are visible on the anterior teeth.

Treatment

- ***How would you treat Tony's bad breath?***

Encourage him. Remember teenagers do not take criticism well! Tell him that he is not alone and lots of 'busy' young people forget twice daily brushing.

Toothbrushing instruction utilizing disclosing tablets or disclosing solution. Brushing twice daily, after breakfast and before school, and then last thing at night with a 2800 ppm fluoride toothpaste based on a high caries risk.

Show him the 'white spot' lesions. Explain that these will progress to decay if the brushing is not corrected.

Daily fluoride mouthwash (0.05% sodium fluoride) used at a separate time to brushing to encourage enamel remineralization.

- ***What factors in children and adolescents are important in halitosis (bad breath)?***

Plaque index.

Bleeding sites in gingiva.

Food impaction.

Nasal infection.

Tonsillar and adenoidal infection.

Furred tongue, especially posterior tongue.

- ***As well as improving his gingival health with improved toothbrushing, what else could be done with the toothbrush?***

Brushing the dorsum of his tongue! Alternative methods can be used to clean the surface of the tongue, and various types of 'tongue scrapers' are available commercially. Very occasionally in a child or adolescent the origin of halitosis can be ulceration of oesophageal or gastric origin. If there are symptoms of this, then a medical referral should be made.

Primary resources and recommended reading

Bharath KP, Subba Reddy VV, Poornima P et al 2014 Comparison of relative efficacy of two techniques of enamel stain removal on fluorosed teeth. An in vivo study. J Clin Pediatr Dent 38:207–213.

Burrows S 2009 A review of the efficacy of tooth bleaching. Dent Update 36:537–538, 541–44, 547–548.

Burrows S 2009 A review of the safety of tooth bleaching. Dent Update 36:604–606, 608–610, 612–614.

Kilpatrick NM, Burbridge L 2012 Anomalies of tooth formation and eruption. In: Welbury RR, Duggal MS, Hosey MT (eds), Paediatric Dentistry, 4th edn. Oxford: Oxford University Press.

Poyser NJ, Kelleher MG, Briggs PF 2004 Managing discoloured non-vital teeth: the inside/outside bleaching technique. Dent Update 31:204–210, 213–214.

For revision, see Mind Map 35, page 256.

36

Mottled teeth

SUMMARY

Sophie is 8 years old. Her main concern is that some of her permanent teeth have white patches, especially the upper central incisors. She is getting teased at school because the upper centrals also have brown patches. What are the causes of the white patches? How may they be treated?

History

Sophie noticed that the permanent teeth came through with the white and brown patches (**Fig. 36.1**). They have not changed in appearance since eruption.

■ ***What important questions would you now ask her mother?***

Were the primary teeth normal?

If the answer to this is yes, then it is unlikely to be an inherited defect and more likely to have a systemic origin.

■ ***Is anyone else in the family affected?***

Unless siblings are subjected to exactly the same systemic diseases and conditions it is likely that an affected sibling will indicate an inherited defect.

Sophie's primary teeth were normal, and she has no siblings. Neither her mother's nor her father's family has anyone with similar dental appearance.

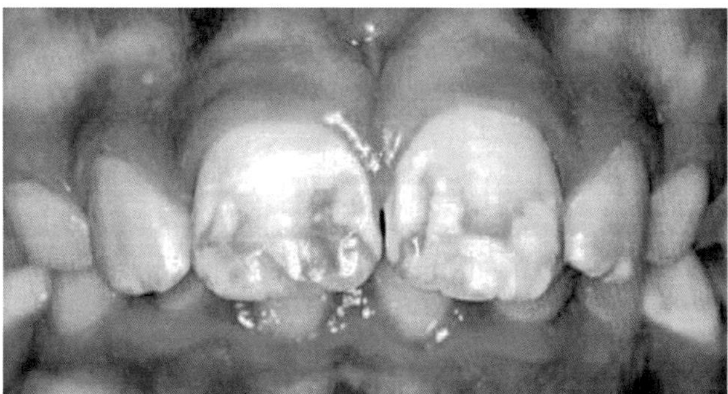

Fig. 36.1 Disfiguring fluorotic mottling affecting upper permanent central incisors.

■ ***What childhood illnesses and infections did she have, and when?***

A chronological hypomineralization or hypoplasia would suggest a systemic origin. There were no significant illnesses.

■ ***What is Sophie's fluoride history?***

This must include where she has lived, any history of supplements, type and amount of toothpaste used and any history of eating toothpaste.

It transpired that Sophie had never received any supplements or used toothpaste excessively. However, she lived on a farm with its own 'well' water supply. This was subsequently analysed and was found to be over 1 ppm fluoride. The diagnosis was one of fluorosis.

Examination

■ ***What is the distribution of the mottling that you can see in*** *Fig. 36.1*?

White and brown mottling of the incisal half of the labial surface of $\underline{1|1}$ and white mottling of the incisal third of the labial surface of $\underline{2|2}$.

■ ***Do you know why the labial surfaces of the upper permanent central incisors are often more affected by mottling?***

Research has shown that these teeth are particularly susceptible to an excess ingestion of fluoride between 24 and 30 months of age.

Mild fluorosis gives a diffuse mottling that may manifest as diffuse lines or patches that merge into the background enamel. When the fluorosis becomes more severe the lines and patches coalesce to produce a confluent white surface. In very severe cases there is also pitting of the enamel. Well-defined or well-demarcated patches (such as molar incisor hypomineralization; see Chapter 34) that do not follow a systemic or chronological distribution, or are localized, are unlikely to be due to fluorosis.

■ ***Which part of the enamel does mild fluorosis affect?***

The outer 200–300 μm.

■ ***How can you use this knowledge to your advantage during your clinical examination?***

Look for areas of the dentition that are subject to erosion or attrition, e.g. the occlusal surfaces of the first permanent molars. If the mottled enamel has been removed on these surfaces then that confirms that the mottling is in the outer aspect of the enamel and the diagnosis is likely to be one of fluorosis.

Key point

History taking in suspected fluorosis:

- Fluoridated water in places of residence.
- Amount of paste and age brushing started.
- Type of toothpaste used and fluoride concentration.
- Flouride supplements.
- Toothpaste eating habits.

■ ***In some cases of fluorosis there is, in addition to white mottling, some brown stain. What is the cause of the brown staining?***

This is usually due to extrinsic agents becoming incorporated into the more porous white mottled areas of enamel. The brown mottling tends to get worse with time.

Treatment

■ ***What treatment options for Sophie would you consider for fluorotic mottling?***

Microabrasion.

Composite veneers.

Vital Bleaching.

Microabrasion can be carried out in a variety of ways and is a controlled removal of the surface layer of enamel in order to improve discolorations that are limited to the outer enamel layer. It is not suitable for deep enamel or dentine discoloration. One of the most reliable methods that has been used extensively since 1986 is the hydrochloric acid (HCl)-pumice microabrasion technique. It is achieved by a combination of abrasion and erosion – the term 'abrosion' is sometimes used. In the clinical technique that will be described, no more than 100 μm of enamel is removed. Once completed the procedure should not be repeated again in the future. Too much enamel removal is potentially damaging to the pulp, and cosmetically the underlying dentine colour will become more evident.

Indications:

- Fluorosis.
- Idiopathic speckling.
- Post-orthodontic treatment demineralization.
- Prior to veneer placement for well-demarcated stains.
- White/brown surface staining, e.g. secondary to primary predecessor infection or trauma (Turner's teeth).

Materials:

- Bicarbonate of soda/water.
- Copalite varnish/Vaseline.
- Fluoridated toothpaste.
- Non-acidulated fluoride (fluoride drops).
- Pumice.
- Rubber dam.
- Rubber prophylaxis cup.
- Sandpaper polishing discs.
- 18% hydrochloric acid.

Technique:

1. Perform pre-operative vitality tests; take radiographs and photographs.
2. Clean the teeth with pumice and water, wash and dry.
3. Isolate the teeth to be treated with rubber dam, and paint Copalite varnish around the necks of the dam (alternatively place Vaseline around the necks of the teeth under the rubber dam).
4. Place a mixture of sodium bicarbonate and water on the dam behind the teeth, as protection in case of spillage.

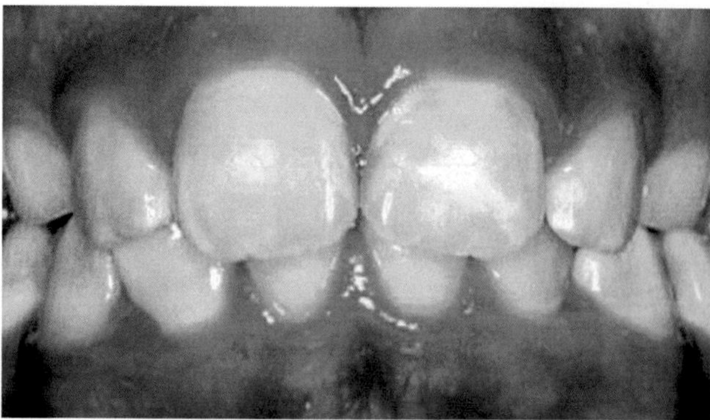

Fig. 36.2 After acid pumice microabrasion.

5. Mix 18% hydrochloric acid with pumice into a slurry and apply a small amount to the labial surface on either a rubber prophylaxis cup rotating slowly or a wooden stick rubbed over the surface for 5 seconds, before washing for 5 seconds directly into an aspirator tip. Repeat until the stain is reduced, up to a maximum of 10 × 5–second applications per tooth. Any improvement that is going to occur will have done so by this time.
6. Apply the fluoride drops to the teeth for 3 minutes.
7. Remove the rubber dam.
8. Polish the teeth with the finest sandpaper discs.
9. Polish the teeth with fluoridated toothpaste for 1 minute.
10. Review in 1 month for vitality tests and clinical photographs (**Fig. 36.2**).
11. Review biannually, checking pulpal status.

Critical analysis of the effectiveness of the technique should not be made immediately but delayed for at least 1 month, as the appearance of the teeth will continue to improve over this time. Experience has shown that brown mottling is removed more easily than white, but even where white mottling is incompletely removed it nevertheless becomes less perceptible. This phenomenon has been attributed to the relatively prismless layer of compacted surface enamel produced by the 'abrosion' technique, which alters the optical properties of the tooth surface.

Long-term studies of the technique have found no association with pulpal damage, increased caries susceptibility or significant prolonged thermal sensitivity. Patient compliance and satisfaction is good, and any dissatisfaction is usually due to inadequate pre-operative explanation. The technique is easy to perform for the operator and patient and is not time consuming. Removal of any mottled area is permanent and achieved with an insignificant loss of surface enamel. Failure to improve appearance by the HCl-pumice microabrasion technique has limited harmful effects but will be less destructive than localized or full-face composite veneers.

Key point

Microabrasion:

- Will improve surface defects, e.g. fluorosis.
- Will not improve deeper defects (full thickness of enamel lesions), e.g. amelogenesis imperfecta.

Fig. 36.2 shows the appearance of Sophie's 1|1 1 month after HCl-pumice microabrasion.

Is vital bleaching legal for children?

Changes in EU legislation in 2012 permit dental bleaching to be undertaken for adults. This guidance specified that the maximum concentration of 6% hydrogen peroxide was permitted for dental bleaching; 10% carbamide peroxide breaks down to 3.4% hydrogen peroxide. For children up to the age of 18 it is illegal. It was only in 2014, that the General Dental Council changed its guidance for dentists. Their statement identified that dentists could bleach children's diseased teeth without fear of disciplinary action. It is always sensible to check with your dental defence organization on the latest position. No matter which treatment option you choose, your discussions with the parents need to be recorded in the patient's clinical records and written consent taken.

Has bleaching of teeth any part to play in the treatment of surface enamel discoloration?

Yes, external vital bleaching has been used as an initial treatment for fluorotic mottling and as a secondary treatment for residual brown staining after microabrasion. It is, however, usually associated with the bleaching of the yellow discoloration of ageing – so-called 'nightguard vital bleaching'. This technique involves the daily placement of 10% carbamide peroxide gel into a custom-fitted tray of either the upper or the lower arch. As the name suggests it is carried out by the patient at home and is initially done on a daily basis.

Materials:

- Upper impression and working model.
- Soft mouthguard – avoiding the gingivae.
- 10% carbamide peroxide gel.

Technique:

1. Take an alginate impression of the arch to be treated and cast a working model in stone.
2. Relieve the labial surfaces of the teeth by about 0.5 mm and make a soft, pull-down, vacuum-formed splint as a mouthguard. The splint should be no more than 2 mm in thickness and should not cover the gingivae. It is only a vehicle for the bleaching gel and not intended to protect the gingivae.
3. Instruct the patient on how to floss the teeth thoroughly. Perform a full mouth prophylaxis and instruct them how to apply the gel into the mouthguard.
4. Note that the length of time the guard should be worn depends on the product used.
5. Review about 2 weeks later to check that the patient is not experiencing any sensitivity, and then at 6 weeks, by which time 80% of any colour change should have occurred. Sensitivity occurs in almost all patients, and reducing the duration of mouthguard wear is effective at minimizing symptoms. However, around 14% may stop this technique owing to the sensitivity it causes.

Carbamide peroxide gel (10%) breaks down in the mouth into 3.4% hydrogen peroxide and 7% urea. Both urea and hydrogen peroxide have low molecular weights, which allow them to diffuse rapidly through enamel and dentine and thus explains the transient pulpal sensitivity occasionally experienced with home bleaching systems.

Pulpal histology with regard to these materials has not been assessed, but no clinical significance has been attributed to the changes seen with 35% hydrogen peroxide over 75 years of usage, except where teeth have been overheated or traumatized. By extrapolation, 3.4% hydrogen peroxide in the home systems is therefore safe.

Although most carbamide peroxide materials contain trace amounts of phosphoric and citric acids as stabilizers and preservatives, no indication of etching or a significant change in the surface morphology of enamel has been demonstrated by scanning electron microscopy analysis. There was early concern that bleaching solutions with a low pH would cause demineralization of enamel when the pH fell below the 'critical' pH of 5.2–5.8. However, no evidence of this process has been noted to date in any clinical trials or laboratory tests, and this may be due to the urea (and subsequently the ammonia) and carbon dioxide released on degradation of the carbamide peroxide elevating the pH.

There is an initial decrease in bond strength of enamel to composite resin immediately after home bleaching, but this returns to normal within 7 days. This effect has been attributed to the residual oxygen in the bleached tooth surface, which inhibits polymerization of the composite resin. The home bleaching systems do not affect the colour of restorative materials. Any perceived effect is probably due to superficial cleansing.

Minor ulceration or irritation may occur during the initial treatment. It is important to check that the mouthguard does not extend on to the gingivae and that the edges of the guard are smooth. If ulceration persists, a decreased exposure time may be necessary. If there is still a problem then allergy is a possibility.

The exact mechanism of bleaching is unknown. Theories of oxidation, photo-oxidation and ion exchange have been suggested. Conversely, the cause of rediscoloration is also unknown. This may be a combination of chemical reduction of the oxidation products previously formed, marginal leakage of restorations allowing ingress of bacterial and chemical byproducts, and salivary or tissue fluid contamination via permeable tooth structure.

What are the indications for composite veneers?

Composite veneers may be required to mask dense white fluorotic plaques that are refractory to microabrasion and bleaching. Most composite veneers placed in children and adolescents are the direct type fashioned at the chairside rather than the indirect or laboratory-made type.

Before proceeding with any veneering technique, the decision must be made whether to reduce the thickness of labial enamel before placing the veneer. Certain factors should be considered:

- Increased labiopalatal bulk makes it harder to maintain good oral hygiene. This may be courting disaster in the adolescent with a dubious oral hygiene technique.
- Composite resin has a better bond strength to enamel when the surface layer of 200–300 μm is removed.

- If a tooth is very discoloured, some sort of reduction will be desirable, as a thicker layer of composite will be required to mask the intense stain.
- If a tooth is already instanding or rotated, its appearance can be enhanced by a thicker labial veneer.

New generation, highly polishable, hybrid composite resins can replace relatively large amounts of missing tooth tissue and be used in thin sections as a veneer. Combinations of shades can be used to simulate natural colour gradations and hues. Within these systems, opaquers can be very useful at blocking out the transmission of the discoloured enamel defect through the composite.

Indications for composite veneers:

- Discoloration.
- Enamel defects.
- Diastemata.
- Malpositioned teeth.
- Large restorations.

Contraindications:

- Insufficient available enamel for bonding.
- Oral habits, e.g. woodwind musicians.

How do you undertake a composite veneer?

The materials required are:

- Rubber dam/contoured matrix strips.
- Preparation and finishing burs.
- New generation, highly polishable, hybrid composite resin.
- Sof-Lex polishing discs and interproximal polishing strips.

Technique:

1. Use a tapered diamond bur to reduce labial enamel by 0.3–0.5 mm. Identify the finish line at the gingival margin and also mesially and distally just labial to the contact points.
2. Clean the tooth with a slurry of pumice in water. Wash and dry and select the shade.
3. Isolate the tooth either with rubber dam or a contoured matrix strip. Hold the latter in place by applying unfilled resin to its gingival side against the gingiva and curing for 10 seconds.
4. Etch the enamel for 60 seconds, wash and dry.
5. Where dentine is exposed, apply dentine primer.
6. Apply a thin layer of bonding resin to the labial surface and roughly shape it into all areas with a plastic instrument, then use a brush lubricated with unfilled resin to 'paddle' and smooth it into the desired shape. Cure for 60 seconds gingivally, 60 seconds mesioincisally, 60 seconds distoincisally, and 60 seconds from the palatal aspect if incisal coverage has been used. Different shades of composite can be combined to achieve good matches with adjacent teeth and a transition from a relatively dark gingival area to a lighter more translucent incisal region. For some darkly stained dentine, a thin layer of composite opaquer is an alternative to removing further enamel and dentine. This is placed as the first layer beneath the incremental composite build-up of different composite shades.
7. Flick away the unfilled resin holding the contour strip and remove the strip.
8. Finish the margins with diamond finishing burs and interproximal strips and the labial surface with graded sandpaper discs. Characterization should be added to improve light reflection properties.

The exact design of the composite veneer will depend on each clinical case, but will usually be one of four types: intra-enamel or window preparation; incisal bevel; overlapped incisal edge; or feathered incisal edge.

Tooth preparation will not usually expose dentine, but this will be unavoidable in some cases of localized hypoplasia or caries. Sound dentine may need to be covered by glass ionomer cement prior to placement of the composite veneer.

Primary resources and recommended reading

Burrows S 2009 A review of the efficacy of tooth bleaching. Dent Update 36:537–538, 541–544, 547–548.

Burrows S 2009 A review of the safety of tooth bleaching. Dent Update 36:604–606, 608–610, 612–614.

Kilpatrick NM, Burbridge LA 2012 Anomalies of tooth formation and eruption. In: Welbury RR, Duggal MS, Hosey MT (eds), Paediatric Dentistry, 4th edn. Oxford University Press, Oxford, pp. 174–198.

Poyser NJ, Kelleher MG, Briggs PF 2004 Managing discoloured non-vital teeth: the inside/outside bleaching technique. Dent Update 31:204–210, 213–214.

For revision, see Mind Map 36, page 257.

37

Multiple missing and abnormally shaped teeth

CASE 1

SUMMARY

Ellen is almost 11 years old. She is very concerned by the gaps between her upper and lower front teeth. She is hoping to become an actress. She is a new patient to your surgery and has been brought by her mother. What are the causes of the problem, and how may it be treated?

History

Ellen is a regular attender with no caries. Her oral hygiene is excellent. There is no history of tooth extraction in either the primary or permanent dentitions.

Medical history

Ellen has no medical problems. She is an active girl who is involved in orienteering with her family as well as participating in the local amateur dramatic society.

■ ***What question do you need to ask Ellen's mother?***

Is there a family history of missing teeth or gaps?

As you are speaking to Ellen's mother you notice that she has a missing upper right lateral incisor and the canine tooth is prominent. She confirms your question that not only has she got a missing tooth but her brother and her nephew (son of her brother) have either missing or very small upper lateral incisors.

■ ***How prevalent are missing teeth in the population?***

0.1–0.9% in the primary dentition.

3.5–6.5% in the permanent dentition (discounting third molars).

More common in females than males (1.4–4×). The most common teeth to be absent are the last teeth in each series (i.e. lateral incisor, second premolar, third molar). The presence of a conical (peg) tooth is frequently associated with a missing tooth on the opposite side of the arch. There is frequently a family history.

■ ***There are a significant number of syndromes of the head and neck that manifest with missing teeth. Can you name some?***

Ectodermal dysplasia.

Cleft lip and/or palate.

Down syndrome.

Chondro-ectodermal dysplasia (Ellis–van Creveld syndrome).

Reiger syndrome.

Incontinentia pigmenti.

Oro-facial-digital syndrome (types I and II).

Ectodermal dysplasia describes a group of inherited disorders involving ectodermally derived structures, i.e. hair, teeth, nails, skin and sweat glands. The most common form is the hypohidrotic X-linked form. The usual presentation is a male child with:

Multiple congenital absence of teeth.

Fine, sparse hair with shaft abnormalities.

Dry skin.

Frontal bossing.

Maxillary hypoplasia.

Thin lips showing little vermilion margin.

Heterozygous females can be identified dentally with microdontia and hypodontia.

Down syndrome affects 1 in 700 births, is commoner in offspring of older mothers and is a result of chromosomal translocation. Apart from the morphological features characteristic of the syndrome, there is commonly delayed eruption and generalized microdontia, as well as hypodontia of some teeth.

The diagnosis and management of all dental anomalies is extremely important and should not be delayed. Genetic consultation is often desirable to not only confirm the diagnosis but also to help parents understand the risk of future offspring and generations being affected. Conversely, geneticists may require help from paediatric dentists to clarify a diagnosis.

Key point

Hypodontia:

- Prevalence is 3.5–6.5% in permanent dentition (excepting third molar).
- May be associated with a number of syndromes.
- Requires interdisciplinary care.

■ ***What factors would you consider important in the management of dental anomalies?***

Reassurance of child and parent.

Elimination of pain.

Prevention of caries and periodontal disease.

Genetic counselling.

Restoration of aesthetics.

Provision of adequate function.

Maintenance of vertical dimension of occlusion.

Interdisciplinary formulation of definitive treatment plan.

Examination

Extraoral

Ellen had a normal facial appearance with a Class 1 skeletal pattern.

Intraoral

The following teeth were present:

$$\begin{array}{r|l} 6\,E\,D\,C\,B\,1 & 1\,B\,C\,D\,E\,6 \\ \hline 6\,E\;\;3\,2\,1 & 2\,3\,4\,E\,6 \end{array}$$

D|D were mobile. The other primary teeth were firm. The primary molars were infraoccluded.

■ ***What special investigations are required?***

A dental panoramic tomogram (**Fig. 37.1**) to check on the presence/absence of other permanent teeth.

■ ***What is visible from the radiograph?***

Absence of: $$\begin{array}{r|l} 8\,7\,5\,3\,2 & 2\,3\,4\,5\,7\,8 \\ \hline 8\,7\,5\,4 & 1\;\;\;\;5\,7 \end{array}.$$

■ ***What is the condition known as?***

It is termed severe hypodontia. This is defined as having six or more permanent teeth missing, not including the missing wisdom teeth.

■ ***What would you do?***

Take impressions and a wax registration for study models. Arrange a joint consultation with paediatric dental/orthodontic/restorative colleagues. Frequently these interdisciplinary teams discuss the cases before they see the patient. Taking facial and intraoral views as well as relevant and justifiable radiographs will all help at this planning meeting.

■ ***What treatment is likely to be required?***

- Attempt to retain the primary molars for as long as possible.
- Management of infraoccluded primary molars (see Chapter 8).
- Assess mesiodistal width 1|1. Probable addition of composite to distal aspect of these teeth to achieve mesiodistal width of 8.5–9 mm.
- Fixed appliance to close the upper median diastema; retain with a palatal bonded retainer.
- Poor prognosis B|B. As the spaces are of concern to Ellen, consider extraction of B|B and replacement with an upper partial denture with prosthetic 2|2. Alternative approaches include the extraction of the B|B and the provision of resin retained cantilever bridges. Another short- to medium-term option is to build up the primary lateral incisors with composite.
- In adulthood there will be the option of implants to replace the missing maxillary and mandibular teeth. Hence the importance of interdisciplinary planning to ensure short-term solutions do not compromise long-term plans.

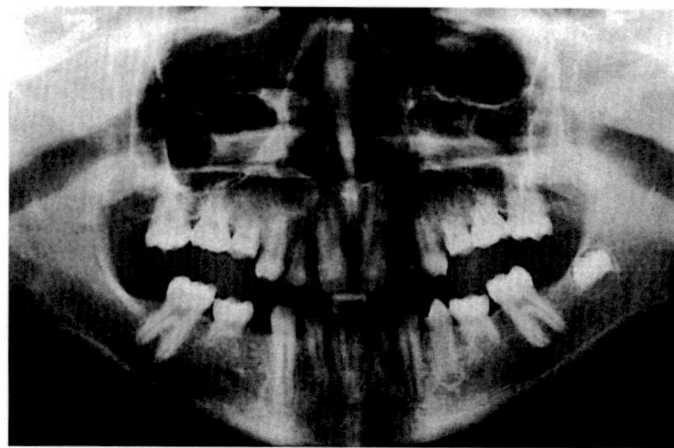

Fig. 37.1 Severe hypodontia. (from Millett and Welbury (2000) with permission).

CASE 2

SUMMARY

Cameron was 3 years old when his mother brought him to the surgery because she was concerned that two of his teeth were joined together (*Fig. 37.2*). What is the cause, and how may it be treated?

Medical and dental history

Cameron is an active child with no medical problems. He has no caries.

■ ***What can you see in*** *Fig. 37.2****?***

The crowns of the upper central and lateral primary incisors are joined together.

A number of different terms have been used to describe the process of the formation of double teeth either on the primary or permanent dentitions: fusion, gemination, dichotomy, synodontia, schizodontia and connation. The mode of development given in older textbooks for the different names are unclear and unproven. The neutral term 'double teeth' is not contentious and describes accurately what the tooth looks like clinically.

■ ***How prevalent do you think double teeth are?***

0.5–1.6% in primary dentition.

0.1–0.2% in permanent teeth.

No clear mendelian trait established.

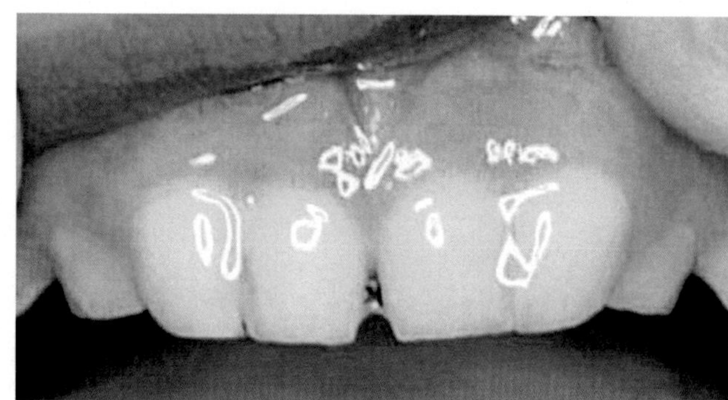

Fig. 37.2 Double incisor teeth.

The clinical manifestation of the anomaly may vary considerably from a minor notch in the incisal edge of an abnormally wide incisor crown to the appearance of two separate crowns. There may be hard tissue continuity between either the crowns or the roots of the two elements or between both. Similarly there may be one unified pulp chamber and radicular pulp or separate ones.

In the primary dentition, double teeth more commonly occur in the labial segments of the arches and most frequently in the mandible. Double permanent teeth can occur anywhere in the arch and frequently involve the incisor teeth.

What are the most important clinical aspects of a double tooth in the primary dentition?

Caries may occur in the 'join' between the two coronal elements if it is not easily accessible to a toothbrush. This risk can be reduced by fissure sealing the groove if there is food stagnation, staining or enamel decalcification.

The presence of a numerical abnormality of the permanent dentition. Counting a double tooth as one unit in the primary dentition, with relation to the total number of teeth present, may be helpful in predicting the type of numerical abnormality of the permanent dentition. Hypodontia is usually followed by missing permanent teeth. A normal number of teeth in the primary dentition is often associated with permanent supernumeraries. The overall frequency of permanent numerical abnormalities following primary double teeth is between 30% and 50% in Caucasians and is 75% in the Japanese population.

Radiography is therefore important at an appropriate time, so the parent can be advised of future treatment and prognosis and a treatment plan formulated. Extraction of double primary teeth may be necessary if physiological root resorption is significantly retarded. Surgical removal of supernumerary teeth may be required to facilitate eruption of normal units. Often treatment planning is most appropriately undertaken within an interdisciplinary team.

Key point

Double primary teeth may:

- Be associated with numerical abnormalities of the permanent dentition.
- Be a caries risk.
- Not undergo normal physiological resorption.

What are the important factors that will dictate whether you retain or extract double permanent teeth?

Space in the arch.

Aesthetics.

Morphology of pulp chambers and roots.

If the coronal parts of the double teeth are joined but the roots are separate, then it may be feasible to divide the crown and extract one portion of the crown and its root, thereby retaining the other portion of the crown with its root. The retained portion will require root canal treatment and subsequent coronal restoration.

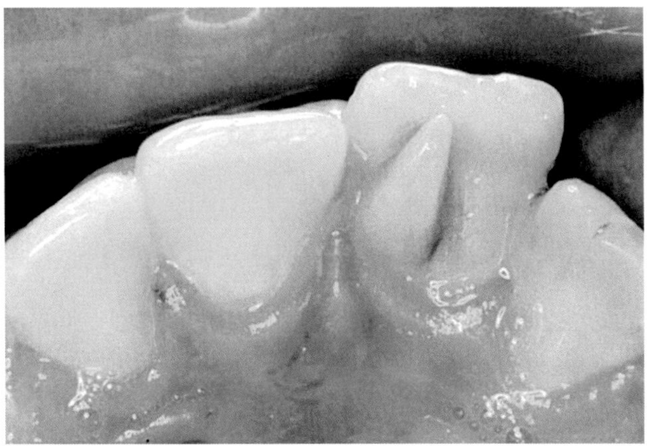

Fig. 37.3 Talon cusp.

What other types of crown abnormalities do you know?

Accessory cusps.

Invaginations.

Evaginations.

Additional primary cusps are seen on the mesiobuccal aspect of maxillary first molars and the mesiopalatal aspect of maxillary second molars.

The commonest additional cusp in permanent teeth is often on the lingual cingulum, more commonly in the maxilla than the mandible. The name 'talon cusp' is often given to the additional cusp (**Fig. 37.3**). The cusp is composed of enamel, dentine and a horn of pulp tissue. Talons in maxillary anterior teeth such as that shown in **Fig. 37.3** can cause a number of problems:

Appearance.

Occlusal interference.

Caries in the deep grooves between the cusp and the tooth.

The commonest accessory cusp in the permanent dentition is the mesiopalatal sited tubercle of Carabelli on the maxillary first molar (10–60%).

What are the treatment options for a talon cusp on a maxillary tooth?

Selective grinding of cusp to encourage obliteration of the pulp horn by secondary dentine.

Aseptic removal of the cusp under rubber dam followed by a limited pulpotomy procedure (immature or mature root).

Aseptic removal of cusp and one-stage endodontic treatment (mature root).

Failure of a pulpotomy technique in an immature tooth will result in the need for induced apical closure with Mineral Trioxide Aggregate. Many clinicians favour waiting until full root formation has occurred prior to removal of the cusp. Invaginations or invagination of the enamel epithelium into the dental papilla of the underlying tooth germ has been described as 'dens in dente', 'gestant composite odontome' and 'dilated composite odontome'. The correct descriptive term is 'dens invaginatus' or 'invaginated tooth'. The anomaly may vary clinically from a deep cingulum pit in a tooth of normal form (**Fig. 37.4**) to a tooth with grossly distorted crown and root. Invaginated teeth are relatively

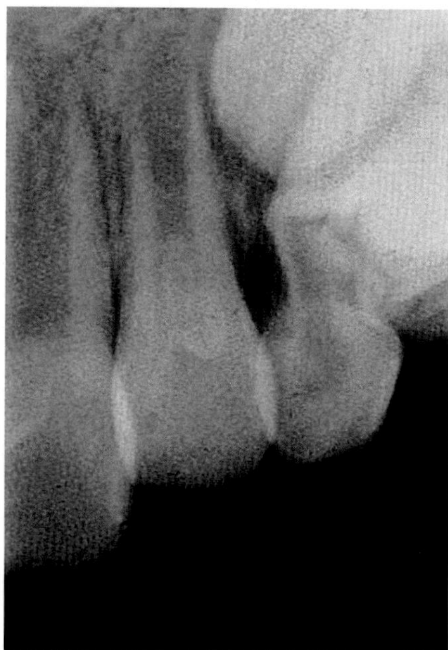

Fig. 37.4 Dens in dente of lateral incisor.

common, occurring in 1–5% of permanent teeth. Primary invaginations are rare.

The main problem with invaginations is infection. The enamel lining of the invagination is either incomplete or very thin and easily breached, resulting in dentinal caries that quickly progresses to involve the pulp causing a rapidly spreading infection presenting with acute facial cellulitis or acute dentoalveolar abscess. Rarely a large invaginated tooth may cause impaction and non-eruption of an adjacent tooth.

There is an association between invaginated teeth and supernumerary teeth. A full radiographic examination is justified if an invaginated tooth is identified.

Invaginations in crowns of normal morphology should be sealed prophylactically as soon as possible after eruption. If these 'high' invaginations do become pulpally involved then root treatment is possible, because the invaginated portion is accessible and can be removed with a crown bur allowing access to the normal root canal. All other invaginations usually require extraction owing to their complex root morphology.

'Evaginated teeth' or 'dens evaginatus' or 'tuberculated teeth' occurs commonly as a conical tubercular projection arising from the occlusal surface of the central fissure or the lingual plane of the buccal cusp. Premolar teeth are the commonest teeth affected, with permanent molars and canines less commonly affected. The condition is mainly seen in people of Mongolian race (1–4%), although rarely it is seen in Caucasians.

Evaginations consist of enamel, dentine and a pulpal extension. Evagination should be suspected if a premolar without caries develops a periapical lesion shortly after eruption.

Treatment is the same as 'talon cusp'.

■ ***What abnormalities of root form do you know?***

Taurodontism.

Accessory roots.

Pyramidal roots.

Taurodontism (bull-like teeth) applies to multirooted teeth in which the body of the tooth is enlarged coronoapically at the expense of the roots. Radiographs show apparent enlargement of the coronal pulp chamber, usually extending below the level of the alveolar crest before root division. The normal constriction at the level of the amelocemental junction is frequently absent in affected teeth. The condition is uncommon in primary teeth but may occur in permanent molars in 6% of the population.

■ ***What conditions may taurodontism be associated with?***

Amelogenesis imperfecta.

Trichodento-osseous syndrome.

Ectodermal dysplasia with hypodontia.

Ellis–van Creveld syndrome.

Achondroplasia.

Klinefelter syndrome.

Accessory roots can occur in almost any tooth. Rarely they may be due to early trauma to a forming root. The majority are likely to be due to genetic factors that remain to be specified.

Pyramidal roots describe the reduction in root number in multirooted teeth. Any molar tooth may be affected.

Primary resources and recommended reading

Holiday R, Lush N, Chapple J et al 2014 Aesthetics and function part 2: management. Dent Update 41:891–898.

Lush N, Holliday R, Chapple J et al 2014 Hypodontia: aesthetics and functions part 1: aetiology and the problems. Dent Update 41:811–815.

Millett D, Welbury R 2000 Orthodontics and Paediatric Dentistry: Colour Guide. Churchill Livingstone, Edinburgh.

Tahmassebi JF, Day PF, Toumba KJ et al 2003 Paediatric dentistry in the new millennium: 6. Dental anomalies in children. Dent Update 30:534–540.

For revision, see Mind Map 37, page 258.

38

Amelogenesis imperfecta

SUMMARY

Mark is 10 years old. He and his parents are concerned because his teeth seem rough. They also stain easily. What is the cause of these problems? What treatment is possible?

■ ***What can you see in** Fig. 38.1**?***

All erupted teeth have pitted hypoplastic enamel.

History

Mark's mother says that she noticed when the teeth first erupted that they were rough. They picked up stain and were difficult to clean. What key questions do you need to ask?

■ ***Was there any systemic illness from birth to early childhood?***

No.

■ ***Were the primary teeth similarly affected?***

There was a slight roughening of the primary teeth, although not as badly affected as the permanent teeth.

■ ***Is anyone else in the family similarly affected?***

Mark's father and his cousin (father's brother's son) have similar roughness of their teeth. After obtaining this history it is most likely that Mark has an inherited enamel defect involving enamel – amelogenesis imperfecta. However, defective enamel formation may be caused by genetic or environmental factors. The defective enamel will exhibit either hypoplasia, due to deficient matrix production, or hypomineralization, from imperfect mineralization of the matrix proteins. In hypoplasia the enamel may be thin, grooved or pitted, whereas in hypomineralization it may appear mottled but of normal thickness. The complete range of causes of developmental abnormalities of enamel are shown in **Box 38.1**.

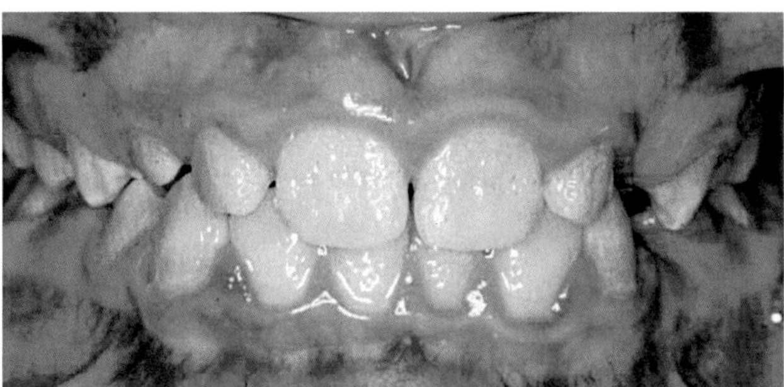

Fig. 38.1 Hypoplastic amelogenesis imperfecta.

Enamel defects of genetic origin may occur either as a phenomenon primarily involving the enamel, with possible secondary effects in other dental tissues (such as delayed eruption, anterior open bite, idopathetic resorption) and craniofacial structures (eye or hearing anomalies), or as a component of a more complex syndrome in which defective enamel is only one of a number of more generalized abnormalities.

Medical history

Mark has no medical problems. He is doing very well at school and is a keen basketball player.

Examination

Intraoral examination revealed that all the surfaces of all the erupted permanent teeth are affected by a roughness or 'pitting' (**Fig. 38.1**). The second primary molar teeth that are still present have a similar roughness that, although not as evident on visual examination, was obvious on tactile examination with a probe. There was no tooth wear.

■ ***Why is this pattern of enamel hypoplasia unlikely to be caused by systemic (chronological) influences?***

Primary and permanent teeth all affected.

All the enamel surface of the teeth is affected.

Positive family history.

Amelogenesis imperfecta (AI) occurs as a result of gene mutations that follow autosomal-dominant, autosomal-recessive or X-linked patterns of inheritance. The prevalence varies around the world with rates of 1 in 718 in northern Sweden and 1 in 14 000 in Michigan, USA. A global quoted figure is often 1 in 10 000.

Box 38.1 Differential diagnosis of enamel defects

General factors

- Genetic:
  - Primarily involving enamel – amelogenesis imperfecta.
  - Associated with generalized defects.
- Systemic (chronological):
  - Nutritional deficiencies.
  - Metabolic or biochemical disorder.
  - Toxic substances.
  - Infectious illnesses: pre-natal; peri-natal; neonatal; infancy; early childhood (see Chapter 34).
  - Excess Fluoride ingestion (see Chapter 36).
- Idiopathic.

Local factors

- Trauma.
- Infection.

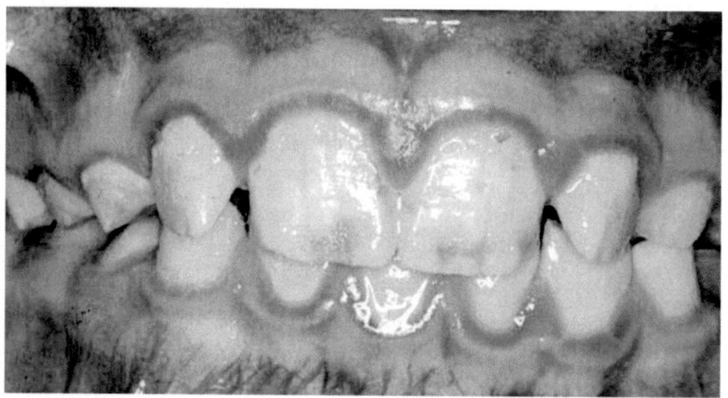

Fig. 38.2 Hypomineralized amelogenesis imperfecta.

Table 38.1 Treatment modalities for amelogenesis imperfecta

	Restoration	Aesthetics
Primary dentition: 0–5 years	Adhesive restorations	Minimal intervention
	Stainless steel crowns (SSCs) especially on E's	Composite veneers
Mixed dentition: 6–16 years	Adhesive restorations/SSCs on primary molars	Composite veneers
	SSCs/adhesive castings on permanent molars	
Permanent dentition: 16+ years	Adhesive castings on premolars	Porcelain veneers
	Full mouth rehabilitation ± crown lengthening	Full crowns

What are the main types of AI?

- Hypoplastic.
- Hypomineralized: hypocalcified or hypomature.
- Mixed pattern of both types.

Although historically, physiological categories of different types of AI were described, there is growing realization the classifications related to the genetic mutation are more appropriate. Consequently, radiographic and clinical phenotypes should simply describe their appearance (for example, hypoplastic, hypomineralized). A good diagnostic guide is to examine radiographs for unerupted teeth to identify the quantity of enamel visible and the differentiation between the enamel and dentine (e.g. the quality of mineralization). Affected teeth, once erupted into the mouth, can quickly pick up pigmentation (for example, change colour from creamy to brown), and the enamel surface can break down (giving the impression of being hypoplastic when it was originally hypomineralized). With a better understanding of the genetic mutations, the pathways through which these genes influence enamel formation is slowly being understood.

Genetic enamel defects can be associated with generalized disorders in a number of uncommon or rare genetically determined diseases and clinical syndromes. These diseases and complex syndromes include epidermolysis bullosa, tuberous sclerosis, pseudohypoparathyroidism, trichodento-osseous syndrome, oculodento-osseous dysplasia, vitamin D-dependent rickets, amelo-cerebrohypohidrotic syndrome, amelo-onychohypohidrotic syndrome and some types of mucopolysaccharidosis.

Mark has a rough, hypoplastic type of AI. An example of a hypominerliazed form of AI is shown in **Fig. 38.2**.

Investigations

What investigations are necessary?

Dental panoramic tomogram This will confirm the presence of all the permanent dentition. In addition, it will diagnose any taurodontism which is associated with some types of AI.

Family examination If it is possible to examine Mark's father's and his cousin's teeth, this will help to confirm your diagnosis.

Referral for genetic testing In the UK testing for different genetic types of AI is now available for NHS patients.

Treatment

The treatment of both amelogenesis and dentinogenesis imperfecta requires early diagnosis in order to improve the long-term prognosis of teeth. Parents need to be educated as to the implications of the condition, and prevention (diet counselling, fluoride supplementation, oral hygiene instruction (OHI)) is a crucial element in the success of any restorative treatment.

There are four main clinical problems associated with inherited enamel and dentine defects:

- Poor aesthetics.
- Chipping and attrition of the enamel.
- Exposure and attrition of the dentine causing sensitivity.
- Poor oral hygiene, gingivitis, calculus and caries.

Long-term treatment needs – this means that treatment should aim to minimize treatment in childhood to reduce burn out and potential dental anxiety.

Although it is impossible to draw up a definitive treatment plan for all cases, it is possible to define the principles of treatment planning for this group of patients. It is important to realize that not all children with amelogenesis imperfecta or dentinogenesis imperfecta are affected equally. Many will not have marked tooth wear or symptoms and will not require advanced intervention. **Table 38.1** describes the principles of treatment in terms of the age of the child/adolescent and with regard to the three aspects of care: prevention, restoration and aesthetics.

Clinicians must be very aware of the impact that AI can have on the affected child and the wider family. The poor appearance of some types of AI, especially those with brown staining, can have a significant impact on children, especially when starting at a new school and making new friends. The impact is not limited to children but also affects their families who need to take time off work to bring them to appointments and may experience possible guilt associated with genetic conditions. For a few adults with AI, the negative impact of their teeth has led them to conclude that they do not want children in case they are also affected.

Key point

Main treatment aims for dental anomalies:

- To alleviate symptoms.
- To maintain/restore occlusal height.
- To improve aesthetics.
- Try to maintain a positive dental attitude, prevent and minimize the likelihood of dental anxiety.

Mark's major concern was the staining and roughness of his front teeth. Fortunately there was no wear of his posterior teeth and his problem, therefore, was solely a cosmetic one. The pitting or hypoplasia on the upper and lower incisors can be masked by a thin, directly applied composite veneer. This should be extended to include the canines and first premolars when the arches are complete. On occasions, if the smile is a very 'wide' one, it may be necessary to include second premolars. Composite veneers can be replaced by porcelain veneers when the gingival contour has matured in late adolescence or early twenties.

If the amelogenesis had been of the hypomineralized variety with more destruction of enamel, it may have been necessary to consider full composite crowns for aesthetics in the anterior teeth and either stainless steel crowns or adhesive castings on the posterior teeth. These will need to be replaced in adolescence/early adulthood by a porcelain-bonded full crown (**Table 38.1**). A randomized controlled trial reporting on the benefits and longevity of two different types of conventional crowns has recently been published showing good efficacy for two types of crown placed in adolescence and early adulthood.

Primary resources and recommended reading

American Academy of Pediatric Dentistry 2013 Guideline on dental management of heritable dental developmental anomalies. Reference Manual 37 (6):266–271.

McDonald S, Arkutu N, Malik K et al 2012 Managing the paediatric patient with amelogenesis imperfecta. Br Dent J 212 (9):425–428.

Parekh S, Almehateb M, Cunningham SJ 2014 How do children with amelogenesis imperfecta feel about their teeth? Int J Paediatr Dent 24 (5):326–335.

Pousette Lundgren G, Morling Vestlund G, Trulsson M et al 2015 A randomized controlled trial of crown therapy in young individuals with amelogenesis imperfecta. J Dent Res 94 (8):1041–1047.

Seow WK 2014 Developmental defects of enamel and dentine: challenges for basic science research and clinical management. Aust Dent J 59 (Suppl. 1):143–154.

For revision, see Mind Map 38, page 259.

39

Dentinogenesis imperfecta

SUMMARY

Siobhan is 9 years old. She and her parents are concerned because her permanent teeth are darker than normal and she is getting teased at school. What is the cause of the discoloration? How would you treat it?

History

Siobhan's mother says she noticed that when the permanent teeth erupted they looked darker. Siobhan is very unhappy at school and refuses to smile for any photographs. When she talks she has the habit of covering her mouth with a hand so it is impossible to see her teeth. What can you see in **Fig. 39.1A**? What key questions do you need to ask?

■ ***Was there any systemic illness from birth until early childhood?***

No. Siobhan had no illness.

■ ***Were the primary teeth similarly affected?***

The primary teeth erupted normally but very quickly chipped away, becoming worn to gum level (see **Fig. 39.1B**).

■ ***Is anyone else in the family similarly affected?***

Siobhan's brother and her father have a problem with their teeth. Siobhan's brother is 14, and he has needed crowns on his back teeth and veneers on his front teeth. Siobhan's father needed a lot of treatment when he was younger and has had some teeth crowned. Many of his posterior teeth, however, were extracted.

Even before you have examined the mouth, the history suggests that Siobhan has an inherited defect. **Fig. 39.1A** confirms your suspicion that this is dentinogenesis imperfecta (DI).

■ ***Why is this DI and not amelogenesis imperfecta (AI)?***

The teeth are translucent.

The enamel is poorly adherent to the underlying dentine and easily chips and wears. The remaining primary canines and molars in **Figs 39.1A and B** are worn to gingival level and have a translucent opalescent appearance.

■ ***What investigations do you need to do to confirm your suspicions?***

Dental panoramic tomogram If this is DI, the dental panoramic radiograph will probably show the following:

- Bulbous crowns with pronounced cervical constriction.
- Shortened roots.
- Progressive pulp chamber and canal obliteration (**Fig. 39.2** (different case)).
- Spontaneous periapical abscess formation.

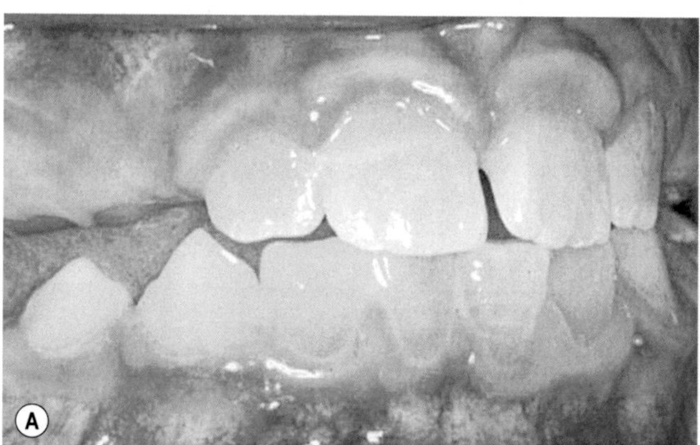

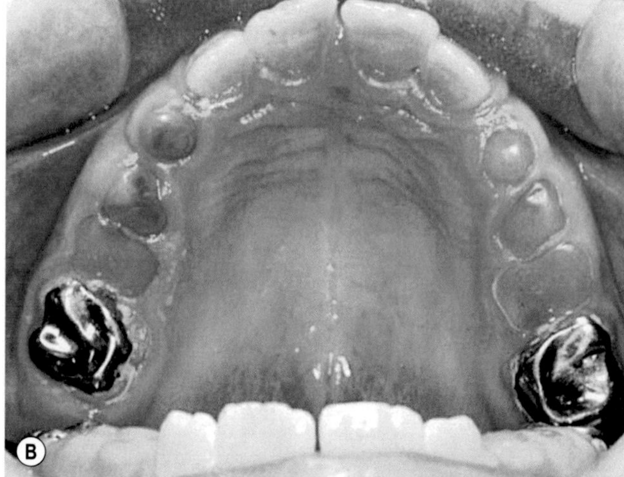

Fig. 39.1 **(A)** Dentinogenesis imperfecta. **(B)** Dentinogenesis imperfecta.

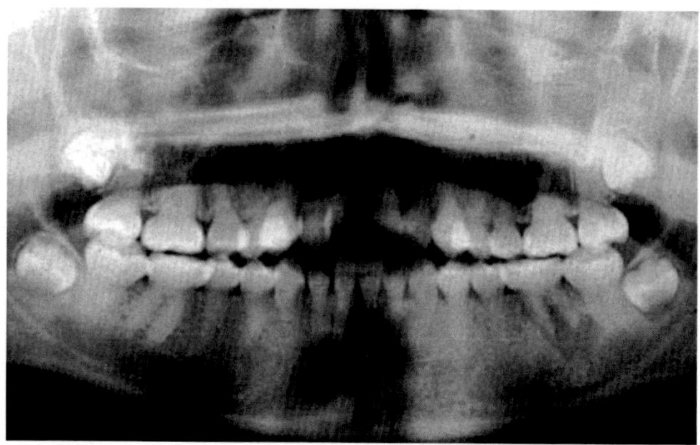

Fig. 39.2 Obliteration of root canals and pulp chambers in dentinogenesis imperfecta.

Box 39.1 Hereditary dentine defects

Limited to the dentine

- Dentinogenesis imperfecta type II (hereditary opalescent dentine).
- Dentine dysplasia type I (radicular dentine dysplasia).
- Dentine dysplasia type II (coronal dentine dysplasia).
- Fibrous dysplasia of dentine.

Associated with generalized disorder

- Osteogenesis imperfecta (dentinogenesis imperfecta type I).
- Ehlers-Danlos syndrome.
- Brachioskeletogenital syndrome.
- Vitamin D resistant rickets.
- Vitamin D dependent rickets.
- Hypophosphatasia.

Family examination

- Family examination of affected members.
- Dentine defects like those of enamel may be subdivided by cause into two main groups based on whether they are of genetic or environmental origin.
- Dentine anomalies that are genetically determined may appear to be limited to the dentition or form part of a more complex generalized disorder (**Box 39.1**).

The most well documented hereditary dentine defects are DI type II (hereditary opalescent dentine), which only affects teeth, and DI type I, in which abnormalities of teeth are associated with osteogenesis imperfecta.

DI type II Both dentitions are usually affected. The severity of the defect varies considerably between families and within families. Primary teeth tend to be more severely affected than permanent teeth, and the later forming permanent teeth may be the least affected. Enamel tends to chip away from the underlying amelodentinal junction (ADJ), exposing the abnormally soft dentine that undergoes rapid wear. This is most marked in the primary dentition where, within 2 years, the crowns may be worn to the gingival margin and appear as amber-coloured remnants (**Fig. 39.1B**), which may be frequently infected and abscessed. In the permanent dentition, following eruption, the enamel may look reasonably normal, but histological studies have shown hypomineralized areas in approximately one-third of cases. Radiographic signs are described previously. Histologically, the ADJ may appear flattened, and while the subadjacent peripheral dentine may approach normality, the remainder is grossly disordered with an amorphous matrix containing areas of interglobular calcification, abnormally shaped and sized tubules and cellular inclusions.

■ ***Is DI more prevalent than AI?***

Possibly, figures of 1 in 8000 have been estimated (AI 1:10 000).

■ ***Has DI got as many inheritance patterns as AI?***

No. Invariably it is autosomal dominant with marked expressivity and good penetrance. Two clinical variants of the condition have been described:

- *Shell teeth.* This is rare and seen in the primary dentition. The pulp remains large and the thin enamel and dentine rapidly fragments to cause pulpal infection.
- *DI type III (brandy wine type).* This was first described in Maryland, USA, and has been traced back to East Anglia in England. It was apparently taken to the USA by one of the sailors who accompanied the Pilgrim Fathers to Maryland. Type III defect has been linked to the same locus on chromosome 4q21 as DI type II.

DI type I associated with osteogenesis imperfecta Osteogenesis imperfecta is a group of connective tissue disorders involving inherited abnormalities of type I collagen. Increased bone fragility is only one aspect of the condition which may include lax joints, blue sclerae, opalescent teeth, hearing loss and a variable degree of bone deformity. The inheritance pattern is either autosomal recessive or dominant. The recessive form is often lethal around birth.

Opalescent teeth are only rarely seen in surviving recessive types. They are commonly a feature of the dominant variety with accompanying bone fragility, bone deformity and blue sclerae. Owing to the bone fragility, frequently children with osteogenesis imperfecta are treated with bisphosphonates. In adults bisphosphonates, especially those given intravenously, are associated with osteonecrosis. Although no cases of osteonecrosis have been reported in children, great care, thought and interdisciplinary working with medical colleagues is required when managing these complex children (see Chapter 28).

The primary teeth in DI type I resemble exactly those in DI type II. However, in the permanent dentition the defect is extremely variable. In many cases the upper anterior teeth may have a normal colour and appearance, whereas the lower incisors and canines are opalescent, discoloured bluish-brown and wear at the incisal edges. In most cases the enamel does not chip away from the underlying dentine as readily as in type II.

Radiographic appearances are as already described with the exception that upper teeth may retain their pulp spaces long after those in the lower jaw. Histological appearances are indistinguishable from type II.

Environmentally determined dentine defects do exist but are less well documented than corresponding anomalies of enamel: trauma, nutritional deficiencies (minerals, proteins and vitamins) and drugs (tetracycline, chemotherapeutic agents – cyclophosphamide) will likely produce increased interglobular dentine, predentine and osteoid.

Key point

Dentinogenesis imperfecta:

- Occurs in 1 in 8000 of the population.
- May be associated with osteogenesis imperfecta.

Treatment

The main clinical problems associated with AI and DI and the key points of treatment objectives are covered in Chapter 38. The principles of treatment for DI are the same as those for AI with the exception that in the permanent dentition from age 16, crown-lengthening procedures are more common in DI and the provision of overdentures and full dentures is not uncommon. The role of implants in these patients has yet to be defined.

Siobhan's major concern was of the colour of her permanent incisors. There was some wear of first permanent molars. The first permanent molars were treated with adhesive castings with micromechanical retention to luting cement (**Fig. 39.1B**). The upper and lower incisors were veneered with composite resin. This can be extended to include the canines and premolars when the arches are complete. The composite veneers can be replaced by porcelain veneers around the age of 18 years.

Young children with DI often pose the greatest problems. The primary teeth undergo such excessive wear that they become worn down to the gingival level and are unrestorable. Teeth affected by DI are also prone to spontaneous abscesses due to the progressive obliteration of the pulp chambers. In these cases pulp therapy is often unsuccessful and extraction of the affected teeth is necessary.

Early consultation with an orthodontist is advisable in inherited abnormalities of enamel and dentine in order to keep the orthodontic requirements simple. Treatment for these patients is possible and in many cases proceeds without problems. The use of removable appliances, where appropriate, and orthodontic bands rather than brackets will minimize the risk of damage to the abnormal enamel. The problem is twofold: there may be frequent bond failure during active treatment or the enamel may be further damaged during debonding. Some orthodontists prefer to use bands even for anterior teeth, while others will use glass ionomer cement as the bonding agent in preference to more conventional resin-based agents. In other instances, cosmetic restorative techniques (veneers and crowns) may be more appropriate than orthodontic treatment.

Primary resources and recommended reading

American Academy of Pediatric Dentistry 2014/2015 Guideline on dental management of heritable dental developmental anomalies. Reference Manual 36 (6):264–269.

Barron MJ, McDonnell ST, Mackie I et al 2008 Hereditary dentine disorders: dentinogenesis imperfecta and dentine dysplasia. Orphanet J Rare Dis 20 (3):31.

Dhaliwal H, McKaig S 2010 Dentinogenesis imperfecta—clinical presentation and management. Dent Update 37 (6):364–366, 369–371.

For revision, see Mind Map 39, page 260.

40

Dental erosion

SUMMARY

Tom is 9 years old. He is a new patient to your practice. On examination you are concerned by the appearance of the occlusal surfaces of his lower primary molars. What has caused this, and how may it be managed?

■ ***What do you see in** Fig. 40.1**?***

There is erosion of the cusps of Tom's primary molars giving cupping or perimolysis of the cusps with loss of enamel and visible underlying dentine.

■ ***How would you define erosion?***

An irreversible loss of tooth substance brought about by a chemical process that does not involve bacterial action.

■ ***What foods and drinks have erosive potential?***

See **Box 40.1**. While a wide range of food and drinks is implicated in the problem, the bulk of the damage is done by soft drinks, especially carbonated drinks, which are increasingly available from vending machines in schools and recreational facilities. All carbonated drinks and fruit-based drinks have lowered pH values, but the direct relationship between pH and erosion is unclear. Other factors such as titratable acidity, the influence of plaque pH and the buffering capacity of saliva will all influence the erosive potential of a substrate. Four things, however, are clear with erosive loss:

- It is worse if consumption is high.
- It is worse if consumption occurs at bedtime.
- It is worse if brushing occurs directly after consumption.
- It is worse if children undertake swishing or holding habits when drinking.

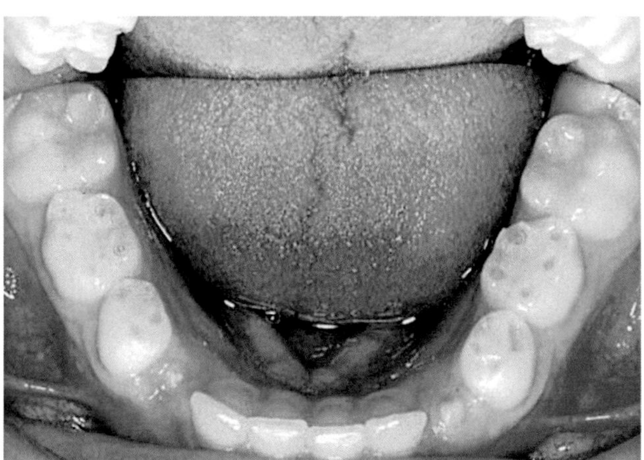

Fig. 40.1 Erosion of cusp tips of primary molars.

History

Tom's only complaint was occasional sensitivity on his back teeth as a result of the visible dentine.

■ ***What is the best way to find out about Tom's diet?***

A 4-day written dietary history is the only way to accurately elucidate constituents of the diet that may be erosive.

■ ***Can the pattern of erosion caused by dietary constituents be related to the manner in which the substrate is consumed?***

This is indeed the case. 'Frothing' of a drink between the upper anterior teeth with its retention labially can lead to palatal, interproximal and labial erosion. Retention of a drink specifically on one side of the mouth can lead to erosion on that side only.

■ ***You have covered Tom's dietary history. Is your history now complete, or are there other questions you need to ask with relation to erosion?***

It is very important to consider gastric acid as a cause of erosion, even in a younger patient. The conditions in children that are associated with chronic regurgitation are shown in **Box 40.2**. The acidity of the stomach contents is below pH 1.0 and therefore any regurgitation or vomiting is damaging to the teeth.

■ ***What question would you ask to give you an indication that regurgitation was occurring?***

'Do you ever have a bitter taste in your mouth?' There is a group of patients who have gastro-oesophageal reflux disease (GORD). This may be either symptomatic, in which the individual knows what provokes the reflux, or more insidiously, asymptomatic GORD, where the patient is unaware of the problem. The latter case is most likely to occur at night when the horizontal sleeping position makes it more likely that acid will reflux through the lower

Box 40.1 Foods and drinks with erosive potential

- Citrus fruits, e.g. lemons, oranges, grapefruits.
- Tart apples.
- Vinegar, pickles, ketchup and brown sauce.
- Yoghurt.
- All fruit juices, including fresh juice and fruit-based squashes.
- Carbonated drinks, including low-calorie varieties, 'sports drinks' and sparkling mineral water.
- Vitamin C tablets and iron preparations (some medication will cause a dry mouth thereby exacerbating other causes).

Box 40.2 Conditions associated with chronic regurgitation in children

- Gastrooesophageal reflux.
- Oesophageal stricture.
- Chronic respiratory disease, e.g. asthma.
- Disease of the liver/pancreas/biliary tree.
- Overfeeding.
- Feeding problems/failure to thrive conditions.
- Learning delay.
- Anorexia.
- Bulimia nervosa.
- Cyclic vomiting syndrome.
- Cerebral palsy.
- Rumination.

oesophageal sphincter. In this case the question about a bitter taste in the mouth should have the suffix 'when you wake up'.

■ ***What is the common pattern of erosive loss when there is chronic gastric regurgitation?***

Initially there is erosion of the palatal surfaces of the upper incisors, canines and premolars. With time this extends to the occlusal and buccal surfaces of the lower molars and premolars.

Whenever there is unexplained erosive loss, an eating disorder should be suspected. There are three such disorders: anorexia nervosa; bulimia nervosa; and rumination. The latter is a condition in which food is voluntarily regurgitated into the oral cavity and either expelled or swallowed again.

■ ***Is there a specific pattern of erosive loss in recurrent vomiting?***

All tooth surfaces can be affected with the relative exception of the lingual surfaces of the lower teeth, which are protected by the tongue and the saliva from the sublingual papillae.

■ ***What would you do if you suspect, after questioning Tom and his parents, that there may be asymptomatic GORD?***

Referral to a paediatrician with an interest in gastrointestinal disease would be appropriate. The paediatrician will seek to eliminate organic disease and then attempt to quantify the problem. The latter may involve 24-hour pH monitoring of the oesophagus, with probes in the lower and upper oesophagus. An additional probe could be added to an intraoral appliance to measure mouth pH. Medical and/or surgical treatment may be required to control GORD. Chronic regurgitation can lead to scarring of the oesophagus and dysplastic change, and this is therefore an important condition to diagnose and treat. In such cases medication or surgery are indicated to prevent regurgitation.

Summary of Tom's history There was no evidence of any gastrointestinal illness, but Tom did consume a number of fizzy drinks, especially between meals and when he was at the local sports centre. In addition to these, he rarely drank water and milk.

■ ***What advice would you give to Tom regarding his high intake of fizzy drinks?***

It is critically important when dealing with children and adolescents not to be too dogmatic in your advice, and it is unrealistic to expect youngsters who have been brought up with a high intake of carbonated beverages to stop altogether.

They should be advised to eradicate between-meal fizzy drink consumption but to have the fizzy drink with meals and preferably to drink it with a straw. The presence of food, and the extra saliva that is generated at mealtimes, will help neutralize the acidity. In addition, a straw will deposit the majority of the carbonated beverage beyond the teeth.

Make sure that the between-meal carbonated drink is not substituted by something with a similar erosive potential, e.g. fresh fruit juice or a juice-based squash.

Milk and water are the most appropriate between-meal drinks. If either of these proves impossible, then an extremely well-diluted 'no added sugar' squash can be accepted.

No carbonated drinks or fruit drinks should be given last thing at night.

Advocate the consumption of a neutral food immediately after a meal, e.g. cheese.

Management

The most important aspect of the management of Tom's erosion was early diagnosis before there had been damage to the permanent teeth, and subsequently to establish the aetiology and eliminate the cause.

Key point

Management of erosion:

- Early diagnosis.
- Establish aetiology.
- Eliminate cause.
- Monitor for further tooth surface loss.

■ ***Tom only has occasional sensitivity. What treatment, if any, does he need?***

Probably none. The following would be realistic initially:

Daily neutral sodium fluoride mouthwash (0.05%) to maximize the resistance to remaining enamel and desensitize the dentine.

High concentration sodium fluoride varnish (Duraphat) to be applied three to four times a year.

High fluoride toothpaste (2800 ppm for children aged 10 years and older, 5000 pmm for children aged 16 years and older).

If there is progressive sensitivity then the areas of enamel loss and dentine exposure could be protected by an adhesive restoration. In many cases, if erosion is diagnosed early then preventive counselling and the above advice may be sufficient. It is a good idea to take photographs and make study casts of all patients with signs of erosion or attrition or abrasion to monitor the rate of progression. In more advanced cases than Tom's, as in **Figs 40.2A and B**, where there are significant sensitivity or cosmetic problems, more active intervention is required. **Table 40.1** shows the merits of the different options available.

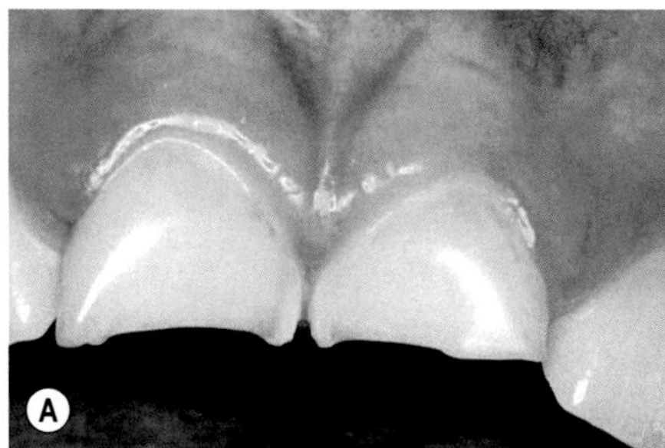

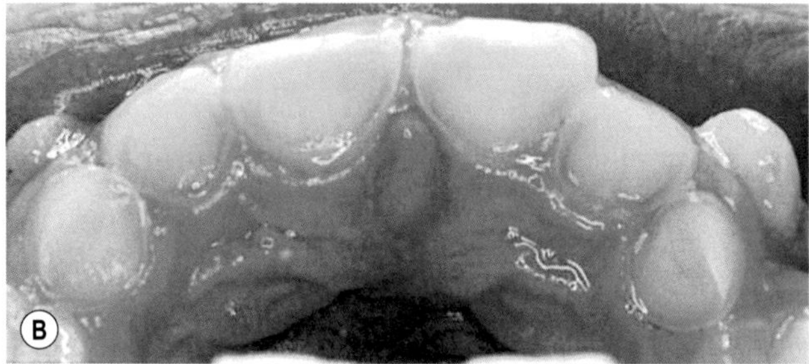

Fig. 40.2 **(A)** Significant erosive tooth surface loss of labial surfaces of upper permanent incisors. **(B)** Significant erosive tooth surface loss of palatal surfaces of upper permanent incisors.

Table 40.1 Treatment techniques for tooth surface loss

Technique	Advantages	Disadvantages
Cast metal (nickel/chrome or gold)	Fabricated in thin section – requires only 0.5 mm space	May be cosmetically unacceptable due to the 'shine through' of metallic grey
	Very accurate fit possible	Cannot be simply repaired or added to intraorally
	Very durable	
	Suitable for posterior restorations in parafunction	
	Does not abrade opposing dentition	
Composite: direct	Least expensive	Technically difficult for palatal veneers
	Can be added to and repaired intraorally	Limited control over occlusal and interproximal contour
	Aesthetically superior to cast metal	Inadequate as a posterior restoration
Composite: indirect	Can be added to and repaired intraorally	Requires more space – minimum of 1.0 mm
	Aesthetically superior to cast metal	Unproven durability
	Control over occlusal contour and vertical dimension	
Porcelain	Best aesthetics	Potentially abrasive to opposing dentition
	Good abrasion resistance	Inferior marginal fit
	Well-tolerated by gingival tissues	Very brittle – has to be used in bulk section
		Hard to repair

Key point

Treatment objectives for erosion:

- Resolve sensitivity.
- Restore missing tooth surface.
- Prevent further tooth tissue loss.
- Maintain a balanced occlusion.

■ *Erosion is only one element of tooth surface loss or wear. What are the other elements?*

Attrition: the wear of the tooth as a result of tooth-to-tooth contact.

Abrasion: physical wear of tooth substance produced by something other than tooth-to-tooth contact.

In children, abrasion is usually due to overzealous toothbrushing, which tends to develop with increasing age. The abnormal brushing technique must be corrected before significant tooth tissue is removed and pulpal exposure occurs. Attrition caused by normal mastication is common, especially with the ageing primary dentition. Almost all primary teeth show signs of attrition by the time they exfoliate.

■ *What categories of patient exhibit more attrition than normal?*

Those with significant parafunctional activity, e.g. cerebral palsy and other physical and developmental disorders with intracranial abnormalities. Controlling attritional wear in these patients can be very difficult. Some drugs act to try to reduce such parafunctional activity, but even if this is successful in the limbs, there is often still residual oral parafunction. This is probably due to the neuronal sensitivity of the mouth and the structures within it. For children with profound neurological conditions who struggle to communicate, grinding is very common. If parents present with an increase in frequency or durations of grinding, a thorough oral examination is essential to eliminate any intraoral pathology and/or pain which may have led to this activity.

■ *What restorative materials are the most durable for attritional wear as a result of parafunction?*

Amalgam and stainless steel crowns. Careful consideration when using these materials is necessary, as occlusal derangement may exacerbate parafuctional habits. One research paper identified higher levels of stainless steel crown failure in children with developmental disabilities, which they suggested may related to bruxist habits.

Primary resources and recommended reading

Kilpatrick NM, Burbridge LA 2012 Anomalies of tooth formation and eruption. In: Welbury RR, Duggal MS, Hosey MT (eds), Paediatric Dentistry, 4th ed. Oxford University Press, Oxford.

Ng MW, Tate AR, Needleman HL et al 2001 The influence of medical history on restorative procedure failure rates following dental rehabilitation. Pediatr Dent 23:487–490.

O'Sullivan E, Barry S, Milosevic A, 2013 Diagnosis, Prevention and Management of Dental Erosion. London: Royal College of Surgeons. Available at: <http://www.rcseng.ac.uk/fds/publications-clinical-guidelines/clinical_guidelines/documents/diagnosis-prevention-and-management-of-dental-erosion.

For revision, see Mind Map 40, page 261.

41

Gingival bleeding and enlargement

SUMMARY

Kayleigh is 15 years old. She is concerned that her upper gums look abnormal, and they bleed whenever she brushes them** (Fig. 41.1)**.

History

Kayleigh has noticed bleeding when she has been brushing for the last year. She is frightened of brushing because of the bleeding and feels that it is getting worse. She is also very socially conscious of her gums because they look very red and are 'bigger' than normal.

Medical history

Kayleigh has insulin-dependent diabetes. She takes her insulin by subcutaneous injection at 07.30 and 17.30 hours. She has a regulated gram intake of carbohydrate at 07.30, 11.00, 13.00, 15.00, 17.30 and 21.00 hours. Apart from this, she is an active girl who plays basketball and hockey at school and has learnt to increase her carbohydrate intake appropriately to cover her sporting activities. Her mum reports that Kayleigh has had the occasional 'rebellion' against her condition and at these times diabetic control has been poor, but generally her control is now good with a stable regimen. She is seen every 2 months by her doctor, and she monitors her blood glucose and urinary glucose at home herself.

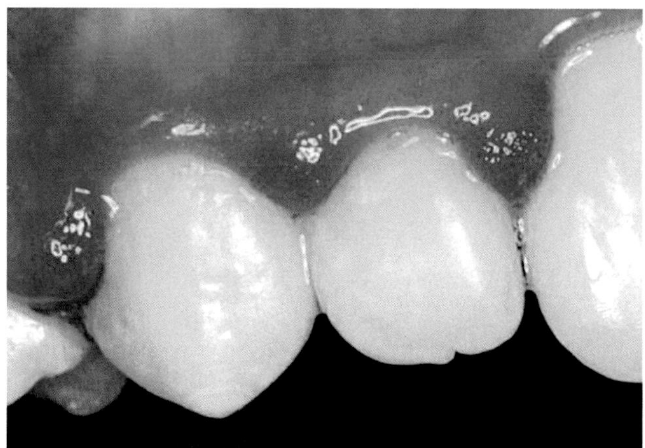

Fig. 41.1 Chronic gingivitis.

Dental history

Kayleigh and her family are regular dental attenders and have just moved to the area with her father's job. This is the first time you have seen her.

Examination

Extraoral examination is normal, with no signs of infection. Intraorally there is widespread marginal gingivitis, which is particularly bad in the upper right quadrant anteriorly (**Fig. 41.1**). Clinical and radiographic examinations of the teeth reveal a low caries rate, with only the need to replace a cracked and deficient restoration in a lower first permanent molar that has recurrent caries.

■ ***What periodontal screening should be undertaken for Kayleigh?***

Periodontal screening should be undertaken for all children over the age of 7 years. For children in the mixed dentition (e.g. 7–12 years old) a simplified basic periodontal examination (BPE) is recommended. BPE is measured at six points (mesiobuccal, buccal, distobuccal, distolingual, lingual and mesiolingual) on six index teeth ($\frac{6\,1\,|\,6}{6\,|\,1\,6}$), and only codes 0, 1 and 2 are used. For older children (13–17 years old) the same index teeth are measured in the same way, but a full range of codes (0, 1, 2, 3 and 4) are used. Any scores over 2 require further investigation, including a full pocket charting for all teeth and, where indicated, referral to specialist care.

■ ***What factors are contributing to the chronic marginal gingivitis?***

Poor oral hygiene.

Hormonal changes of puberty.

Poorly controlled diabetes mellitus.

> **Key point**
>
> Gingival bleeding can be as a result of:
> - Local causes.
> - Systemic causes.

The commonest local and systemic causes of gingival bleeding in childhood/adolescence are shown in **Box 41.1**.

■ ***What do you think may have precipitated the initial gingivitis?***

This is likely to have coincided with one of the periods where diabetic control was poor. Further questioning revealed that about a year ago Kayleigh was struggling to come to terms with her insulin-dependent diabetes. She refused to take her insulin regularly and ended up being admitted to hospital in coma with ketoacidosis. Her blood

Box 41.1 Commonest causes of gingival bleeding in childhood and adolescence

Local causes

- Eruption gingivitis.
- Acute/chronic gingivitis.
- Chronic periodontitis.
- Foreign body entrapment.
- Acute necrotizing ulcerative gingivitis.
- Haemangioma.
- Reactive hyperplasias, such as pyogenic granuloma.
- Factitial injury.

Systemic causes

- Hormonal changes such as pregnancy or puberty.
- Diabetes mellitus – poor control.
- Anaemia.
- Leukaemia.
- Any platelet disorder.
- Clotting defects.
- Drugs (e.g. anticoagulants).
- Scurvy.
- Human immunodeficiency virus-associated periodontal disease.

sugar at that time was very high and her breath smelt of 'pear drops' due to ketone bodies. This was a hyperglycaemic coma. She was resuscitated with intravenous fluids, as she was severely dehydrated, prior to restabilization on an insulin regimen.

■ ***What is the other cause of diabetic coma and what are its signs?***

Hypoglycaemic coma occurs due to inadequate carbohydrate intake (missed meal), exercise or excess insulin. The onset is quicker than the hyperglycaemic coma. The signs of hypoglycaemic coma are very similar to having 'a drink too many', and can be summarized into those caused by adrenaline release and cerebral hypoglycaemia:

Adrenaline release:

- Sweaty warm skin.
- Rapid bounding pulse.
- Dilated (reacting pupils).
- Anxiety, tremor.
- Tingling around mouth.

Cerebral hypoglycaemia:

- Confusion, disorientation.
- Headache.
- Dysarthria.
- Unconsciousness.
- Focal neurological signs, e.g. fits.

If an individual having a hypoglycaemic episode is conscious, they should be given sugar orally – 25 g glucose. In many emergency drug boxes are sachets of thick glucose syrup, which can be slowly squirted under the tongue. If comatosed, they require 20 mg of 20% dextrose intravenously, followed by 25 g orally on arousal. Alternatively, if intravenous access is difficult, give 1 mg intramuscularly of glucagon. In practical terms, 10 g glucose approximates to:

2 tsp sugar.

3 lumps sugar.

3 Dextrosol tablets.

60 ml Lucozade.

15 ml Ribena (full sugar type).

90 ml cola (not diet variety).

⅓ pint of milk.

Treatment

Kayleigh's gingivitis probably started as a result of poor diabetic control and unfortunately has been compounded by poor oral hygiene and the hormonal changes of puberty.

■ ***Why is the gingivitis worst in the anterior part of the upper right quadrant?***

She is right-handed, and this is often the case when a right-handed person changes their brushing action from the left hand side of the mouth to the right hand side. The opposite would be true for the left-hander.

■ ***What other generalized causes of gingival enlargement do you know?***

There are a number of causes, which can be classified into congenital and acquired (**Box 41.2**).

■ ***Why is it important to eradicate Kayleigh's gingivitis?***

Poor oral hygiene in combination with diabetes can result in rapid periodontal destruction and attachment loss. An example of this in another subject with diabetes is shown in **Fig. 41.2**. There is some evidence that significant periodontitis can upset glycaemic control.

Kayleigh needs reassurance that the bleeding will reduce and stop when her oral hygiene improves. She needs to appreciate the importance of good oral hygiene and the problems that will occur if oral hygiene is poor.

■ ***Why is it important not to leave caries in a diabetic?***

Infection of any origin can result in an increased need for insulin. Without an insulin increase there will be a rise in blood sugar resulting in ketosis. Therefore all infections in a diabetic, including those in the orofacial region, should be treated vigorously with antibiotics. Caries should be treated early to prevent pulpal necrosis and subsequent infection.

Key point

In diabetics:

- Poor oral hygiene will accelerate attachment loss.
- Infection can interfere with diabetic control.

■ ***Why is the timing of the appointment to restore Kayleigh's first permanent molar important?***

To not interfere with Kayleigh's carbohydrate intake and precipitate hypoglycaemia, it is probably best to give her an

Box 41.2 Systemic causes of gingival enlargement

Congenital

- Hereditary gingival fibromatosis.
- Mucopolysaccharidoses.
- Infantile systemic hyalinosis.

Acquired

- Puberty/pregnancy gingivitis.
- Plasma cell gingivitis.
- Infections: herpes simplex virus.
- Haematological: acute myeloid leukaemia, preleukaemic leukaemia, aplastic anaemia, vitamin C deficiency (scurvy).
- Drugs: phenytoin, cyclosporin, calcium-channel blockers, vigabatrin.
- Deposits: mucocutaneous amyloidosis.
- Chronic granulomatous disorders: sarcoidosis, Crohn disease, orofacial granulomatosis.

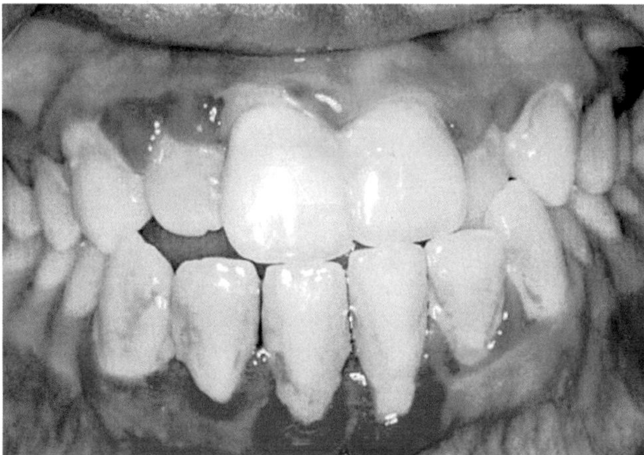

Fig. 41.2 Gingival and periodontal disease.

appointment either first thing in the morning or directly after lunch. For any prolonged surgical procedure in a diabetic person, or any treatment that requires general anaesthesia (GA), a referral to hospital is required. GA will require admission pre-operatively to stabilize insulin and glucose requirements via a drip so that hypoglycaemic coma does not occur with pre-operative GA starvation.

■ ***What dietary advice should you give to diabetic patients?***

Do not change your required carbohydrate intakes, as these are critical to diabetic control.

Tailor the dental advice to the specific needs of the patient, i.e. take your toothbrush to school if possible. Try to clean your teeth after snacks and at lunchtime. Try to take snacks that provide the necessary sugar but do not remain stuck to the teeth. Use sugar-free gum if it is not possible to brush the teeth during the day. In summary, changing dietary sugar intake or frequency is difficult and therefore attention should be concentrated on increasing the frequency of toothbrushing, strength of fluoride toothpaste (e.g. 2800 ppm for Kayleigh, increasing to 5000 ppm when she is 16 years old) and the effectiveness of brushing.

■ ***What other oral manifestations can occur in diabetes?***

Dry mouth.

Swelling of salivary glands (sialosis).

Glossitis.

Burning of tongue.

Oral candidosis if control is poor.

These manifestations are more commonly seen in adults.

Primary resources and recommended reading

Chapple ILC, Wilson NHF 2014 Manifesto for a paradigm shift: periodontal health for a better life. Br Dent J 216:159–162.

Clerehugh V 2008 Periodontal diseases in children and adolescents. Br Dent J 204:469–471.

Clerehugh V, Kindelan S 2011 Guidelines for periodontal screening and management of children and adolescents under 18 years of Age. London. Available at: http://www.bsperio.org.uk/publications/downloads/54_090016_bsp_bspd-perio-guidelines-for-the-under-18s-2012.pdf.

Firatli E, Yilmaz O, Onan U 1996 The relationship between clinical attachment loss and the duration of insulin dependent diabetes mellitus (IDDM) in children and adolescents. J Clin Periodontol 23:362–366.

Karjalainen KM, Knuuttila MLE, Kaar M-L 1997 Relationship between caries and level of metabolic balance in children and adolescents with insulin-dependent diabetes mellitus. Caries Res 31:13–18.

For revision, see Mind Map 41, page 262.

42

Oral ulceration

SUMMARY

Alan is 8 years old. He has been brought to the surgery by his mother because his mouth is so painful he cannot eat (*Fig. 42.1*). What could cause this problem? How would you treat it?

History

Alan has not been well for a couple of weeks. He had a 'virus' that resulted in his being put to bed and missing school. Just as he was improving, his mouth became very sore. He has been unable to eat solid food for 3 days and has been on liquids only. He feels hot and lethargic. His gums bleed when he tries to brush them.

Medical history

Alan is generally a healthy boy. He has had a couple of courses of antibiotics for ear infections but has had no real illnesses. He has never been in hospital and is not on any tablets or medicines from his doctor.

■ ***Describe the appearance of the upper and lower gingivae in* Fig. 42.1*.***

There is erythematous gingival enlargement with small ulcerations of the gingival margin.

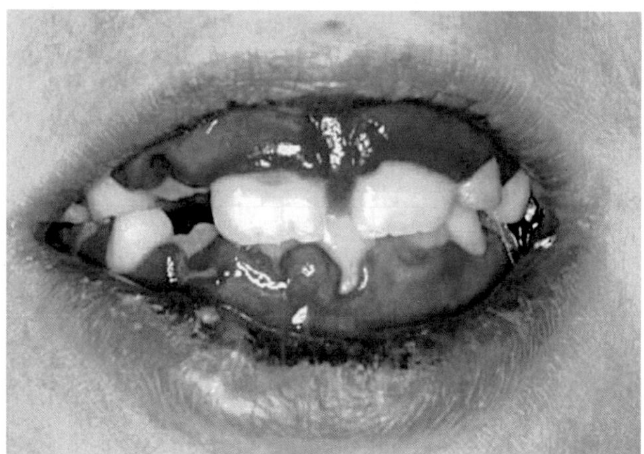

Fig. 42.1 Gingival enlargement and ulceration.

■ ***What is the diagnosis?***

Primary herpetic gingivostomatitis.

There are two types of herpes simplex virus: herpes simplex type 1 (HSV-1) and herpes simplex type 2 (HSV-2). Classically HSV-1 causes oral disease and HSV-2 causes genital disease. The viruses, however, are very similar, and both can cause both oral and genital disease, although there are differences in recurrence rates. Primary exposure to HSV in the mouth causes acute primary herpetic gingivostomatitis (**Fig. 42.1**). The virus causes a viraemia, fever, malaise and lymphadenopathy. All the surfaces of the mouth, including the hard palate and attached gingiva, can be involved initially with a vesicular rash that ulcerates and can become superinfected. The illness lasts for 10–14 days before resolving spontaneously. Diagnosis is usually made on clinical grounds but can be confirmed by a threefold rise in the convalescent antibody titre over that seen in the acute phase or by direct immunofluorescence of vesicular fluid using specific antisera.

Key point

Systemic signs in HSV:

- Fever.
- Malaise.
- Lymphadenopathy.
- Difficulty eating and drinking.

The primary infection may be mild and subclinical in the majority of young children who are exposed to it, though the condition may be severe and debilitating. In an immunocompromised individual, it may lead to severe illness and sometimes herpetic hepatitis or encephalitis, which may be fatal in the absence of treatment.

Oral infection arises from direct contact with secretions from an individual who has either primary or recurrent HSV infection. Direct inoculation of the fingers or skin with virally contaminated secretions or fluid can lead to local infection, e.g. herpetic whitlow of the finger.

HSV is a neurogenic virus, and on recovery from the primary infection the virus may become latent within the trigeminal ganglion or basal ganglia of the brain and may subsequently be reactivated to cause a secondary infection. The secondary infection may cause a 'cold sore' on the lip or Bell's palsy. Best practice for patients presenting with a cold sore for regular dental treatment (e.g. not in acute pain) is to rebook them once the lesion has disappeared. When a cold sore is present, there is increased risk to the patient of exacerbating the infection and infecting one or more members of the dental team (eye infection).

Treatment

Alan responded well to rehydration and analgesia such as paracetamol, which is also antipyretic, and an antiseptic mouthwash such as chlorhexidine (Corsodyl) or benzydamine hydrochloride (Difflam). Had Alan not been able to maintain hydration, he would have had to be admitted for intravenous fluid therapy. There is no evidence that systemic aciclovir is of any benefit at the relatively late stage of the condition that he presented. If he had been seen within 72 hours of the onset of the infection and the clinical severity warranted it, aciclovir could have been prescribed. The dose is 200 mg five times daily for 5 days in patients over 2 years of age and 100 mg five times daily for 2 days in patients under 2 years of age. Although aciclovir can shorten the course of the primary infection, there is no evidence that it reduces the incidence of recurrent herpetic lesions.

What are the reasons given for the reactivation of HSV to produce a cold sore (herpes labialis) (Fig. 42.2)?

See **Box 42.1**.

How should herpes labialis be treated?

Apply aciclovir 5% cream to the lip lesion as soon as tingling or prickling of the prodromal phase is felt. This is usually 24 hours prior to vesiculation and pain.

What other viral infection can occur in the mouths of paediatric patients?

Varicella zoster virus (VZV). VZV is a neurogenic DNA virus that causes a primary infection in the form of chickenpox. Thereafter it remains dormant until reactivation as shingles.

Epstein–Barr virus (EBV). EBV is a herpes virus with a predilection for infecting B lymphocytes. This infection causes the B lymphocytes to become activated and produce their own antibodies. A primary infection with EBV causes glandular fever or infectious mononucleosis.

Cytomegalovirus. This is associated with a glandular fever-like illness in childhood. On occasion it is found in severe atypical oral ulceration in human immunodeficiency virus (HIV).

Herpes virus type 8. This has been demonstrated in Kaposi sarcoma in HIV infection.

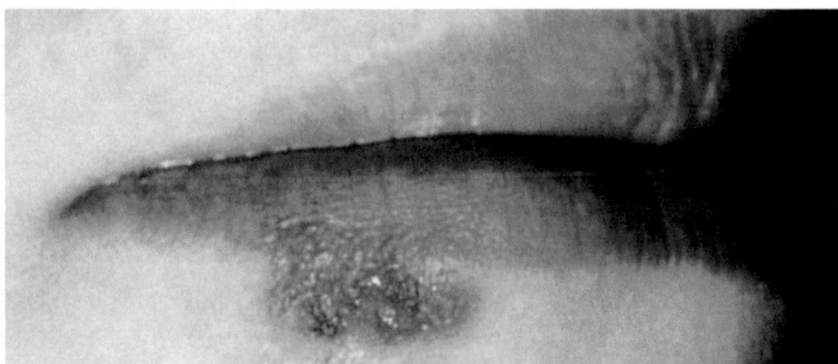

Fig. 42.2 Recurrent herpes 'cold sore'.

Box 42.1 Reactivation of HSV

- Trauma.
- Chemicals.
- Heat.
- Hormones.
- Sunlight.
- Emotion.
- Immunosuppression.
- Concurrent infection.

Coxsackie viruses. These are RNA viruses and responsible for herpangina and hand, foot and mouth disease.

Herpangina is a Coxsackie A virus that causes a herpes-like oropharyngitis where the ulceration is predominantly on the tonsil, soft palate and uvula. The mild illness is associated with fever and malaise but only persists for a few days.

Hand, foot and mouth disease is also Coxsackie A virus and occurs predominantly in children and their families. The condition is characterized by ulceration affecting the gingiva, tongue, cheeks and palate. It is associated with vesicles and ulcers on the palms and soles. It may persist for 2 weeks.

Human papilloma virus (HPV). An increasing number of HPV types have been identified. Types 2 and 4, the common wart, occur in children usually due to autoinoculation by biting fingers or hand warts. Condyloma acuminata or venereal warts can occur on the oral mucosa and are associated with HPV types 6, 11 and 60.

There are a number of other causes of oral ulceration in children and adolescents that are not associated with infections. These are shown in **Box 42.2**.

What types of aphthae are there?

Minor.

Major.

Herpetiform.

Behçet syndrome.

Recurrent aphthae affect up to 20% of the population.

Minor aphthae are commonest and account for 85% of recurrent aphthae. Ulcers are less than 1 cm in diameter, usually only 2–3 mm. They occur singly or in crops of up to 10, last 3 days to 3 weeks and heal without scarring. Ulcers are round or oval with a yellowish-grey base and surrounded by an erythematous halo. They affect only non-keratinized mucosa.

Major aphthae are more severe and usually more than 1 cm in diameter with an irregular outline. They are usually single and often affect the fauces. They are often deeper and bleed, and may last for several weeks or months before healing with scarring. Again, they tend to affect non-keratinized mucosa.

Herpetiform aphthae look similar to primary herpes. The ulcers are 1–2 mm in diameter and large numbers may occur simultaneously. They last from 2 days to 2 weeks before healing without scar formation. Again they affect only non-keratinized mucosa.

Box 42.2 Other causes of oral ulceration

- Aphthae.
- Gastrointestinal disease.
- Haematological disease.
- Infections.
- Mucocutaneous disorders.
- Radiotherapy.
- Trauma.
- Carcinoma.

Box 42.3 Common aetiological factors in recurrent aphthae in children

Host factors

- Genetics.
- Nutrition.
- Systemic disease.
- Immunity.

Environmental factors

- Trauma.
- Allergy.
- Infection.
- Stress.

Box 42.4 Dietary allergens in recurrent aphthae

- Cheese.
- Chocolate.
- Nuts.
- Tomatoes.
- Citrus fruits.
- Benzoates.
- Cinnamon aldehyde.

Behçet syndrome describes the triad of oral and genital ulceration and anterior uveitis. It is rare in the UK and USA.

What aetiological factors are important in recurrent aphthae?

See **Box 42.3**. Although only 20% of the population experience recurrent aphthae, there is a positive family history in 50% of fathers and 60% of mothers. There is, in addition, a weak human leucocyte antigen (HLA) association with HLA types A2 and B12.

Nutritional deficiencies of iron, folic acid and B_{12} can occur singly or in combination. Many of these are latent and have a normal peripheral blood picture. It is necessary to assay individual levels of ferritin, folic acid and vitamin B_{12}, as well as do a full blood count (FBC).

What systemic diseases in children are commonly associated with aphthae?

Coeliac disease.

Crohn disease.

Ulcerative colitis.

In older patients and less commonly in children, aphthae may also be associated with pernicious anaemia, HIV infection and malabsorption.

There is an increasing awareness of the role of dietary allergens in recurrent aphthae in children. Dietary allergens implicated in recurrent aphthae are shown in **Box 42.4**.

Box 42.5 Therapy for recurrent aphthae

Topical

- Coating agents (Gelclair, Orabase).
- Antimicrobials (chlorhexidene mouthwash, tetracycline mouthwash).
- Corticosteroids (beclomethasone inhaler spray, betamethasone mouthwash, triamcinolone dental paste).
- Local analgesics (lidocaine spray, lidocaine ice lolly, topical benzocaine (20%).

Systemic

- Systemic corticosteroids.
- Colchicine.
- Thalidomide.

Patients usually develop fresh ulceration within 12–24 hours of ingesting the suspect food. Foods may be identified more objectively by patch testing. Dietary avoidance is often attended by clinical improvement.

Key point

Aetiological factors in recurrent aphthae:

- Host related.
- Environment related.

Treatment of recurrent aphthae can be grouped into topical and systemic medication depending on the severity and frequency of the ulceration (**Box 42.5**).

Primary resources and recommended reading

Al Johani KA, Moles DR, Hodgson TA et al 2010 Orofacial granulomatosis: clinical features and long-term outcome of therapy. J Am Acad Dermatol 62:611–620.

Montgomery-Cranny JA, Wallace A, Rogers HJ et al 2015 Management of recurrent aphthous stomatitis in children. Dent Update 42:564–566, 69–72.

Scully C, Welbury R, Flaitz C, et al 2002 A Color Atlas of Orofacial Health and Disease in Children and Adolescents, 2nd ed. Martin Dunitz, London.

Scottish Dental Clinical Effectiveness Program (SDCEP) 2011 Drug Prescribing for Dentistry, 2nd ed. SDCEP, Dundee. Available at: http://www.sdcep.org.uk/published-guidance/drug-prescribing/.

For revision, see Mind Map 42, page 263.

43

Mind maps

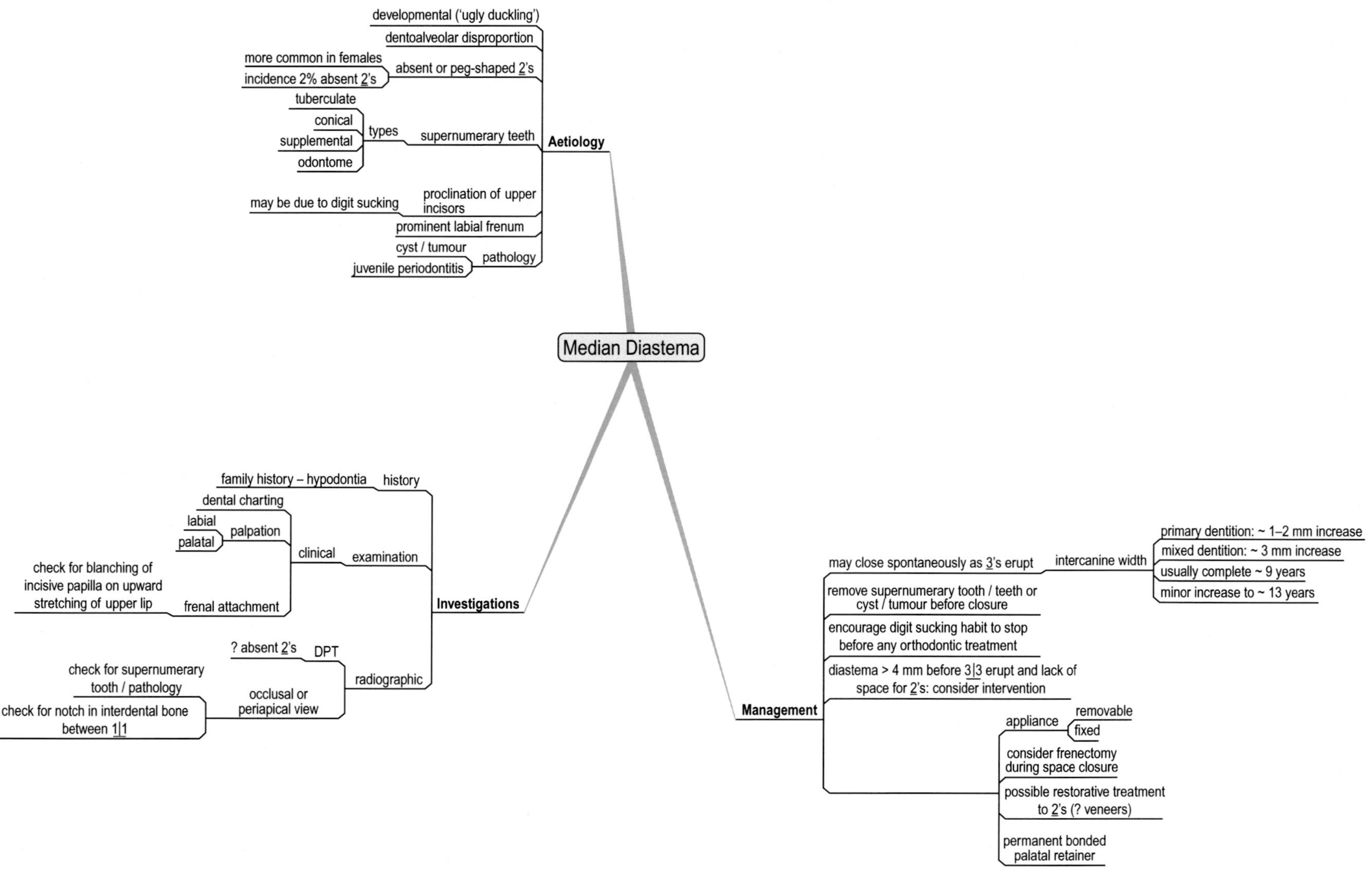
Median Diastema
Aetiology
developmental ('ugly duckling')
dentoalveolar disproportion
absent or peg-shaped 2's
more common in females
incidence 2% absent 2's
supernumerary teeth
types
tuberculate
conical
supplemental
odontome
proclination of upper incisors
may be due to digit sucking
prominent labial frenum
pathology
cyst / tumour
juvenile periodontitis
Investigations
history
family history – hypodontia
examination
clinical
dental charting
palpation
labial
palatal
frenal attachment
check for blanching of incisive papilla on upward stretching of upper lip
radiographic
DPT
? absent 2's
occlusal or periapical view
check for supernumerary tooth / pathology
check for notch in interdental bone between 1|1
Management
may close spontaneously as 3's erupt
intercanine width
primary dentition: ~ 1–2 mm increase
mixed dentition: ~ 3 mm increase
usually complete ~ 9 years
minor increase to ~ 13 years
remove supernumerary tooth / teeth or cyst / tumour before closure
encourage digit sucking habit to stop before any orthodontic treatment
diastema > 4 mm before 3|3 erupt and lack of space for 2's: consider intervention
appliance
removable
fixed
consider frenectomy during space closure
possible restorative treatment to 2's (? veneers)
permanent bonded palatal retainer

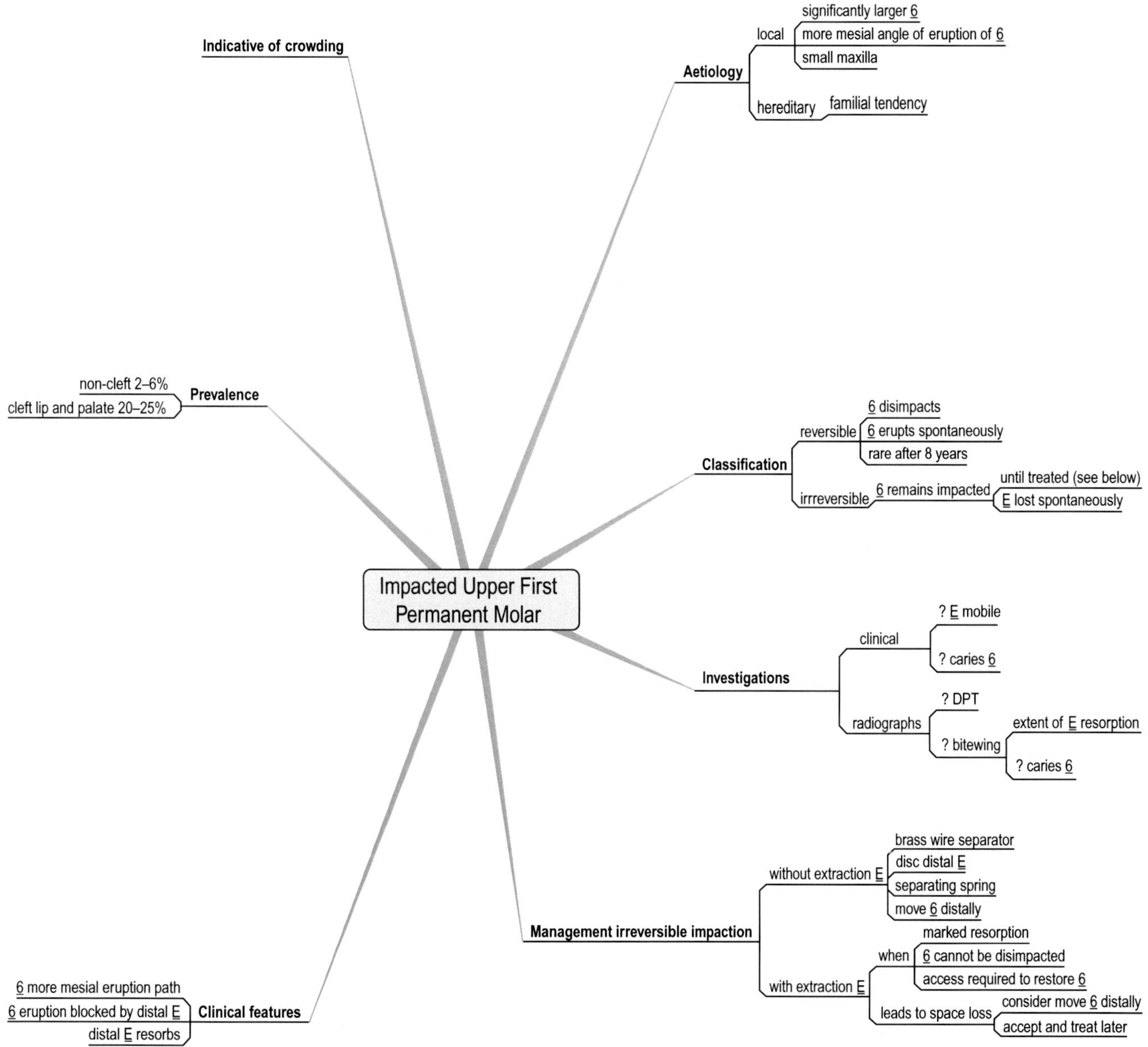
Impacted Upper First Permanent Molar
Indicative of crowding
Aetiology
local
significantly larger 6
more mesial angle of eruption of 6
small maxilla
hereditary
familial tendency
Prevalence
non-cleft 2–6%
cleft lip and palate 20–25%
Classification
reversible
6 disimpacts
6 erupts spontaneously
rare after 8 years
irrreversible
6 remains impacted
until treated (see below)
E lost spontaneously
Investigations
clinical
? E mobile
? caries 6
radiographs
? DPT
? bitewing
extent of E resorption
? caries 6
Management irreversible impaction
without extraction E
brass wire separator
disc distal E
separating spring
move 6 distally
with extraction E
when
marked resorption
6 cannot be disimpacted
access required to restore 6
leads to space loss
consider move 6 distally
accept and treat later
Clinical features
6 more mesial eruption path
6 eruption blocked by distal E
distal E resorbs

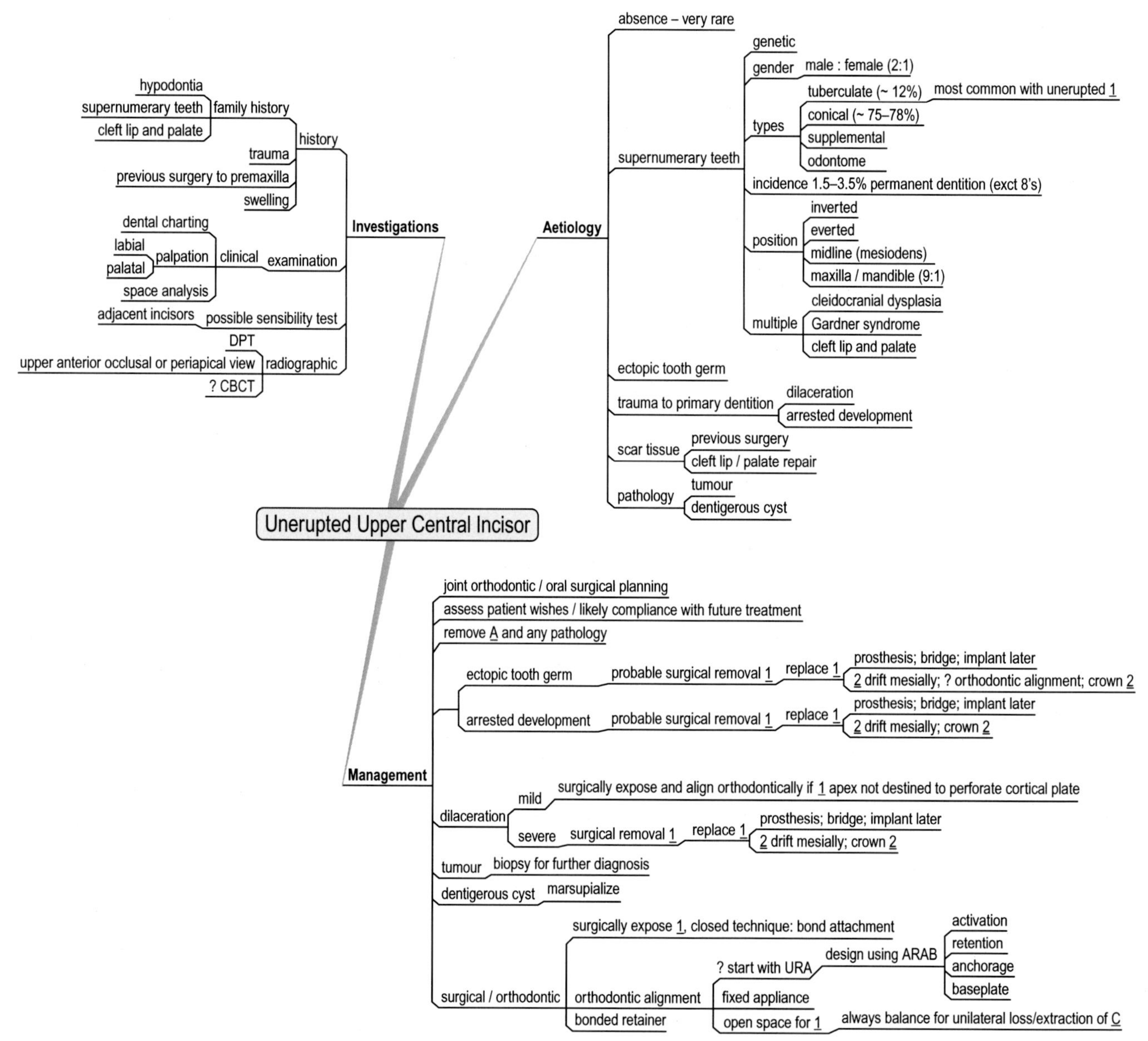
Unerupted Upper Central Incisor
Investigations
history
family history
hypodontia
supernumerary teeth
cleft lip and palate
trauma
previous surgery to premaxilla
swelling
examination
clinical
dental charting
palpation
labial
palatal
space analysis
possible sensibility test
adjacent incisors
radiographic
DPT
upper anterior occlusal or periapical view
? CBCT
Aetiology
absence – very rare
supernumerary teeth
genetic
gender
male : female (2:1)
types
tuberculate (~ 12%)
most common with unerupted 1
conical (~ 75–78%)
supplemental
odontome
incidence 1.5–3.5% permanent dentition (exct 8's)
position
inverted
everted
midline (mesiodens)
maxilla / mandible (9:1)
multiple
cleidocranial dysplasia
Gardner syndrome
cleft lip and palate
ectopic tooth germ
trauma to primary dentition
dilaceration
arrested development
scar tissue
previous surgery
cleft lip / palate repair
pathology
tumour
dentigerous cyst
Management
joint orthodontic / oral surgical planning
assess patient wishes / likely compliance with future treatment
remove A and any pathology
ectopic tooth germ
probable surgical removal 1
replace 1
prosthesis; bridge; implant later
2 drift mesially; ? orthodontic alignment; crown 2
arrested development
probable surgical removal 1
replace 1
prosthesis; bridge; implant later
2 drift mesially; crown 2
dilaceration
mild
surgically expose and align orthodontically if 1 apex not destined to perforate cortical plate
severe
surgical removal 1
replace 1
prosthesis; bridge; implant later
2 drift mesially; crown 2
tumour
biopsy for further diagnosis
dentigerous cyst
marsupialize
surgical / orthodontic
surgically expose 1, closed technique: bond attachment
orthodontic alignment
? start with URA
design using ARAB
activation
retention
anchorage
baseplate
fixed appliance
open space for 1
always balance for unilateral loss/extraction of C
bonded retainer

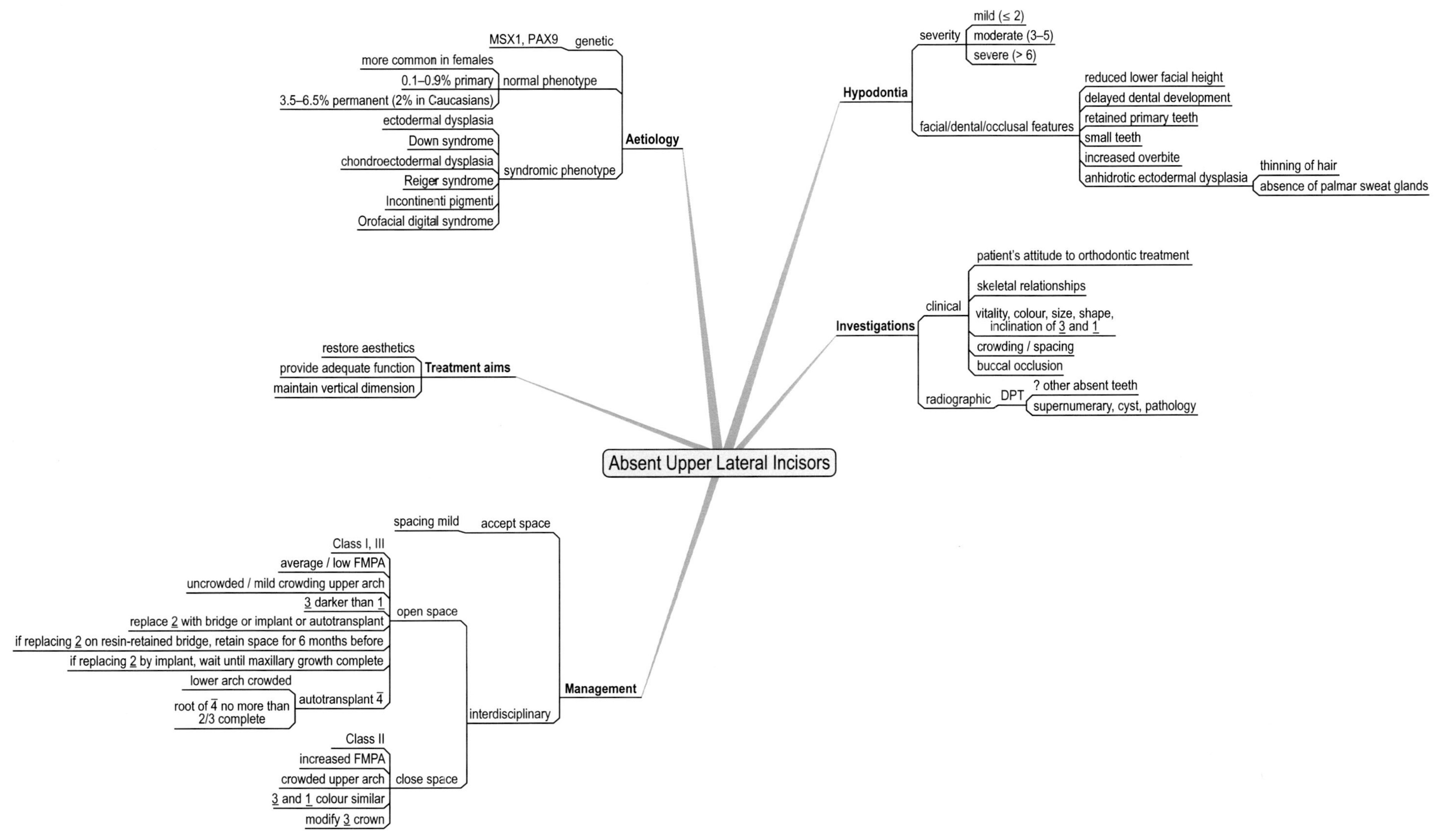
Absent Upper Lateral Incisors
Aetiology
genetic
MSX1, PAX9
normal phenotype
more common in females
0.1–0.9% primary
3.5–6.5% permanent (2% in Caucasians)
syndromic phenotype
ectodermal dysplasia
Down syndrome
chondroectodermal dysplasia
Reiger syndrome
Incontinenti pigmenti
Orofacial digital syndrome
Hypodontia
severity
mild (≤ 2)
moderate (3–5)
severe (> 6)
facial/dental/occlusal features
reduced lower facial height
delayed dental development
retained primary teeth
small teeth
increased overbite
anhidrotic ectodermal dysplasia
thinning of hair
absence of palmar sweat glands
Investigations
clinical
patient's attitude to orthodontic treatment
skeletal relationships
vitality, colour, size, shape, inclination of 3 and 1
crowding / spacing
buccal occlusion
radiographic
DPT
? other absent teeth
supernumerary, cyst, pathology
Treatment aims
restore aesthetics
provide adequate function
maintain vertical dimension
Management
accept space
spacing mild
interdisciplinary
open space
Class I, III
average / low FMPA
uncrowded / mild crowding upper arch
3 darker than 1
replace 2 with bridge or implant or autotransplant
if replacing 2 on resin-retained bridge, retain space for 6 months before
if replacing 2 by implant, wait until maxillary growth complete
autotransplant 4
lower arch crowded
root of 4 no more than 2/3 complete
close space
Class II
increased FMPA
crowded upper arch
3 and 1 colour similar
modify 3 crown

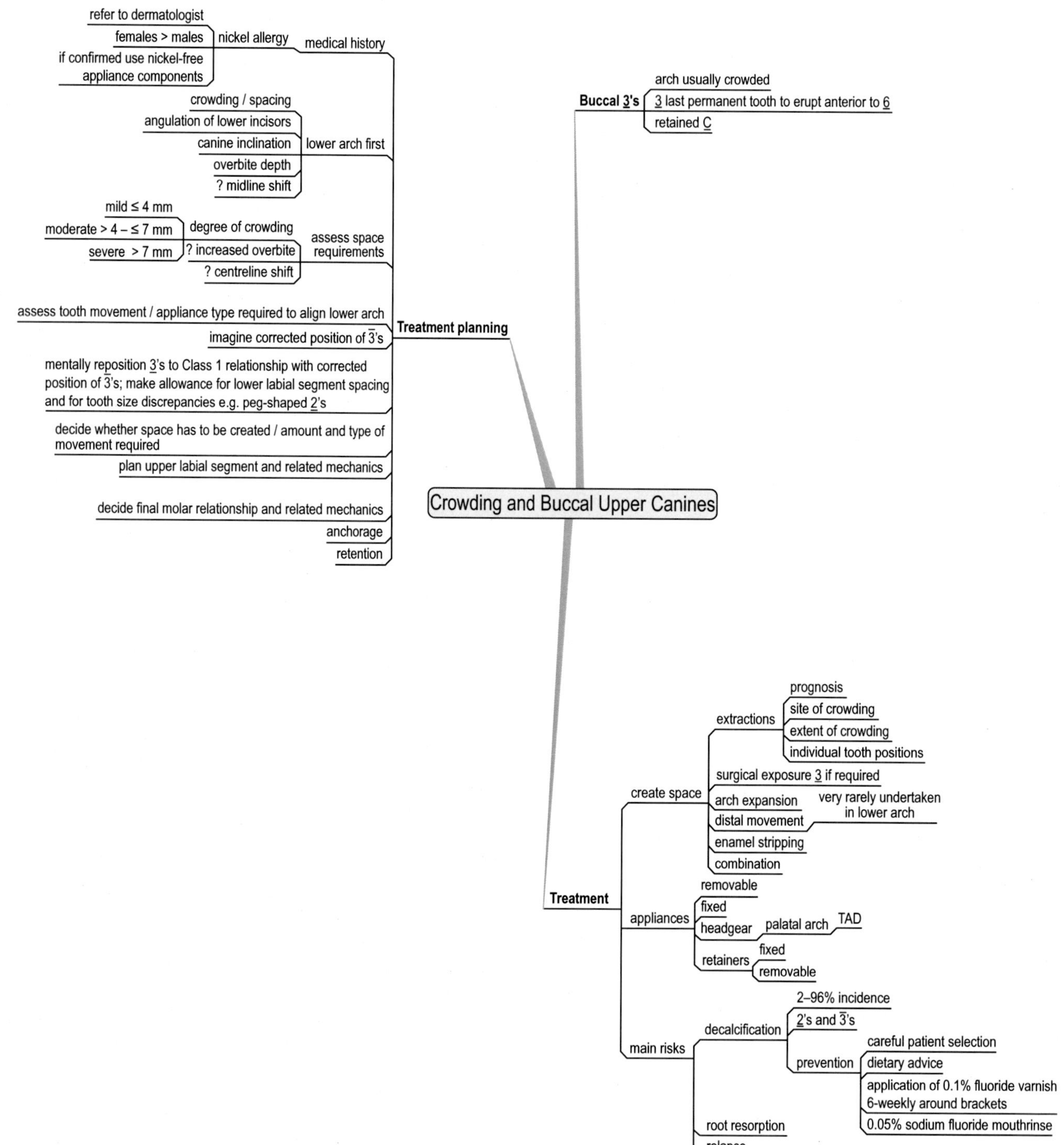
Crowding and Buccal Upper Canines
Buccal 3's
arch usually crowded
3 last permanent tooth to erupt anterior to 6
retained C
Treatment planning
medical history
nickel allergy
refer to dermatologist
females > males
if confirmed use nickel-free appliance components
lower arch first
crowding / spacing
angulation of lower incisors
canine inclination
overbite depth
? midline shift
assess space requirements
degree of crowding
mild ≤ 4 mm
moderate > 4 – ≤ 7 mm
severe > 7 mm
? increased overbite
? centreline shift
assess tooth movement / appliance type required to align lower arch
imagine corrected position of 3's
mentally reposition 3's to Class 1 relationship with corrected position of 3's; make allowance for lower labial segment spacing and for tooth size discrepancies e.g. peg-shaped 2's
decide whether space has to be created / amount and type of movement required
plan upper labial segment and related mechanics
decide final molar relationship and related mechanics
anchorage
retention
Treatment
create space
extractions
prognosis
site of crowding
extent of crowding
individual tooth positions
surgical exposure 3 if required
arch expansion
distal movement
very rarely undertaken in lower arch
enamel stripping
combination
appliances
removable
fixed
headgear
palatal arch
TAD
retainers
fixed
removable
main risks
decalcification
2–96% incidence
2's and 3's
prevention
careful patient selection
dietary advice
application of 0.1% fluoride varnish 6-weekly around brackets
0.05% sodium fluoride mouthrinse
root resorption
relapse

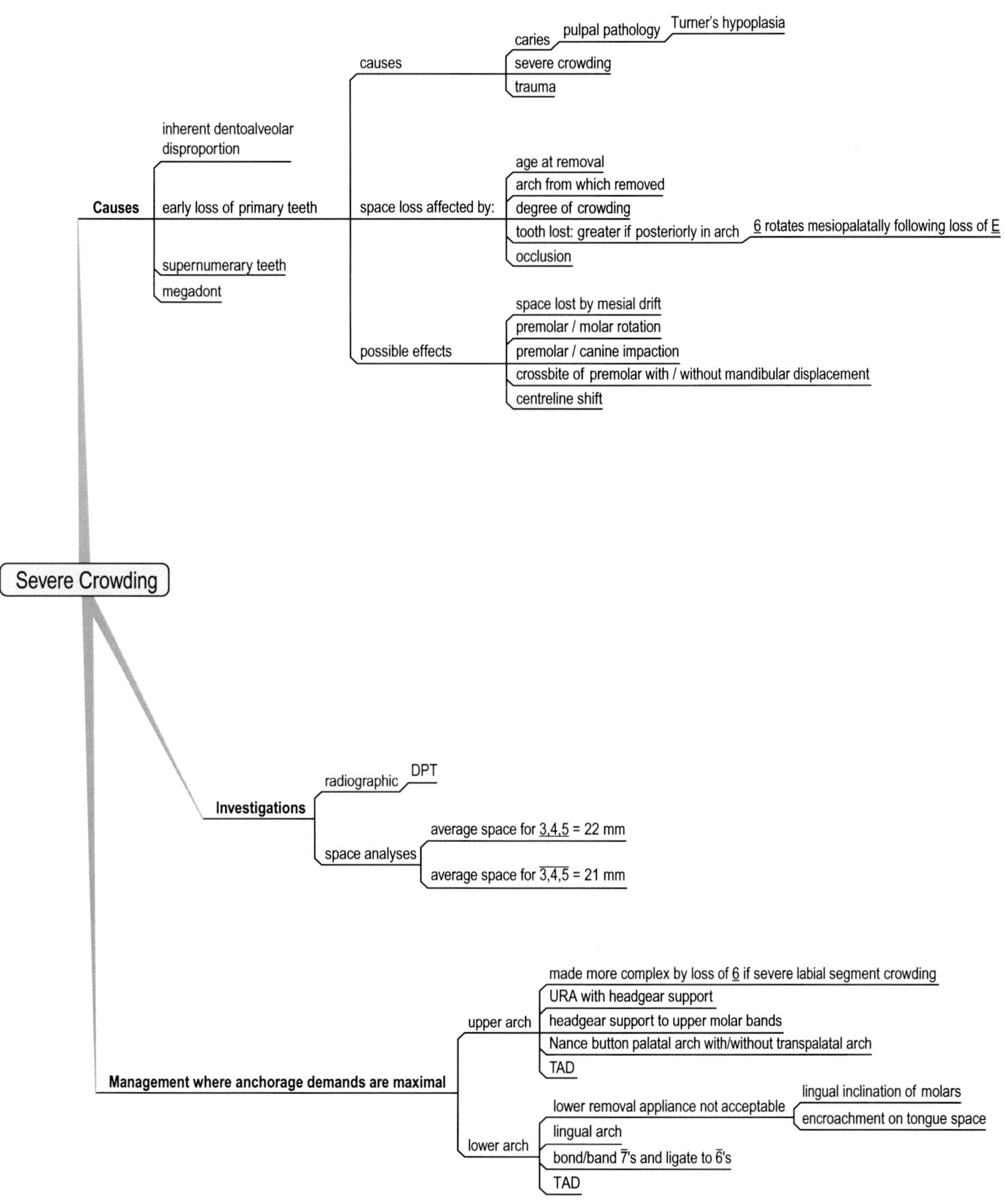
Severe Crowding
Causes
inherent dentoalveolar disproportion
early loss of primary teeth
supernumerary teeth
megadont
causes
caries
pulpal pathology
Turner's hypoplasia
severe crowding
trauma
space loss affected by:
age at removal
arch from which removed
degree of crowding
tooth lost: greater if posteriorly in arch
6 rotates mesiopalatally following loss of E
occlusion
possible effects
space lost by mesial drift
premolar / molar rotation
premolar / canine impaction
crossbite of premolar with / without mandibular displacement
centreline shift
Investigations
radiographic
DPT
space analyses
average space for 3,4,5 = 22 mm
average space for 3,4,5 = 21 mm
Management where anchorage demands are maximal
upper arch
made more complex by loss of 6 if severe labial segment crowding
URA with headgear support
headgear support to upper molar bands
Nance button palatal arch with/without transpalatal arch
TAD
lower arch
lower removal appliance not acceptable
lingual inclination of molars
encroachment on tongue space
lingual arch
bond/band 7's and ligate to 6's
TAD

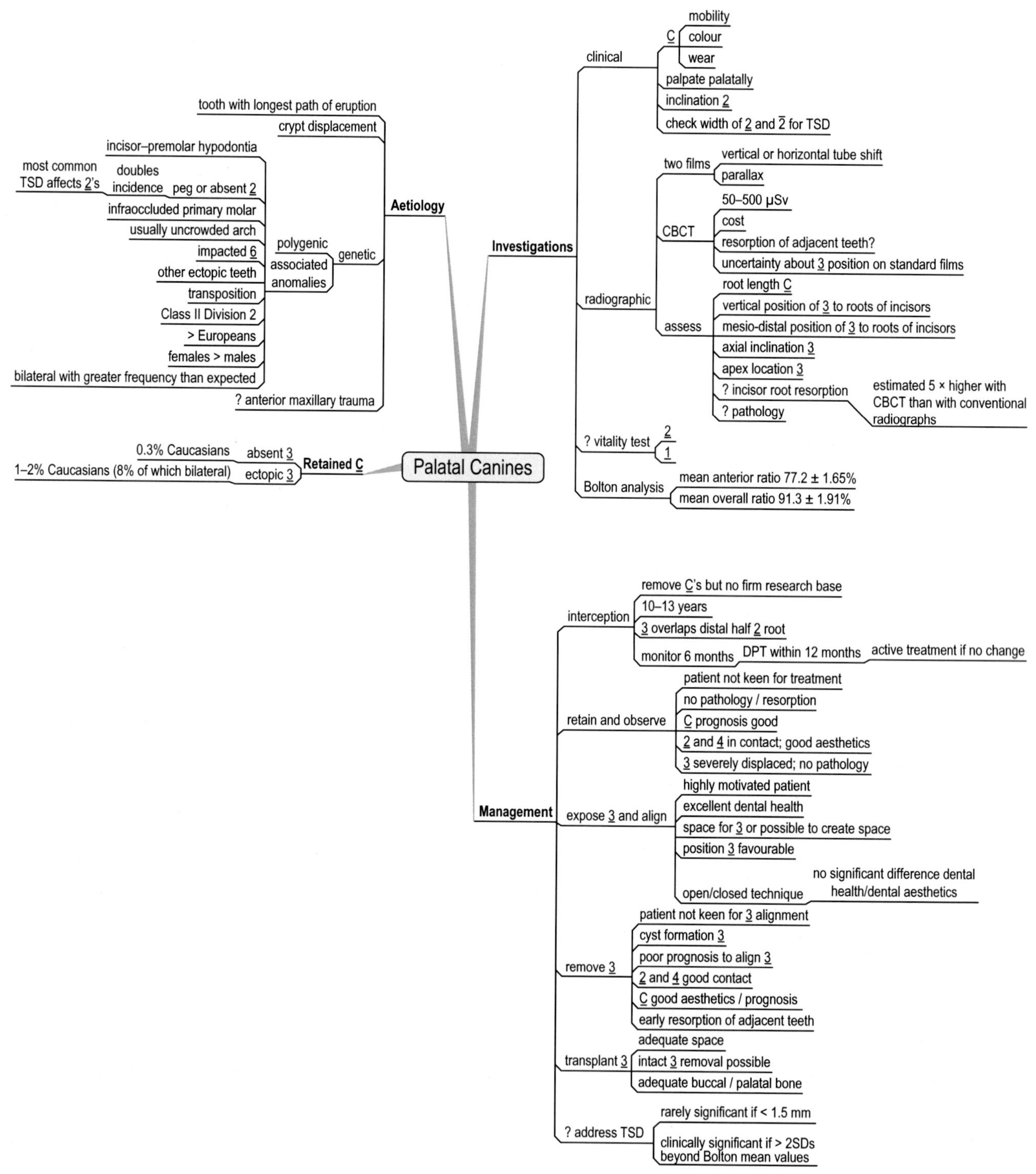
Palatal Canines
Aetiology
tooth with longest path of eruption
crypt displacement
genetic
polygenic
associated anomalies
incisor–premolar hypodontia
most common TSD affects 2's
doubles incidence
peg or absent 2
infraoccluded primary molar
usually uncrowded arch
impacted 6
other ectopic teeth
transposition
Class II Division 2
> Europeans
females > males
bilateral with greater frequency than expected
? anterior maxillary trauma
Retained C
absent 3
0.3% Caucasians
ectopic 3
1–2% Caucasians (8% of which bilateral)
Investigations
clinical
C
mobility
colour
wear
palpate palatally
inclination 2
check width of 2 and 2 for TSD
radiographic
two films
vertical or horizontal tube shift
parallax
CBCT
50–500 μSv
cost
resorption of adjacent teeth?
uncertainty about 3 position on standard films
assess
root length C
vertical position of 3 to roots of incisors
mesio-distal position of 3 to roots of incisors
axial inclination 3
apex location 3
? incisor root resorption
estimated 5 × higher with CBCT than with conventional radiographs
? pathology
? vitality test
2
1
Bolton analysis
mean anterior ratio 77.2 ± 1.65%
mean overall ratio 91.3 ± 1.91%
Management
interception
remove C's but no firm research base
10–13 years
3 overlaps distal half 2 root
monitor 6 months
DPT within 12 months
active treatment if no change
retain and observe
patient not keen for treatment
no pathology / resorption
C prognosis good
2 and 4 in contact; good aesthetics
3 severely displaced; no pathology
expose 3 and align
highly motivated patient
excellent dental health
space for 3 or possible to create space
position 3 favourable
open/closed technique
no significant difference dental health/dental aesthetics
remove 3
patient not keen for 3 alignment
cyst formation 3
poor prognosis to align 3
2 and 4 good contact
C good aesthetics / prognosis
early resorption of adjacent teeth
transplant 3
adequate space
intact 3 removal possible
adequate buccal / palatal bone
? address TSD
rarely significant if < 1.5 mm
clinically significant if > 2SDs beyond Bolton mean values

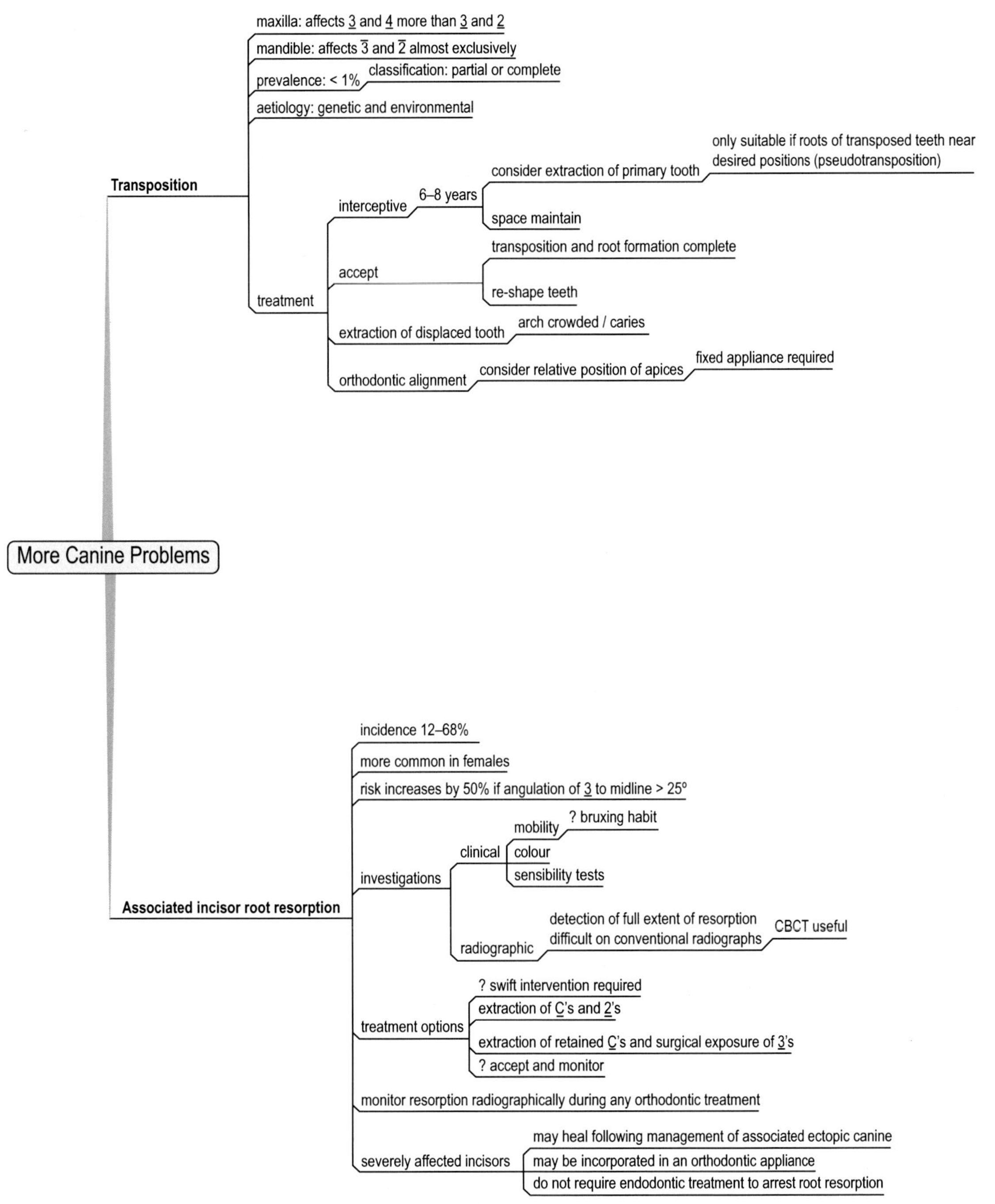
More Canine Problems
Transposition
maxilla: affects 3 and 4 more than 3 and 2
mandible: affects 3 and 2 almost exclusively
prevalence: < 1%
classification: partial or complete
aetiology: genetic and environmental
treatment
interceptive
6–8 years
consider extraction of primary tooth
only suitable if roots of transposed teeth near desired positions (pseudotransposition)
space maintain
accept
transposition and root formation complete
re-shape teeth
extraction of displaced tooth
arch crowded / caries
orthodontic alignment
consider relative position of apices
fixed appliance required
Associated incisor root resorption
incidence 12–68%
more common in females
risk increases by 50% if angulation of 3 to midline > 25°
investigations
clinical
mobility
? bruxing habit
colour
sensibility tests
radiographic
detection of full extent of resorption difficult on conventional radiographs
CBCT useful
treatment options
? swift intervention required
extraction of C's and 2's
extraction of retained C's and surgical exposure of 3's
? accept and monitor
monitor resorption radiographically during any orthodontic treatment
severely affected incisors
may heal following management of associated ectopic canine
may be incorporated in an orthodontic appliance
do not require endodontic treatment to arrest root resorption

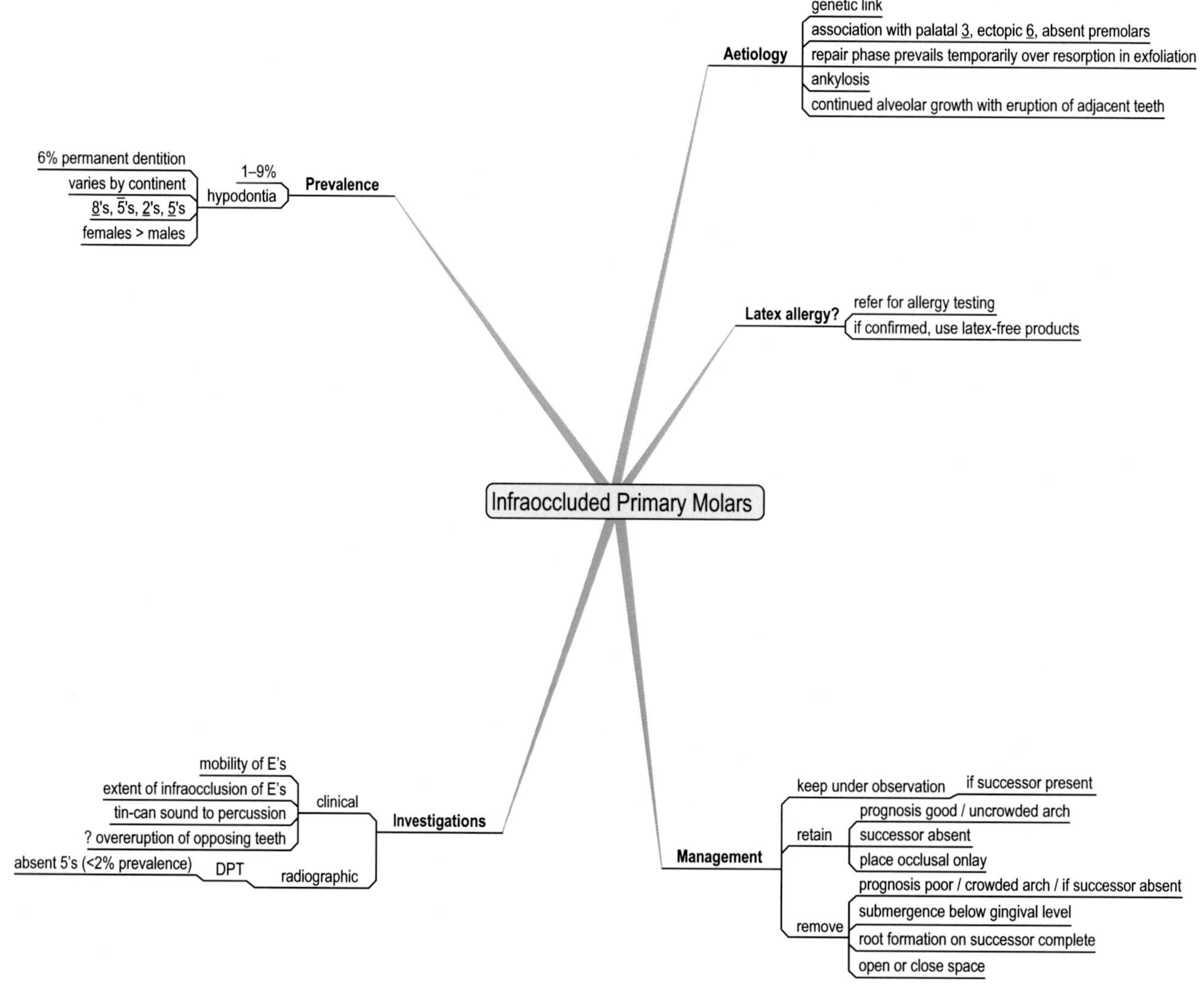
Infraoccluded Primary Molars
Aetiology
genetic link
association with palatal 3, ectopic 6, absent premolars
repair phase prevails temporarily over resorption in exfoliation
ankylosis
continued alveolar growth with eruption of adjacent teeth
Prevalence
1–9%
hypodontia
6% permanent dentition
varies by continent
8's, 5's, 2's, 5's
females > males
Latex allergy?
refer for allergy testing
if confirmed, use latex-free products
Investigations
clinical
mobility of E's
extent of infraocclusion of E's
tin-can sound to percussion
? overeruption of opposing teeth
radiographic
DPT
absent 5's (<2% prevalence)
Management
keep under observation
if successor present
retain
prognosis good / uncrowded arch
successor absent
place occlusal onlay
remove
prognosis poor / crowded arch / if successor absent
submergence below gingival level
root formation on successor complete
open or close space

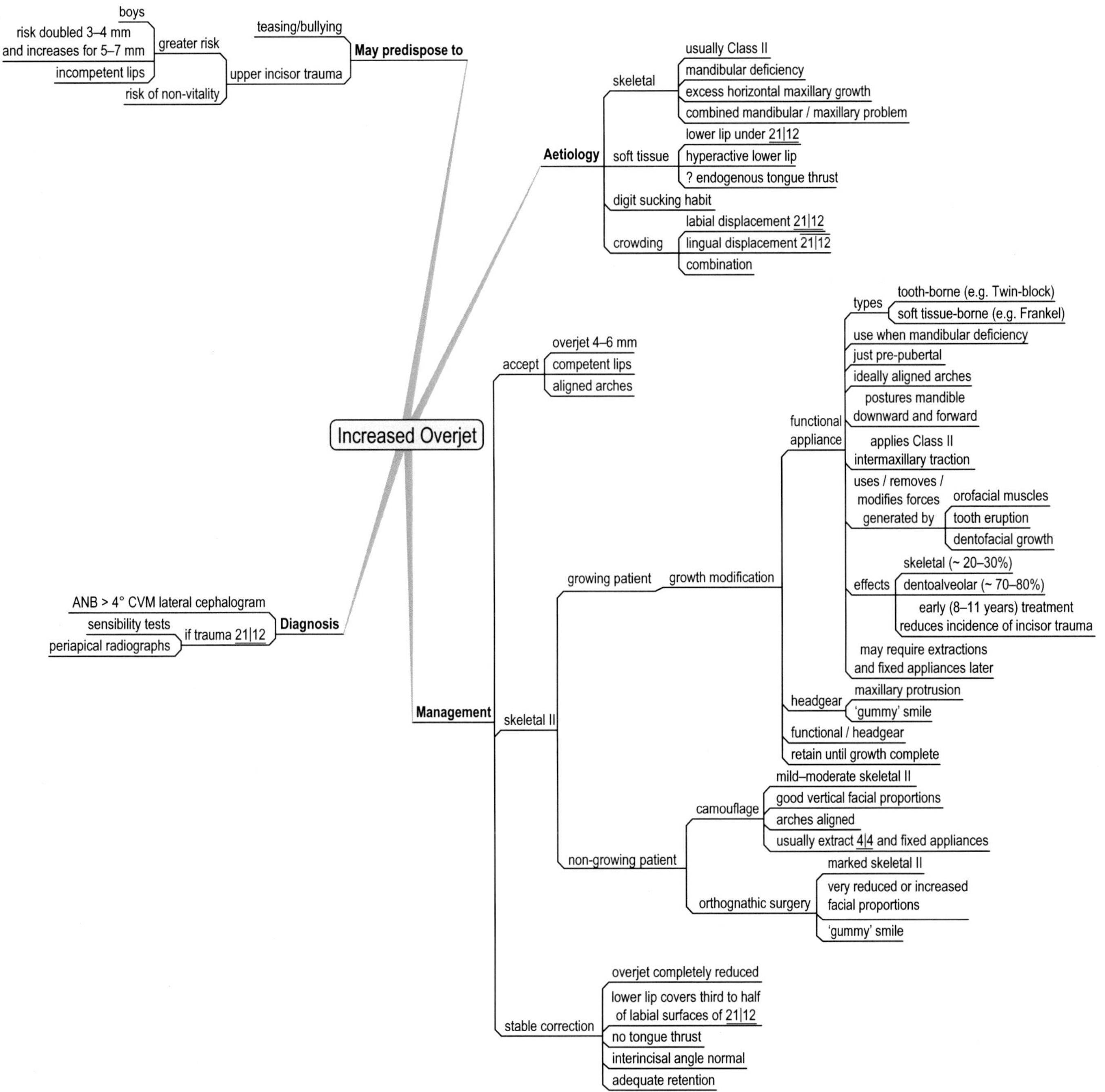
Increased Overjet
May predispose to
teasing/bullying
upper incisor trauma
greater risk
boys
risk doubled 3–4 mm
and increases for 5–7 mm
incompetent lips
risk of non-vitality
Aetiology
skeletal
usually Class II
mandibular deficiency
excess horizontal maxillary growth
combined mandibular / maxillary problem
soft tissue
lower lip under 21|12
hyperactive lower lip
? endogenous tongue thrust
digit sucking habit
crowding
labial displacement 21|12
lingual displacement 21|12
combination
Diagnosis
ANB > 4° CVM lateral cephalogram
if trauma 21|12
sensibility tests
periapical radiographs
Management
accept
overjet 4–6 mm
competent lips
aligned arches
skeletal II
growing patient
growth modification
functional appliance
types
tooth-borne (e.g. Twin-block)
soft tissue-borne (e.g. Frankel)
use when mandibular deficiency
just pre-pubertal
ideally aligned arches
postures mandible
downward and forward
applies Class II
intermaxillary traction
uses / removes /
modifies forces
generated by
orofacial muscles
tooth eruption
dentofacial growth
effects
skeletal (~ 20–30%)
dentoalveolar (~ 70–80%)
early (8–11 years) treatment
reduces incidence of incisor trauma
may require extractions
and fixed appliances later
headgear
maxillary protrusion
'gummy' smile
functional / headgear
retain until growth complete
non-growing patient
camouflage
mild–moderate skeletal II
good vertical facial proportions
arches aligned
usually extract 4|4 and fixed appliances
orthognathic surgery
marked skeletal II
very reduced or increased
facial proportions
'gummy' smile
stable correction
overjet completely reduced
lower lip covers third to half
of labial surfaces of 21|12
no tongue thrust
interincisal angle normal
adequate retention

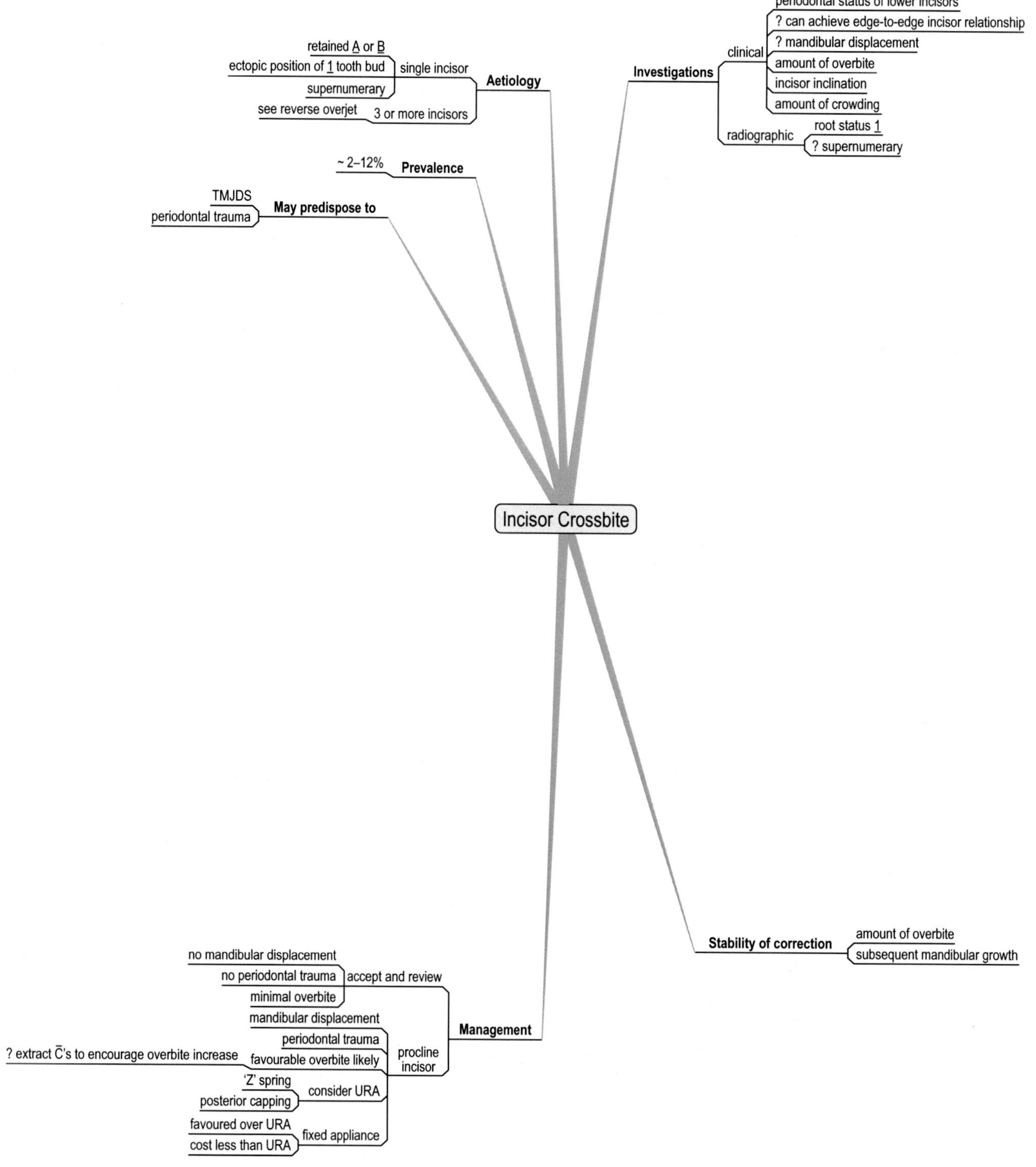
Incisor Crossbite
Aetiology
single incisor
retained A or B
ectopic position of 1 tooth bud
supernumerary
3 or more incisors
see reverse overjet
Prevalence
~ 2–12%
May predispose to
TMJDS
periodontal trauma
Investigations
clinical
periodontal status of lower incisors
? can achieve edge-to-edge incisor relationship
? mandibular displacement
amount of overbite
incisor inclination
amount of crowding
radiographic
root status 1
? supernumerary
Stability of correction
amount of overbite
subsequent mandibular growth
Management
accept and review
no mandibular displacement
no periodontal trauma
minimal overbite
procline incisor
mandibular displacement
periodontal trauma
favourable overbite likely
? extract C̄'s to encourage overbite increase
consider URA
'Z' spring
posterior capping
fixed appliance
favoured over URA
cost less than URA

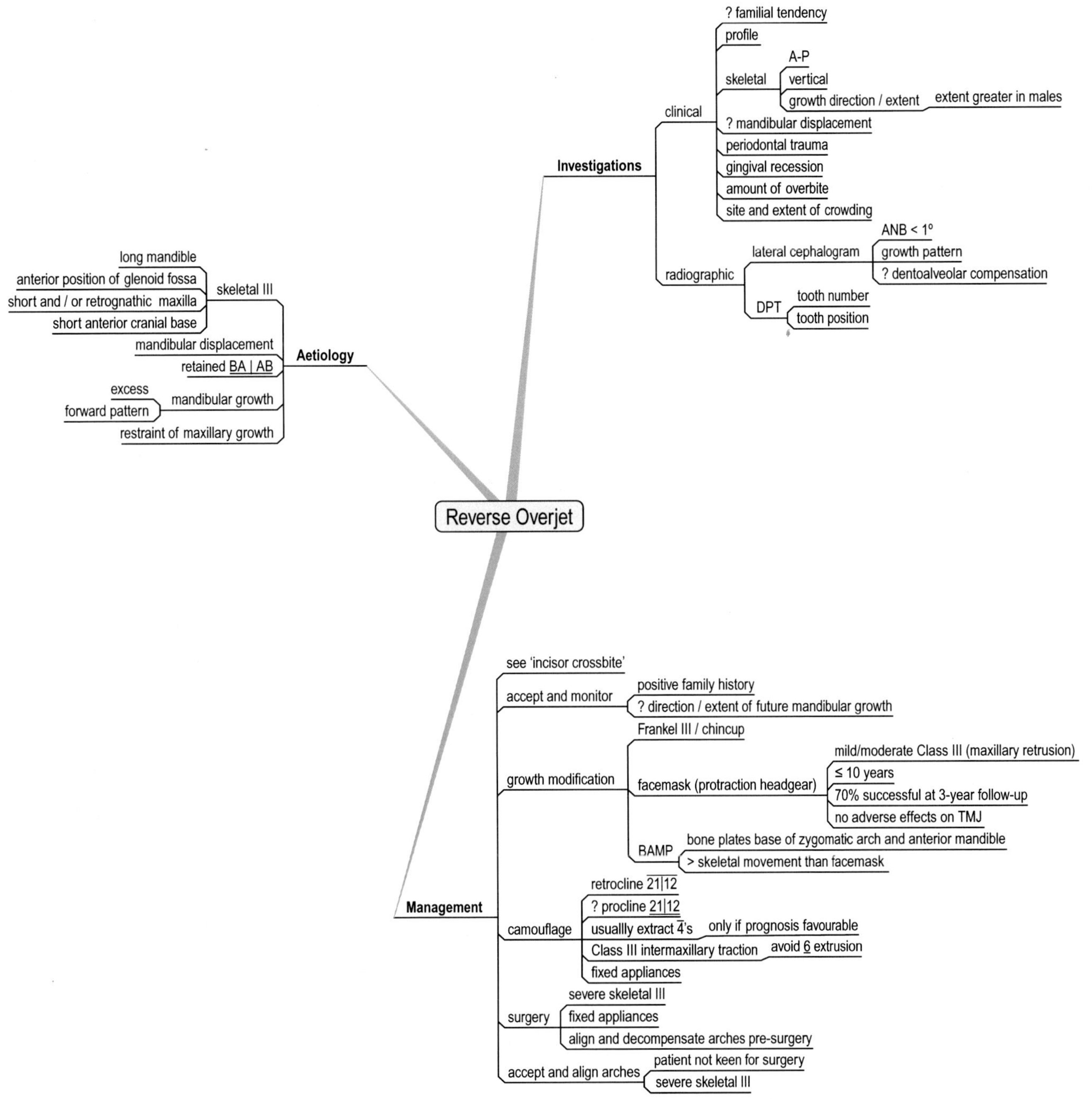
Reverse Overjet
Investigations
clinical
? familial tendency
profile
skeletal
A-P
vertical
growth direction / extent
extent greater in males
? mandibular displacement
periodontal trauma
gingival recession
amount of overbite
site and extent of crowding
radiographic
lateral cephalogram
ANB < 1º
growth pattern
? dentoalveolar compensation
DPT
tooth number
tooth position
Aetiology
skeletal III
long mandible
anterior position of glenoid fossa
short and / or retrognathic maxilla
short anterior cranial base
mandibular displacement
retained BA | AB
mandibular growth
excess
forward pattern
restraint of maxillary growth
Management
see 'incisor crossbite'
accept and monitor
positive family history
? direction / extent of future mandibular growth
growth modification
Frankel III / chincup
facemask (protraction headgear)
mild/moderate Class III (maxillary retrusion)
≤ 10 years
70% successful at 3-year follow-up
no adverse effects on TMJ
BAMP
bone plates base of zygomatic arch and anterior mandible
> skeletal movement than facemask
camouflage
retrocline 21|12
? procline 21|12
usuallly extract 4's
only if prognosis favourable
Class III intermaxillary traction
avoid 6 extrusion
fixed appliances
surgery
severe skeletal III
fixed appliances
align and decompensate arches pre-surgery
accept and align arches
patient not keen for surgery
severe skeletal III

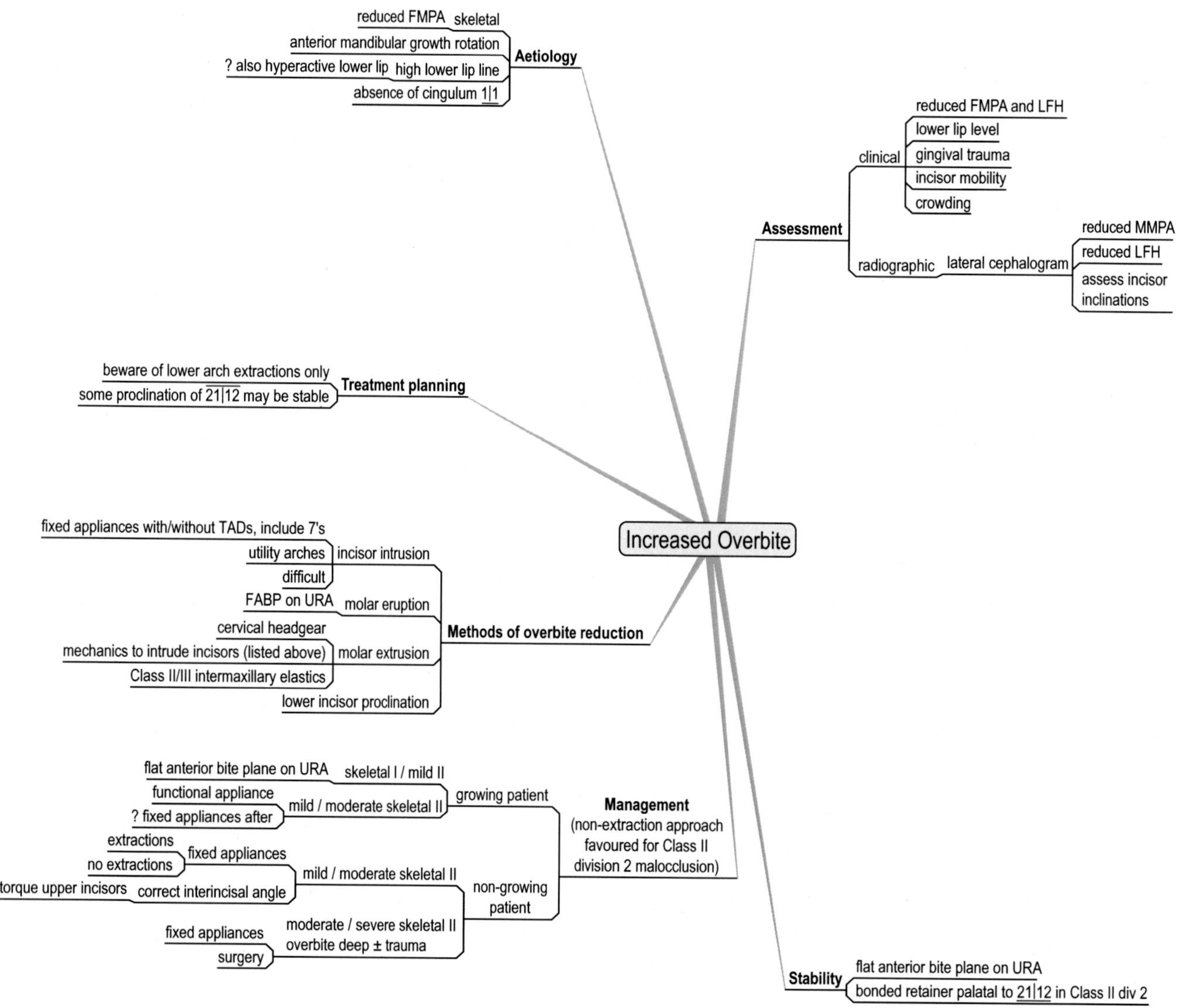
Increased Overbite
Aetiology
reduced FMPA
skeletal
anterior mandibular growth rotation
? also hyperactive lower lip
high lower lip line
absence of cingulum 1|1
Assessment
clinical
reduced FMPA and LFH
lower lip level
gingival trauma
incisor mobility
crowding
radiographic
lateral cephalogram
reduced MMPA
reduced LFH
assess incisor inclinations
Treatment planning
beware of lower arch extractions only
some proclination of 21|12 may be stable
Methods of overbite reduction
incisor intrusion
fixed appliances with/without TADs, include 7's
utility arches
difficult
molar eruption
FABP on URA
molar extrusion
cervical headgear
mechanics to intrude incisors (listed above)
Class II/III intermaxillary elastics
lower incisor proclination
Management
(non-extraction approach favoured for Class II division 2 malocclusion)
growing patient
skeletal I / mild II
flat anterior bite plane on URA
mild / moderate skeletal II
functional appliance
? fixed appliances after
non-growing patient
mild / moderate skeletal II
fixed appliances
extractions
no extractions
correct interincisal angle
torque upper incisors
moderate / severe skeletal II
overbite deep ± trauma
fixed appliances
surgery
Stability
flat anterior bite plane on URA
bonded retainer palatal to 21|12 in Class II div 2

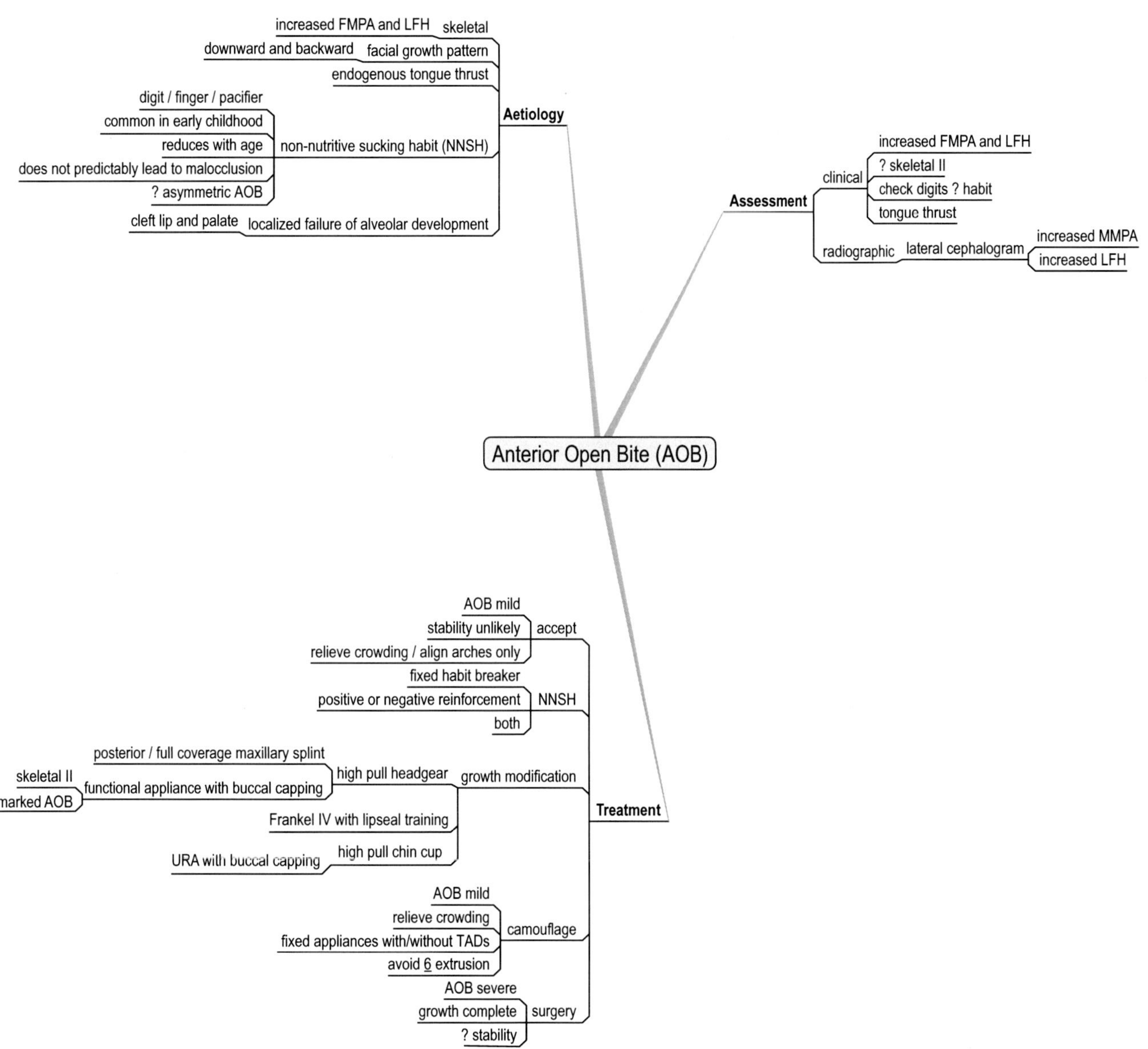
Anterior Open Bite (AOB)
Aetiology
increased FMPA and LFH
skeletal
downward and backward
facial growth pattern
endogenous tongue thrust
digit / finger / pacifier
common in early childhood
reduces with age
non-nutritive sucking habit (NNSH)
does not predictably lead to malocclusion
? asymmetric AOB
cleft lip and palate
localized failure of alveolar development
Assessment
clinical
increased FMPA and LFH
? skeletal II
check digits ? habit
tongue thrust
radiographic
lateral cephalogram
increased MMPA
increased LFH
Treatment
AOB mild
stability unlikely
accept
relieve crowding / align arches only
fixed habit breaker
positive or negative reinforcement
NNSH
both
posterior / full coverage maxillary splint
high pull headgear
growth modification
skeletal II
functional appliance with buccal capping
marked AOB
Frankel IV with lipseal training
URA with buccal capping
high pull chin cup
AOB mild
relieve crowding
camouflage
fixed appliances with/without TADs
avoid 6 extrusion
AOB severe
growth complete
surgery
? stability

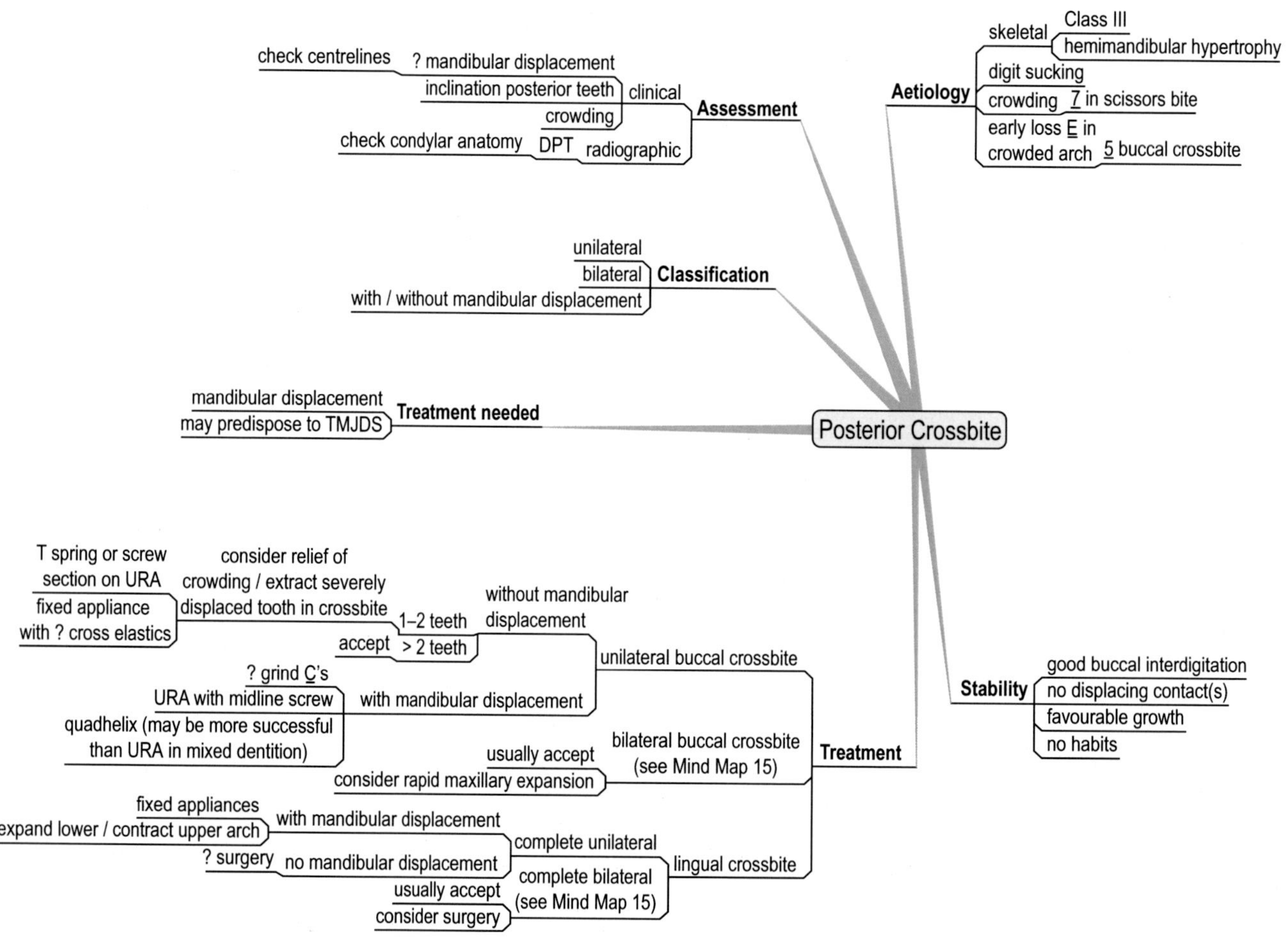
Posterior Crossbite
Assessment
clinical
? mandibular displacement
check centrelines
inclination posterior teeth
crowding
radiographic
DPT
check condylar anatomy
Classification
unilateral
bilateral
with / without mandibular displacement
Treatment needed
mandibular displacement
may predispose to TMJDS
Aetiology
skeletal
Class III
hemimandibular hypertrophy
digit sucking
crowding 7 in scissors bite
early loss E in
crowded arch 5 buccal crossbite
Treatment
unilateral buccal crossbite
without mandibular
displacement
1–2 teeth
consider relief of
crowding / extract severely
displaced tooth in crossbite
T spring or screw
section on URA
fixed appliance
with ? cross elastics
> 2 teeth
accept
with mandibular displacement
? grind C's
URA with midline screw
quadhelix (may be more successful
than URA in mixed dentition)
bilateral buccal crossbite
(see Mind Map 15)
usually accept
consider rapid maxillary expansion
lingual crossbite
complete unilateral
with mandibular displacement
fixed appliances
expand lower / contract upper arch
no mandibular displacement
? surgery
complete bilateral
(see Mind Map 15)
usually accept
consider surgery
Stability
good buccal interdigitation
no displacing contact(s)
favourable growth
no habits

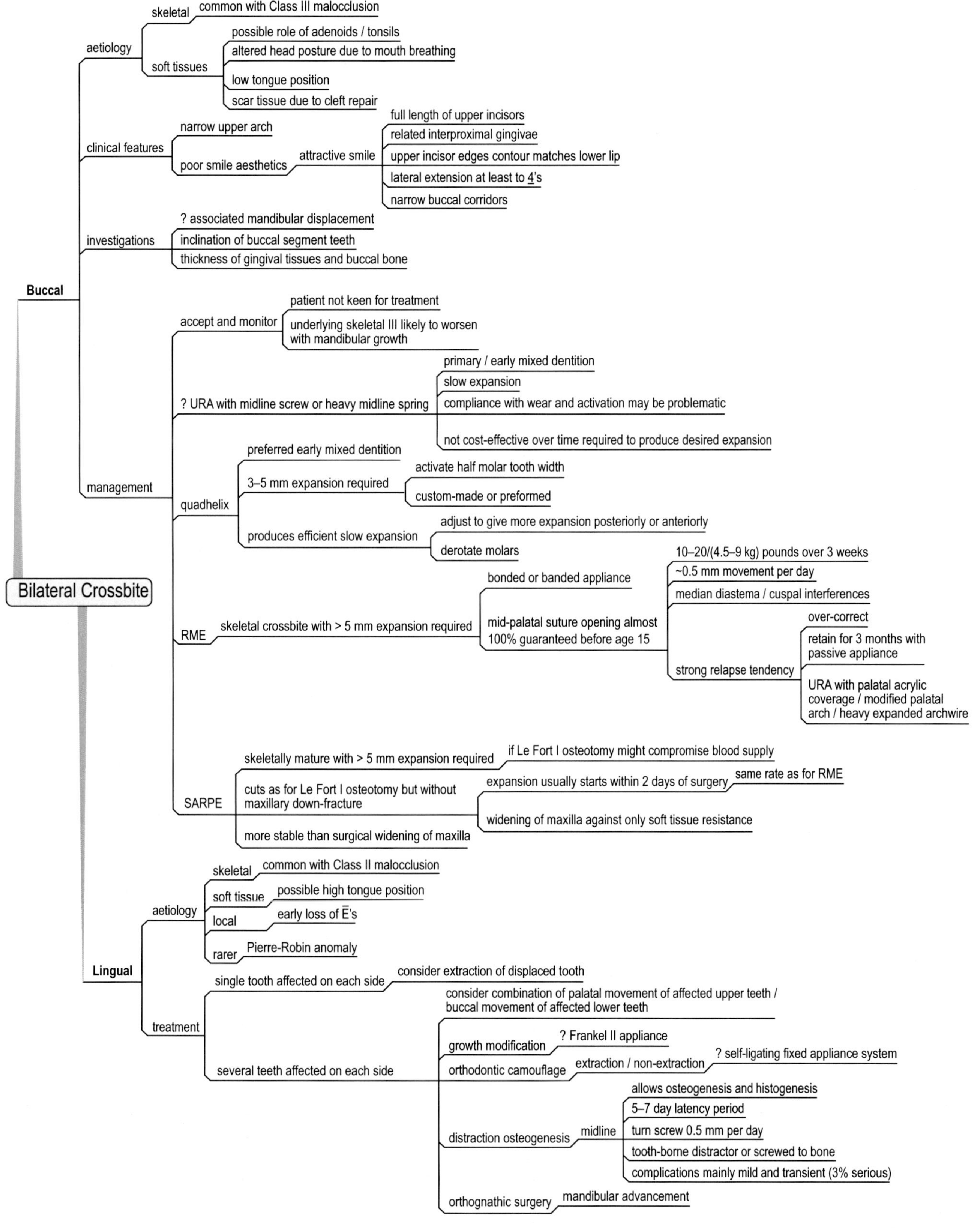
Bilateral Crossbite
Buccal
aetiology
skeletal
common with Class III malocclusion
soft tissues
possible role of adenoids / tonsils
altered head posture due to mouth breathing
low tongue position
scar tissue due to cleft repair
clinical features
narrow upper arch
poor smile aesthetics
attractive smile
full length of upper incisors
related interproximal gingivae
upper incisor edges contour matches lower lip
lateral extension at least to 4's
narrow buccal corridors
investigations
? associated mandibular displacement
inclination of buccal segment teeth
thickness of gingival tissues and buccal bone
management
accept and monitor
patient not keen for treatment
underlying skeletal III likely to worsen with mandibular growth
? URA with midline screw or heavy midline spring
primary / early mixed dentition
slow expansion
compliance with wear and activation may be problematic
not cost-effective over time required to produce desired expansion
quadhelix
preferred early mixed dentition
3–5 mm expansion required
activate half molar tooth width
custom-made or preformed
produces efficient slow expansion
adjust to give more expansion posteriorly or anteriorly
derotate molars
RME
skeletal crossbite with > 5 mm expansion required
bonded or banded appliance
mid-palatal suture opening almost 100% guaranteed before age 15
10–20/(4.5–9 kg) pounds over 3 weeks
~0.5 mm movement per day
median diastema / cuspal interferences
strong relapse tendency
over-correct
retain for 3 months with passive appliance
URA with palatal acrylic coverage / modified palatal arch / heavy expanded archwire
SARPE
skeletally mature with > 5 mm expansion required
if Le Fort I osteotomy might compromise blood supply
cuts as for Le Fort I osteotomy but without maxillary down-fracture
expansion usually starts within 2 days of surgery
same rate as for RME
widening of maxilla against only soft tissue resistance
more stable than surgical widening of maxilla
Lingual
aetiology
skeletal
common with Class II malocclusion
soft tissue
possible high tongue position
local
early loss of Ē's
rarer
Pierre-Robin anomaly
treatment
single tooth affected on each side
consider extraction of displaced tooth
several teeth affected on each side
consider combination of palatal movement of affected upper teeth / buccal movement of affected lower teeth
growth modification
? Frankel II appliance
orthodontic camouflage
extraction / non-extraction
? self-ligating fixed appliance system
distraction osteogenesis
midline
allows osteogenesis and histogenesis
5–7 day latency period
turn screw 0.5 mm per day
tooth-borne distractor or screwed to bone
complications mainly mild and transient (3% serious)
orthognathic surgery
mandibular advancement

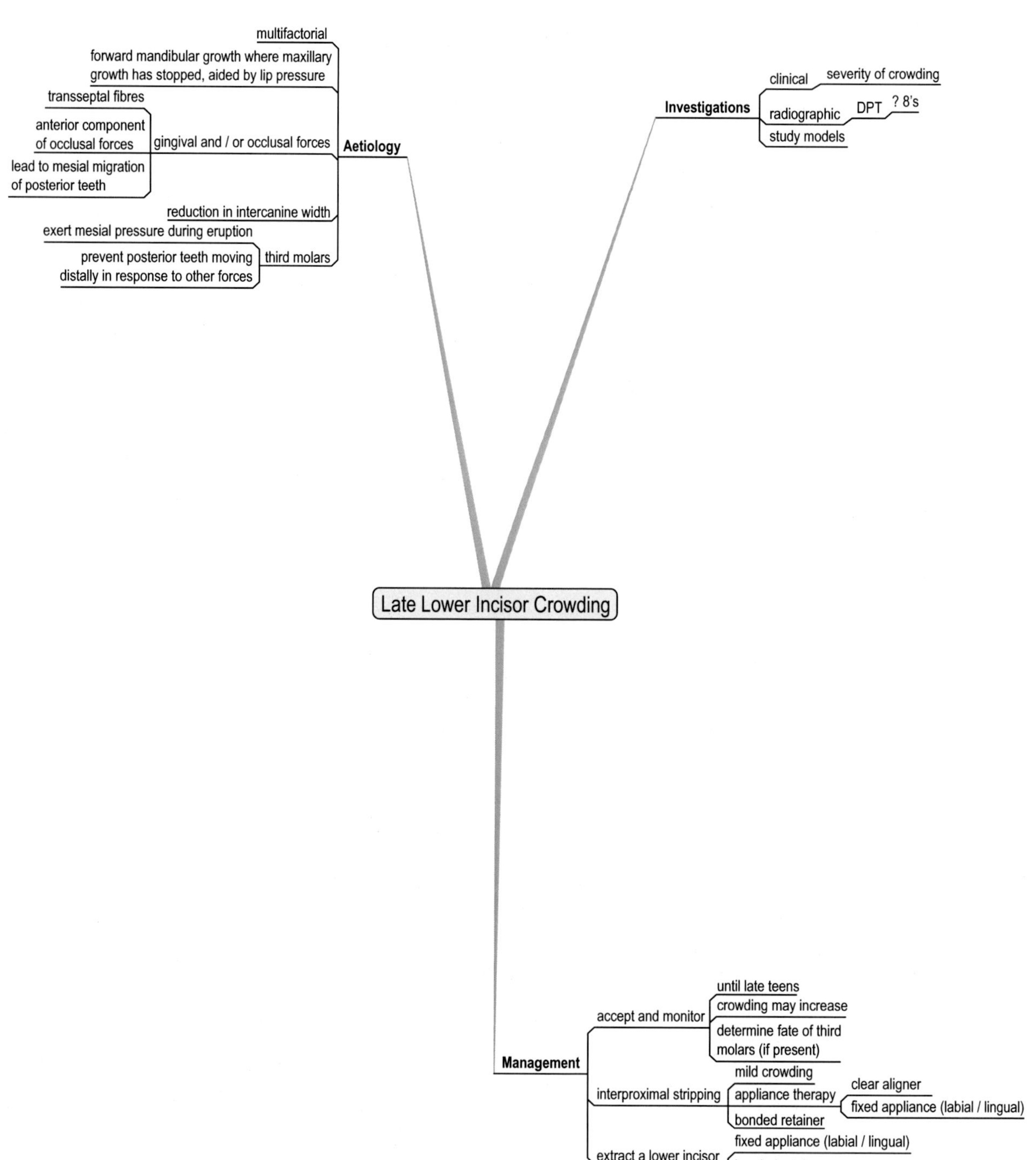
Late Lower Incisor Crowding
Aetiology
multifactorial
forward mandibular growth where maxillary growth has stopped, aided by lip pressure
gingival and / or occlusal forces
transseptal fibres
anterior component of occlusal forces
lead to mesial migration of posterior teeth
reduction in intercanine width
third molars
exert mesial pressure during eruption
prevent posterior teeth moving distally in response to other forces
Investigations
clinical
severity of crowding
radiographic
DPT
? 8's
study models
Management
accept and monitor
until late teens
crowding may increase
determine fate of third molars (if present)
interproximal stripping
mild crowding
appliance therapy
clear aligner
fixed appliance (labial / lingual)
bonded retainer
extract a lower incisor
fixed appliance (labial / lingual)
bonded retainer

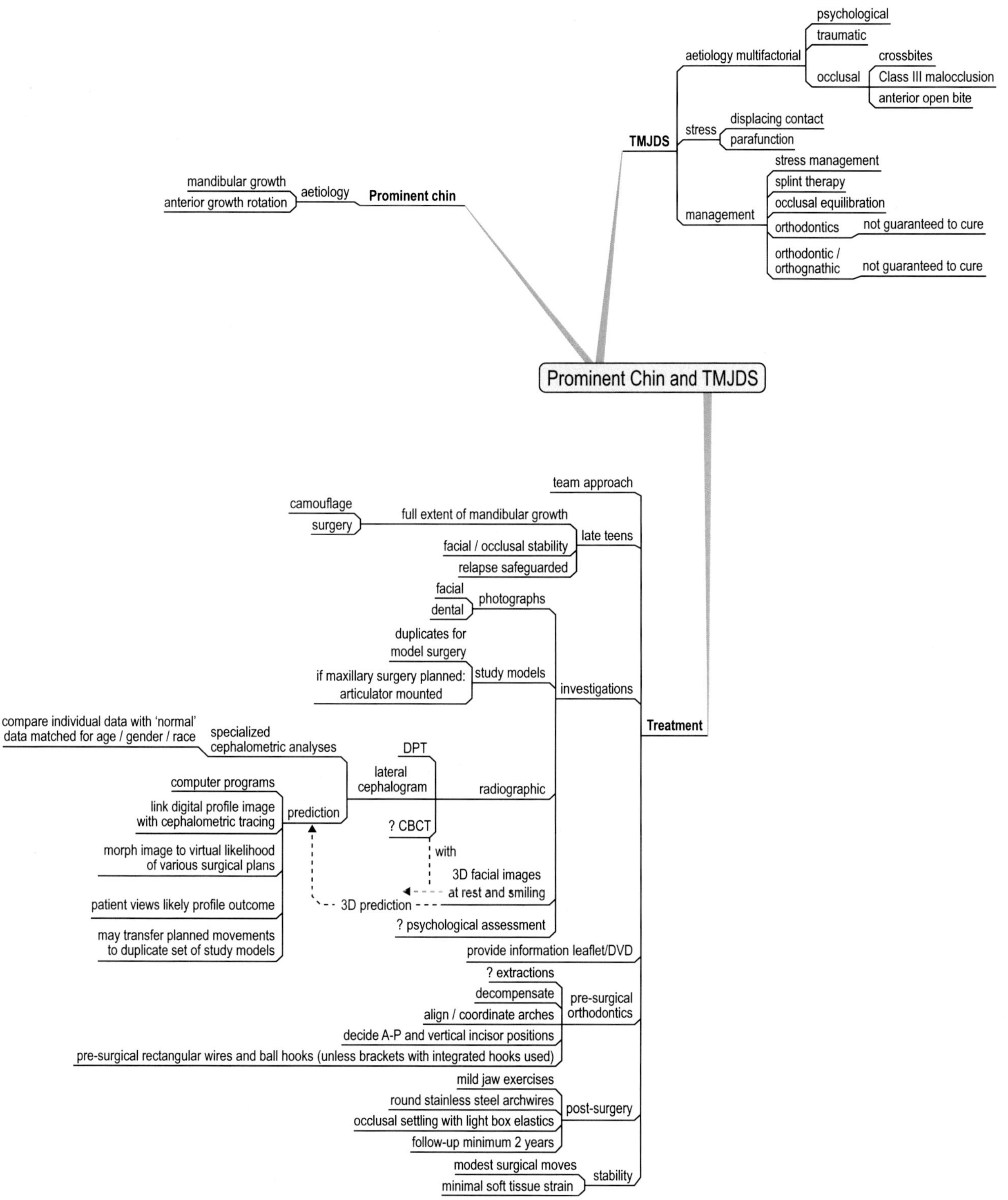
Prominent Chin and TMJDS
Prominent chin
aetiology
mandibular growth
anterior growth rotation
TMJDS
aetiology multifactorial
psychological
traumatic
occlusal
crossbites
Class III malocclusion
anterior open bite
stress
displacing contact
parafunction
management
stress management
splint therapy
occlusal equilibration
orthodontics
not guaranteed to cure
orthodontic / orthognathic
not guaranteed to cure
Treatment
team approach
late teens
full extent of mandibular growth
camouflage
surgery
facial / occlusal stability
relapse safeguarded
investigations
photographs
facial
dental
study models
duplicates for model surgery
if maxillary surgery planned: articulator mounted
radiographic
DPT
lateral cephalogram
? CBCT
with
3D facial images at rest and smiling
3D prediction
specialized cephalometric analyses
compare individual data with 'normal' data matched for age / gender / race
prediction
computer programs
link digital profile image with cephalometric tracing
morph image to virtual likelihood of various surgical plans
patient views likely profile outcome
may transfer planned movements to duplicate set of study models
? psychological assessment
provide information leaflet/DVD
pre-surgical orthodontics
? extractions
decompensate
align / coordinate arches
decide A-P and vertical incisor positions
pre-surgical rectangular wires and ball hooks (unless brackets with integrated hooks used)
post-surgery
mild jaw exercises
round stainless steel archwires
occlusal settling with light box elastics
follow-up minimum 2 years
stability
modest surgical moves
minimal soft tissue strain

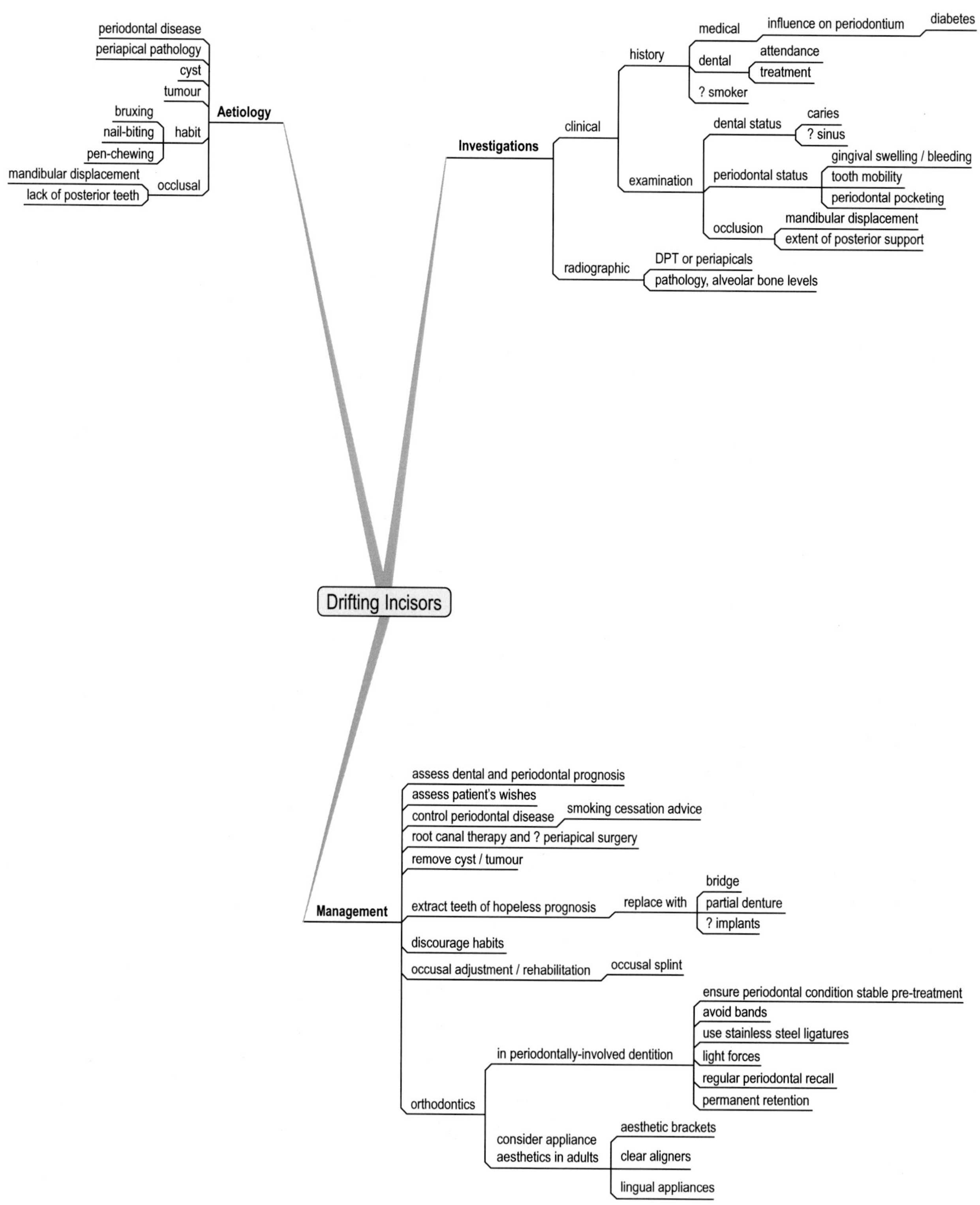
Drifting Incisors
Aetiology
periodontal disease
periapical pathology
cyst
tumour
habit
bruxing
nail-biting
pen-chewing
occlusal
mandibular displacement
lack of posterior teeth
Investigations
clinical
history
medical
influence on periodontium
diabetes
dental
attendance
treatment
? smoker
examination
dental status
caries
? sinus
periodontal status
gingival swelling / bleeding
tooth mobility
periodontal pocketing
occlusion
mandibular displacement
extent of posterior support
radiographic
DPT or periapicals
pathology, alveolar bone levels
Management
assess dental and periodontal prognosis
assess patient's wishes
control periodontal disease
smoking cessation advice
root canal therapy and ? periapical surgery
remove cyst / tumour
extract teeth of hopeless prognosis
replace with
bridge
partial denture
? implants
discourage habits
occusal adjustment / rehabilitation
occusal splint
orthodontics
in periodontally-involved dentition
ensure periodontal condition stable pre-treatment
avoid bands
use stainless steel ligatures
light forces
regular periodontal recall
permanent retention
consider appliance
aesthetics in adults
aesthetic brackets
clear aligners
lingual appliances

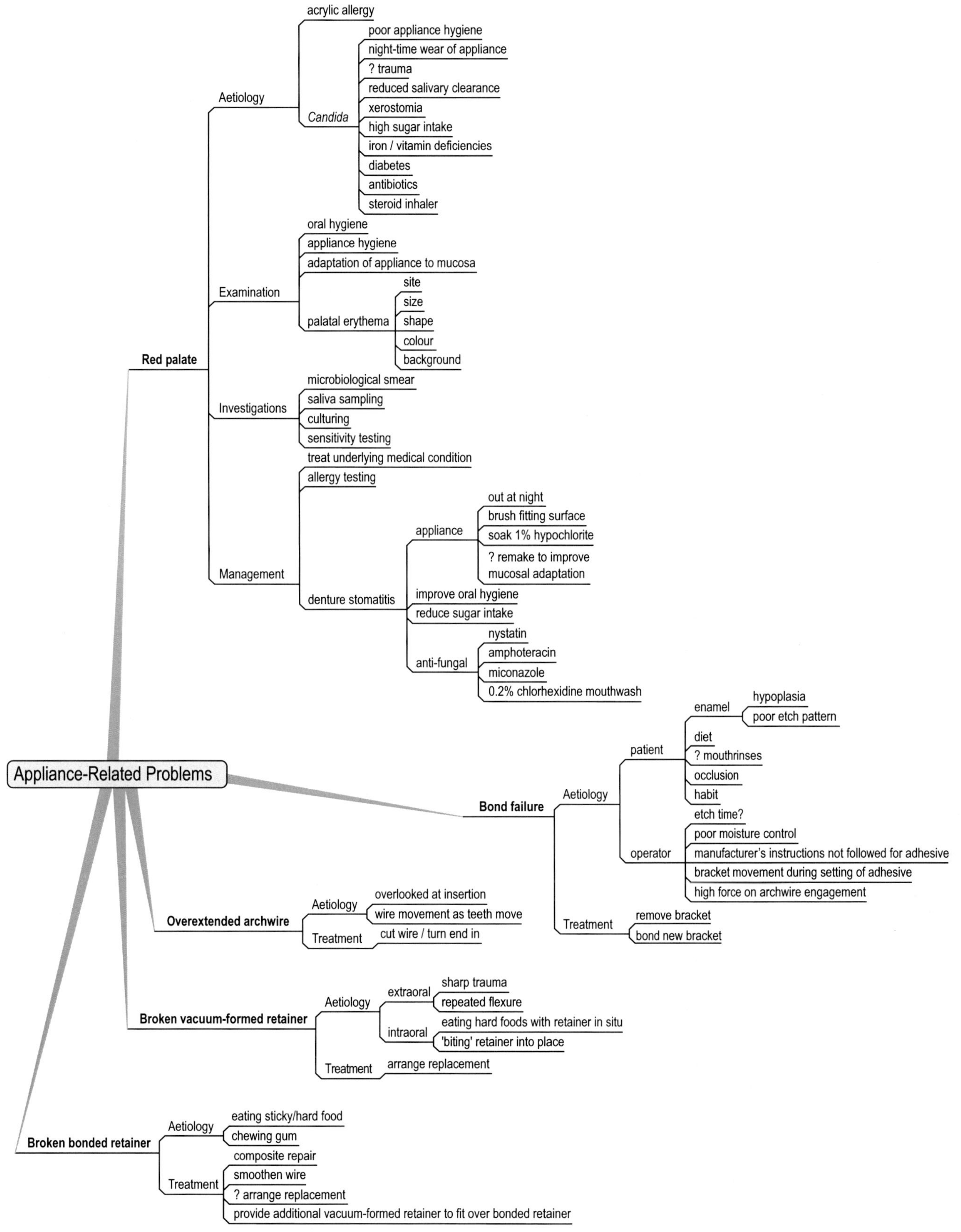
Appliance-Related Problems
Red palate
Aetiology
acrylic allergy
Candida
poor appliance hygiene
night-time wear of appliance
? trauma
reduced salivary clearance
xerostomia
high sugar intake
iron / vitamin deficiencies
diabetes
antibiotics
steroid inhaler
Examination
oral hygiene
appliance hygiene
adaptation of appliance to mucosa
palatal erythema
site
size
shape
colour
background
Investigations
microbiological smear
saliva sampling
culturing
sensitivity testing
Management
treat underlying medical condition
allergy testing
denture stomatitis
appliance
out at night
brush fitting surface
soak 1% hypochlorite
? remake to improve mucosal adaptation
improve oral hygiene
reduce sugar intake
anti-fungal
nystatin
amphoteracin
miconazole
0.2% chlorhexidine mouthwash
Bond failure
Aetiology
patient
enamel
hypoplasia
poor etch pattern
diet
? mouthrinses
occlusion
habit
operator
etch time?
poor moisture control
manufacturer's instructions not followed for adhesive
bracket movement during setting of adhesive
high force on archwire engagement
Treatment
remove bracket
bond new bracket
Overextended archwire
Aetiology
overlooked at insertion
wire movement as teeth move
Treatment
cut wire / turn end in
Broken vacuum-formed retainer
Aetiology
extraoral
sharp trauma
repeated flexure
intraoral
eating hard foods with retainer in situ
'biting' retainer into place
Treatment
arrange replacement
Broken bonded retainer
Aetiology
eating sticky/hard food
chewing gum
Treatment
composite repair
smoothen wire
? arrange replacement
provide additional vacuum-formed retainer to fit over bonded retainer

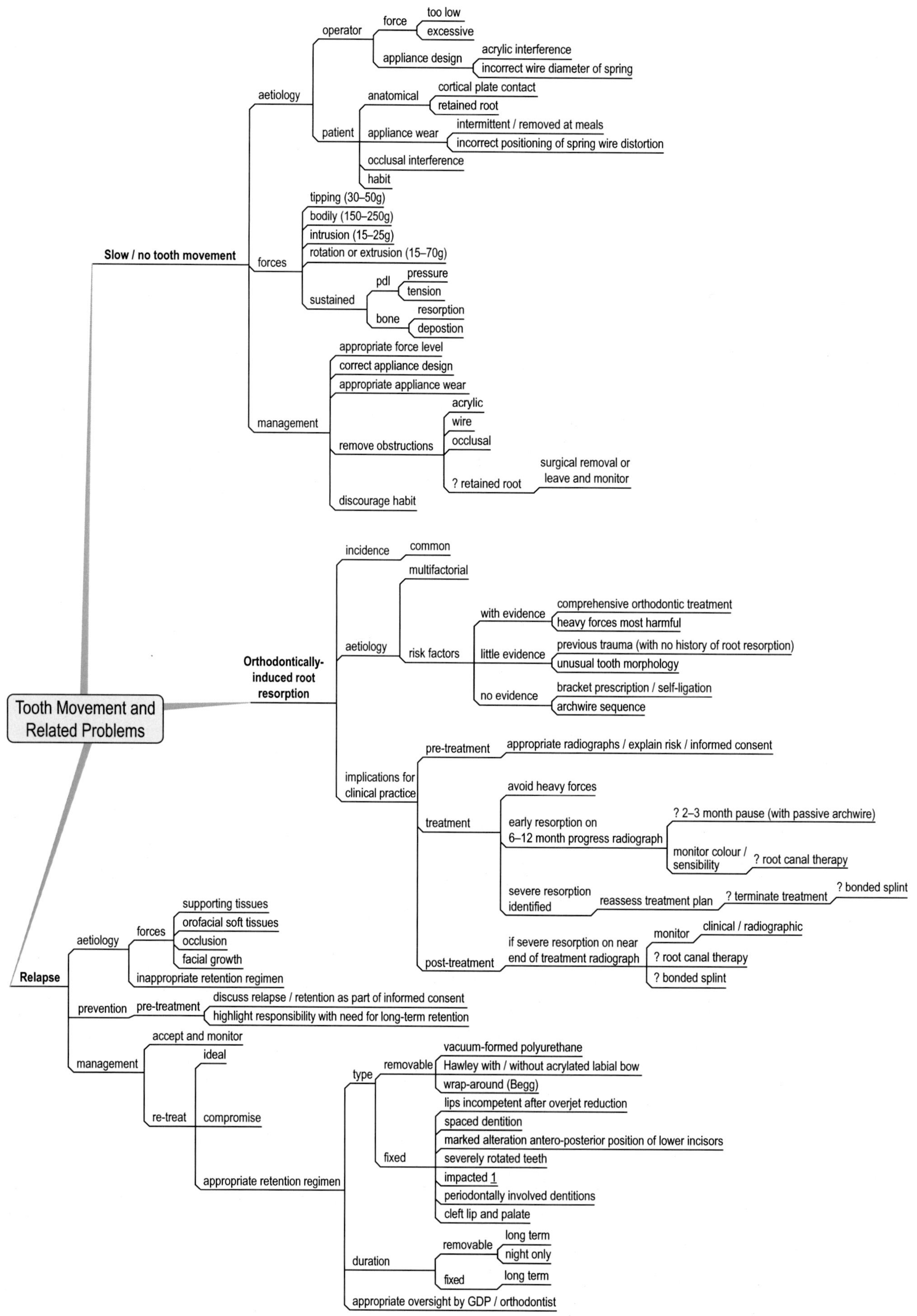
Tooth Movement and Related Problems
Slow / no tooth movement
aetiology
operator
force
too low
excessive
appliance design
acrylic interference
incorrect wire diameter of spring
patient
anatomical
cortical plate contact
retained root
appliance wear
intermittent / removed at meals
incorrect positioning of spring wire distortion
occlusal interference
habit
forces
tipping (30–50g)
bodily (150–250g)
intrusion (15–25g)
rotation or extrusion (15–70g)
sustained
pdl
pressure
tension
bone
resorption
depostion
management
appropriate force level
correct appliance design
appropriate appliance wear
remove obstructions
acrylic
wire
occlusal
? retained root
surgical removal or leave and monitor
discourage habit
Orthodontically-induced root resorption
incidence
common
aetiology
multifactorial
risk factors
with evidence
comprehensive orthodontic treatment
heavy forces most harmful
little evidence
previous trauma (with no history of root resorption)
unusual tooth morphology
no evidence
bracket prescription / self-ligation
archwire sequence
implications for clinical practice
pre-treatment
appropriate radiographs / explain risk / informed consent
treatment
avoid heavy forces
early resorption on 6–12 month progress radiograph
? 2–3 month pause (with passive archwire)
monitor colour / sensibility
? root canal therapy
severe resorption identified
reassess treatment plan
? terminate treatment
? bonded splint
post-treatment
if severe resorption on near end of treatment radiograph
monitor
clinical / radiographic
? root canal therapy
? bonded splint
Relapse
aetiology
forces
supporting tissues
orofacial soft tissues
occlusion
facial growth
inappropriate retention regimen
prevention
pre-treatment
discuss relapse / retention as part of informed consent
highlight responsibility with need for long-term retention
management
accept and monitor
re-treat
ideal
compromise
appropriate retention regimen
type
removable
vacuum-formed polyurethane
Hawley with / without acrylated labial bow
wrap-around (Begg)
fixed
lips incompetent after overjet reduction
spaced dentition
marked alteration antero-posterior position of lower incisors
severely rotated teeth
impacted 1
periodontally involved dentitions
cleft lip and palate
duration
removable
long term
night only
fixed
long term
appropriate oversight by GDP / orthodontist

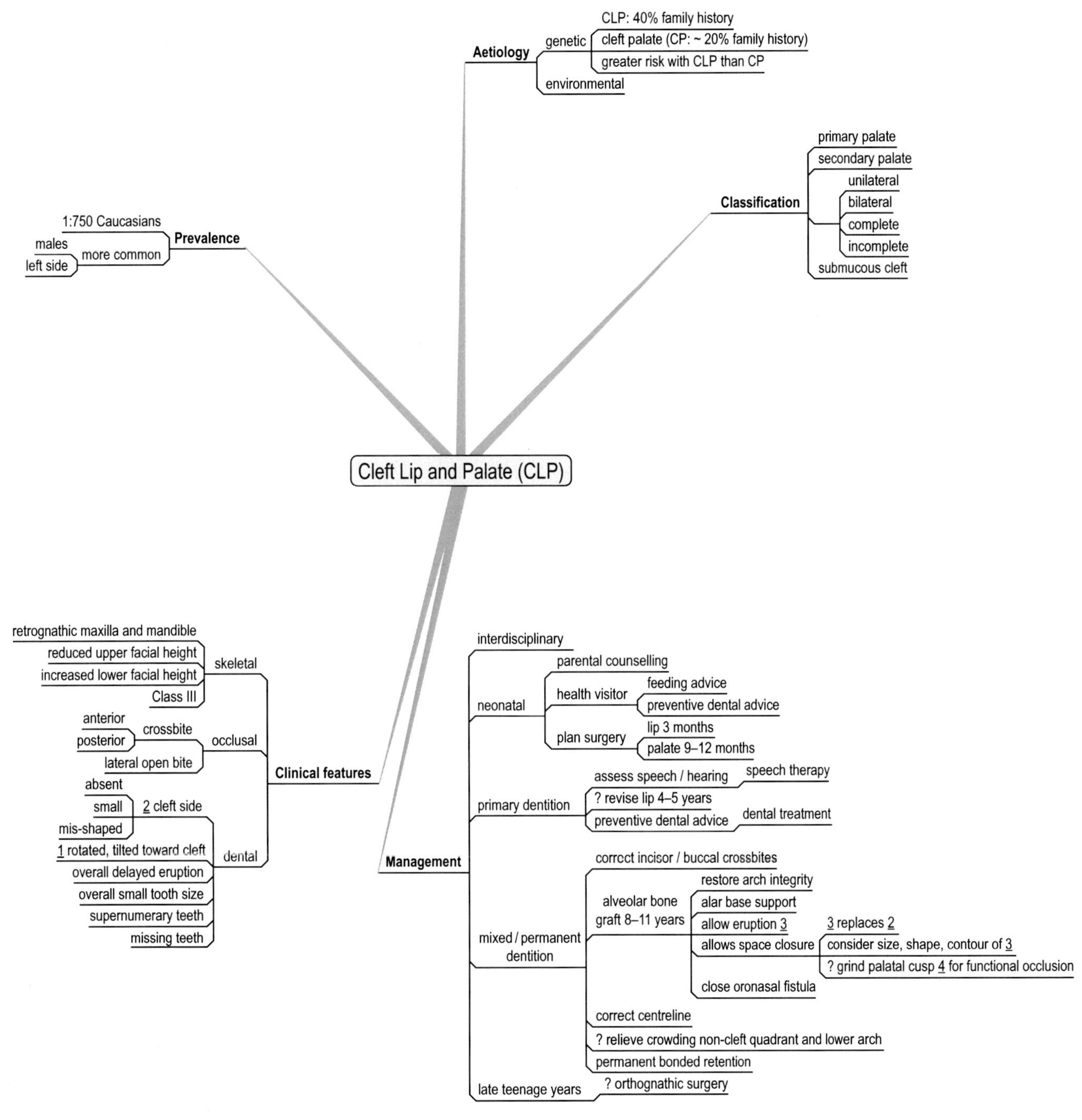
Cleft Lip and Palate (CLP)
Aetiology
genetic
CLP: 40% family history
cleft palate (CP: ~ 20% family history)
greater risk with CLP than CP
environmental
Classification
primary palate
secondary palate
unilateral
bilateral
complete
incomplete
submucous cleft
Prevalence
1:750 Caucasians
more common
males
left side
Clinical features
skeletal
retrognathic maxilla and mandible
reduced upper facial height
increased lower facial height
Class III
occlusal
crossbite
anterior
posterior
lateral open bite
dental
2 cleft side
absent
small
mis-shaped
1 rotated, tilted toward cleft
overall delayed eruption
overall small tooth size
supernumerary teeth
missing teeth
Management
interdisciplinary
neonatal
parental counselling
health visitor
feeding advice
preventive dental advice
plan surgery
lip 3 months
palate 9–12 months
primary dentition
assess speech / hearing
speech therapy
? revise lip 4–5 years
preventive dental advice
dental treatment
mixed / permanent dentition
correct incisor / buccal crossbites
alveolar bone graft 8–11 years
restore arch integrity
alar base support
allow eruption 3
3 replaces 2
allows space closure
consider size, shape, contour of 3
? grind palatal cusp 4 for functional occlusion
close oronasal fistula
correct centreline
? relieve crowding non-cleft quadrant and lower arch
permanent bonded retention
late teenage years
? orthognathic surgery

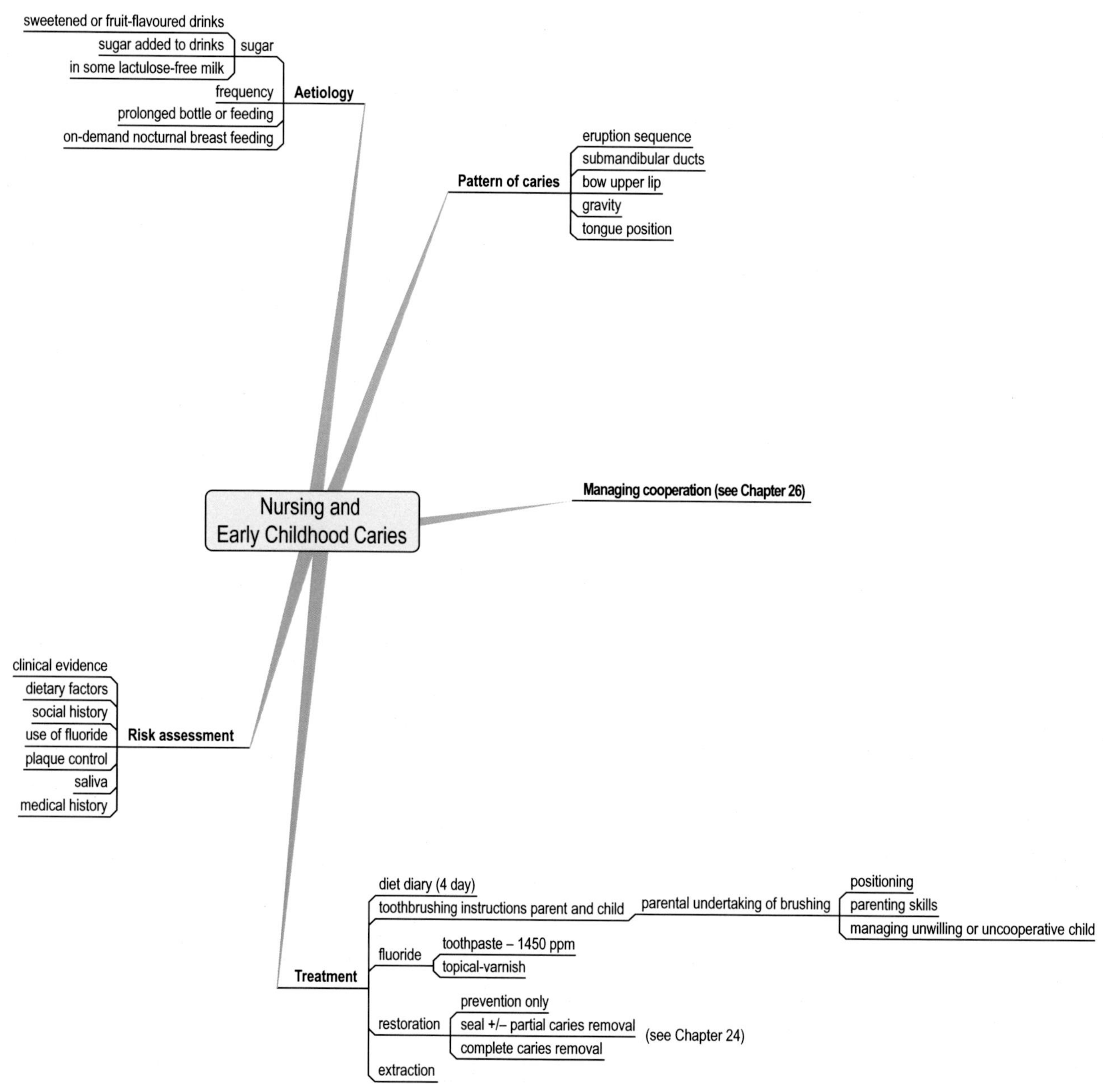
Nursing and Early Childhood Caries
Aetiology
sugar
sweetened or fruit-flavoured drinks
sugar added to drinks
in some lactulose-free milk
frequency
prolonged bottle or feeding
on-demand nocturnal breast feeding
Pattern of caries
eruption sequence
submandibular ducts
bow upper lip
gravity
tongue position
Managing cooperation (see Chapter 26)
Risk assessment
clinical evidence
dietary factors
social history
use of fluoride
plaque control
saliva
medical history
Treatment
diet diary (4 day)
toothbrushing instructions parent and child
parental undertaking of brushing
positioning
parenting skills
managing unwilling or uncooperative child
fluoride
toothpaste – 1450 ppm
topical-varnish
restoration
prevention only
seal +/– partial caries removal
complete caries removal
(see Chapter 24)
extraction

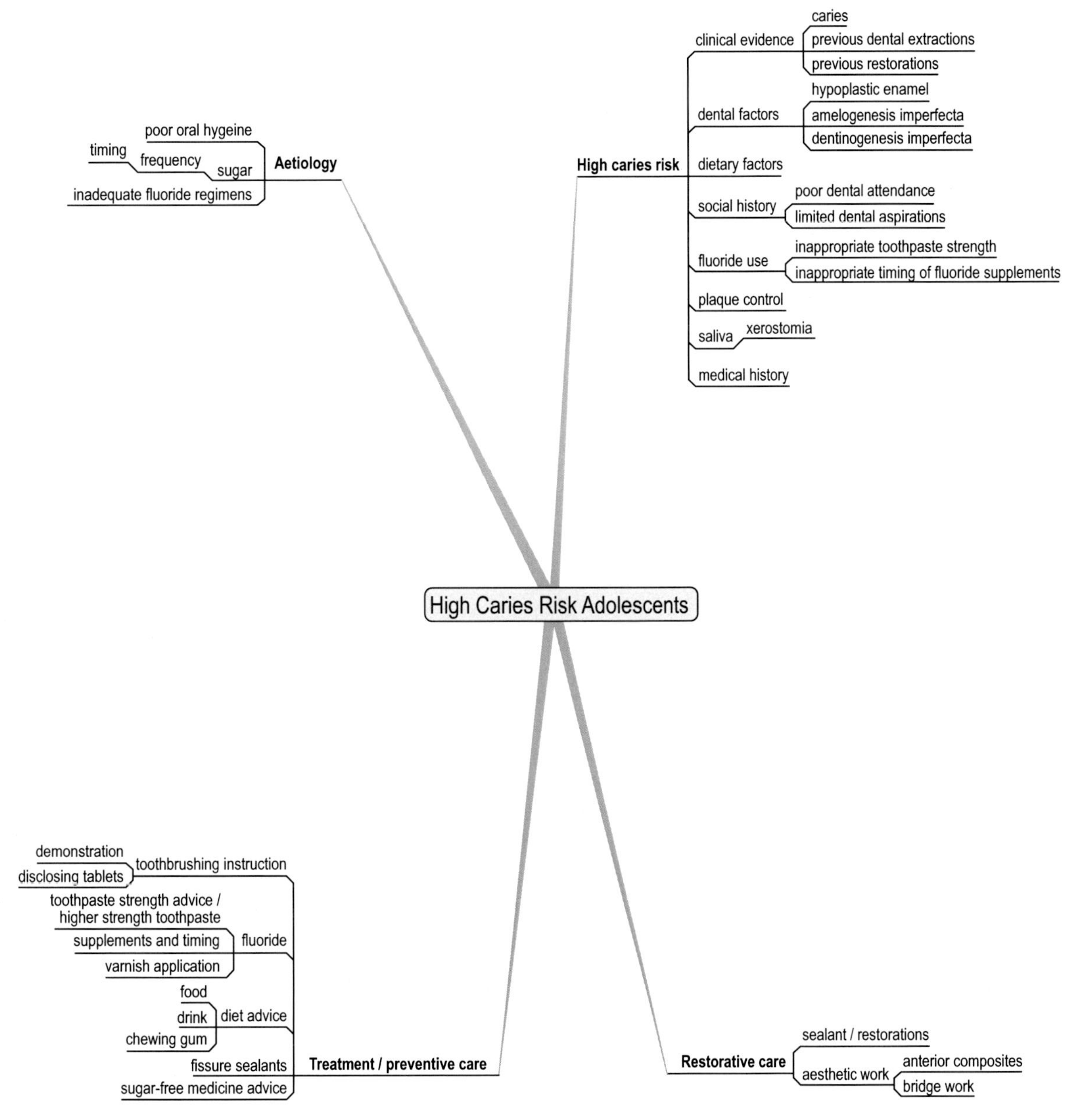
High Caries Risk Adolescents
Aetiology
poor oral hygeine
timing
frequency
sugar
inadequate fluoride regimens
High caries risk
clinical evidence
caries
previous dental extractions
previous restorations
dental factors
hypoplastic enamel
amelogenesis imperfecta
dentinogenesis imperfecta
dietary factors
social history
poor dental attendance
limited dental aspirations
fluoride use
inappropriate toothpaste strength
inappropriate timing of fluoride supplements
plaque control
saliva
xerostomia
medical history
Treatment / preventive care
toothbrushing instruction
demonstration
disclosing tablets
fluoride
toothpaste strength advice / higher strength toothpaste
supplements and timing
varnish application
diet advice
food
drink
chewing gum
fissure sealants
sugar-free medicine advice
Restorative care
sealant / restorations
aesthetic work
anterior composites
bridge work

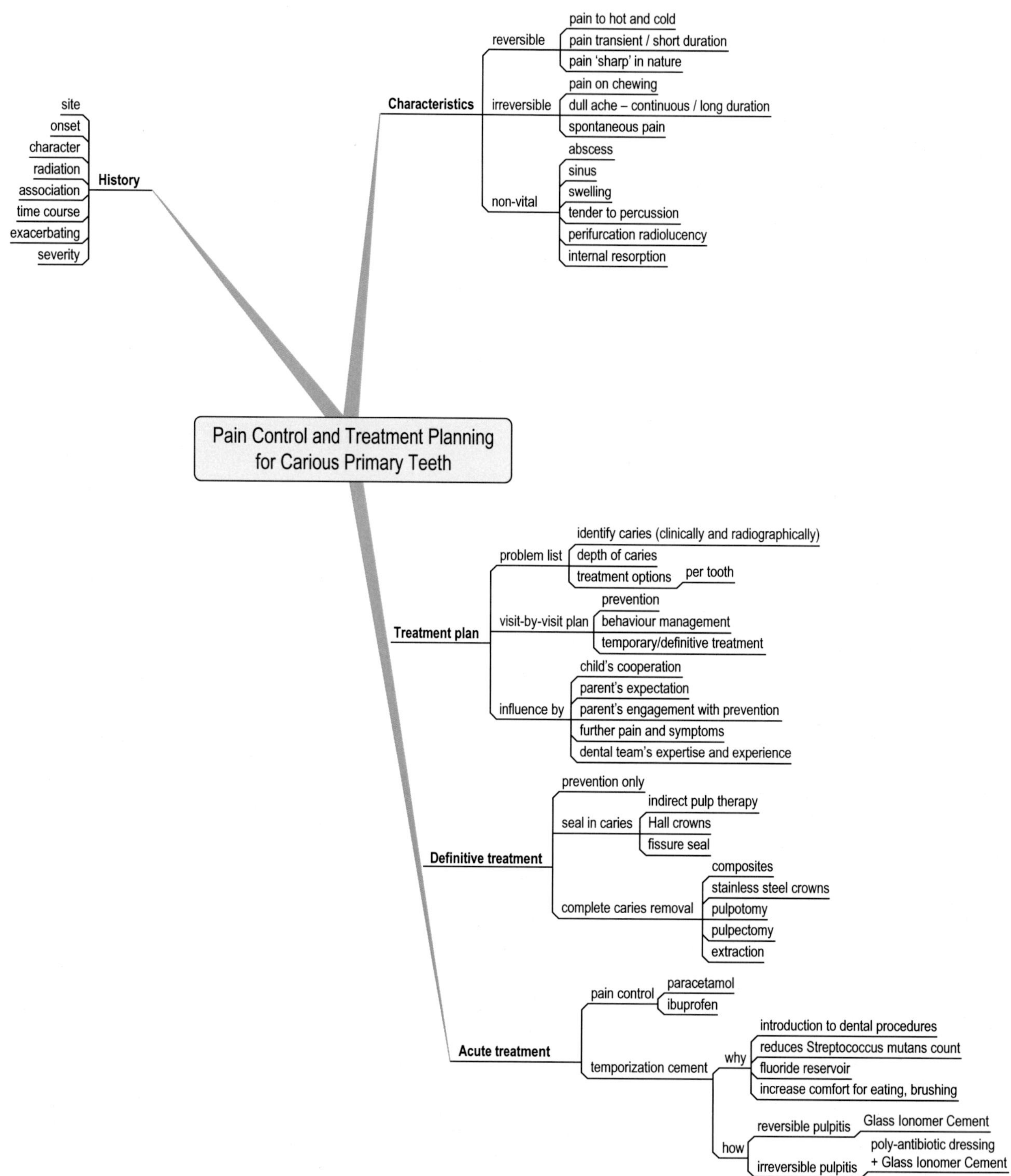
Pain Control and Treatment Planning for Carious Primary Teeth
History
site
onset
character
radiation
association
time course
exacerbating
severity
Characteristics
reversible
pain to hot and cold
pain transient / short duration
pain 'sharp' in nature
irreversible
pain on chewing
dull ache – continuous / long duration
spontaneous pain
non-vital
abscess
sinus
swelling
tender to percussion
perifurcation radiolucency
internal resorption
Treatment plan
problem list
identify caries (clinically and radiographically)
depth of caries
treatment options
per tooth
visit-by-visit plan
prevention
behaviour management
temporary/definitive treatment
influence by
child's cooperation
parent's expectation
parent's engagement with prevention
further pain and symptoms
dental team's expertise and experience
Definitive treatment
prevention only
seal in caries
indirect pulp therapy
Hall crowns
fissure seal
complete caries removal
composites
stainless steel crowns
pulpotomy
pulpectomy
extraction
Acute treatment
pain control
paracetamol
ibuprofen
temporization cement
why
introduction to dental procedures
reduces Streptococcus mutans count
fluoride reservoir
increase comfort for eating, brushing
how
reversible pulpitis
Glass Ionomer Cement
irreversible pulpitis
poly-antibiotic dressing
+ Glass Ionomer Cement

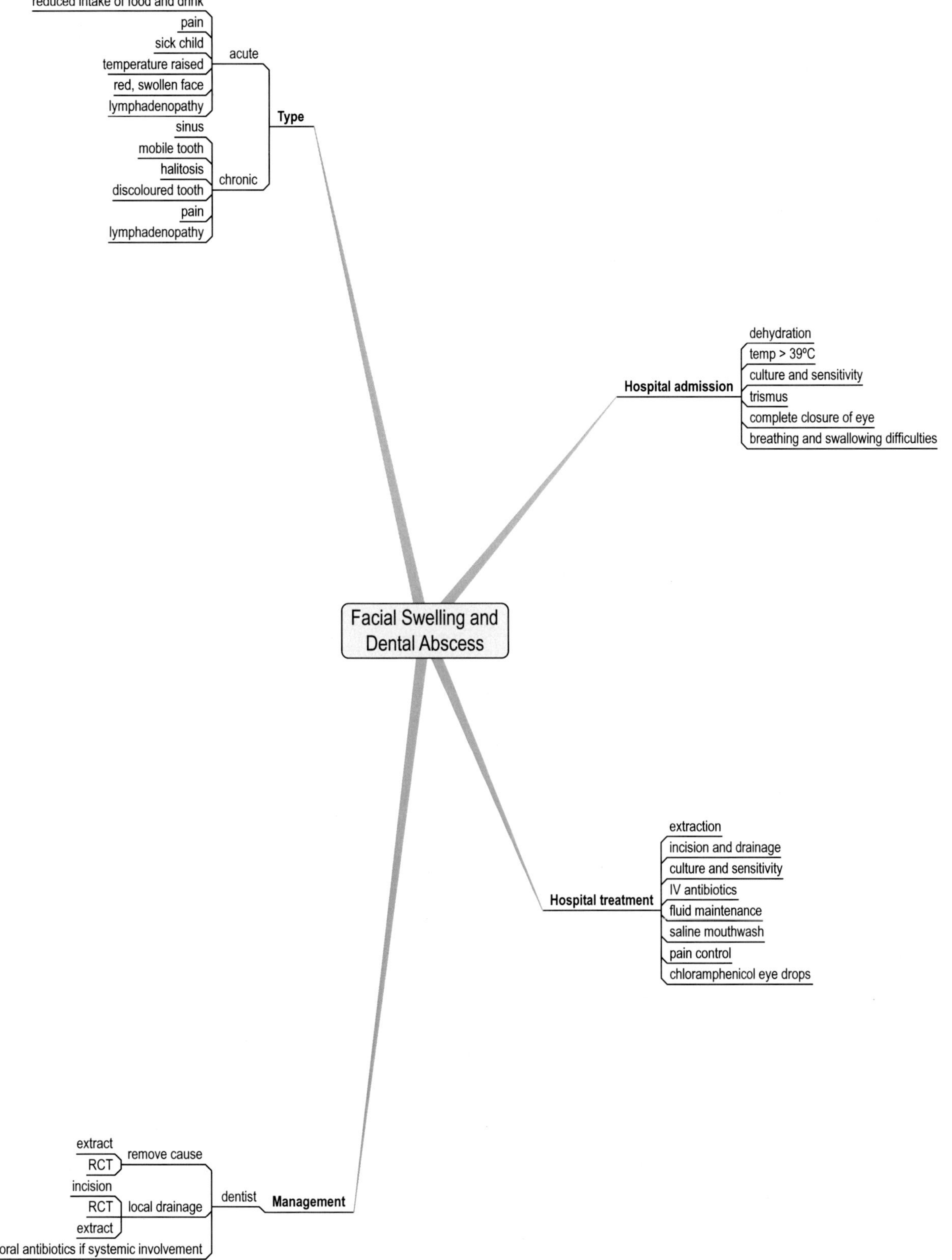
Facial Swelling and Dental Abscess
Type
acute
reduced intake of food and drink
pain
sick child
temperature raised
red, swollen face
lymphadenopathy
chronic
sinus
mobile tooth
halitosis
discoloured tooth
pain
lymphadenopathy
Hospital admission
dehydration
temp > 39ºC
culture and sensitivity
trismus
complete closure of eye
breathing and swallowing difficulties
Hospital treatment
extraction
incision and drainage
culture and sensitivity
IV antibiotics
fluid maintenance
saline mouthwash
pain control
chloramphenicol eye drops
Management
dentist
remove cause
extract
RCT
local drainage
incision
RCT
extract
oral antibiotics if systemic involvement

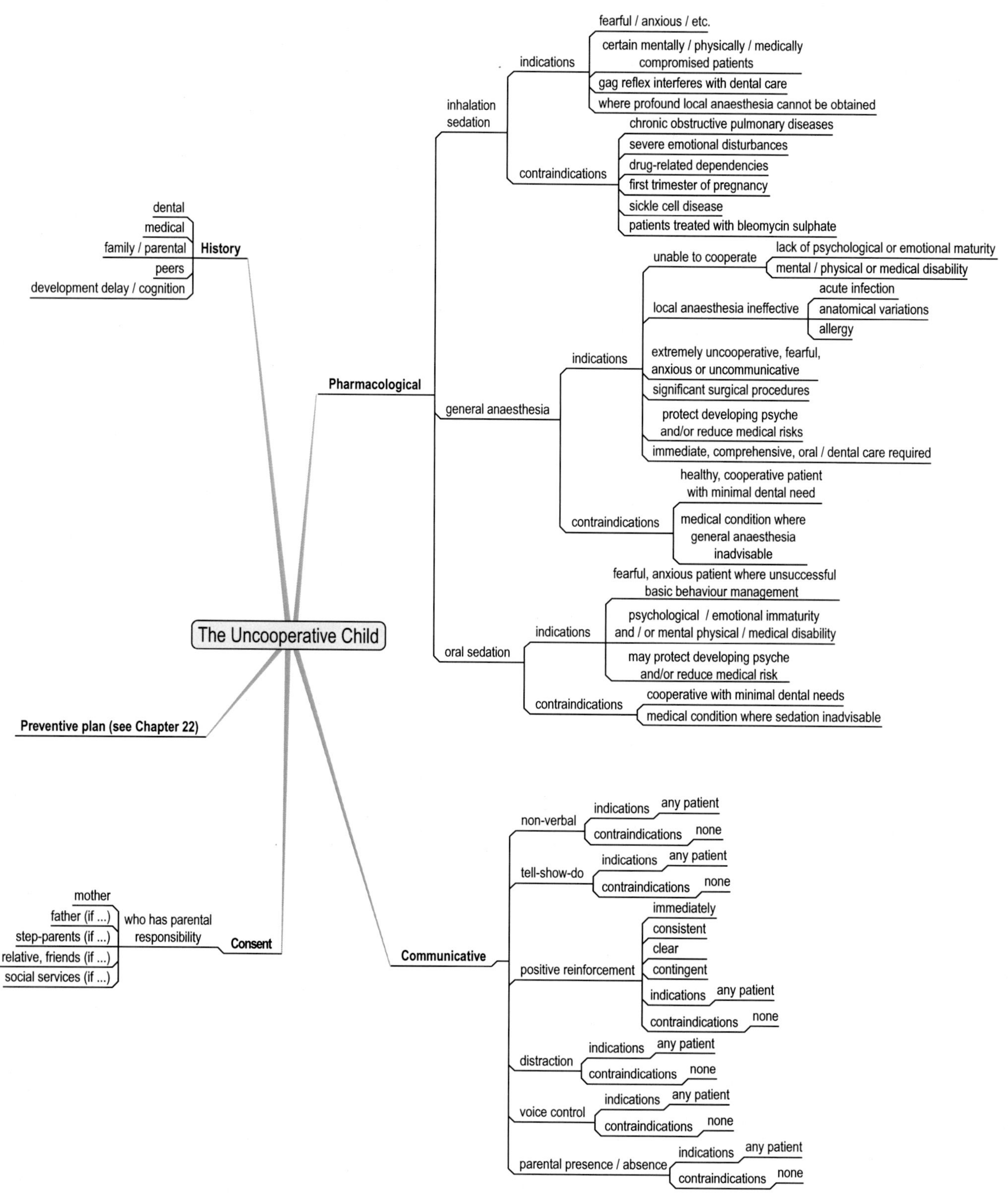
The Uncooperative Child
History
dental
medical
family / parental
peers
development delay / cognition
Pharmacological
inhalation sedation
indications
fearful / anxious / etc.
certain mentally / physically / medically compromised patients
gag reflex interferes with dental care
where profound local anaesthesia cannot be obtained
contraindications
chronic obstructive pulmonary diseases
severe emotional disturbances
drug-related dependencies
first trimester of pregnancy
sickle cell disease
patients treated with bleomycin sulphate
general anaesthesia
indications
unable to cooperate
lack of psychological or emotional maturity
mental / physical or medical disability
local anaesthesia ineffective
acute infection
anatomical variations
allergy
extremely uncooperative, fearful, anxious or uncommunicative
significant surgical procedures
protect developing psyche and/or reduce medical risks
immediate, comprehensive, oral / dental care required
contraindications
healthy, cooperative patient with minimal dental need
medical condition where general anaesthesia inadvisable
oral sedation
indications
fearful, anxious patient where unsuccessful basic behaviour management
psychological / emotional immaturity and / or mental physical / medical disability
may protect developing psyche and/or reduce medical risk
contraindications
cooperative with minimal dental needs
medical condition where sedation inadvisable
Preventive plan (see Chapter 22)
Consent
who has parental responsibility
mother
father (if ...)
step-parents (if ...)
relative, friends (if ...)
social services (if ...)
Communicative
non-verbal
indications
any patient
contraindications
none
tell-show-do
indications
any patient
contraindications
none
positive reinforcement
immediately
consistent
clear
contingent
indications
any patient
contraindications
none
distraction
indications
any patient
contraindications
none
voice control
indications
any patient
contraindications
none
parental presence / absence
indications
any patient
contraindications
none

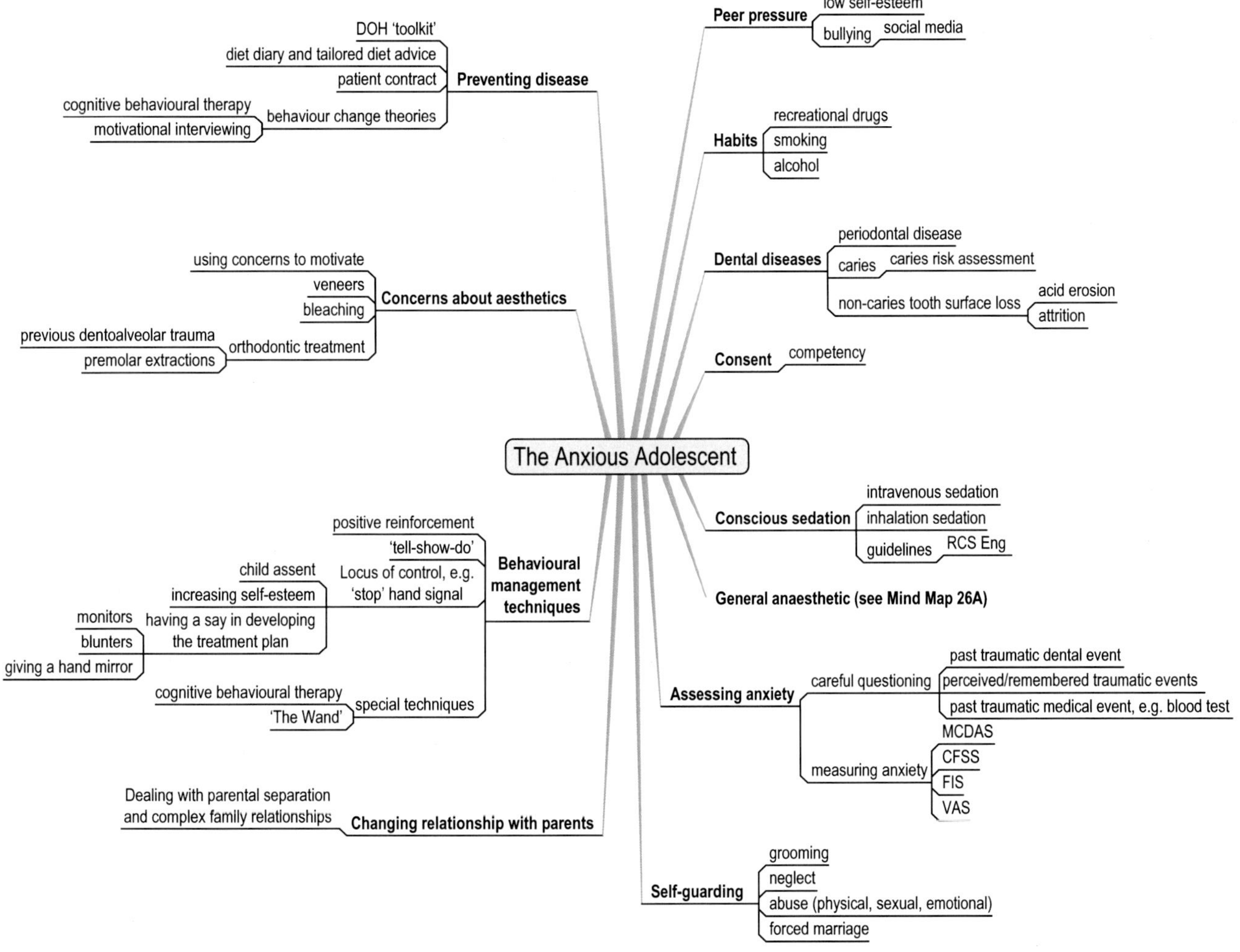
The Anxious Adolescent
Preventing disease
DOH 'toolkit'
diet diary and tailored diet advice
patient contract
behaviour change theories
cognitive behavioural therapy
motivational interviewing
Concerns about aesthetics
using concerns to motivate
veneers
bleaching
orthodontic treatment
previous dentoalveolar trauma
premolar extractions
Behavioural management techniques
positive reinforcement
'tell-show-do'
Locus of control, e.g. 'stop' hand signal
child assent
increasing self-esteem
having a say in developing the treatment plan
monitors
blunters
giving a hand mirror
special techniques
cognitive behavioural therapy
'The Wand'
Changing relationship with parents
Dealing with parental separation and complex family relationships
Peer pressure
low self-esteem
bullying
social media
Habits
recreational drugs
smoking
alcohol
Dental diseases
periodontal disease
caries
caries risk assessment
non-caries tooth surface loss
acid erosion
attrition
Consent
competency
Conscious sedation
intravenous sedation
inhalation sedation
guidelines
RCS Eng
General anaesthetic (see Mind Map 26A)
Assessing anxiety
careful questioning
past traumatic dental event
perceived/remembered traumatic events
past traumatic medical event, e.g. blood test
measuring anxiety
MCDAS
CFSS
FIS
VAS
Self-guarding
grooming
neglect
abuse (physical, sexual, emotional)
forced marriage

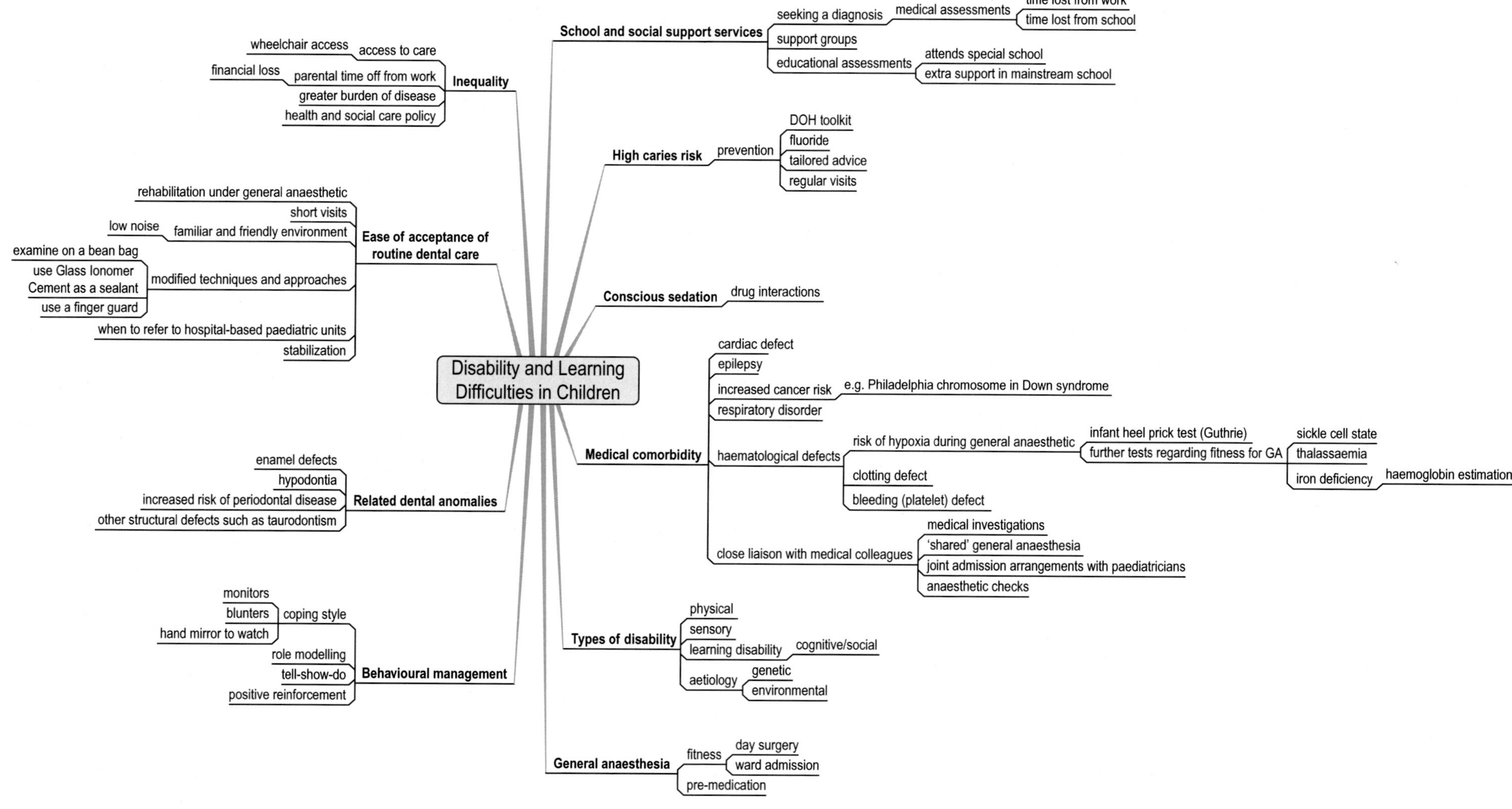
Disability and Learning Difficulties in Children
School and social support services
seeking a diagnosis
medical assessments
time lost from work
time lost from school
support groups
educational assessments
attends special school
extra support in mainstream school
High caries risk
prevention
DOH toolkit
fluoride
tailored advice
regular visits
Conscious sedation
drug interactions
Medical comorbidity
cardiac defect
epilepsy
increased cancer risk
e.g. Philadelphia chromosome in Down syndrome
respiratory disorder
haematological defects
risk of hypoxia during general anaesthetic
infant heel prick test (Guthrie)
further tests regarding fitness for GA
sickle cell state
thalassaemia
iron deficiency
haemoglobin estimation
clotting defect
bleeding (platelet) defect
close liaison with medical colleagues
medical investigations
'shared' general anaesthesia
joint admission arrangements with paediatricians
anaesthetic checks
Types of disability
physical
sensory
learning disability
cognitive/social
aetiology
genetic
environmental
General anaesthesia
fitness
day surgery
ward admission
pre-medication
Inequality
wheelchair access
access to care
financial loss
parental time off from work
greater burden of disease
health and social care policy
Ease of acceptance of routine dental care
rehabilitation under general anaesthetic
short visits
low noise
familiar and friendly environment
examine on a bean bag
use Glass Ionomer Cement as a sealant
use a finger guard
modified techniques and approaches
when to refer to hospital-based paediatric units
stabilization
Related dental anomalies
enamel defects
hypodontia
increased risk of periodontal disease
other structural defects such as taurodontism
Behavioural management
monitors
blunters
hand mirror to watch
coping style
role modelling
tell-show-do
positive reinforcement

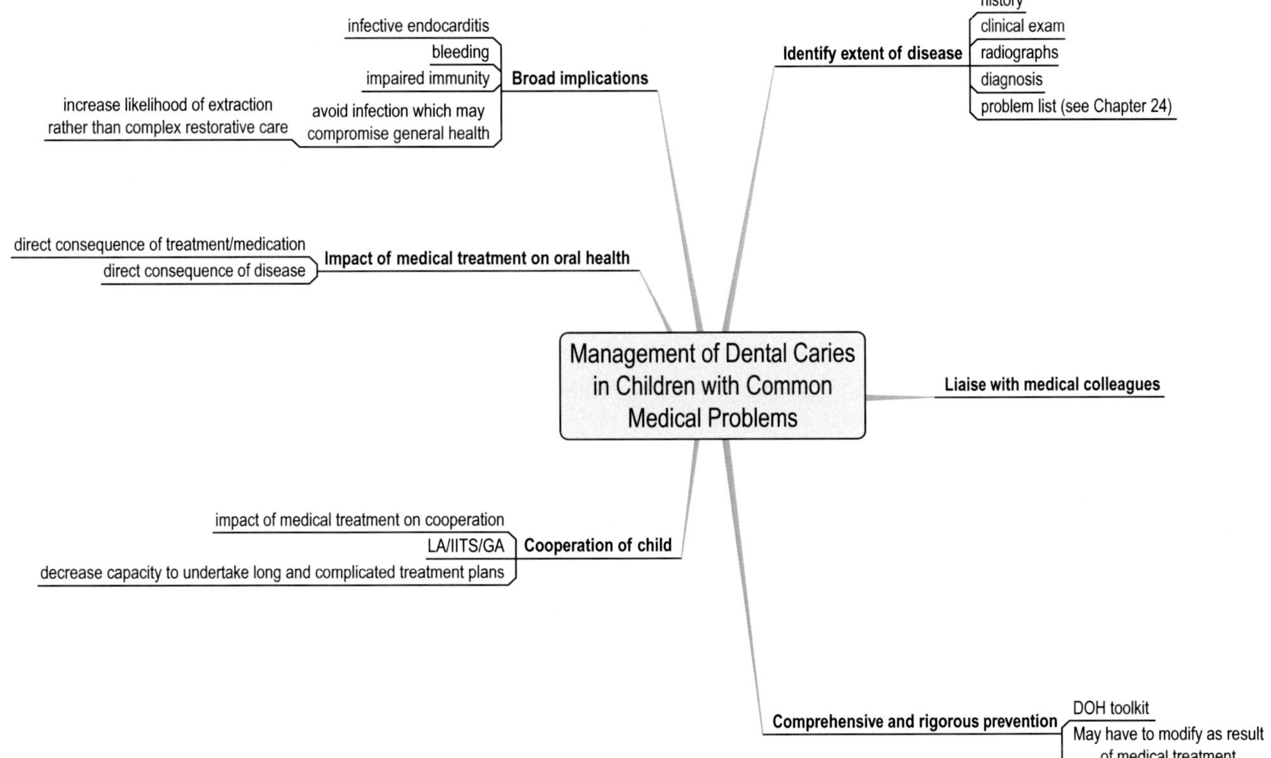
Management of Dental Caries in Children with Common Medical Problems
Broad implications
infective endocarditis
bleeding
impaired immunity
avoid infection which may compromise general health
increase likelihood of extraction rather than complex restorative care
Impact of medical treatment on oral health
direct consequence of treatment/medication
direct consequence of disease
Cooperation of child
impact of medical treatment on cooperation
LA/IITS/GA
decrease capacity to undertake long and complicated treatment plans
Identify extent of disease
history
clinical exam
radiographs
diagnosis
problem list (see Chapter 24)
Liaise with medical colleagues
Comprehensive and rigorous prevention
DOH toolkit
May have to modify as result of medical treatment

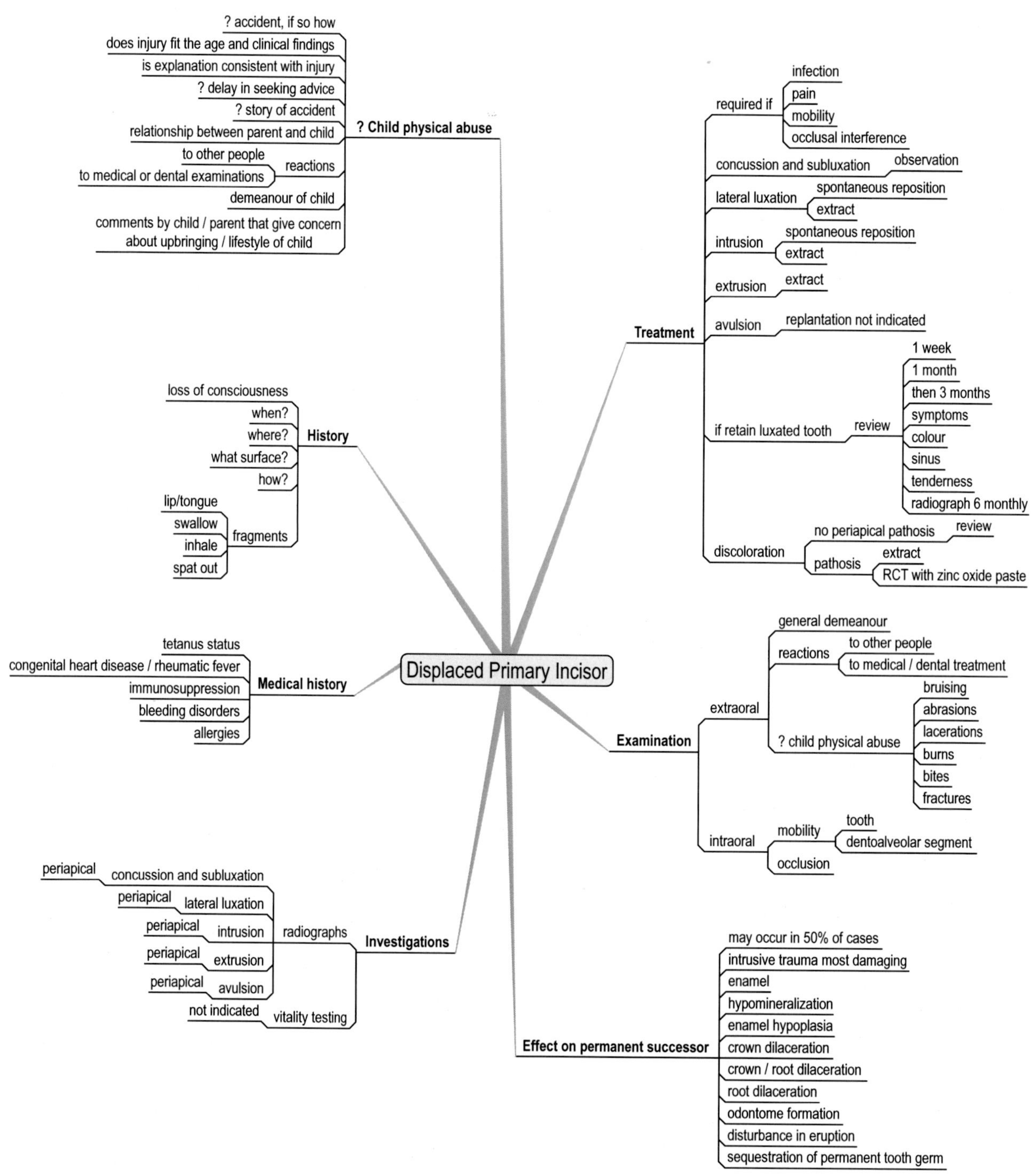
Displaced Primary Incisor
? Child physical abuse
? accident, if so how
does injury fit the age and clinical findings
is explanation consistent with injury
? delay in seeking advice
? story of accident
relationship between parent and child
reactions
to other people
to medical or dental examinations
demeanour of child
comments by child / parent that give concern about upbringing / lifestyle of child
History
loss of consciousness
when?
where?
what surface?
how?
fragments
lip/tongue
swallow
inhale
spat out
Medical history
tetanus status
congenital heart disease / rheumatic fever
immunosuppression
bleeding disorders
allergies
Investigations
radiographs
concussion and subluxation
periapical
lateral luxation
periapical
intrusion
periapical
extrusion
periapical
avulsion
periapical
vitality testing
not indicated
Treatment
required if
infection
pain
mobility
occlusal interference
concussion and subluxation
observation
lateral luxation
spontaneous reposition
extract
intrusion
spontaneous reposition
extract
extrusion
extract
avulsion
replantation not indicated
if retain luxated tooth
review
1 week
1 month
then 3 months
symptoms
colour
sinus
tenderness
radiograph 6 monthly
discoloration
no periapical pathosis
review
pathosis
extract
RCT with zinc oxide paste
Examination
extraoral
general demeanour
reactions
to other people
to medical / dental treatment
? child physical abuse
bruising
abrasions
lacerations
burns
bites
fractures
intraoral
mobility
tooth
dentoalveolar segment
occlusion
Effect on permanent successor
may occur in 50% of cases
intrusive trauma most damaging
enamel
hypomineralization
enamel hypoplasia
crown dilaceration
crown / root dilaceration
root dilaceration
odontome formation
disturbance in eruption
sequestration of permanent tooth germ

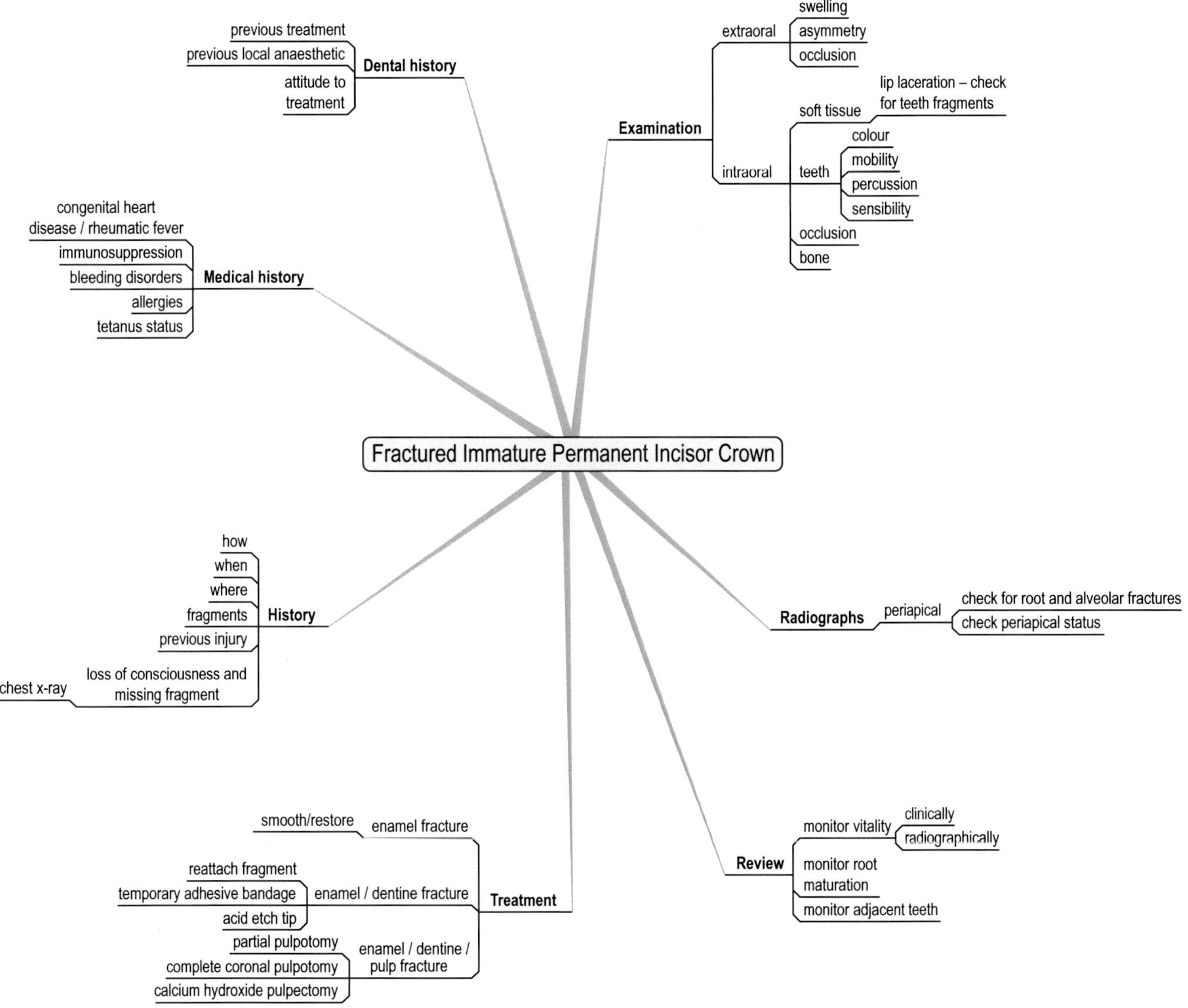
Fractured Immature Permanent Incisor Crown
Dental history
previous treatment
previous local anaesthetic
attitude to treatment
Medical history
congenital heart disease / rheumatic fever
immunosuppression
bleeding disorders
allergies
tetanus status
History
how
when
where
fragments
previous injury
loss of consciousness and missing fragment
chest x-ray
Treatment
enamel fracture
smooth/restore
enamel / dentine fracture
reattach fragment
temporary adhesive bandage
acid etch tip
enamel / dentine / pulp fracture
partial pulpotomy
complete coronal pulpotomy
calcium hydroxide pulpectomy
Examination
extraoral
swelling
asymmetry
occlusion
intraoral
soft tissue
lip laceration – check for teeth fragments
teeth
colour
mobility
percussion
sensibility
occlusion
bone
Radiographs
periapical
check for root and alveolar fractures
check periapical status
Review
monitor vitality
clinically
radiographically
monitor root maturation
monitor adjacent teeth

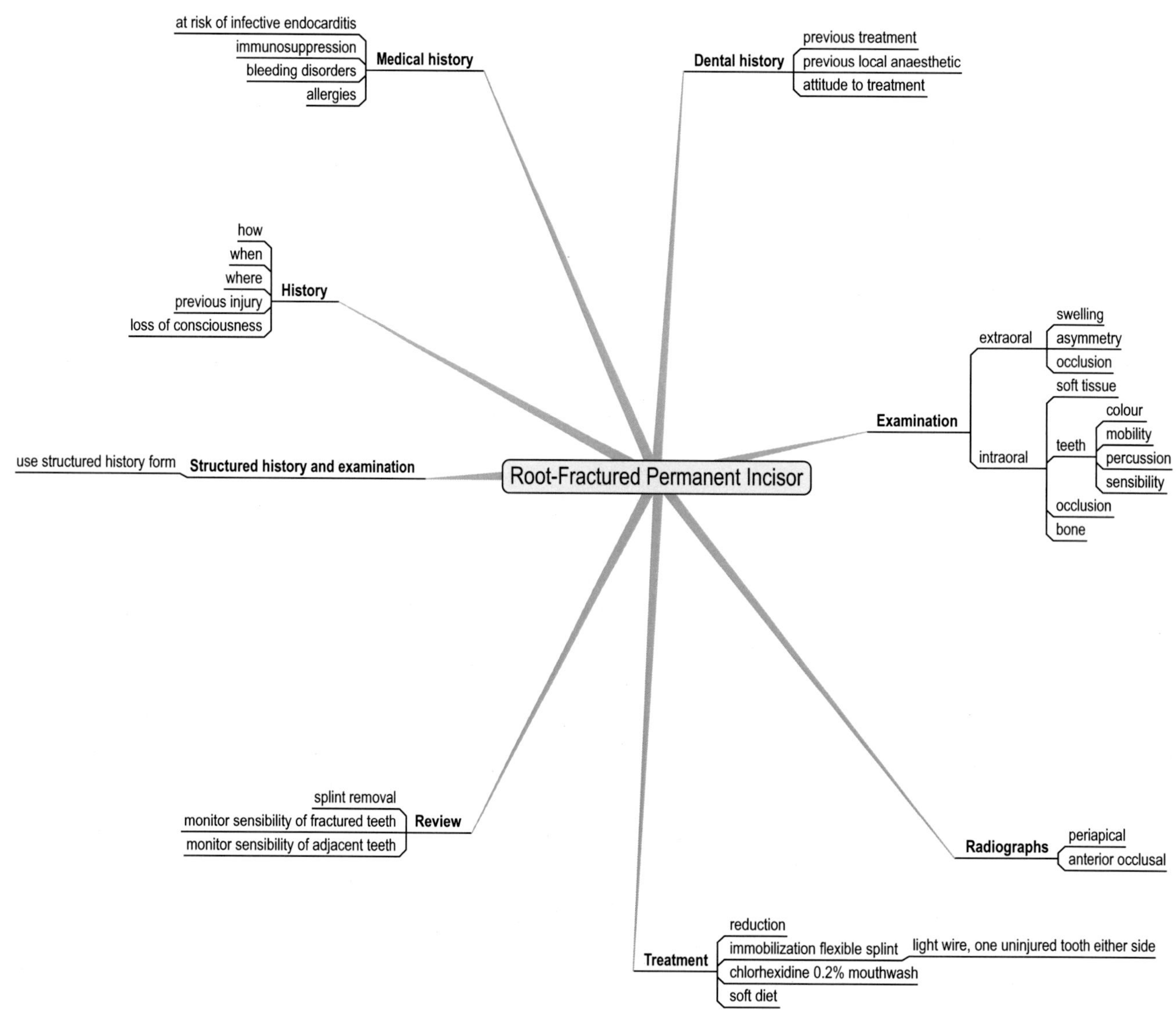
Root-Fractured Permanent Incisor
Medical history
at risk of infective endocarditis
immunosuppression
bleeding disorders
allergies
Dental history
previous treatment
previous local anaesthetic
attitude to treatment
History
how
when
where
previous injury
loss of consciousness
Structured history and examination
use structured history form
Examination
extraoral
swelling
asymmetry
occlusion
intraoral
soft tissue
teeth
colour
mobility
percussion
sensibility
occlusion
bone
Radiographs
periapical
anterior occlusal
Treatment
reduction
immobilization flexible splint
light wire, one uninjured tooth either side
chlorhexidine 0.2% mouthwash
soft diet
Review
splint removal
monitor sensibility of fractured teeth
monitor sensibility of adjacent teeth

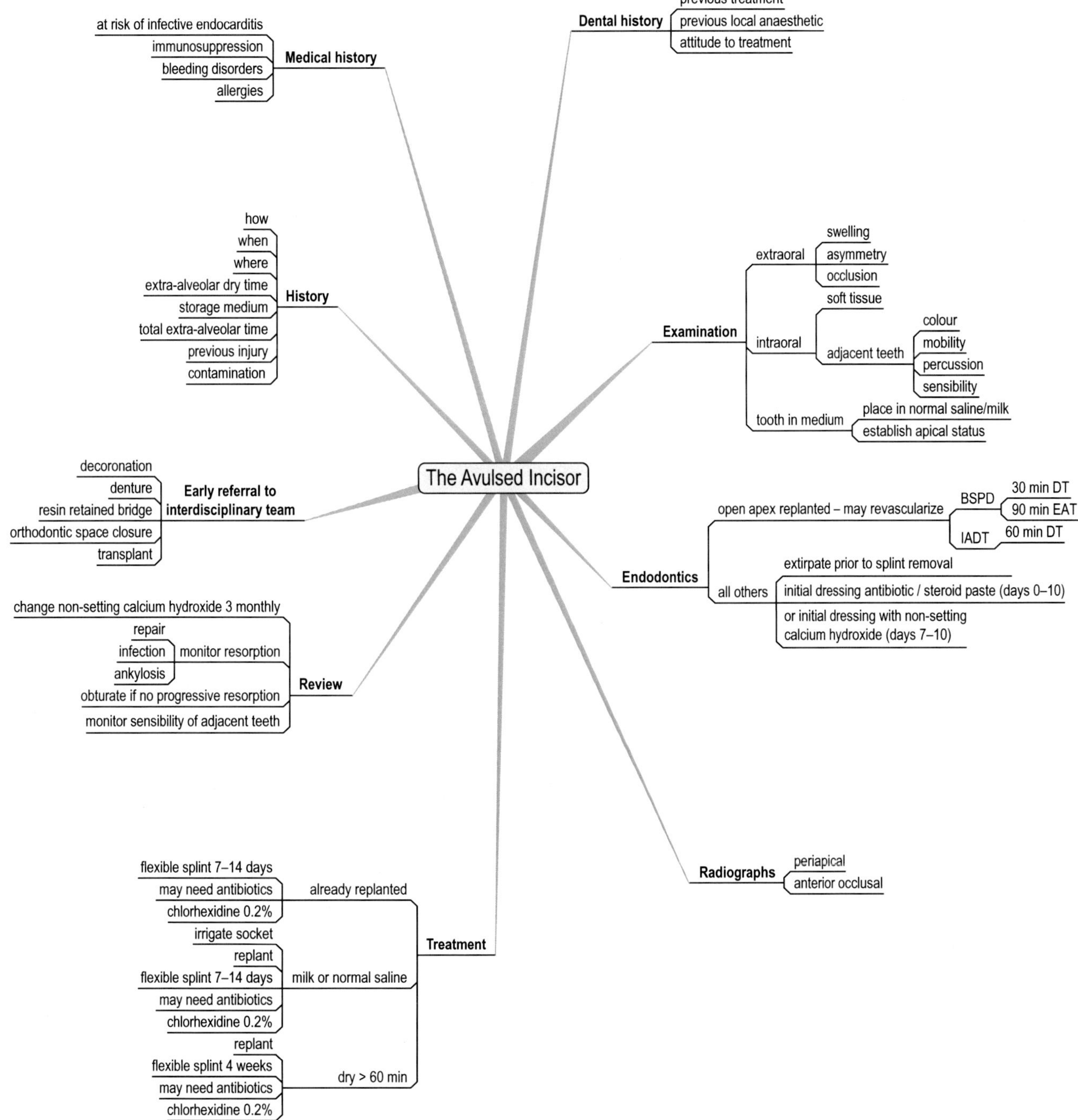
The Avulsed Incisor
Medical history
at risk of infective endocarditis
immunosuppression
bleeding disorders
allergies
Dental history
previous treatment
previous local anaesthetic
attitude to treatment
History
how
when
where
extra-alveolar dry time
storage medium
total extra-alveolar time
previous injury
contamination
Examination
extraoral
swelling
asymmetry
occlusion
intraoral
soft tissue
adjacent teeth
colour
mobility
percussion
sensibility
tooth in medium
place in normal saline/milk
establish apical status
Early referral to interdisciplinary team
decoronation
denture
resin retained bridge
orthodontic space closure
transplant
Endodontics
open apex replanted – may revascularize
BSPD
30 min DT
90 min EAT
IADT
60 min DT
all others
extirpate prior to splint removal
initial dressing antibiotic / steroid paste (days 0–10)
or initial dressing with non-setting calcium hydroxide (days 7–10)
Review
change non-setting calcium hydroxide 3 monthly
repair
infection
ankylosis
monitor resorption
obturate if no progressive resorption
monitor sensibility of adjacent teeth
Radiographs
periapical
anterior occlusal
Treatment
already replanted
flexible splint 7–14 days
may need antibiotics
chlorhexidine 0.2%
milk or normal saline
irrigate socket
replant
flexible splint 7–14 days
may need antibiotics
chlorhexidine 0.2%
dry > 60 min
replant
flexible splint 4 weeks
may need antibiotics
chlorhexidine 0.2%

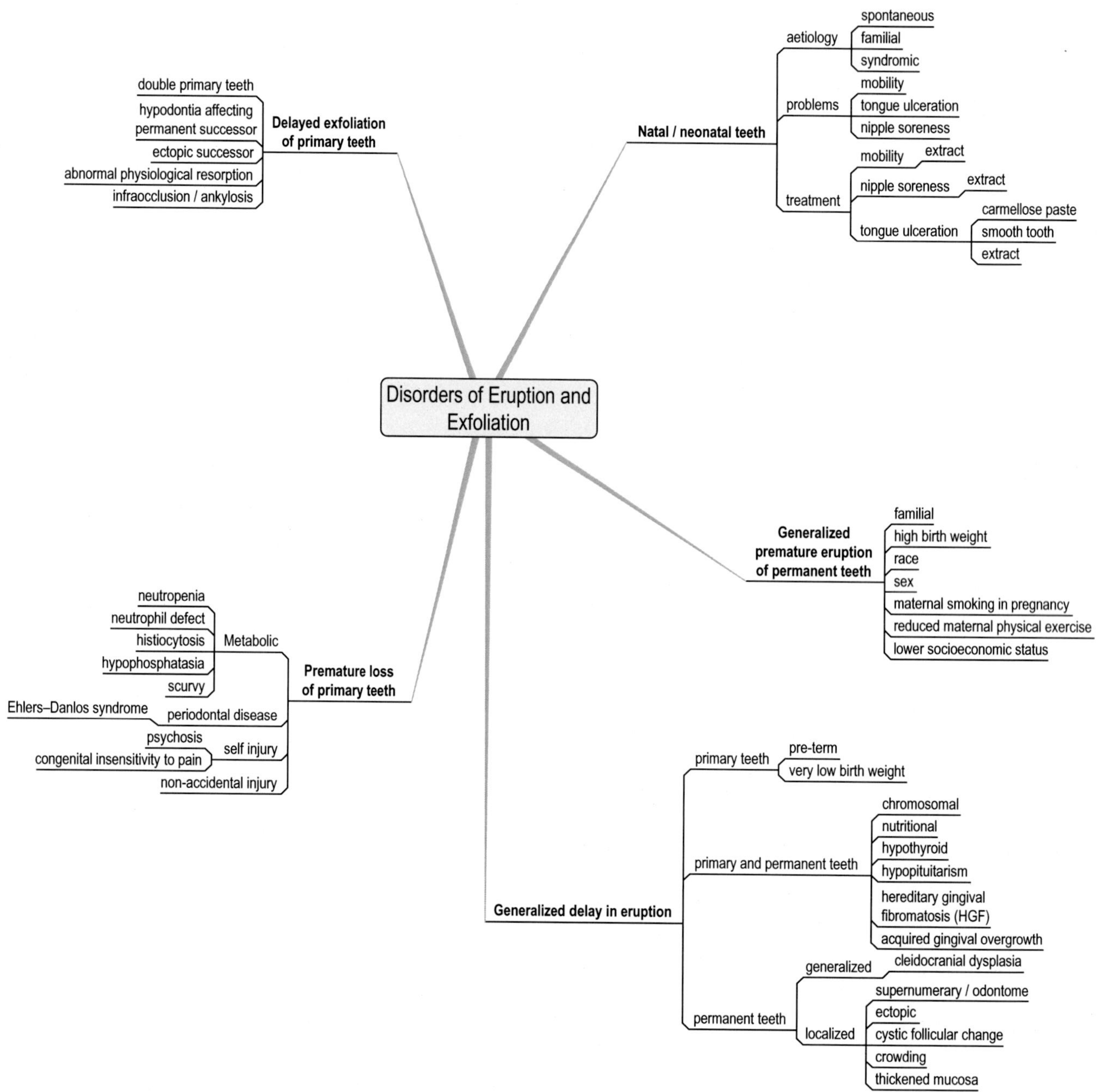
Disorders of Eruption and Exfoliation
Delayed exfoliation of primary teeth
double primary teeth
hypodontia affecting permanent successor
ectopic successor
abnormal physiological resorption
infraocclusion / ankylosis
Natal / neonatal teeth
aetiology
spontaneous
familial
syndromic
problems
mobility
tongue ulceration
nipple soreness
treatment
mobility
extract
nipple soreness
extract
tongue ulceration
carmellose paste
smooth tooth
extract
Generalized premature eruption of permanent teeth
familial
high birth weight
race
sex
maternal smoking in pregnancy
reduced maternal physical exercise
lower socioeconomic status
Premature loss of primary teeth
Metabolic
neutropenia
neutrophil defect
histiocytosis
hypophosphatasia
scurvy
periodontal disease
Ehlers–Danlos syndrome
self injury
psychosis
congenital insensitivity to pain
non-accidental injury
Generalized delay in eruption
primary teeth
pre-term
very low birth weight
primary and permanent teeth
chromosomal
nutritional
hypothyroid
hypopituitarism
hereditary gingival fibromatosis (HGF)
acquired gingival overgrowth
permanent teeth
generalized
cleidocranial dysplasia
localized
supernumerary / odontome
ectopic
cystic follicular change
crowding
thickened mucosa

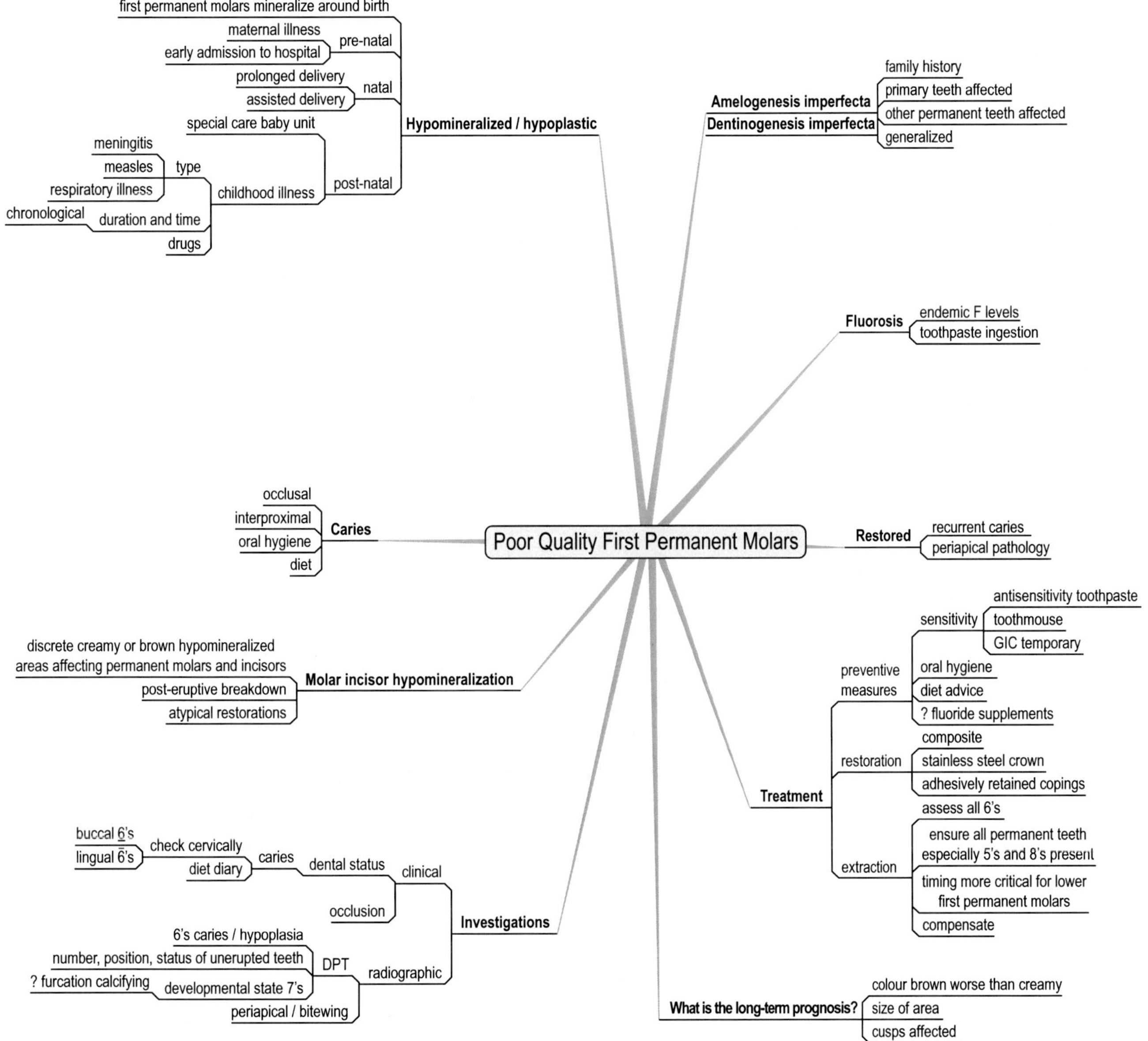
Poor Quality First Permanent Molars
Hypomineralized / hypoplastic
first permanent molars mineralize around birth
pre-natal
maternal illness
early admission to hospital
natal
prolonged delivery
assisted delivery
post-natal
special care baby unit
childhood illness
type
meningitis
measles
respiratory illness
duration and time
chronological
drugs
Amelogenesis imperfecta
Dentinogenesis imperfecta
family history
primary teeth affected
other permanent teeth affected
generalized
Fluorosis
endemic F levels
toothpaste ingestion
Caries
occlusal
interproximal
oral hygiene
diet
Restored
recurrent caries
periapical pathology
Molar incisor hypomineralization
discrete creamy or brown hypomineralized areas affecting permanent molars and incisors
post-eruptive breakdown
atypical restorations
Treatment
preventive measures
sensitivity
antisensitivity toothpaste
toothmouse
GIC temporary
oral hygiene
diet advice
? fluoride supplements
restoration
composite
stainless steel crown
adhesively retained copings
extraction
assess all 6's
ensure all permanent teeth especially 5's and 8's present
timing more critical for lower first permanent molars
compensate
Investigations
clinical
dental status
caries
check cervically
buccal 6's
lingual 6's
diet diary
occlusion
radiographic
DPT
6's caries / hypoplasia
number, position, status of unerupted teeth
developmental state 7's
? furcation calcifying
periapical / bitewing
What is the long-term prognosis?
colour brown worse than creamy
size of area
cusps affected

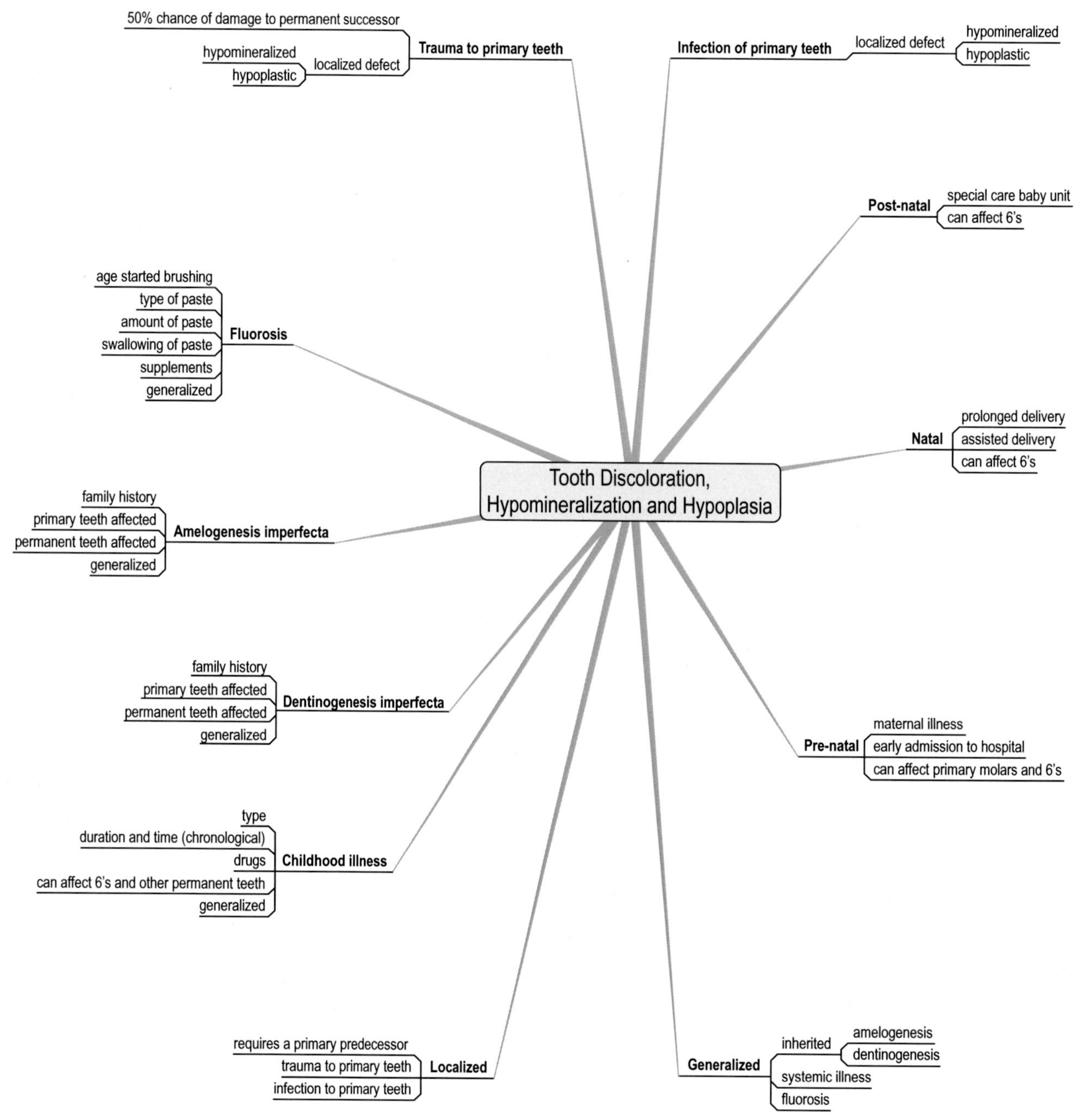
Tooth Discoloration, Hypomineralization and Hypoplasia
Trauma to primary teeth
50% chance of damage to permanent successor
localized defect
hypomineralized
hypoplastic
Infection of primary teeth
localized defect
hypomineralized
hypoplastic
Post-natal
special care baby unit
can affect 6's
Fluorosis
age started brushing
type of paste
amount of paste
swallowing of paste
supplements
generalized
Natal
prolonged delivery
assisted delivery
can affect 6's
Amelogenesis imperfecta
family history
primary teeth affected
permanent teeth affected
generalized
Dentinogenesis imperfecta
family history
primary teeth affected
permanent teeth affected
generalized
Pre-natal
maternal illness
early admission to hospital
can affect primary molars and 6's
Childhood illness
type
duration and time (chronological)
drugs
can affect 6's and other permanent teeth
generalized
Localized
requires a primary predecessor
trauma to primary teeth
infection to primary teeth
Generalized
inherited
amelogenesis
dentinogenesis
systemic illness
fluorosis

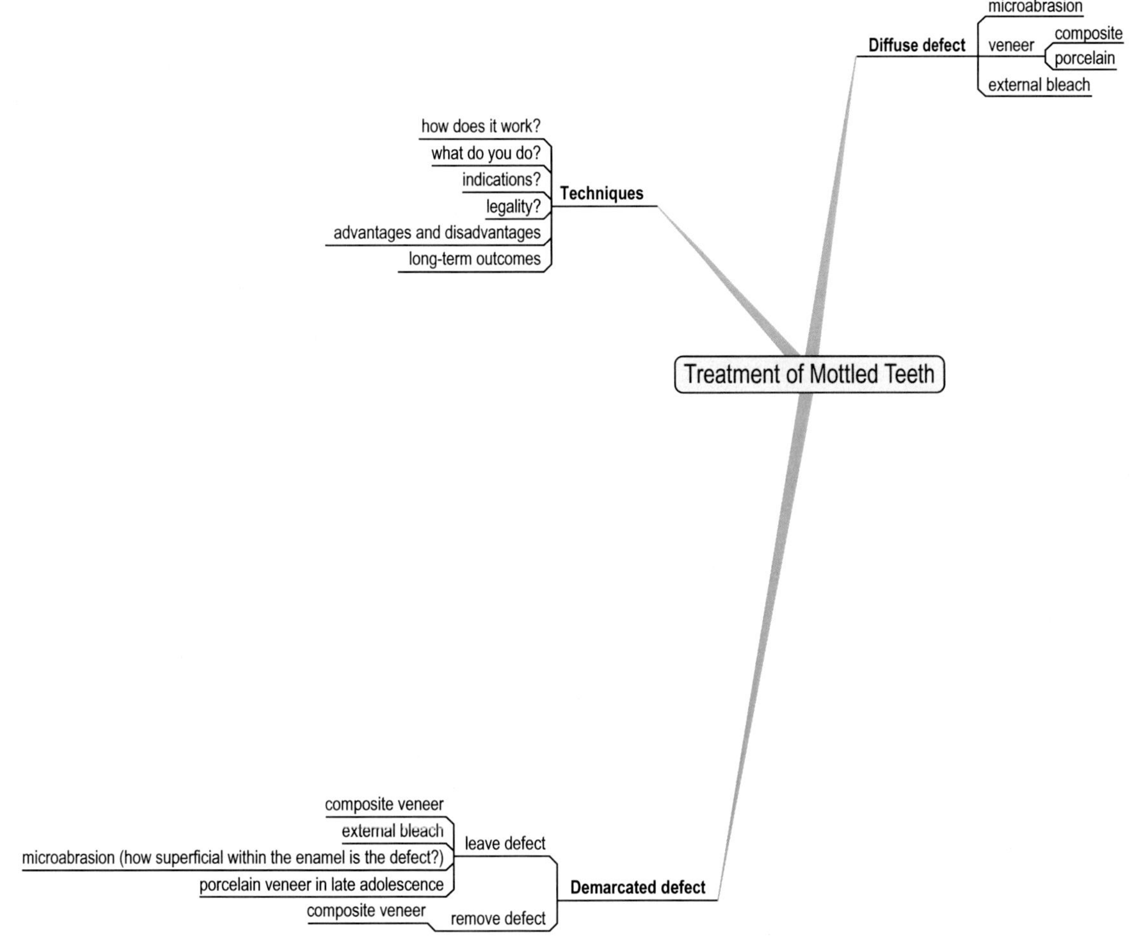
Treatment of Mottled Teeth
Diffuse defect
microabrasion
veneer
composite
porcelain
external bleach
Techniques
how does it work?
what do you do?
indications?
legality?
advantages and disadvantages
long-term outcomes
Demarcated defect
leave defect
composite veneer
external bleach
microabrasion (how superficial within the enamel is the defect?)
porcelain veneer in late adolescence
remove defect
composite veneer

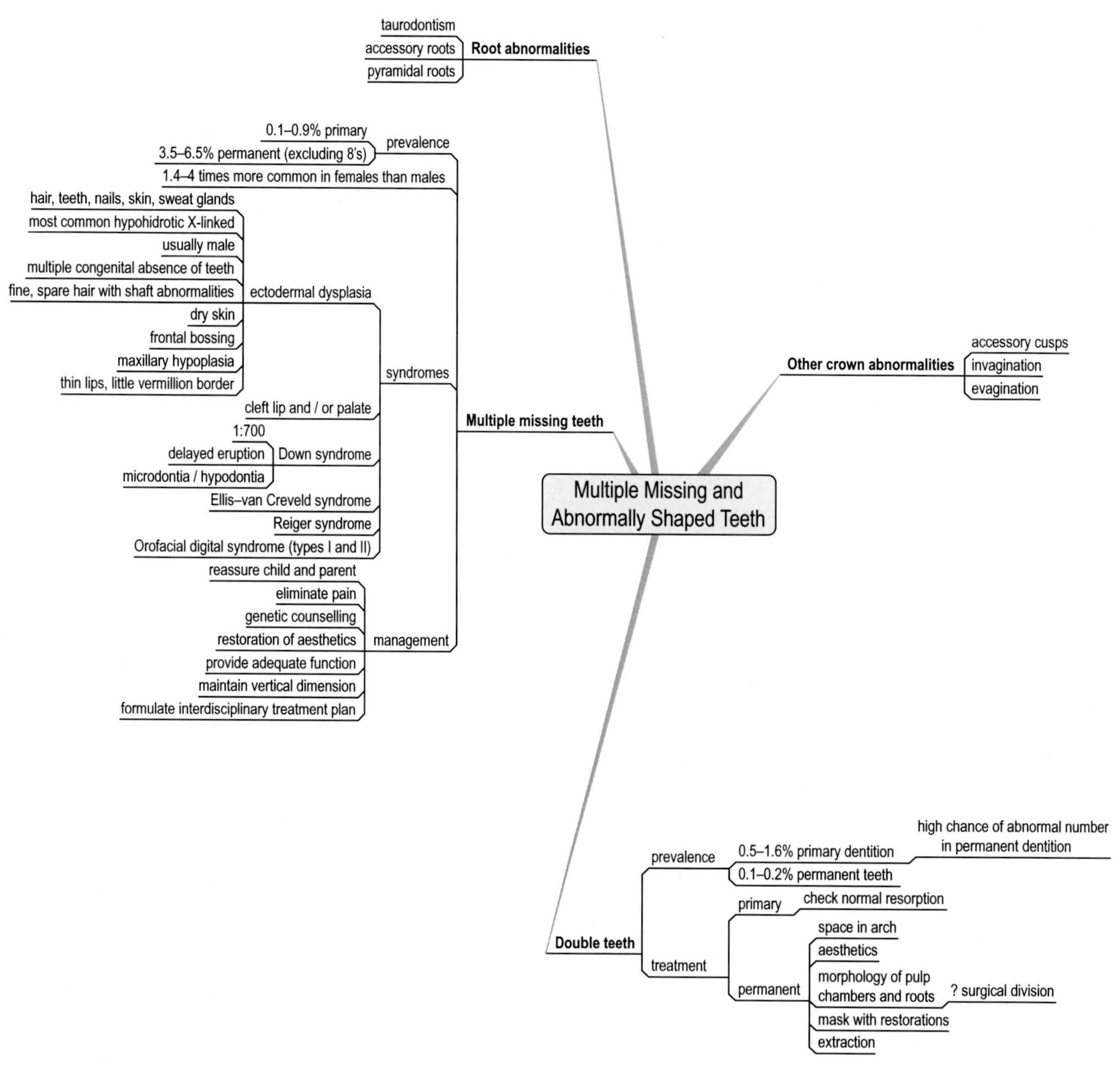
Multiple Missing and Abnormally Shaped Teeth
Root abnormalities
taurodontism
accessory roots
pyramidal roots
Multiple missing teeth
prevalence
0.1–0.9% primary
3.5–6.5% permanent (excluding 8's)
1.4–4 times more common in females than males
syndromes
ectodermal dysplasia
hair, teeth, nails, skin, sweat glands
most common hypohidrotic X-linked
usually male
multiple congenital absence of teeth
fine, spare hair with shaft abnormalities
dry skin
frontal bossing
maxillary hypoplasia
thin lips, little vermillion border
cleft lip and / or palate
Down syndrome
1:700
delayed eruption
microdontia / hypodontia
Ellis–van Creveld syndrome
Reiger syndrome
Orofacial digital syndrome (types I and II)
management
reassure child and parent
eliminate pain
genetic counselling
restoration of aesthetics
provide adequate function
maintain vertical dimension
formulate interdisciplinary treatment plan
Other crown abnormalities
accessory cusps
invagination
evagination
Double teeth
prevalence
0.5–1.6% primary dentition
high chance of abnormal number in permanent dentition
0.1–0.2% permanent teeth
treatment
primary
check normal resorption
permanent
space in arch
aesthetics
morphology of pulp chambers and roots
? surgical division
mask with restorations
extraction

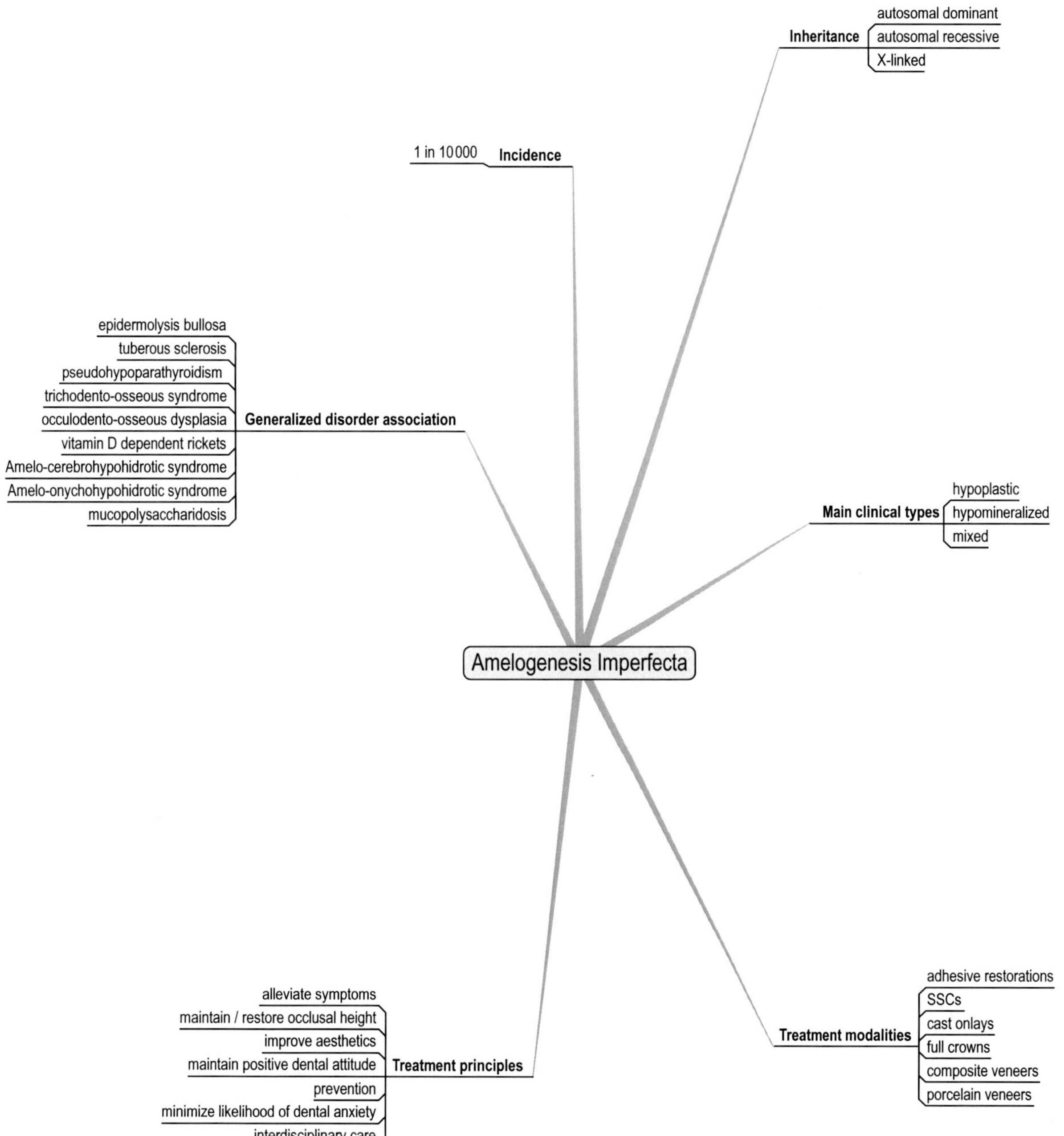
Amelogenesis Imperfecta
Inheritance
autosomal dominant
autosomal recessive
X-linked
Incidence
1 in 10000
Generalized disorder association
epidermolysis bullosa
tuberous sclerosis
pseudohypoparathyroidism
trichodento-osseous syndrome
occulodento-osseous dysplasia
vitamin D dependent rickets
Amelo-cerebrohypohidrotic syndrome
Amelo-onychohypohidrotic syndrome
mucopolysaccharidosis
Main clinical types
hypoplastic
hypomineralized
mixed
Treatment principles
alleviate symptoms
maintain / restore occlusal height
improve aesthetics
maintain positive dental attitude
prevention
minimize likelihood of dental anxiety
interdisciplinary care
Treatment modalities
adhesive restorations
SSCs
cast onlays
full crowns
composite veneers
porcelain veneers

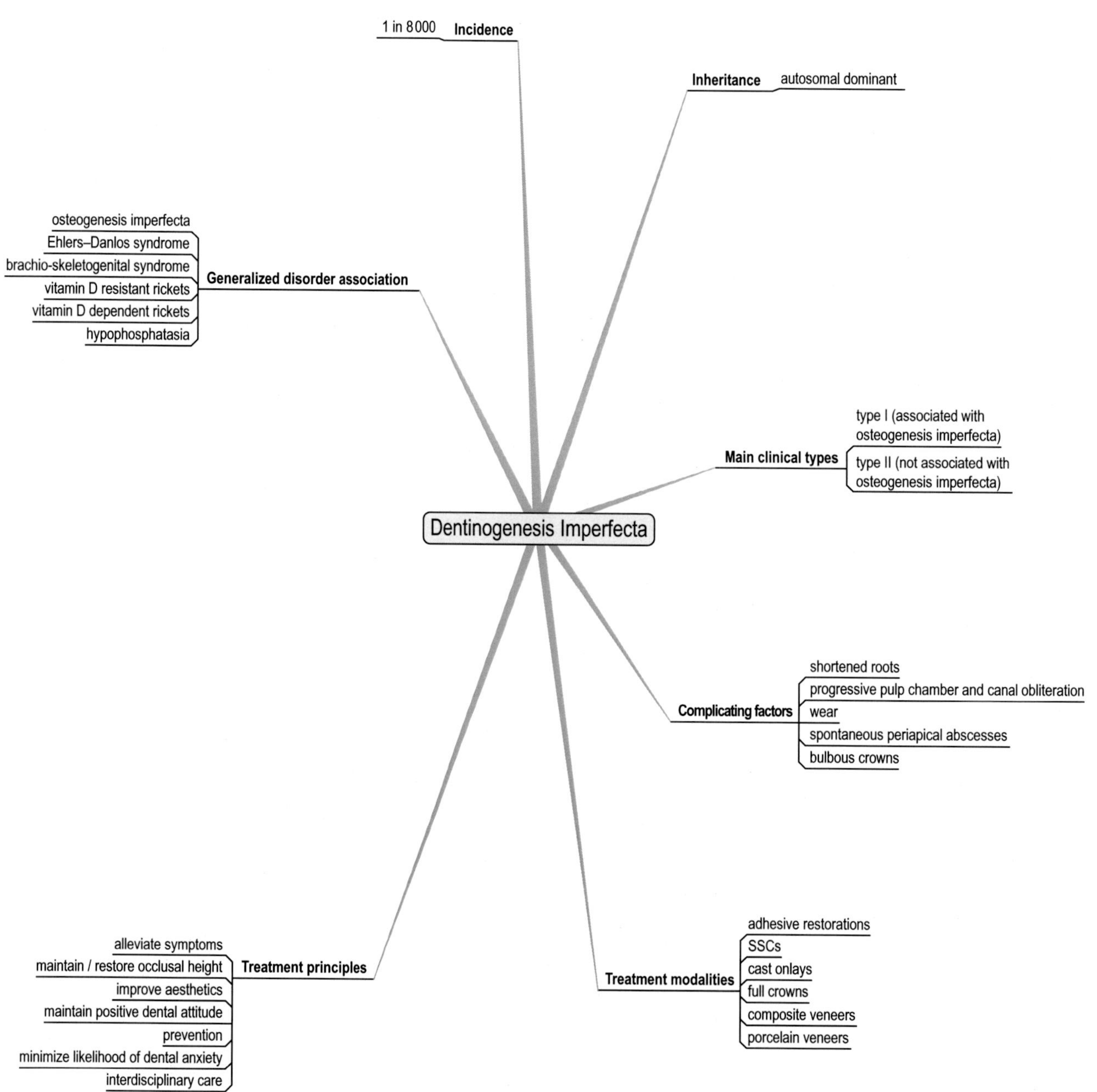
Dentinogenesis Imperfecta
Incidence
1 in 8000
Inheritance
autosomal dominant
Generalized disorder association
osteogenesis imperfecta
Ehlers–Danlos syndrome
brachio-skeletogenital syndrome
vitamin D resistant rickets
vitamin D dependent rickets
hypophosphatasia
Main clinical types
type I (associated with osteogenesis imperfecta)
type II (not associated with osteogenesis imperfecta)
Complicating factors
shortened roots
progressive pulp chamber and canal obliteration
wear
spontaneous periapical abscesses
bulbous crowns
Treatment modalities
adhesive restorations
SSCs
cast onlays
full crowns
composite veneers
porcelain veneers
Treatment principles
alleviate symptoms
maintain / restore occlusal height
improve aesthetics
maintain positive dental attitude
prevention
minimize likelihood of dental anxiety
interdisciplinary care

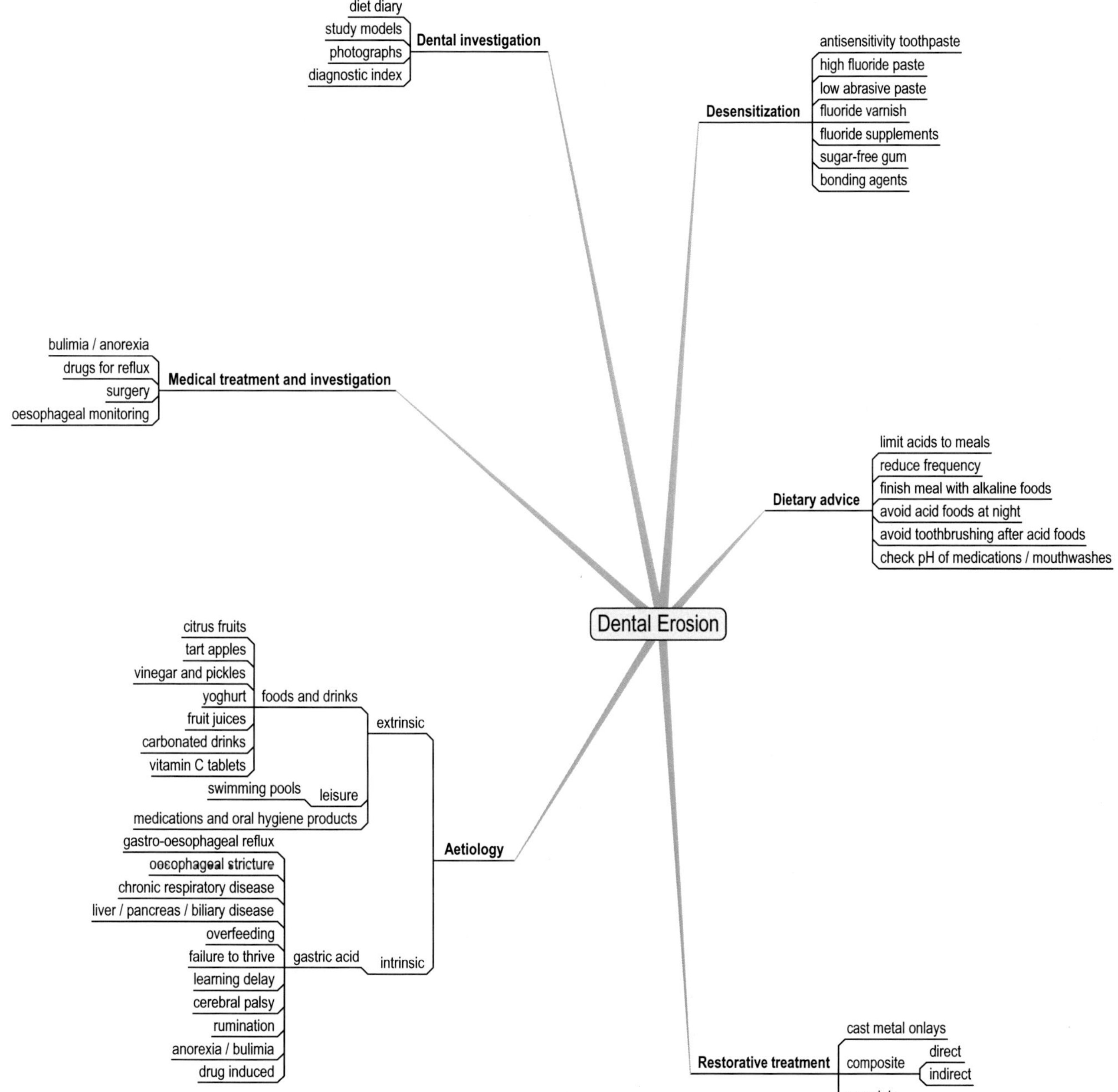
Dental Erosion
Dental investigation
diet diary
study models
photographs
diagnostic index
Desensitization
antisensitivity toothpaste
high fluoride paste
low abrasive paste
fluoride varnish
fluoride supplements
sugar-free gum
bonding agents
Medical treatment and investigation
bulimia / anorexia
drugs for reflux
surgery
oesophageal monitoring
Dietary advice
limit acids to meals
reduce frequency
finish meal with alkaline foods
avoid acid foods at night
avoid toothbrushing after acid foods
check pH of medications / mouthwashes
Aetiology
extrinsic
foods and drinks
citrus fruits
tart apples
vinegar and pickles
yoghurt
fruit juices
carbonated drinks
vitamin C tablets
leisure
swimming pools
medications and oral hygiene products
intrinsic
gastric acid
gastro-oesophageal reflux
oesophageal stricture
chronic respiratory disease
liver / pancreas / biliary disease
overfeeding
failure to thrive
learning delay
cerebral palsy
rumination
anorexia / bulimia
drug induced
Restorative treatment
cast metal onlays
composite
direct
indirect
porcelain

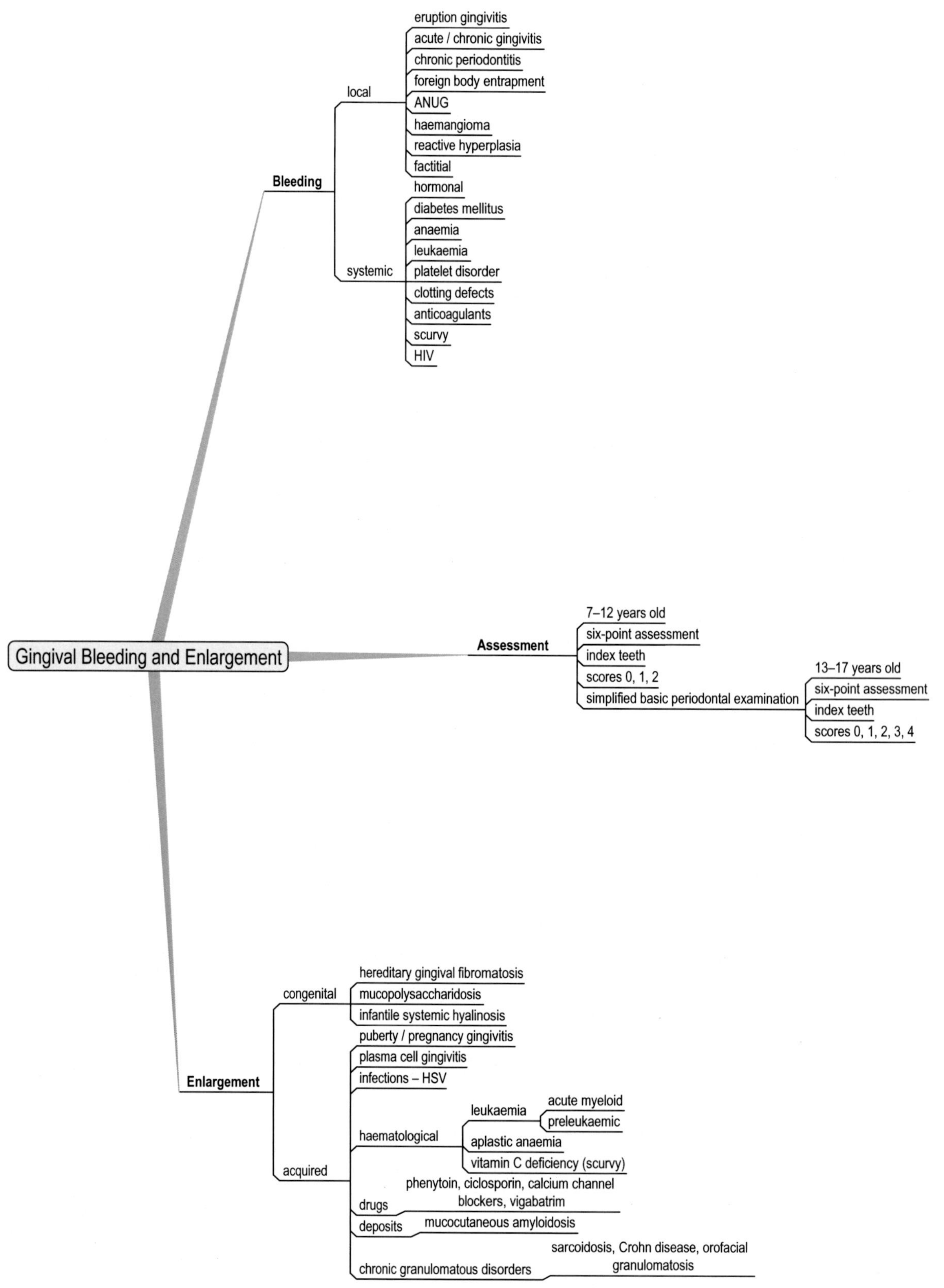
Gingival Bleeding and Enlargement
Bleeding
local
eruption gingivitis
acute / chronic gingivitis
chronic periodontitis
foreign body entrapment
ANUG
haemangioma
reactive hyperplasia
factitial
systemic
hormonal
diabetes mellitus
anaemia
leukaemia
platelet disorder
clotting defects
anticoagulants
scurvy
HIV
Assessment
7–12 years old
six-point assessment
index teeth
scores 0, 1, 2
simplified basic periodontal examination
13–17 years old
six-point assessment
index teeth
scores 0, 1, 2, 3, 4
Enlargement
congenital
hereditary gingival fibromatosis
mucopolysaccharidosis
infantile systemic hyalinosis
acquired
puberty / pregnancy gingivitis
plasma cell gingivitis
infections – HSV
haematological
leukaemia
acute myeloid
preleukaemic
aplastic anaemia
vitamin C deficiency (scurvy)
drugs
phenytoin, ciclosporin, calcium channel blockers, vigabatrim
deposits
mucocutaneous amyloidosis
chronic granulomatous disorders
sarcoidosis, Crohn disease, orofacial granulomatosis

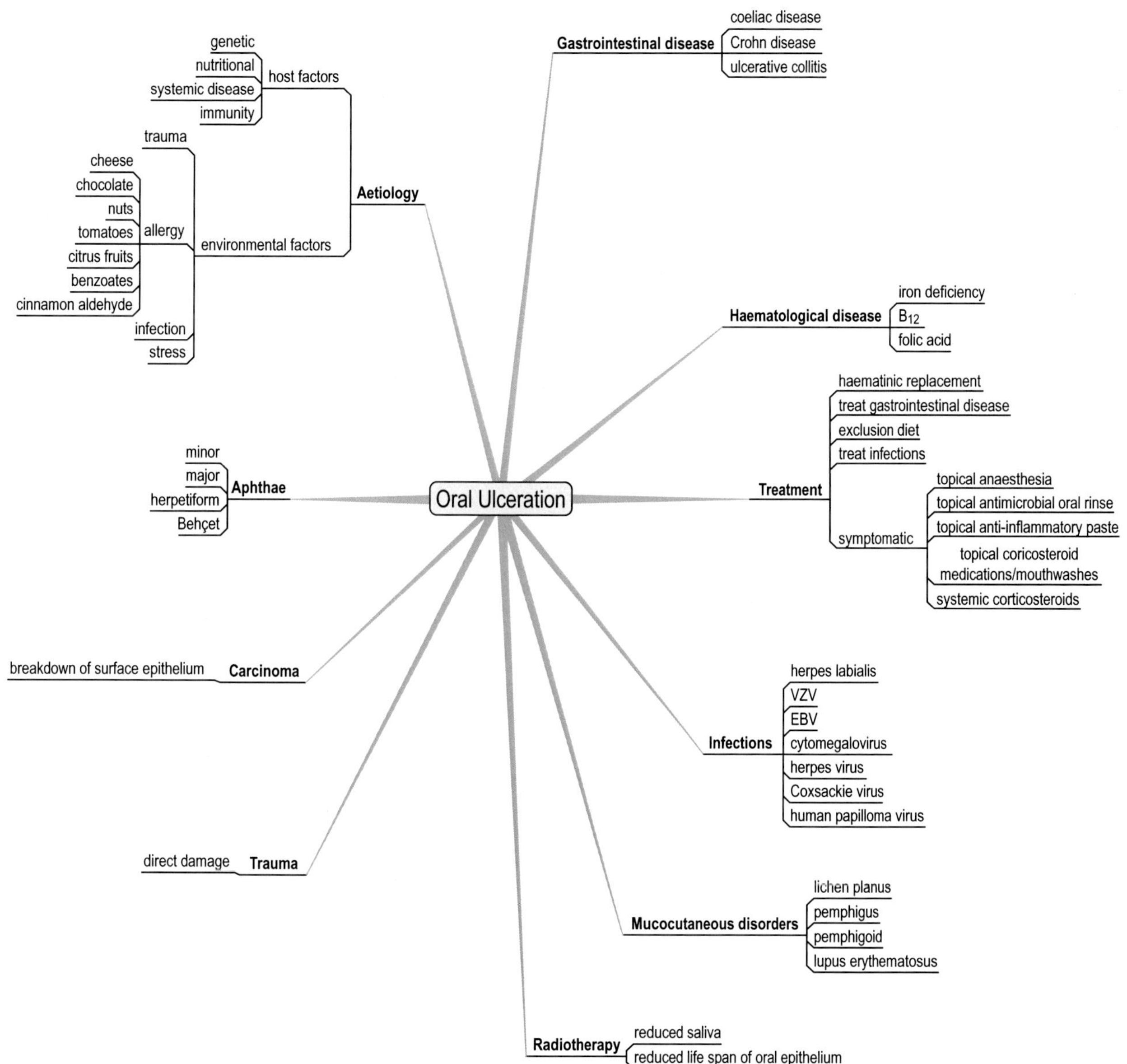

From Heasman P 2008 Master Dentistry Vol. 2, Restorative Dentistry, Paediatric Dentistry and Orthodontics, 2nd Edn. Edinburgh, Churchill Livingstone. Fig. 110, with permission.

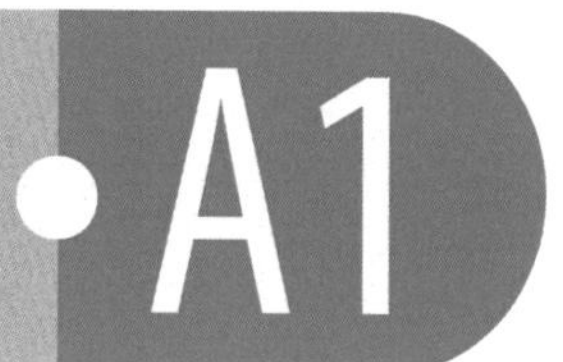

The index of orthodontic treatment need: dental health component

Grade	Characteristics
1. None	Extremely minor malocclusions including displacements <1 mm
2. Little	a. Increased overjet >3.5 mm but ≤6 mm with competent lips b. Reverse overjet >0 mm but ≤1 mm c. Anterior or posterior crossbite with ≤1 mm discrepancy between retruded contact position and intercuspal position d. Displacement of teeth >1 mm but ≤2 mm e. Anterior or posterior open bite >1 mm but ≤2 mm f. Increased overbite ≥3.5 mm without gingival contact g. Prenormal or postnormal occlusions with no other anomalies; includes up to half a unit discrepancy
3. Moderate	a. Increased overjet >3.5 mm but ≤6 mm with incompetent lips b. Reverse overjet >1 mm but ≤3.5 mm c. Anterior or posterior crossbites with >1 mm but ≤2 mm discrepancy between retruded contact position and intercuspal position d. Displacement of teeth >2 mm but ≤4 mm e. Lateral or anterior open bite >2 mm but ≤4 mm f. Increased and complete overbite without gingival or palatal trauma
4. Great	a. Increased overjet >6 mm but ≤9 mm b. Reverse overjet >3.5 mm with no masticatory or speech difficulties c. Anterior or posterior crossbite with >2 mm discrepancy between retruded contact position and intercuspal position d. Severe displacements of teeth >4 mm e. Extreme lateral or anterior open bites >4 mm f. Increased and complete overbite with gingival or palatal trauma h. Less extensive hypodontia, requiring prerestorative orthodontics or orthodontic space closure to obviate the need for a prosthesis l. Posterior lingual crossbite with no functional occlusal contact in one or both buccal segments m. Reverse overjet >1 mm but <3.5 mm, with recorded masticatory and speech difficulties t. Partially erupted teeth, tipped and impacted against adjacent teeth x. Supplemental teeth
5. Very great	a. Increased overjet >9 mm h. Extensive hypodontia with restorative implications (more than one tooth missing in any quadrant) requiring prerestorative orthodontics i. Impeded eruption of teeth (with the exception of third molars) owing to crowding, displacement, the presence of supernumerary teeth, retained deciduous teeth and any pathological cause m. Reverse overjet >3.5 mm with reported masticatory and speech difficulties p. Defects of cleft lip and palate s. Submerged deciduous teeth

From Heasman P 2013 Master Dentistry Vol. 2, Restorative Dentistry, Paediatric Dentistry and Orthodontics, 3rd edn. Churchill Livingstone, Edinburgh, with permission.

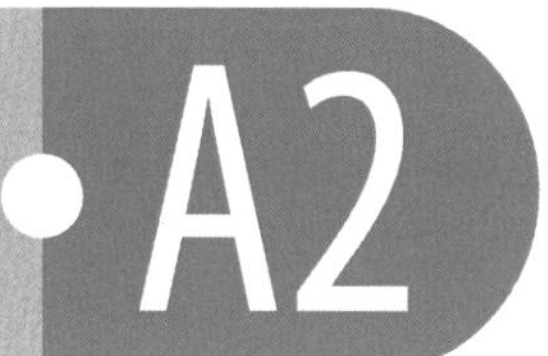

Classification and definitions

Extraoral	Skeletal pattern (Anteroposterior)	Class I	Mandible 2–4 mm behind maxilla
		Class II	Mandible >4 mm behind maxilla
		Class III	Mandible <2 mm behind maxilla
	Skeletal pattern (Vertical: FMPA)	Average	Frankfort plane (FP; superior aspect of external auditory meatus to lower border of orbit) and mandibular plane (MP; lower border of mandible) intersect at occiput (back of head)
		Increased	FP and MP intersect in front of occiput
		Reduced	FP and MP intersect behind occiput
	Skeletal pattern (Transverse)	Symmetrical	Midpoint of eyebrows, nasal tip, middle of upper lip at vermillion border and chinpoint coincident with facial midline
		Asymmetrical	Midpoint of eyebrows, nasal tip, middle of upper lip and chinpoint non-coincident with facial midline
	Skeletal pattern	Retrognathia	Retrusion of maxilla and/or mandible relative to cranial base
		Prognathism	Protrusion of maxilla and/or mandible relative to cranial base
	Nasolabial/lips/smile	Nasolabial angle	Angle between line drawn through midpoint of nostril aperture and line perpendicular to FP while intersecting subnasale
		Competent	Upper and lower lips contact without muscular activity at rest
		Incompetent	Some muscular activity required for lips to meet together
		Posed smile	Voluntary smile, with no emotional link and fairly reproducible
		Spontaneous smile	Involuntary smile, linked with emotion, maximal elevation of upper lip
		Smile arc	Relationship between curvature of maxillary incisal edges and canine tips to curvature of lower lip during posed smile.
	TMJ/mandibular position	Centric relation	Condyle in most superior anterior position in glenoid fossa
		Rest position (RP) of the mandible	Position in which muscles acting on mandible show minimal activity; determined by resting lengths of muscles of mastication
		Postured position	Position in which mandible habitually maintained to facilitate anterior oral seal or aesthetics
		Freeway space	Space between occlusal surfaces of the teeth when the mandible is in RP or a position of habitual posture
		Premature contact	Occlusal contact during centric path of closure of mandible before maximum intercuspation; may produce mandibular displacement, tooth movement or both
		Mandibular displacement	When closing from RP, mandible displaces (either laterally or anteriorly) to avoid premature contact
		Mandibular deviation	Closure path of mandible starts from a postured position
Incisor relationship (British Standards Institute classification)	Class I	Lower incisor edges occlude with or lie immediately below cingulum plateau of upper central incisors	
	Class II	Lower incisor edges lie posterior to cingulum plateau of upper incisors	
	Division 1	Upper central incisors are proclined or of average inclination; overjet increased	
	Division 2	Upper central incisors are retroclined; overjet usually minimal or may be increased	
	Class III	Lower incisor edges lie anterior to cingulum plateau of upper incisors; overjet reduced or reversed	

Continued

Molar relationship (Angle's classification)	Class I		Mesiobuccal cusp of $\underline{6}$ occludes with buccal groove of $\overline{6}$
	Class II		Mesiobuccal cusp of $\underline{6}$ occludes anterior to buccal groove of $\overline{6}$
	Class III		Mesiobuccal cusp of $\underline{6}$ occludes posterior to buccal groove of $\overline{6}$
Dental	Malocclusion		Variation from ideal occlusion with dental health and/or psychosocial implications; division between normal occlusion and malocclusion debatable
	Cingulum plateau		Convexity of cervical third of lingual/palatal aspect of incisors and canines
	Angulation		Degree of tip of a tooth in mesiodistal plane
	Inclination		Degree of tip of a tooth in labio-palatal plane
	Proclined		Upper or lower incisors incline labially to a greater degree than normal
	Retroclined		Upper or lower incisors incline palatally/lingually to a greater extent than normal
	Overjet		Distance between upper and lower incisors in horizontal plane; normal = 2–4 mm
	Reverse		Lower incisors lie anterior to upper incisors; if one or two incisors are involved, term anterior crossbite used
	Overbite		Vertical overlap of upper and lower incisors when viewed anteriorly: normal = $\frac{1}{3}$ – $\frac{1}{2}$ coverage of lower incisors; $>\frac{1}{2}$ = increased; $<\frac{1}{3}$ = reduced
	Curve of Spee		Curvature of occlusal plane in sagittal plane
	Complete		Lower incisors occlude with upper incisors or palatal mucosa
	Traumatic		Occlusion of lower incisors with palatal mucosa with ulceration
	Incomplete		Lower incisors do not occlude with opposing upper incisors or palatal mucosa when buccal segment teeth are in occlusion
	Open bite	Anterior	No vertical overlap of incisors when buccal segment teeth are in occlusion
		Posterior	When teeth are in occlusion, there is space between posterior teeth
	Bimaxillary	Proclination	Upper and lower incisors are proclined relative to skeletal base
		Retroclination	Upper and lower incisors are retroclined relative to skeletal base
	Dentoalveolar compensation		Inclination of teeth compensates for underlying skeletal pattern, so occlusal relationship less marked
	Bolton (tooth size) discrepancy		Mismatch between sum of m-d widths of maxillary and mandibular dentition
	Dilaceration		Abnormal bend or curve in root or crown often following trauma
	Supernumerary teeth		Teeth in excess of normal series
Occlusion	Centric		Position of maximum interdigitation
	Ideal		Anatomically perfect arrangement of the teeth; rare
	Normal		Acceptable variation from ideal occlusion
Crossbite	Buccal		Buccal cusps of lower premolars and/or molars occlude buccally to buccal cusps of upper premolars and/or molars
	Lingual (scissors bite)		Buccal cusps of lower premolars and/or molars occlude lingually to palatal cusps of upper premolars or molars
Crowding/spacing	Crowding		Insufficient space to accommodate teeth in perfect alignment in arch, or segment of arch
	Rotation		Tooth twisted around long axis
	Impaction		Impeded tooth eruption, may be as a result of displacement of tooth, crowding or supernumerary
	Leeway space		Difference in diameter between C, D, E and 3, 4, 5
	Midline diastema		Space between 1–1; more common in upper arch
	Spacing		Teeth do not touch interproximally; localized or generalized
	Hypodontia		One or more permanent teeth (excluding third molars) congenitally absent
Anchorage/tooth movement	Anchorage		Source of resistance to forces generated in reaction to active components of an appliance
	Intermaxillary		Between arches
	Intramaxillary		Within same arch
	Tilting		Movement of root apex and crown of tooth in opposite directions around a fulcrum
	Bodily		Equal movement of root apex and crown of tooth in same direction
	Uprighting		Mesial or distal movement of root apex so root and crown of tooth are at ideal angulation
	Torque		Movement of root apex buccolingually, with no or minimal movement of crown in same direction
	Centroid		Imaginary point in root, ~ $\frac{1}{3}$ from apex, about which a tooth will tip when force applied to crown
	Moment (of a force)		Tendency of a force to cause rotation
	Migration		Physiological (minor) movement of tooth
	Relapse		Return, following correction, of features of original malocclusion
	Hyalinization		Loss of cells from an area as per light microscopy
	Transseptal fibres		Periodontal fibres interconnecting adjacent teeth
	Camouflage		Occlusal compensation by orthodontic tooth movement for skeletal discrepancies

Extractions	Balancing	Extraction of same (or adjacent) tooth on opposite side of arch to maintain symmetry	
	Compensating	Extraction of same tooth in opposing arch	
	Serial	Extract C's at 8.5–9.5 years, D's ~1 year later, 4's as 3's erupting	
Functional occlusion	Working side	Side to which mandible shifts during normal masticatory function	
	Non-working side	Side away from which mandible moves during normal masticatory function	
	Non-working side interferences	Occlusal contacts present on non-working side during lateral excursion of mandible	
	Disclusion	Dynamic separation of opposing teeth during mandibular movements	
	Canine guided	Contact maintained on working side canine teeth during lateral excursion of mandible	
	Group function	Contacts maintained between several teeth on working side during lateral excursion of mandible	
Appliances	Removable	Appliance removable from mouth consisting primarily of wire and acrylic components; may be active or passive; used almost exclusively in upper arch; most functional appliances are removable	
	Fixed	Appliance fixed to teeth by attachments through which force application is by archwires or auxiliaries	
	Archwire	Wire engaged into orthodontic brackets to provide active forces for tooth movement or to stabilize teeth	
	Anchorage	Lingual arch	Mandibular fixed anchorage reinforcing appliance, wire soldered onto 6|6 bands extends forward to contact lingual surfaces of incisors, to maintain arch length
		Nance palatal arch	Maxillary fixed anchorage reinforcing appliance, wire soldered onto the 6|6 bands connected to acrylic button contacting anterior vault of palatal.
		Quadhelix	Maxillary expansion appliance, stainless steel wire, four helices, attached to 6|6 bands
		Transpalatal arch	Maxillary fixed anchorage appliance, wire connecting 6|6 bands, to maintain intermolar width
	Two-by-four	Fixed appliance to 6|6 and 21|12	
	Couple	Pair of equal and opposite parallel forces applied to a body	
	Functional	Appliance using, removing or modifying forces generated by orofacial musculature, tooth eruption and dentofacial growth	
	Headgear	Extraoral appliance using cervical or cranial anchorage (or both) to apply forces to teeth or jaws for tooth movement or growth modification	
	Facemask	Extraoral appliance using anchorage from chin and forehead to apply anterior forces to maxillary dentition and/or maxilla; frequently used in class III malocclusion	
Cephalometric analysis	Cephalometric analysis	Evaluation and interpretation of both lateral and p-a radiographs of head (usually confined to former)	
	Ricketts' E-Line	Tangent to chin and nose used to assess lip fullness; see Appendix 5, Fig. A5.3	
Orthofgnathic surgery (OGS)	Pre-surgical orthodontics	Orthodontic treatment in preparation for OGS	
	Decompensation	Removal of dentoalveolar compensation prior to OGS	
	OGS	Surgical repositioning of mandible and/or maxilla for correction of dentofacial deformity	
	Osteotomy	Bilateral sagittal split (BSSO)	Surgical mandibular procedure, ramus split parallel to sagittal plane, used to advance, setback or rotate mandible
		Le Fort 1	Surgical maxillary procedure, maxilla osteotomised above tooth apices, used to advance or vertically reposition maxilla
	Autorotation	Rotation of mandible around condylar axis after vertical maxillary repositioning	
	Distraction osteogenesis	Surgical technique for lengthening bones and their associated soft tissue envelope, involving corticotomy, followed by gradual separation (distraction) of bone segments (1 mm/day) and osseous infill	
	Genioplasty	Surgical chin procedure to reposition bony chin point a-p, vertically and/or transversely	
Tooth surface loss	Abrasion	Loss of tooth substance as a result of wear caused by dissimilar materials	
	Attrition	Loss of tooth substance as a result of tooth wear	
	Erosion	Loss of tooth substance as a result of chemical dissolution	
Growth	Growth rotation	Rotation of core of mandible and maxilla in relation to cranial base; occurs with normal growth; may be clockwise or anticlockwise	
	Functional matrix theory	Theory suggesting skeletal growth determined by functional spaces and soft tissues associated with skeletal unit	

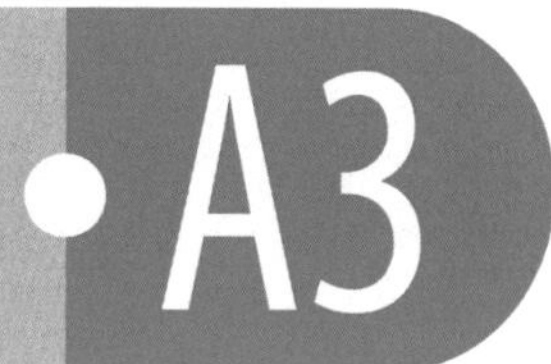

Orthodontic problems: referral guide

When to refer	What to refer
Primary dentition	• Gross skeletal discrepancy • Markedly slow dental development (see Chapters 1 and 33) • Craniofacial anomalies, especially cleft lip and/or palate (unless care provided already by specialist team) (see Chapter 21)
Mixed dentition	• Increased overjet with associated severe teasing or marked lip incompetence (greater trauma risk[1]) (see Chapter 9) • Severe reverse overjet[2] (see Chapter 11) • Anterior crossbite with marked mandibular displacement, with or without associated periodontal trauma (see Chapter 10) • Posterior crossbite with marked mandibular displacement (see Chapter 14) • Unerupted upper permanent incisor(s) (see Chapter 2) • Ectopic eruption of 6 (see Chapter 1) • Poor-quality first permanent molars (see Chapter 34) • Developmentally absent permanent teeth (see Chapter 8) • Palatal/ectopic canine (see Chapter 6) • Pathology, e.g. root resorption of 2's by 3's (see Chapter 6) • Medically compromised (see Appendix 4)
Permanent dentition	• Manifest malocclusion with or without skeletal problem (see Chapter 5) • Drifting incisors (see Chapter 18) • Temporomandibular joint problem (see Chapter 17) • Complex combined orthodontic-restorative or orthodontic-orthognathic problems (see Chapter 17)

[1]Early growth modification indicated

[2]Likely to benefit from early orthopaedic intervention

Adapted by permission from Scott JK & Atack NE, 2015 The developing occlusion of children and young people in general practice: when to watch and when to refer. Br Dent J. Macmillan Publishers Ltd.

Adapted with permission of BOS.

Primary resources and recommended reading

British Orthodontic Society 2010 Managing the Developing Occlusion – A Guide for Dental Practitioners, London.

Cobourne M 2014 National clinical guidelines for the extraction of first permanent molars in children. Br Dent J 217:643–648.

Scott JE, Atack NE 2015 The developing occlusion of children and young people in general practice: when to watch and when to refer. Br Dent J 218:151–156.

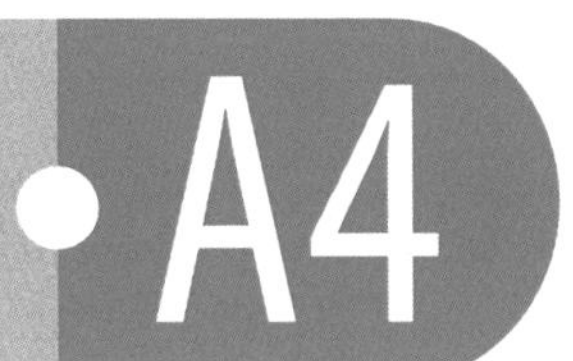

Implications of some medical problems for orthodontics

Problem	Implications
Asthma	• Risk of intraoral candidiasis with steroid-based inhalers • Maintain excellent oral and appliance hygiene, especially with URA
Allergy	
Latex	• Refer for testing to confirm • Avoid latex gloves and latex-containing orthodontic products • Treat early morning to avoid exposure to airborne latex products
Nickel	• Uncommon for intraoral allergy • Place plastic sleeving on headgear to avoid extraoral dermatitis; if intraoral atopy confirmed, use nickel-free appliance components
Bleeding diathesis	• Liaise with medical specialist regarding extractions/surgery • May usually proceed with orthodontic treatment • Avoid mucosal/gingival irritation from appliances
Biphosphonates	• Discuss potential treatment with physician, especially if extraction is likely • Assess risk of osteonecrosis and advise on slow tooth movement/reduced bone healing
Cardiac defect with IE risk	• Current guidelines indicate ABC is not recommended routinely for procedures likely to produce bacteraemia • Consult patient's cardiologist if any concern
Diabetes	• Only consider treatment if diabetes is well controlled • Greater risk of periodontal disease • Time appointment to minimize interference with control regime and possible hypoglycaemic attack
Drugs Steroids NSAIDs TSADs	• Slow orthodontic tooth movement
Epilepsy	• Treat only if epilepsy is well controlled • Avoid headgear and removable appliances due to risks associated with seizure • Phenytoin-induced gingival hyperplasia • Ensure patient has rested, eaten and taken antiepileptic medication before appointment to reduce risk of seizure
Juvenile rheumatoid arthritis	• Steroid injections into TMJ may reduce jaw growth • Prone to periodontal breakdown due to long-term steroids • Controversy with regard to role of functional appliances • Avoid prolonged orthodontic treatment
Leukaemia	• Delay treatment to >2 years post BMT • May have short blunt roots and increased risk of root resorption • Reduced resistance to oral infections • Growth modification guarded prognosis, as growth may be suppressed

URA, upper removable appliance; *IE*, infective endocarditis; *ABC*, antibiotic cover; *NSAIDs*, non-steroid anti-inflammatory drugs; *TSADs*, tricyclic antidepressants; *BMT*, bone marrow transplant.

Primary sources and recommended reading

Patel A, Burden DJ, Sandler J 2009 Medical disorders and orthodontics. J Orthod 36:1–21.

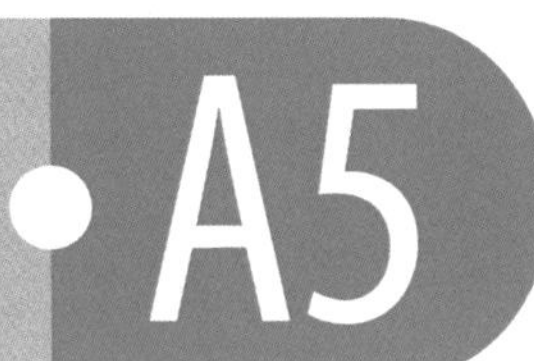

A5 Lateral cephalometric analysis

Aim and objective of cephalometric analysis

Aim: To assess the anteroposterior and vertical relationships of the upper and lower teeth with supporting alveolar bone to their respective maxillary and mandibular bases and to the cranial base.

Objective: To compare the patient to normal population standards appropriate to his or her racial group, identifying any differences between the two.

Practice of cephalometric analysis

Ensure that teeth are in occlusion and that the patient is not postured forward.

In a darkened room, by tracing or digitizing, identify the points and planes listed in **Table A5.1** (**Fig. A5.1**); always trace the most prominent image. For bilateral landmarks, unless directly superimposed, take the average. Calculate angular and linear measurements.

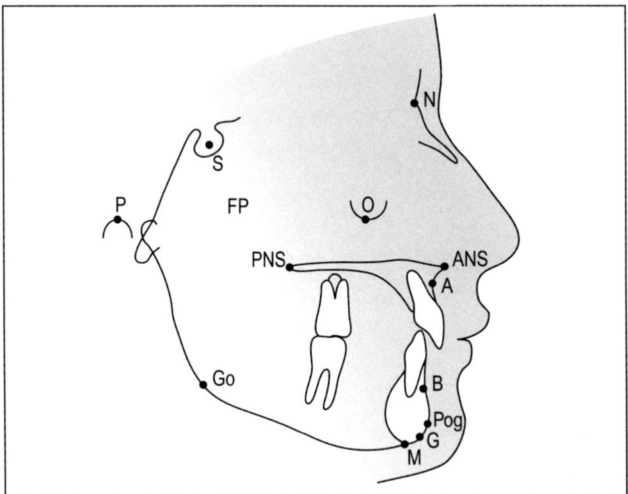

Fig. A5.1 Standard cephalometric points.
(From Heasman P 2013 Master Dentistry Vol. 2, Restorative Dentistry, Paediatric Dentistry and Orthodontics, 3rd edn. Churchill Livingstone, Edinburgh, with permission).

Cephalometric interpretation

For Caucasians, compare individual values with Eastman norms (**Table A5.2**).

Skeletal relationships

- *A-P.* If SNA is < or >81° and S–N/maxillary plane is within 8° ± 3°, correct ANB as follows: for every degree SNA is >81°, subtract 0.5° from the ANB value and vice versa.
- *Vertical.* MMPA and facial proportion should lend support to each other usually.

Tooth position

- To assess if overjet reduction is possible by tipping movement, do a prognosis tracing (**Fig. A5.2**), or for every 1 mm of overjet reduction, subtract 2.5° from 1 angulation. If the final angulation is not <95° to maxillary plane, tipping is acceptable.

Table A5.1 Definition of commonly used cephalometric points and planes

Points and planes	Definition
S	Sella: midpoint of sella turcica
N	Nasion: most anterior point of the frontonasal suture (may use the deepest point at the junction of the frontal and nasal bones instead)
P	Porion: uppermost, outermost point on the bony external auditory meatus (upper border of the condylar head is at the same level, which helps location)
O	Orbitale: most inferior anterior point on the margin of the orbit (use average of the left and right orbital shadows)
ANS	Tip of the anterior nasal spine
PNS	Tip of the posterior nasal spine (pterygomaxillary fissure is directly above, which helps location)
A	A point: most posterior point of the concavity on the anterior surface of the premaxilla in the midline below ANS
B	B point: most posterior point of the concavity on the anterior surface of the mandible in the midline above pogonion
Pog	Pogonion: most anterior point on the bony chin
Me	Menton: lowermost point on the mandibular symphysis in the midline
Go	Gonion: most posterior-inferior point at the angle of the mandible (bisect the angle between tangent to the posterior ramus and inferior body of the mandible to locate)
Planes S–N line	Line drawn through S and N
Frankfort plane	Line connecting porion and orbitale
Maxillary plane	Line joining PNS and ANS
Mandibular plane	Line joining Go and Me
Functional occlusal plane	Line drawn between the cusp tips of the first permanent molars and premolars/primary molars

From Heasman P 2013 Master Dentistry Vol. 2, Restorative Dentistry, Paediatric Dentistry and Orthodontics, 3rd edn. Churchill Livingstone, Edinburgh, with permission.

Table A5.2 Normal Eastman cephalometric values for Caucasians

Parameter	Value (± SD)
SNA	81 ± 3°
SNB	78 ± 3°
ANB	3 ± 2°
S–N/Max	8 ± 3°
$\overline{1}$ to maxillary plane	109 ± 6°
$\overline{1}$ to mandibular plane	93 ± 6°
Interincisal angle	135 ± 10°
MMPA	27 ± 4°
Facial proportion	55 ± 2%

From Heasman P 2013 Master Dentistry Vol. 2, Restorative Dentistry, Paediatric Dentistry and Orthodontics, 3rd edn. Churchill Livingstone, Edinburgh, with permission.

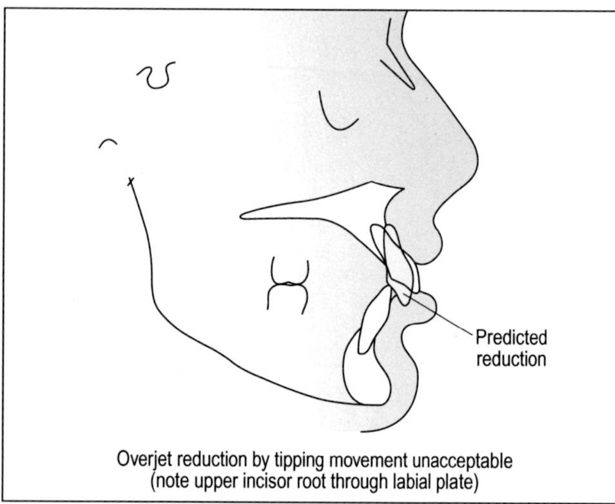

Predicted
reduction
Overjet reduction by tipping movement unacceptable
(note upper incisor root through labial plate)

Fig. A5.2 Prognosis training.

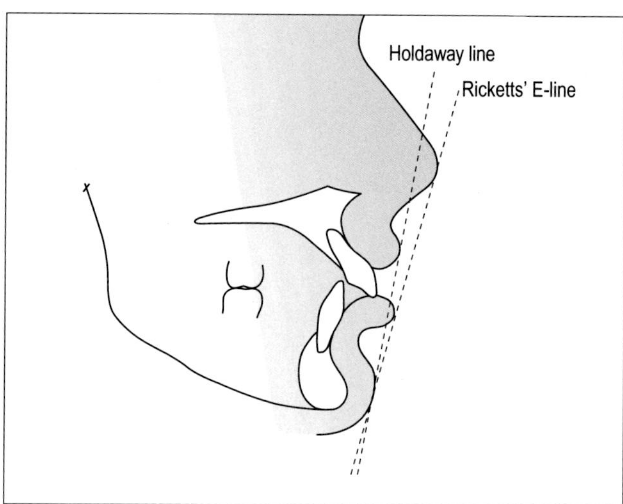

Fig. A5.3 Soft tissue lines.

- Check $\overline{1}$ angle to mandibular plane in conjunction with ANB and MMPA. There is an inverse relationship between $\overline{1}$ angle and MMPA.
- Interincisal angle: as this increases, overbite deepens.
- $\overline{1}$ to APo: this is an aesthetic reference line, but it is unwise to use for treatment planning purposes.

Soft tissue analysis

- *Holdaway line.* Lower lip should be ±1 mm to this line.
- *Ricketts' E-line.* Lower lip should be 2 mm (±2 mm) in front of this with the upper lip slightly behind (**Fig. A5.3**).

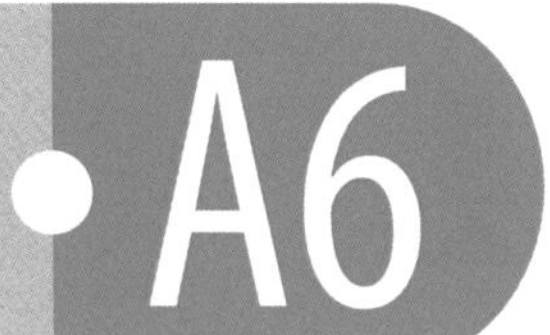

A structured dental trauma history form

THE LEEDS TEACHING HOSPITALS

Leeds Dental Institute

Department of Paediatric Dentistry

Trauma History & Diagnosis Form

WUN178

Name .... Hospital No. ..../.................................

Date ..../........../......... Referral Source ....

History of Injury

Date of injury ..../........../.......... Time ....

Location ....

Cause ....

Nature of Dental Injury

Other injuries? .... KO'd? Yes ☐ No ☐

Previous dental opinion/treatment?

Radiographs? ....

Symptoms now?

Nausea/dizziness/diplopia? ....

PDH **Relevant PMH**

EXAMINATION

Extraoral ....

Soft tissues ....

Facial skeleton ....

Mandibular movement/occlusion ....

Intraoral ....

Soft tissues ....

Oral hygiene/perio status ....

Teeth Present

8	7	6	5	4	3	2	1	1	2	3	4	5	6	7	8
8	7	6	5	4	3	2	1	1	2	3	4	5	6	7	8

A STRUCTURED DENTAL TRAUMA HISTORY FORM

Teeth Injured

Tooth	Clinical Injury	Vitality Tests Eth. Cl	ETP	Mobility	TTP	Transillu-mination	Root dev stage

Vitality
- = no resp
N = normal
+ = hypersens

Mobility
Grade 0–3

TTP
0 = nil
+ = yes
++ = severe
ANK = ankylosis

Transillumination
N = normal

Root Dev Stage
1 = < 2/3
2 = > 2/3
3 = complete (apex open)
4 = complete (apex closed)

For Avulsion Only

1. Extra Alv Period .... 2. Method of Storage ....

Radiographs Views

Report ....
....
....
....

Diagnosis

Tooth	Diagnosis

Treatment Plan

....
....
....
....
....
....

Signed Student .... Staff ....

Form reproduced courtesy of Monty Duggal, Leeds Dental Institute.

Index

Page numbers followed by "*f*" indicate figures, "*t*" indicate tables, and "*b*" indicate boxes.

A

Abnormally shaped teeth, multiple, 199–202
Abscess, 146–148
Absent upper lateral incisors, 11–15, 11*f*–12*f*, 223*f*
  treatment options for, 13, 13*b*
Acceptance
  of infraoccluded primary molar, 53
  of root resorption, 49–50
  of transposition of canines, 47
Accessory cusp, 201
Accessory roots, 202
Aciclovir, for primary herpetic gingivostomatitis, 216–217
Acrylated labial bow, lower incisor crowding, 101
Acrylic allergy, 114
Activator-type functional appliance, for increased overbite, 75
Active ligatures, 54
Acute lymphoblastic leukaemia, dental care and, 163
ADHD. *see* Attention deficit hyperactivity disorder (ADHD)
Adhesively retained copings, 189
Adolescent
  anxious, 247*f*
  consent for, 155
  gingival bleeding in, 214*b*
  high caries risk, 135–139, 135*f*–136*f*, 136*t*
    preventive care for, 137–138, 138*b*, 138*f*
  uncooperative child and, 149–156, 152*b*
Aesthetics
  for amelogenesis imperfecta, 204*t*
  appliances, drifting incisors, 111
AI. *see* Amelogenesis imperfecta (AI)
Alignment
  minor shifts in, 117, 117*f*
  in transposition, 47
  of upper canine, 118
Allergens, in recurrent aphthae, 218*b*
Allergy
  acrylic, 114
  implications of, 269
Alveolar bone grafting, for cleft lip and palate, 128, 129*b*
Alveolar development, localized failure of, in anterior open bite, 82*t*
Amelogenesis imperfecta (AI), 188, 203–205, 259*f*
  compared with dentinogenesis imperfecta (DI), 206, 206*f*
Analgesics, for carious primary teeth, 141*t*
Anchorage
  in bilateral crossbite, 93
  with crowding, 27, 28*b*
    temporary, 28–29
  with incisor drifting, 112
  in increased overbite, 75
  with palatal canines, 41
  with upper and lower arches, 34, 34*f*–35*f*
Angulation, canines/incisors, 13
Ankylosis-related resorption, 180
Anterior occlusion, 25*f*, 36*f*
Anterior open bite (AOB), 81–86, 81*f*–82*f*, 233*f*
  causes of, 82, 82*b*, 82*t*, 83*f*
  diagnosis of, 84
  examination of, 81–83, 81*f*–82*f*
  treatment of, 84–86, 84*b*, 86*b*
Antibiotics
  intravenous, 147, 147*t*
  oral, 146–147, 147*t*
  prophylaxis, 166
Antifungals, palatal stomatitis, 114
Anxiety
  dental, 152
  management, 152–153
Aphthae
  recurrent. *see* Recurrent aphthae
  types of, 217–218
Apical periodontitis, acute, 140
Appliance-related problems, 239*f*
Appliances
  in anterior open bite, 84
  ARAB (activation, retention, anchorage, baseplate), 9, 9*b*
  in bilateral crossbite, 93–94, 93*t*, 94*f*
  with canine transposition, 47–48
  with crowding, 28–29, 28*f*
  demineralization in, 19–20, 20*b*
  fixed
    for absent upper lateral incisors, 13
    with crowding and buccal upper canines, 17–18
  hygiene, 114
  for incisor crossbite, 64
  with increased overbite, 73, 75
  in lingual crossbite, 97–98, 97*f*
  lower incisor crowding, 101
  orthodontic, 112*t*
  for posterior crossbite, 89–90
  quadhelix, for buccal upper canines, 23, 24*f*
  related problems, 113–117
  removable, with absent upper lateral incisors, 14, 14*b*, 14*f*
  removable problems, 113*f*
    upper, 113
  removal of, in unerupted upper permanent central incisor, 9, 9*f*
  repair of, 115
  risk of, 19
  upper fixed, 111*f*
Arch
  affected by transposition of canines, 47
  crowding, treatment options for, 23
  expansion, in buccal upper canines, 23
  length discrepancy, 37
  upper, severe crowding and, 26
Archwire
  adjustment of, 115*f*
  projection of, 116
Arrested caries, 193
Asperger's syndrome, 158*b*
Asthma, implications of, 269
Attention deficit hyperactivity disorder (ADHD), 158*b*
Attrition
  in late lower incisor crowding,
    approximal, lack in modern diet, 100
  wear due to, 211
Autism, 158*b*
Avulsed incisor, 169, 179–183, 179*f*, 253*f*
  long-term treatment options for, 182

B

Bacteria, chromogenic, 193
Bad breath, 194
BAMP. *see* Bone anchored maxillary protraction (BAMP)
Bands
  avoidance with periodontal disease, 112
  for dentinogenesis imperfecta, 208
Baseplate
  in bilateral crossbite, 93
  in increased overbite, 75
  with palatal canines, 41
Begg retainer, 122, 123*f*
Behaviour management, 149–150
  nonpharmacological, 152
Behçet syndrome, 218
Bilateral crossbite, 91–98, 91*f*, 92*t*, 235*f*
Biphosphonates, implications of, 269
Bitewing radiographs
  of caries, in adolescents, 136*f*
  for carious primary teeth, 141, 141*f*
Bleaching, for enamel discoloration, 197
Bleeding diathesis, implications of, 269
Bolton discrepancy, 37, 38*b*
Bonded retention, for cleft lip and palate, 128
Bone anchored maxillary protraction (BAMP), 72
  advantages and disadvantages of, 72
Brackets
  bond failure, 115*f*, 115*t*
  drifting incisors, 112*t*
Brandy wine type (DI type III), 207
Breastfeeding, and caries, 130
Breath, bad, 194
Brown staining, fluorosis, 196
Buccal crossbite, bilateral, 91, 91*f*, 92*t*
Buccal eruption, of upper permanent canines, 16–20, 16*f*–17*f*, 17*b*, 19*f*
Buccal occlusion, right, 46, 46*f*

Buccal segment
of absent upper lateral incisors, 13–14
crossbite, 87, 87*f*, 90, 90*b*
Bullying
compared to teasing, 55
consequences of, 55
prominent teeth and, 55

C

Candida, and palatal stomatitis, 114, 114*b*
Canine fossa infection, maxillary, 146, 146*f*
Canines
eruption dates, 2*t*
palatal, 36–45
primary, unilateral loss of, 6, 6*b*
problems, 227*f*
removal of, 27–28
retraction and alignment of, 35, 35*b*, 35*f*
transposition in, 46
upper, crowding and buccal, 16–20, 16*f*–17*f*, 17*b*, 19*f*
Carbamide peroxide gel, 197
Carbonated drinks, causing erosion, 209, 209*b*
Cardiac defect with IE risk, implications of, 269
Caries, 188
in adolescents, 135–139, 135*f*–136*f*, 136*t*
risk assessment of, 136*b*
arrested, 193
in diabetic patient, 214
early childhood, 130–134, 131*f*
diet advice for, 132
high-risk factors for, 132*t*
home based advice for, 131
medication for, 133
professional interventions for, 133
removal of, 133
management of, for incisor crossbite, 64
Carious primary teeth, pain control and treatment planning for, 140–145, 140*f*
Carisolv, for early childhood caries, 133
Cast metal, with tooth surface loss, 211*t*
Cavernous sinus thrombosis, 146
Cavitation, in early childhood caries, 130*f*, 133
Cellulitis, facial, 146
Centerline, lower, monitor of, for incisor crossbite, 64
Central incisors, trauma to, 171*f*
Centreline shift
with buccal upper canines, 21, 22*f*
in posterior crossbite, 88, 88*b*
with unerupted upper central incisors, 6
correction of, 10, 10*b*
prevention of, 6
Cephalometric analysis, lateral, 271–272
aim and objective of, 271
interpretation of, 271, 272*t*
practice of, 271, 271*f*, 271*t*
Cephalometric findings, 34
Cephalometric radiograph
in bilateral crossbite, 92
for increased overjet, 57
for reverse overjet, 67, 70
Cephalometric values, TMJ pain and prominent chin and, 104, 104*t*
Cephalometry
in anterior open bite, 83
of buccal upper canines, 22
in increased overbite, 74, 77
Cervical pulpotomy, for fractured permanent incisor crown, 172
Cervical vertebral maturation (CVM) index, 57
Cheek mucosa, 115
Chemotherapy
dental care and, 163, 163*f*
side effects of, 164*b*
Chewing gum, sugar-free, for adolescents, with caries, 138
Child physical abuse, 169
Children
with disabilities and learning difficulties, 157–162, 161*t*
communication with, 160–161, 161*b*
dental management for, 159
general anaesthetic for, 160
medical comorbidities in, 160, 160*b*
nitrous oxide inhalation sedation for, 159–160
nonpharmacological management of, 159, 159*b*
radiographic investigation for, 158–160
treatment plan for, 160
medical problems in, 163–167, 167*b*, 167*t*
acute lymphoblastic leukaemia as, 163, 163*f*–164*f*
congenital heart defect as, 166, 166*f*
haemophilia A as, 165, 165*f*
vital bleaching for, 197
Chin, prominent, and TMJ pain, 102–108, 102*f*
Chronic moderate periodontitis, 111, 111*b*
Chronic periodontal disease, 109
Chronological hypoplasia, in childhood illnesses, 191
Class II division 2 malocclusion, 42
Class III malocclusion
diagnosis of, 105
TMJ pain and prominent chin and, 103–104
Classification and definitions, 265–267
Cleft lip and palate (CLP), 125–129, 125*f*, 241*f*
diagnosis of, 128
examination of, 126–127
extraoral, 126, 127*f*
intraoral, 125*f*, 126–127, 127*f*
genetic risk of, 125, 125*b*
investigations of, 127
prevalence of, 125, 125*b*
sex and side variation and, 125
treatment of, 128–129
Cleidocranial dysplasia, 185
CLP. *see* Cleft lip and palate (CLP)
Cold sore, 216, 217*f*
Colour, canines/incisors, 13
Coma, diabetic, 214
Combined orthodontic-surgical approach, TMJ pain and prominent chin and, 104–105, 105*b*
Combined orthodontic-surgical planning, 104*t*
Communication, with children with disabilities, 160–161, 161*b*
Communication passport, 157, 157*f*
Communicative management, 149–150
Composite, poor quality first permanent molars and, 189
Composite direct/indirect, with surface loss, 211*t*
Composite veneers, fluorotic mottling, 197–198
Computational method, of tooth-size discrepancy, 37–38
Computed tomography, of palatal canines, 38, 38*b*, 39*f*
Cone beam computed tomographic (CBCT) view, for unerupted upper permanent central incisor, 8
Consent, informed, 155, 155*b*
Copings, adhesively retained, 189
Coronal portion, of non-vital, root fractured tooth, 177
Coxsackie virus, 217
Crossbite, 32
bilateral, 91–98, 91*f*, 92*t*–93*t*
buccal segment, 87, 87*f*, 90, 90*b*
in cleft lip and palate, 126*b*, 127
with palatal canines, correction of, 41
posterior, 87–90
Crowding
buccal upper canines and, 224*f*
in increased overjet aetiology, 57*t*
lack of, 53
late lower incisor, 99–101
causes of, 100
diagnosis of, 100–101
management of, 100–101
lower and upper arch, 42–44, 44*f*–45*f*
severe, 25–35, 26*f*
Crown, shape abnormalities of, 201
Crown fragments, partial pulpotomy for, 173, 173*f*
Crypt displacement, 37
Cusp, accessory, 201
Cyclic neutropenia, 185*f*
Cytomegalovirus, 217

D

Deep overbite, 77–78
Delaire-type facemask, 70, 70*f*
Delayed development, 149
Dens evaginatus, 202
Dens invaginatus, 201–202, 202*f*
Dental anomalies, treatment for, 205*b*
Dental anxiety, 152, 152*b*
Dental caries, in children with common medical problems, management of, 249*f*
Dental erosion, 209–212, 261*f*
Dental health component, 264
Dental management, for children with disabilities, 159
Dental panoramic tomogram (DPT), 31, 31*f*, 100*f*
in amelogenesis imperfecta, 204
of dentinogenesis imperfecta, 206, 206*f*
Dentine defects, environmentally determined, 207
Dentinogenesis imperfecta (DI), 206–208, 207*b*, 260*f*
treatment of, 204
Dentoalveolar injury, splinting of, 176, 176*b*
'Denture' stomatitis, with fixed appliances, 114
causes of, 114*t*
prognosis of, 114
treatment of, 114
Developmental abnormalities
of enamel, 203*b*
in upper premolar rotations, 27
DI. *see* Dentinogenesis imperfecta (DI)

Diabetes
gingival bleeding and enlargement in, 213
implications of, 269
periodontal pathology and drifting incisor, 111
Diastema, median
causes of, 2*t*
ectopic eruption and, 1–4, 1*f*
labial segment problems in, 3, 3*f*
upper first permanent molar of, 1–4, 1*f*
Dietary advice, for diabetic patients, 215
Dietary allergens, in recurrent aphthae, 218*b*
Dietary causes (food and drinks)
of erosion, 209, 209*b*
staining due to, 193–194, 194*f*
Dietary constituents, causing erosion, 209
Dietary history, of adolescents, with caries, 136
Digit-sucking habit, 121
anterior open bite due to, 83, 83*f*, 85*b*
in buccal segment, 91
in increased overjet aetiology, 57*t*
with posterior crossbite, 88*b*, 88*t*, 89
Direct pulp capping, 172
Direction of displacement, in displaced primary incisor, 169
Disability, in children, 248*f*
Discoloration/staining, 187
extrinsic, 193–194
restorative techniques in, 193*b*
Displaced primary incisor, 168–170, 250*f*
Displacement, in posterior crossbite, 88
Distraction, 150
Distraction osteogenesis, in lingual crossbite, 97*t*, 98
Double permanent teeth, 201
Double primary teeth, 201, 201*b*
Double teeth, 200–201
Down syndrome, 199
DPT. *see* Dental panoramic tomogram (DPT)
Drainage of pus, 147
Dressing, for open cavities, 140, 140*f*, 141*b*
Drifting
incisors, 109–112, 238*f*
specifically relation to history, 110
of lower second premolars into contact with second molars, 103
Drugs
dentinogenesis imperfecta due to, 207
implications of, 269
staining due to, 194
Dry time, teeth with, 180
Dummy sucking, anterior open bite due to, 83*f*

E

EADT. *see* Extraalveolar dry time (EADT)
Eating disorder, 210
EBV. *see* Epstein-Barr virus (EBV)
Ectodermal dysplasia, 199
Ectopic eruption
clinical features of, 3–4
treatment of, 4, 4*b*, 4*f*
upper canines, buccal, 16–20, 16*f*–17*f*, 17*b*, 19*f*
upper first permanent molar of, 1–4, 1*f*. *see also* Impacted upper first molars
Elastic traction, 41, 42*f*
Electric pulp testing (EPT), 177
for fractured incisor crown, 172
for root resorption, 49
Emergency care, appliance related problems, 116, 116*b*
Enamel, fluorosis-related, 195
Enamel defects, developmental causes of, 203, 203*b*
Enamel microabrasion, 190
Enamel-dentine fracture, 172
Endocarditis, infective, risk of, 25
Environmental causes, dentine defects, 207
Epilepsy, implications of, 269
Epstein-Barr virus (EBV), 217
EPT. *see* Electric pulp testing (EPT)
Erosion, dental, 209–212
management of, 210–211, 210*b*
treatment for, 211*b*, 211*t*
Eruption
dates of, 2*b*, 2*t*
exfoliation and, disorders of, 254*f*
premature, 184
Essix retainers, 28–30
lower vacuum-formed, 116, 116*f*
Evaginated teeth, 202
Exfoliation, 185, 185*b*
eruption and, 184–186
External inflammatory resorption, 180
Extirpated tooth, intracanal medicament in, 182
Extraalveolar dry time (EADT), 180
Extraction
in buccal upper canines, 23
with canine transposition (of most displaced tooth), 47
of carious primary teeth, 141–142
with crowding, 27
of first premolars, 27
of upper canines, 27–28
with crowding and buccal upper canines, 17–18
of first premolars, 18–19, 19*b*
of infraoccluded primary molar, 53
in lingual crossbite, 97*t*
with poor quality first permanent molars, 189–190, 190*b*
with root resorption, 50
of upper canines, 119
Extraction-only plan, 32, 32*f*
Extraoral examination
in bilateral crossbite, 91
in increased overbite, 73, 73*f*, 76–77, 77*f*
in late lower incisor crowding, 99
in lingual crossbite, 97–98
in posterior crossbite, 87, 87*b*
TMJ pain and prominent chin and, 102–103
Extrinsic staining, 193–194, 193*f*
Eye swelling, root fractured permanent incisors and, 175

F

Facemask, 70, 72*b*
design of, 70, 70*f*–71*f*
effects of, 71, 71*f*–72*f*
psychological benefits of, 71
success of, 72
long-term, 72
Facial asymmetry, mild, in buccal upper canines, 16
Facial convexity, 56
Facial growth, post-treatment, 122
Facial height, lower, in increased overjet, 56
Facial profile, in anterior open bite, 81, 81*f*
Facial swelling, dental abscess and, 146–148, 245*f*
Fissure sealants, for adolescents, with caries, 137–138, 137*f*, 137*t*
Fixation, with TMJ pain and prominent chin, 107
Fixed appliances
for absent upper lateral incisors, 13
in anterior open bite, 85
in bilateral crossbite, 93
for cleft lip and palate, 128
with crowding and buccal upper canines, 17–18
with deep overbite, 80*f*
drifting incisors, 109
for incisor crossbite, 64–65
with increased overbite, 73, 75–76
for infraoccluded primary molar, 53–54, 53*f*–54*f*
in lingual crossbite, 97–98, 97*f*
problems, 114
in tooth movement, 121, 121*f*–122*f*
for transposition of canines, 47–48, 48*f*
Fixed bonded retainer, 123, 123*b*–124*b*
Fixed retainers, 122
Fizzy (carbonated drinks), causing erosion, 210
Fluoride
for adolescents, 151–152
history, 192*b*
of adolescents, with caries, 136
mottling, 195
toothpaste, for children, 152
Fluoride mouthwash
of adolescents, with caries, 136
for early childhood caries, 133
for eroded teeth, 210
Fluoride supplements
for adolescents, with caries, 137, 137*t*
for early childhood caries, 132–133
Fluoride toothpaste
for adolescents, with caries, 137–138, 137*t*
for early childhood caries, 131–132
Fluoride varnish
application, for adolescents, with caries, 137, 137*t*
for eroded teeth, 210
Fluorosis, 188, 192, 195, 195*b*
FMPA. *see* Frankfort-mandibular planes angle (FMPA)
Forces, gingival/occlusal, 100
Formocresol, for pulpotomy, of carious primary teeth, 144
Fracture
clean-cut, 116
incisor root, 109
root, drifting incisors and, 109
Fractured incisor crown, 171–174
immature permanent, 251*f*
Fractured permanent incisor, root, 175–178
Frankel II appliance, for lingual crossbite, 97, 97*f*
Frankel III appliance for reversed overjet, 67–68, 68*f*
Frankfort-mandibular planes angle (FMPA), with increased overjet, 56
Functional appliances
in anterior open bite, 84–85
with increased overbite, 75, 75*b*
for increased overjet, 58, 58*b*–60*b*, 60*f*
types for, 58

Functional appliances *(Continued)*
for reverse overjet, 67–68, 68*f*
effects of, 68
wear of, 68

G

Gastric acid, causing erosion, 209
Gastro-oesophageal reflux disease (GORD), gastric regurgitation and, 209–210
GDP. *see* General dental practitioner (GDP)
Gender, affected by transposition of canines, 47
General anaesthesia
for children with disabilities, 160
contraindications for, 154
indications for, 154
General dental practitioner (GDP), 116–117
Generalised slight gingival erythema, 42, 43*f*
Generalized marginal gingival erythema, 30, 31*f*
Genetic enamel defects, 203–204
Genetic factors, in palatal canine ectopia, 36–37
GICs. *see* Glass ionomer cement (GICs)
Gingiva
bleeding of, 213*b*
enlargement, oral ulceration and, 216, 216*f*
pressure from, causing late lower incisor crowding, 100
Gingival bleeding and enlargement, 213–215, 262*f*
Gingival enlargement, systemic causes of, 214, 215*b*
Gingival health, with toothbrushing, 194
Gingival recession, 62–63
Gingival third root fractures, 177
Gingivitis, chronic, 213, 213*f*
Gingivoplasty, labial, 10
Gingivostomatitis, primary herpetic, 216, 216*f*
Glass ionomer cement (GICs), 189
GORD. *see* Gastro-oesophageal reflux disease (GORD)
Grafting, alveolar bone, for cleft lip and palate, 128, 129*b*
Greater maxillary protraction, for reverse overjet, 72
Growth modification, in lingual crossbite, 97*t*

H

Haemophilia A, 165, 165*f*
Halitosis, 194
Hall crown technique, for children with medical problems, 166–167
Hall crowns
for carious primary teeth, 143–144
for children with disabilities, 159
Hand, foot and mouth disease, 217
Hawley retainer
for severe crowding, 29–30
in tooth movement, 122, 123*f*
Head and neck syndromes, associated with missing teeth, 199
Headgear
with severe crowding, 28
wear, for absent upper lateral incisors, 14
Herbst appliance, increased overbite, 75
Hereditary dentine defects, 207*b*
Herpangina, 217
Herpes labialis, 217
Herpes simplex virus (HSV), 216, 216*b*
reactivation of, 217*b*
Herpes virus type 8, 217
Herpetic gingivostomatitis, primary, 216, 216*f*
Herpetiform aphthae, 217
High caries risk adolescents, 243*f*
Hospital admission, for orofacial infection, 147, 147*b*
HPV. *see* Human papilloma virus (HPV)
HSV. *see* Herpes simplex virus (HSV)
Human papilloma virus (HPV), 217
Hydrochloric acid (HCl)-pumice microabrasion technique, 196, 196*f*
Hyperglycaemic coma, 213–214
Hypodontia, 199*b*, 201
facial/dental/occlusal associated with, 13
genes associated with, 13
prevalence of, 52–53, 53*b*
upper incisors, 11–15, 11*f*–12*f*
Hypoglycaemic coma, 214
Hypomineralization
early childhood caries and, 131*f*
enamel, hypoplasia and, 187*b*, 187*f*, 188
treatment for, 190
Hypomineralized amelogenesis imperfecta, 204*f*
Hypoplasia
early childhood caries and, 131*f*
enamel
cause of, 26
hypomineralization and, 187*b*, 187*f*, 188
systemic (chronological) influences in, 203
Hypoplastic amelogenesis imperfecta, 203, 203*f*

I

Ibuprofen, for carious primary teeth, 141*t*
Impacted upper first molars
causes, 3, 4*t*
frequency/prevalence, 3
management of, 4
permanent, 221*f*
treatment of, 4, 4*b*, 4*f*
Impressions
of dental arches, in posterior crossbite, 88
upper and lower, 100
Incisor crossbite, 62–65, 62*f*, 230*f*
diagnosis of, 64
extraoral examination of, 62
features of, 63, 63*b*
intraoral examination of, 62, 62*f*
IOTN DHC grade of, 64
labial recession in, prognosis for, 64
prevalence of, 63
special investigations for, 63
treatment for, 64–65, 64*b*
Incisors
angulations of, 21–22
central, unerupted upper, 5–10, 5*f*
crown, permanent, fractured, 171–174
double (crowns are joined), primary teeth, 200, 200*f*
drifting, 109–112
intrusion, in overbite reduction, 78, 78*b*, 78*f*
lateral, upper, absent, 11–15, 11*f*–12*f*
maxillary, severely reabsorbed, 50*b*
permanent
central, affected by mottling, 195
eruption dates, 2*t*
root fractured, 175–178
rotations, median diastema and, 2
upper, space creation in development, 2, 2*b*
primary, eruption dates, 2*t*
resorption
detection of, 49*b*
by ectopic maxillary canine, 49*b*
upper
with increased overbite, 75
trauma of, 58
Increased overbite, 232*f*
Increased overjet, 229*f*
Index of orthodontic treatment need, 264
Infection-related resorption, 180
Infective endocarditis
dental care and, 166, 166*f*
risk of, 25
Inferior alveolar block injection, 166
Infiltration injection, 166
Informed consent, 155, 155*b*
Infraoccluded primary molar, 51–54, 228*f*
aetiology of, 51
cause of, 52, 52*b*
dental history, 51
diagnosis of, 53
examination of, 51–52
extraoral, 51
intraoral, 51–52, 51*f*–52*f*
family history, 51
history of, 51
complaint, 51
investigations for, 52–53
clinical, 52, 52*b*
radiographic, 52–53, 53*f*
IOTN DHC grade, 53
medical history, 51
prevalence of, 51
treatment of, 53–54, 53*f*–54*f*, 54*b*
Infraocclusion, 186, 186*b*
Infraorbital floor, fracture of, 175
Infraorbital margin, fracture of, 175
Inhalational sedation, 150, 151*b*
Insulin-dependent diabetes, gingival bleeding and enlargement in, 213–214
Intercanine width
in developing dentition, 2*b*
reduced, causing late lower incisor crowding, 100
Interceptive measure, for absent upper lateral incisors, 13–14, 14*b*
Interceptive treatment, for transposition of canines, 47
Intermaxillary fixation, with TMJ pain and prominent chin, 106
Interproximal stripping, late lower incisor crowding, 101
Intracanal medicament, in extirpated tooth, 182
Intraoral examination
in bilateral crossbite, 91–92, 92*f*
in increased overbite, 73–74, 73*f*–74*f*, 74*b*
in late lower incisor crowding, 99–100
in posterior crossbite, 87–88, 87*f*–88*f*
TMJ pain and prominent chin and, 103–104, 103*f*
Intraoral periapical radiographs, root fractures in, 175, 176*f*

Intravenous antibiotics, 147, 147*t*
Intrinsic discoloration, 191*f*
Invaginations, 201–202
Invisalign, drifting incisors and, 111
IOTN DHC grade, 100, 105
Irreversible pulpitis, 140, 140*t*

J

Joint periodontal, referral for, 111
Juvenile rheumatoid arthritis, implications of, 269

K

Kim mechanics, in anterior open bite, 85

L

Labial bow
with absent upper permanent central incisor, 9
with increased overbite, 75
with lower incisor crowding (late presentation), 101
Labial gingivoplasty, 10
Labial segment crowding, 26, 29, 29*b*, 29*f*
Labial segment problems, in median diastema, 3, 3*f*
Labial segment spacing
drifting incisors and, 111
upper, causes of, 12, 12*b*, 12*t*
Labial surface, of upper permanent incisors, affected by mottling, 195
Lain's dentition, prognosis of, 111
Lateral cephalometric analysis, 271–272
aim and objective of, 271
interpretation of, 271, 272*t*
practice of, 271, 271*f*, 271*t*
Latex
allergy, 51
implications of, 269
Le Fort I advancement, TMJ pain and prominent chin, 107
Learning difficulties, in children, 248*f*
Left buccal occlusion, 99*f*
Lesions, in palate, 113
Leukaemia, implications of, 269
Lingual appliances, of late lower incisor crowding, 101
Lingual crossbite, bilateral, 97*b*, 97*t*
Lip swelling, fractured permanent incisor crown and, 171
Lower arch
crowding, 32, 42–44, 44*f*–45*f*
eruption pattern in, 30
Lower bonded retainer, 123*f*
Lower centreline shift, 30, 31*b*
Lower incisor
crowding, late presentation, 99*f*, 236*f*
extraction of, 101
in overbite reduction, 78
Luxated primary tooth, 170

M

Major aphthae, 217
MAKATON, for children with disabilities, 160–161
Mandibular displacement on closure, 63
in posterior crossbite, 88, 88*b*
prominent chin and TMJ pain, 103
reverse overjet and, 67
Mandibular growth, 24, 24*f*
in late, lower incisor crowding causation, 100
in posterior crossbite, 88*t*
Mandibular infections, 146
Mandibular midline distraction, in lingual crossbite, 98
Mandibular path of closure, prominent chin and TMJ pain, 103
Mandibular setback osteotomy, TMJ pain and prominent chin, 107
Maxillary canine fossa infections, 146, 146*f*
Maxillary expansion, rapid, in bilateral crossbite, 93–94, 93*b*–94*b*, 93*t*, 94*f*
Maxillary tooth, talon cusp in, 201–202
MCDAS. *see* Modified Child Dental Anxiety Scale (MCDAS)
Median diastema, 220*f*
causes of, 2*t*
labial segment problems in, 3, 3*f*
upper first permanent molar of, 1–4, 1*f*
Medical comorbidities, in children with disabilities, 160, 160*b*
Medical condition, staining due to, 194
Medical problems, in children, 163–167, 167*b*, 167*t*
acute lymphoblastic leukaemia as, 163, 163*f*–164*f*
congenital heart defect as, 166, 166*f*
haemophilia A as, 165, 165*f*
Microabrasion, fluorotic mottling for, 196*b*, 197
Midazolam
intravenous sedation, 154
for oral sedation, 154
Middle third root fractures, 176*f*
Midline distraction osteogenesis, in lingual crossbite, 97*t*
Mid-palatal suture, in bilateral crossbite, 93
MIH. *see* Molar incisor hypomineralization (MIH)
Mild marginal gingival erythema, 32, 33*f*
Millard repair, 126
Mind maps, 219
Mineralization times, for permanent dentition, 188*t*
Minor aphthae, 217
Missing shaped teeth, multiple, 199–202
Missing teeth, 199
Mixed dentition, referral guide for, 268
Mobility, of natal teeth, 184
Modified Child Dental Anxiety Scale (MCDAS), 152, 153*f*
Modified palatal arch, in anterior open bite, 84–85, 84*f*
Molar eruption, in overbite reduction, 78
Molar extrusion, in overbite reduction, 78
Molar incisor hypomineralization (MIH), 188, 188*b*–189*b*
Molar intrusion, in anterior open bite, 85*f*
Molars
erosion in, 209, 209*f*
permanent
eruption dates, 2*t*
poor quality first, 187–190
upper first, ectopic eruption of, 1–4, 1*f*
primary
early loss, space loss following, 26, 26*t*, 27*b*
first, infraocclusion of, 186, 186*b*
third
in late lower incisor crowding, 100, 100*b*
removal of, 101, 101*b*
Mottled teeth, 195–198
treatment of, 257*f*
Mottling, 195, 195*f*
Mouth
breathing, in bilateral crossbite, 91, 91*b*
in increased overbite, appearance of, 73–74
Multiple missing and abnormally shaped teeth, 258*f*
Multistrand wire retainer, 122, 123*f*

N

Natal teeth, 184, 184*b*, 184*f*
Neonates
cleft lip and palate in, 126
teeth, 184, 184*b*
Neutropenia, cyclic, 185*f*
Nickel, implications of, 269
Nickel allergy, 20–21, 20*b*, 21*f*
Nickel titanium archwires, advantages of, 45
Nickel-titanium (NiTi) springs, 54, 54*f*
Nightguard vital bleaching, 197
Night-time feeding, early childhood caries and, 131
Nitrous oxide, 151, 151*b*
inhalation sedation, 153
for children with disabilities, 159–160
NNSHs. *see* Nonnutritive sucking habits (NNSHs)
Nonextraction approach, in deep overbite, 78–79, 79*f*–80*f*, 80*b*
Nonnutritive sucking habits (NNSHs), 83, 83*b*
Nonpharmacological behaviour management, 152
for children with disabilities, 159, 159*b*
Non-verbal communication, 149
Non-vital bleaching, 192
NSAIDs, implications of, 269
Nursing caries, 130–134, 130*f*, 131*b*
early childhood and, 242*f*

O

Occlusal radiograph
of cleft lip and palate, 127, 128*f*
of palatal canines, 38
unerupted upper permanent central incisor, 7, 8*f*
Occlusion
anterior, 94, 95*f*–96*f*
buccal, 96, 96*f*
final, with drifting incisors, 112*f*
forces, causing late lower incisor crowding, 100
posttreatment
in bilateral crossbite, 95, 96*f*
in increased overbite, 76, 76*f*
in lingual crossbite, 98, 98*f*
in posterior crossbite, 89, 90*f*
at presentation, with drifting incisors, 109*f*–110*f*
relapsed in, in increased overbite, 76, 76*b*
TMJ pain and prominent chin, 107, 107*f*
Opalescent dentine, hereditary (DI type II), 207

Open bite, anterior, 81–86, 81*f*
Oral hygiene
in bilateral crossbite, 93
diabetes due to, 214*b*
with drifting incisors, 109
instruction, for incisor crossbite, 64
poor, chromogenic staining due to, 194
severe crowding and, 25
Oral manifestations, diabetes, 215
Oral sedation, 154
Oral ulceration, 216–218, 217*b*, 263*f*
Orbital flow (blow out) fractures, 175
Orofacial infection, 147, 147*b*
Orofacial soft tissues, forces from, 121–122
Orthodontic alignment, 42
Orthodontic camouflage, 60
in lingual crossbite, 97*t*
Orthodontic consultation, referral for, 111
Orthodontic movement, of root fractured teeth, 177
Orthodontic problems, referral guide for, 268
Orthodontic treatment
need, index of, 264
for unerupted teeth, risks of, 9
Orthodontics, implications of some medical problems for, 269–270
Orthognathic surgery
in lingual crossbite, 97*t*
TMJ pain and prominent chin, 105
Osteogenesis imperfecta, DI type I associated with, 207
Overbite
amount of, 63
increased, 73–80
reduction, 78*b*
traumatic, 73, 73*f*, 74*t*
Overjet
increased, 55–61, 55*f*
aims of treatment for, 58
causes of, 56, 57*t*
diagnosis of, 57–58
early, treatment for, 58
extraoral examination of, 55–56, 56*f*
intraoral examination of, 56, 57*f*
options for treatment of, 60
radiographs for, 57
risk of trauma with, 55
reverse, 66–72, 66*f*, 70*f*
causes of, 67*t*
diagnosis of, 67, 70
extraoral examination of, 66, 66*f*
intraoral examination of, 66–67, 67*f*
IOTN DHC grade of, 67
prognosis of, 69
treatment for, 67–72, 67*b*–68*b*, 68*f*–69*f*, 68*t*, 71*b*

P

Pain
control
for carious primary teeth, 140–145, 140*f*
and treatment planning for carious primary teeth, 244*f*
poor quality first permanent molars and, 188–189
relief, for nursing caries, 133
TMJ, and prominent chin, 102–108, 102*f*
Palatal canine ectopia, 36–37, 37*b*, 37*f*
Palatal canines, 226*f*
exposure, surgery of, 40*t*, 41, 41*b*
Palatal crib, in anterior open bite, 84–85, 84*f*
Palatal luxation, of primary incisor, 168*f*
Palatal mucosa, as diagnosis of appliance, 114
Palatal stomatitis, management of, 114*b*
Palatally displaced canines, 39–40, 40*b*, 40*t*
Palate, appearance of, 113
Panoramic tomogram
acute lymphoblastic leukaemia and, 164, 164*f*
in anterior open bite, 83
in bilateral crossbite, 92
for children with disabilities, 158
for cleft lip and palate, 127, 128*f*
crowding and buccal upper canines, 17, 17*f*
in increased overbite, 74
of late lower incisor crowding, 100
median diastema, 3, 3*f*
nickel allergy and, 20, 20*f*
of palatal canines, 38, 39*f*
of permanent teeth, 200, 200*f*
poor quality first permanent molars and, 189, 189*f*
in posterior crossbite, 88–89, 89*f*
of severe crowding, 27
of tooth movement, 119, 120*f*
of unerupted upper permanent central incisor, 7, 8*f*
Paracetamol, for carious primary teeth, 141*t*
Parafunctional activity, attritional wear with, 211
Parental involvement, early childhood caries and, 132
Parental presence/absence, in behavioural management, 150
Partial pulpotomy, for fractured permanent incisor crown, 172, 173*b*, 173*f*
Periapical periodontitis, drifting incisors, 109
Periapical radiograph
for canine transposition, 47
of fractured incisor crown, 172
full-mouth, drifting incisors and, 110–111, 110*f*
intraoral, root fractures in, 175, 176*f*
of root fractures, 172
of tooth movement, 119, 119*f*–120*f*
Periodontal assessment, for root resorption, 49
Periodontal disease, gingival and, 215*f*
Periodontal healing, 181–182, 181*f*
Periodontal ligament, damaged, 182
Periodontal probing depths, in increased overbite, 74
Periodontal treatment, 111
Periodontally compromised dentition, 112, 112*b*
Periodontitis
chronic moderate, 111, 111*b*
periapical, drifting incisors, 109
Permanent dentition
delayed or failed eruption of teeth in, 185
mineralization times for, 188*t*
referral guide for, 268
Permanent incisor
crown, fractured immature, 171–174
erosive tooth surface loss of, 211*f*
Permanent teeth
double, 201
premature exfoliation of, 185*b*
treatment modalities for, in amelogenesis imperfecta, 204, 204*t*
Permanent tooth pulpotomy, 172–173
Physical abuse, 169
Plaque control
in adolescents, 136
in caries, 132*t*
Polyurethane powerchain, 54
Poor quality first permanent molar, 255*f*
Porcelain, for tooth surface loss, 211*t*
Position, tooth, cephalometric analysis for, 271–272, 272*f*
Positive reinforcement, 149–150, 150*b*
Posterior crossbite, 87–90, 234*f*
Posterior open bite, 59
Post-surgical orthodontics, phase of, 107
Post-surgical stability, influence of, 107, 107*b*
Pre-adjusted edgewise appliance, 53–54, 53*f*–54*f*
Pregnancy, first permanent molars (FPMs) in, 191
Premature eruption, 184
Premaxilla, anterior, vertical parallax of, 7
Premolars
eruption dates, 2*t*
first, extraction of, 18–19, 19*b*
lower, extraction of, 101
rotations, causes of, 27
TMJ pain and prominent chin, 105
transplant, avulsed incisor and, 183*f*
Pressure zones, in tooth movements, 118, 118*f*
Pre-surgical orthodontics, phase of, 106, 107*b*
Primary dentition
in cleft lip and palate, 126, 126*b*
delayed or failed eruption of teeth in, 185
referral guide for, 268
Primary incisors
discoloured, 170, 170*f*
displaced, 168–170
palatal luxation of, 168*f*
Primary teeth
amelogenesis imperfecta affecting, 203
carious, 140–145, 140*f*, 143*b*
examination of, 141, 141*f*
restorative treatment of, 142*t*, 143*b*
treatment planning for, 142–143, 142*t*
delayed eruption of, 184
delayed exfoliation of, 186
dentinogenesis imperfecta affecting, 206
double, 201, 201*b*
luxated, 170
trauma, 169, 170*b*
treatment modalities for, in amelogenesis imperfecta, 204, 204*t*
Prominent chin and TMJDS, 237*f*
Protraction (reverse-pull) headgear, 70, 72*b*
design of, 70, 70*f*–71*f*
effects of, 71, 71*f*–72*f*
long-term, 72
psychological benefits of, 71
success of, 72
Pulp capping, direct, 172
Pulp chambers, obliteration of, in dentinogenesis imperfecta, 206*f*, 208
Pulp survival, 182
Pulp tester, electric, for fractured incisor crown, 172
Pulp therapy, indirect, for carious primary teeth, 143–144
Pulpal exposure, of fractured permanent incisor crown, 172

Pulpectomy, for carious primary teeth, 142
Pulpitis, 140–141, 140*t*
Pulpotomies
for carious primary teeth, 144
for fractured permanent incisor crown, 173
Pyramidal roots, 202

Q

Quadhelix
appliance, for buccal upper canines, 23, 24*f*
in bilateral crossbite, 93*t*
for cleft lip and palate, 128, 128*f*
in posterior crossbite, 89–90, 90*f*
Quick-check method, of tooth-size discrepancy, 37

R

Radiographic investigations
for children with disabilities, 158–160, 159*b*
in increased overbite, 74
Radiography
of absent upper lateral incisors, 12
for adolescents, with caries, 136–138, 136*f*
in amelogenesis imperfecta, 204
in anterior open bite, 83
in bilateral crossbite, 92
of buccal upper canines, 22
for cleft lip and palate, 127
in dentinogenesis imperfecta, 206
for displaced primary incisor, 169–170
in double teeth, 201
for incisor crossbite, 63
for increased overjet, 57
for infraoccluded primary molar, 52–53
intraoral, poor quality first permanent molars and, 189
of late lower incisor crowding, 100
for reverse overjet, 67, 69–70
root fractures and, 175
root resorption, 48–49, 49*f*
of severe crowding, 27
transposition of canines, 47
unerupted teeth, 7, 7*b*
Radiology, in posterior crossbite, 89
Radiotherapy, side effects of, 165*b*
Rapid maxillary expansion (RME), in bilateral crossbite, 93–95, 93*b*–94*b*, 93*t*, 94*f*, 96*b*, 96*f*
not feasible, 95
surgically assisted, 93*t*
Recession, labial, 64
Recurrent aphthae
aetiological factors in, 218, 218*b*
dietary allergens in, 218*b*
therapy for, 218*b*
Reduction
of deep overbite, 78, 78*b*
procedure in, of root fractured incisor, 176
Referral letter, to orthodontist, 18*f*
Regurgitation, gastric, 210
Reinforcement, positive, 149–150
Removable appliances
with absent upper lateral incisors, 14, 14*b*, 14*f*
in bilateral crossbite, 93*t*
in increased overbite, 75
with palatal canines, 41
in posterior crossbite, 89
with severe crowding, 29, 30*f*
therapy, tooth movements and, 118
Removable retainers, 122–123, 123*b*
Repair-related resorption, 180
Replacement resorption, 180
Replantation, avulsed incisor and, 180, 181*f*
Resin-retained bridge, for absent upper lateral incisors, 14, 14*b*, 15*f*
Resorption (root), 49*f*
avulsed incisor and, 180, 180*b*
causes of, 49
drifting incisors, 109
incidence of, 49
orthodontically induced, 119, 120*b*
prevention of, 120, 120*b*
radiographs of, 49
short- to medium-term prognosis with, 50, 50*f*
treatment options for, 49–50, 50*b*
Restoration
for amelogenesis imperfecta, 204*t*
of first permanent molar, 214–215
surface tooth loss and, 211
Retainer, type of, 45, 45*f*
Retaining, 41
Retention
in bilateral crossbite, 94
in crowding, 28
in increased overbite, 75
orthodontic, role of general dental practitioner (GDP) in, 123, 124*t*
in palatal canines, 41
plan, in tooth movement, 122, 122*b*
Retraction, of upper canines, 119
Reverse overjet, 231*f*
Reversible pulpitis, 140, 140*t*
RME. *see* Rapid maxillary expansion (RME)
Root
filled incisor, non-vital bleaching for, 192
filling material, orthodontic tooth movement, 9
fractured permanent incisor, 175–178, 252*f*
in incisor trauma, fracture, 109
resorption, monitoring of, 49–50
shape abnormalities of, 202
Root canal
obliteration of, in dentinogenesis imperfecta, 206*f*
treatment, avulsed incisor and, 179–180
Rotational correction, in increased overbite, 76
Rotations, upper premolar, causes of, 27

S

SARPE. *see* Surgically assisted rapid maxillary expansion (SARPE)
Screw turning, with palatal canines, 41
Sedation, oral, 154
Sensibility testing, 177, 177*b*
of incisor, 7
for root resorption, 49
Sensitivity
with erosive loss, treatment of, 210–211
with poor quality first permanent molars, 189
Severe class III skeletal pattern, as interpretation of findings, in TMJ pain and prominent chin, 104
Severe crowding, 225*f*
Severe hypodontia, 200, 200*f*
Shape, canines/incisors, 13
Shaped teeth, abnormally, 199–202
Shell teeth, 207
Size
canines/incisors, 13
discrepancy, 37, 38*b*
Skeletal pattern
in anterior open bite, 82*t*, 84
in bilateral crossbite, 91, 92*t*
of buccal upper canines, 22
in increased overbite, 73, 74*t*, 76–77
in increased overjet, 55–56, 57*t*
in lingual crossbite, 97
in posterior crossbite, 87, 88*t*
Skeletal relationships, cephalometric analysis for, 271
Smile, attractive, 95, 95*b*
Smoking
cessation of, 111
periodontal disease and, 111
SOCRATES, 140
Soft tissues
analysis, cephalometric analysis for, 272, 272*f*
increased overbite in, 73–74, 74*t*
in increased overjet aetiology, 57*t*
Space
closure (therapeutic), absent upper lateral incisors, 13
creation
absent upper lateral incisors, 13
for crowding and buccal upper canines, 18, 18*b*–19*b*
for upper permanent incisors, 2, 2*b*
Speech
with anterior open bite, 81–82
with cleft lip and palate, 126
Splinting
in root fractures, 176
with TMJ pain and prominent chin, 107
Stability
of corrected overjet, 60
of crossbite correction, 64, 64*f*
Stainless steel crowns, poor quality first permanent molars, 189
Steroids, implications of, 269
Stomach, acidity of, and regurgitation, 209, 210*b*
Stomatitis, palatal (red palate), with fixed appliances, 114
Stress, TMJ pain and, 103
Structured history form, 273, 273*f*–274*f*
Study models, of late lower incisor crowding, 100
Subluxed incisor, 179*f*
Sugar intake, reduce, 114
Sugar-free chewing gum, for adolescents, with caries, 138
Supernumerary teeth
aetiology of, 7, 7*b*
treatment plan for, 8
unerupted upper permanent central incisor due to, 6, 6*b*, 7*f*
Surface
resorption, 180
tooth, loss or wear
erosion in, 211
in increased overbite, 74
Surgically assisted rapid maxillary expansion (SARPE), in bilateral crossbite, 93*t*, 95, 95*f*–96*f*, 96*b*

Suture splint, avulsed incisor and, 181, 182*f*
Swallowing pattern, in anterior open bite, 81
Sweetened drink, early childhood caries and, 130
Syndromes, associated with missing teeth, 199
Systemic diseases, associated with aphthae, 218

T

TADs. *see* Temporary anchorage devices (TADs)
Talon cusp, 201, 201*f*
Taurodontism, 202
Teasing
  compared to bullying, 55
  history of, and incisor trauma, 55
Teens
  late, lower incisor crowding in, 99–100
  prominent chin and TMJ pain, reassessed in, 103–104, 104*b*
Teeth, affected by transposition of canines, 47
Tell-show-do technique, 149
Temporary anchorage devices (TADs)
  in anterior open bite, 85–86, 85*f*
  in overbite reduction, 78
  in severe crowding, 28–29
Temporomandibular joint dysfunction syndrome, 103
Temporomandibular joint pain and prominent chin, 102–108, 102*f*
  aims of treatment of, 105
  case manage and, 105
  surgical planning and, 105–106, 106*b*, 106*f*
Ten Hove appliance, in deep overbite, 79, 79*f*
Tension zones, in tooth movements, 118, 118*f*, 119*b*
Thrombosis, cavernous sinus, 146
Thumb sucking, anterior open bite due to, 83*f*
Tipping movement, 118, 118*b*, 118*f*
Titanium trauma splint, avulsed incisor with, 179, 179*f*
Tomogram
  of incisor crossbite, 63, 63*f*
  for increased overjet, 57
  of infraoccluded primary molar, 52, 53*f*
  for reverse overjet, 67, 69
Tongue
  scrapers, 194
  swallowing pattern in, with anterior open bite, 81
Tooth discoloration, hypomineralization, and hypoplasia, 191–194, 192*b*, 256*f*
Tooth fragments, in fractured permanent incisor crown and, 171, 171*b*, 172*f*
Tooth mousse, for adolescents, with caries, 138
Tooth movement, 118–124
  mechanism for, 119
  and related problems, 240*f*
  slow rate of, 118
Toothbrushing, 194
  for adolescents, 151–152
    with caries, 137, 137*t*
  early childhood caries and, 131–132
  overzealous, 211
Tooth-size discrepancy (TSD), 37, 38*b*
Transpalatal arch, 28–29
Transposition, canines, 46, 47*b*
  aetiology of, 47
  arch and teeth affected by, 47
  classification of, 47
  incidence of, 47
  positions of, correction of, 48
  treatment for
    factors to consider in, 47, 47*t*
    options in, 47, 47*b*
Trauma
  infection-related resorption and, 180–181
  risk of, with increased overjet, 55, 55*b*
  upper incisor, 58
Traumatic overbite, 73, 73*f*, 74*t*
TSADs, implications of, 269
TSD. *see* Tooth-size discrepancy (TSD)
Tuberculated teeth, 202
Turner's tooth/hypoplasia, 26
Twin-Block appliance, 59, 59*f*
  in anterior open bite, 84
  effects of, and other functional appliances, 59
  fabrication of, 58
  in increased overbite, 75
  instructions for, 58–59

U

Ulceration, oral, 216–218, 217*b*
Uncooperative child, 246*f*
  and adolescents, 149–156, 152*b*
    anxiety management for, 152–154
    behavior management for, 149
    communicative management for, 149–150
    dental anxiety in, 152
    informed consent for, 155
    inhalation sedation for, 150–151
    treatment plan for, 153–154
Unerupted teeth
  upper canines, 21–24, 22*f*
  upper central incisor, 5–10, 5*f*, 222*f*
    causes of, 6, 6*b*
    management of, 10*b*
Upper arch crowding, 32, 42–44, 44*f*–45*f*
Upper permanent central incisors, affected by mottling, 195
Upper removable appliance therapy, 118, 119*b*
  to procline, for incisor crossbite, 64, 64*f*

V

Vacuum formed retainers, 30, 117, 122, 123*f*
Varicella zoster virus (VZV), 217
Veneers, composite, 192
  dentinogenesis imperfecta and, 208
  fluorotic mottling, 197–198
Vertical parallax, of anterior premaxilla, 7
Vital bleaching, for fluorotic mottling, 197
Vital pulpectomy, for carious primary teeth, 144
Vitality
  of root fractured teeth, maintain, 177, 178*f*
  tests, 175
    for fractured incisor crown, 172
Voice control, 150
Vomiting, recurrent, erosive loss, 210
VZV. *see* Varicella zoster virus (VZV)

W

Water, adolescent consumption, 136
Wax registration
  for functional appliances, reverse overjet, 68
  of late lower incisor crowding, 100
  in posterior crossbite, 88
White spot demineralization lesions, 194
Wire
  composite, 117
  spurs, with absent upper lateral incisors, 14, 14*b*, 14*f*

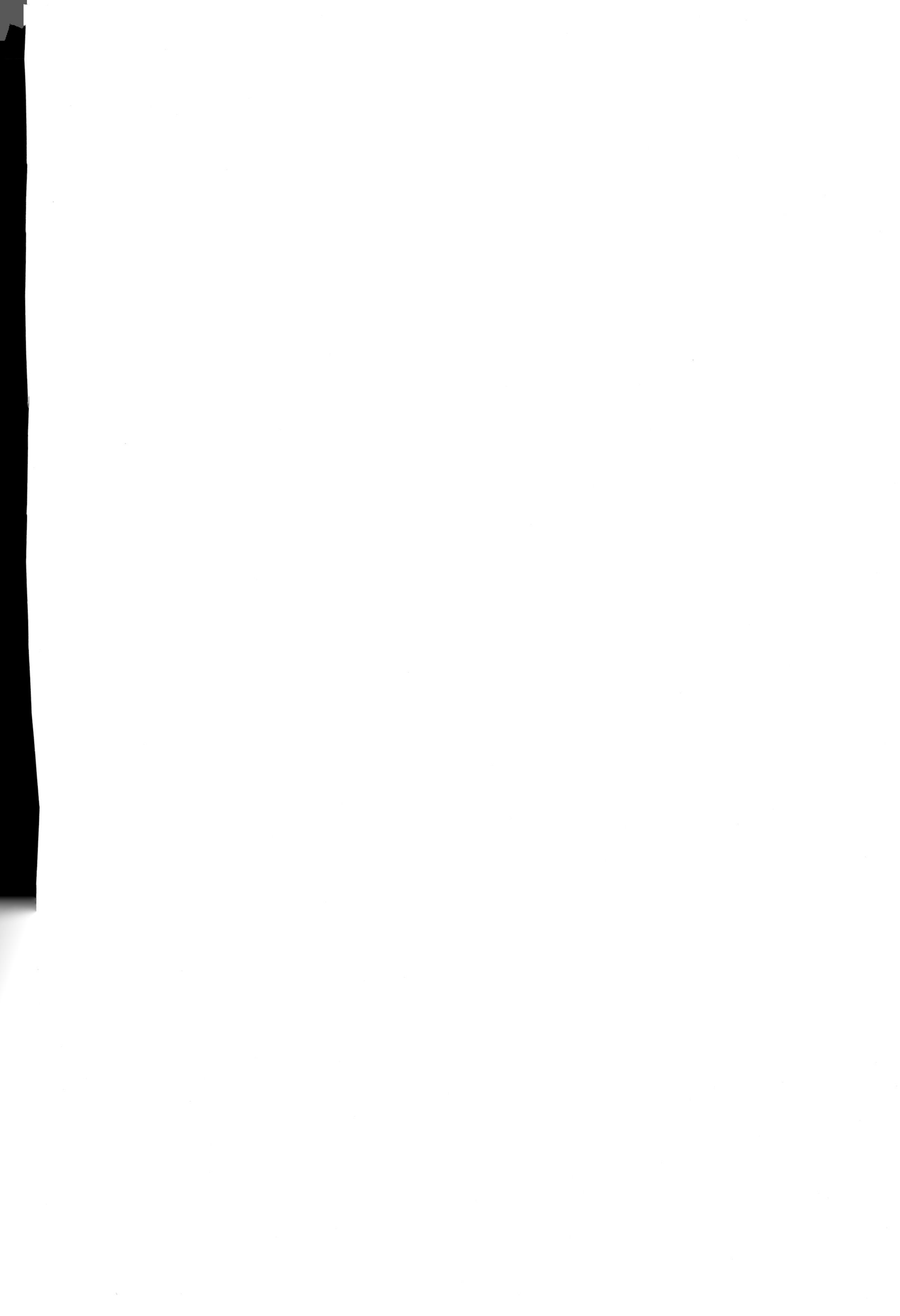